The Whole Nurse Catalog

The Whole Nurse Catalog

Jane Jackson, R.N., C.N.M., B.S.N., M.S.N.

Churchill Livingstone
New York, Edinburgh, London, and Melbourne

1980

© Churchill Livingstone Inc. 1980

All rights reserved. No part of this publication may be reproduced, stored in a retrieval system, or transmitted in any form or by any means, electronic, mechanical, photocopying, recording or otherwise, without prior permission of the publishers (Churchill Livingstone Inc., 19 West 44th Street, New York, N.Y. 10036).

Distributed in the United Kingdom by Churchill Livingstone, Robert Stevenson House, 1-3 Baxter's Place, Leith Walk, Edinburgh EH1 3AF and by associated companies, branches and representatives throughout the world.

First published 1980

Printed in USA

ISBN 0-443-08062-3 Churchill Livingstone

7 6 5 4 3 2 1

Library of Congress Cataloging in Publication Data

Jackson, Jane, 1948–
   The whole nurse catalog.

Bibliography: p.
   Includes index.
   1. Nursing—Handbooks, manuals, etc. 2. Nursing—Information services—United States—Directories.
3. Nursing—Bibliography. 4. Nursing—Equipment and supplies—Catalogs. I. Title.
RT51.J32   610.73'02'02   80-24005
ISBN 0-443-08062-3

This book is dedicated with love

To my husband, Blyden, in appreciation for his constant support and encouragement

To my son, Aaron, my teacher, and source of much joy

To Alberta Hunter, an inspiration to nurses and survivors of all ages

and to
All Nurses

Introduction

The Whole Nurse Catalog is intended as a resource in itself and as a guide to other resources for nurses in all fields of nursing. It is not a textbook and is not necessarily meant to be read from cover to cover. Directed to the practicing nurse, it can be used to provide answers to specific questions or as a reference to the vast stores of resource material and organizations available. Several excerpts from other sources are included in this one reference in order to provide a handy reference book on a variety of topics, thus avoiding the need to scan several bulky references.

In this age of specialization in nursing it is important that nurses maintain a broad knowledge base, because we are all called upon occasionally for information relating to other nursing specialties. This knowledge is becoming increasingly important as the need for a "holistic" view of health and health care becomes more apparent. It is not enough to treat a specific condition of a client without concern for other factors in his or her life which have a bearing on health status. For this reason *The Whole Nurse Catalog* not only provides a ready reference for an individual nurse's field, but also contains key information from other fields of nursing as well. It is meant for use by individual nurses and for placement on clinical units in hospitals and health agencies as a general reference. Although it is particularly aimed at nurses, other allied health professionals will be able to make use of this book as well.

There is no one source available to date which contains clinical information as well as information on resource agencies and other health resources, including educational materials, publications, nursing organizations, and sources for nursing equipment for all fields of nursing. Nurses seeking resource information must depend on specialized publications, conferences and workshops. *The Whole Nurse Catalog* provides this information so that nurses can have a ready resource guide for themselves and their clients. In researching this book the author was continually impressed with the vast number of organizations and publications available to health professionals and the general public having to do with health care. It is heartening to know of the many groups and

INTRODUCTION

individuals working for better health. One of the aims of this book is to give nurses access to these resources and materials.

It is also impressive to learn of the many innovative practices nurses are involved with. Another feature of *The Whole Nurse Catalog* is the inclusion of articles describing some of these innovations, so that nurses may learn from what their colleagues are doing.

The Whole Nurse Catalog is divided into sections according to subject matter. Each section is subdivided into a clinical data component, followed by information on resources for each topic, including resource agencies, periodicals and other publications, and films related to the particular topic. Addresses are given with the descriptive material on each resource except in cases where the resource is listed several times, as with film resources and publishers. The addresses for these are listed alphabetically in the appendix to avoid repetition.

The material on sources for nursing equipment and uniforms has been listed separately and not categorized by topic since many of these materials are of use to nurses in several areas of practice.

Nursing organizations are also listed alphabetically in a separate section rather than categorized by field of interest since many of the organizations are open to nurses in several fields.

The inclusion in *The Whole Nurse Catalog* of any source for equipment, any resource organization, periodical, or film does not necessarily constitute an endorsement by the author or publisher. It has been impossible to evaluate everything listed, and it is not the intention of this book to endorse certain materials. Rather it is intended as a guide so that nurses can decide for themselves what is useful to them. Selected reviews of particularly useful resources are included to draw special attention to them.

There has been some selectivity in the listing of specific materials available from each resource due to limited space. Only the materials deemed the most useful to nurses have been included. Information on other materials available may be obtained by contacting the sources given.

Since the scope of this book is quite large, some useful resources may have been unintentionally overlooked. The author regrets this and welcomes information on any such resources. The address to which such suggestions may be sent is given at the end of this Introduction.

The same is true of the clinical data material. There may be clinical data in the form of charts and tables which other nurses find helpful to refer to, in addition to the material included here. And surely there are innovative practices in nursing beyond those described in this book. Again, it has been necessary to be selective in the material included since the amount of clinical data available to nurses is so extensive. An attempt has been made to include material which the nurse often needs at his/her fingertips but which is not readily committed to memory.

The information on specific drugs is current at the time of publication, but, due to rapid changes in medical knowledge and practice, it is

INTRODUCTION

advised that before giving any medications, nurses read the product information which accompanies medicines for the most up-to-date information on dosages, safety, side effects, contraindications, etc.

For the most part the cost of specific items listed has not been included, since this is subject to change. For information on current prices, contact the sources listed.

The Whole Nurse Catalog owes its existence to many individuals who have contributed their time and ideas. I would like to thank all of the individuals and organizations who responded to inquiries into their functions as resources for nurses and their clients. Their positive responses have been most encouraging. Much of the material on resources is adapted from the brochures and letters received in response to these inquiries. I would also like to thank the publishers of the clinical data excerpted from other sources for their kind permission to reprint these materials.

Especially helpful have been the nurses who have given of their time and expertise as consultants for this work. Thanks go to Bethea Brost, R.N., B.S., Judy Despirito, R.N., C.N.M., M.S., Suzanne Lego, R.N., Ph.D., Susan MacKenzie, R.N., B.S., Janice Shapiro, R.N., C.N.M., and Marie Smith, R.N., M.S.N. for their contributions and support.

Thanks also to Ann Clark, M.S.W., and Bonnie Gordon, B.A., for their support and assistance; to Stephanie Katz for her typing expertise; to my Mom, Cecile Clark, and Sharon, Stephanie, Diane and Jessica for their much needed babysitting assistance; and a very special thanks to Blyden.

Finally, I would like to express my gratitude to Churchill Livingstone for all the support and encouragement that has been extended me. In particular, thanks go to Lewis Reines, Carole Baker, Michiko Davis, and Laura Papach.

As mentioned previously, this book only begins to compile all of the valuable resources available to nurses. Readers are encouraged to share any special resources which they utilize. Kindly send any comments and suggestions for future editions to:

The Whole Nurse Catalog
P.O. Box 630
Bloomfield, N.J. 07003

Credit will be given for suggestions used.

Jane Jackson

Nursing Defined

Nursing is as old as mankind, although the origins of the profession as we know it today go back less than a century and a half. The word *nurse* is a reduced form of the Middle English *nurice,* which was derived, through the Old French *norrice,* from the Latin *nutricius* (nourishing). In Roman mythology, the goddess Fortuna, in addition to her usual function as goddess of fate, was also worshipped as Jupiter's nurse (Fortuna Praeneste) and prayed to for hygiene in the public baths (Fortuna Balnearis). From the dawn of civilization mankind has sought to acquire a knowledge of pain-relieving remedies and to discover additional means of preventing disease. To alleviate human suffering, man has also developed nursing roles.

The Advance of American Nursing, by Philip Kalisch and Beatrice Kalisch. Copyright 1978, Little, Brown and Company. Reprinted with permission.

Contents

1. **PATIENTS' RIGHTS** — 1
   - The American Nurses' Association's "Code for Nurses" — 1
   - A Patient's Bill of Rights — 2
   - Resources on Patients' Rights — 3

2. **DIAGNOSTICS AND PHYSICAL ASSESSMENT** — 4
   - Taking the Health History — 5
   - Outline Guide for the Collection of a Health History — 6
   - Normal Values—Hematology — 11
   - Normal Chemistries—Serum, Plasma, Whole Blood — 12
   - Normal Values—Urine Chemistry — 15
   - Hematocrit — 17
   - Hemoglobin — 17
   - Some Pediatric Laboratory Values the Intensive Care Nurse Must Know — 18
   - Hematologic Values During Infancy and Childhood — 19
   - Tests of Fetal Status — 20
   - Oral Glucose Tolerance Test (GTT) — 22
   - Methods of Urine Testing for Sugar — 23
   - Liver Function Tests — 24
   - Chromosome Number and Karyotype in Various Clinical Conditions — 25
   - ABO System of Antigens and Antibodies for Determining Blood Compatibility — 26
   - Drugs that May Cause Color Changes in Stool — 26
   - Drugs that May Alter Urine Color — 27
   - Summary of Basic Components of Neurological Examination — 28
   - Neurological Examination for Testing Cranial Nerves — 31

CONTENTS

Deep Tendon Reflexes	33
Pathological Reflexes	34
Average Pulse Rates at Rest	35
Pulse Points	36
Sequence of Auscultating Heart Sounds	37
Placement of the Bell of the Stethoscope	38
Placement of Electrocardiographic Leads	38
Summary of Basic Arrhythmias	39
Effect of Drugs and Electrolytes on the ECG	41
Guidelines for Adult Coronary Risk Assessment and Health Maintenance	42
Abnormalities in Rate and Rhythm of Breathing	44
Adventitious Sounds in the Chest Examination	45
Location of Major Structures in Each Abdominal Quadrant	46
Summary of Procedures of Biopsy or Aspiration	46
Summary of Common Radiological Procedures	48
Summary of Common Isotopic Procedures	52
Summary of Signs and Symptoms of Shock	55
Diseases Associated with Unusual Odors	56
Summary of Assessment of Acid-Base Imbalance	57
Differential Diagnosis of High Fever	59
Differential Diagnosis of Abdominal Pain	61
Differential Diagnosis of Cardiac and Pulmonary Dyspnea	64
What to Expect in Seven Types of Cerebrovascular Accidents	65
A Comparison of Juvenile Diabetes and Adult-Onset Diabetes	67
Comparison of Clinical Features in Insulin Reactions and Diabetic Coma	68
Clinical Appraisal of Thrombophlebitis	69
Categories of Seizure Types	70
Differentiation of Common Breast Nodules	71
A Comparison of the Characteristics of Benign and Malignant Neoplasms	73
Recommended Sources on Physical Assessment for Nurses	75
Audiovisual Materials on Physical Assessment	76
3. PHARMACOLOGY	77
Formulas Used for Computation of Correct Dosage for Administration	78

Calculating Drops per Minute	79
Intramuscular Injection Sites	81
Drug Administration in Relation to Meals	84
Specific Antidotes for Toxic Agents	85
Selected Drug Incompatibilities with Intravenous 5 Per Cent Glucose	86
Summary of Drug Interactions	88
Analgesics	90
Agents Used in Anesthesia Administration	93
Antianemics	96
Antihypertensive Agents	98
Commonly Used Antipsychotic Agents	99
Barbiturates	100
Cardiac Glycosides	104
Drugs Used in Cardiac Emergencies	107
Major Drugs (Used in Chemotherapy)	108
Diuretics	113
Antibiotic Therapy in Gonorrhea	115
Insulins	116
Radioisotopes and Their Therapeutic Uses	117
The Penicillins	118
Examples of Drugs Known to Cause Blood Dyscrasias, by Disorder	120
Drug Effects on Human Sexual Behavior	121
Characteristics of Abused Drugs and Their Acute Reactions in Adolescents	124
Publications on Pharmacology	126
Audiovisual Materials on Pharmacology	126
4. MEDICAL-SURGICAL NURSING	**127**
Nurses—The Caring Link	129
A Mother's Letter	129
Methods of Patient Teaching	130
First Aid in Cardiopulmonary Resuscitation	131
The Heimlich Maneuver	132
First Aid for Choking	134
Position to Dislodge Foreign Objects from Child's Airway	136
Equipment for an Emergency Cart for Cardiopulmonary Resuscitation	137
Body Water Balance in the Adult over a 24-hour Period	138
Operation and Exam Positions	139

CONTENTS

Examples of Exercises to Help Maintain Joint Range in Motion	140
Which Wounds to Watch	141
How Wounds Heal	142
Pain	143
Comparative Uses of Hot and Cold Applications	143
Methods of Oxygen Administration	144
General Nursing Assessment, Intervention and Evaluation During IV Therapy	145
Superficial Veins, Dorsal Aspect of Hand	148
Superficial Veins, Forearm	148
Prevention, Assessment and Intervention Methods for Complications of IV Therapy	149
Summary of Bedside Intravascular Monitoring Techniques in Critically Ill Patients	151
Nursing Interventions for Patients on Chemotherapy	153
Hemolytic Transfusion Reaction	153
Nursing Assessment, Intervention, and Evaluation During Peritoneal Dyalysis	155
Bladder Elimination	157
Acute Head Injury: A Plan for Assessment	161
Nursing Interventions for Patients on Chemotherapy	162
Burn Care	165
Management of Chemical Burns Care	165
Methods of Burn Care	166
Educational Programs and Materials in Burn Care Research	166
Phases of Hypertension	167
Orthopaedics	168
Possible Complications from Fractures	169
Spinal Cord Injury Rehabilitation: A Message to Helping Professionals	170
Functional Goals and Potential Equipment in Spinal Cord Lesions	172
Plan of a Coronary Care Unit	176
The ABGs of Radiation	177
"In the Event of Radiation Exposure..."	178
Effects of Some Common Industrial Agents Upon the Worker	180
Preoperative Assessment Guidelines	182
Innovation in Surgical Nursing	184

General Medical-Surgical Resources	185
Publications on Medical-Surgical Nursing and Related Topics	191
General Nursing Periodicals	196
Audiovisual Materials	200
Resources on Burns and Burn Care	203
Resources on Cancer	204
Sources on Mastectomy Information	208
Resources on Communicable Diseases	210
Resources on Diabetes	211
Resources in Environmental and Occupational Health	213
Resources on the Handicapped	218
National Spinal Cord Injury Foundation	219
Bibliography on Higher Education and the Handicapped	223
Resources on Self-Help and Consumer-Oriented Health Care	226
Resources on Smoking	229
NCI Makes Available Smokers "Quit Kit"	230
Resources on Speech and Hearing Disorders	231
Resources on Vision and Blindness	232
5. NUTRITION	**235**
Nutrients for Health	237
Other Important Nutrients	240
Recommended Daily Dietary Allowances	242
Safety of Common Food Additives	243
Liquid Diets	247
Restricted Sodium Diet	250
Low- or Minimal-Fiber Diet	250
Bland Diet	251
Restricted Fat Diets (Hyperlipoproteinemia Diets)	252
Dietary Strategies for the Two Main Types of Diabetes	253
Quantities of Food Needed During Pregnancy and Lactation	254
Vegetarian Diets	254
Some Sound Guidelines for Vegetarians	256
Food Guide for Pregnant Vegetarians	257
The Calorie—A Brief Summary of Basic Facts	258
Summary of Treatments for Obesity	259
Compulsive Eating Cycle	261

CONTENTS

The Protein Sparing Modified Fast—What Is It?	262
Protein Quality	263
Dietary Habits of Two Ethnic Groups	271
Oriental Dietary Habits	271
Jewish Dietary Laws	272
6. MATERNITY NURSING	**280**
The Pregnant Patient's Bill of Rights	283
Family-Centered Maternity Care	286
Diagnosis of Pregnancy	289
Weight Gain in Pregnancy	290
Fundal Height at Various Times During Pregnancy	291
Childbirth Educator's Role	293
Innovations in Prenatal Education	294
Recommended References on Adolescent Pregnancy	301
Alcohol and Pregnancy	302
Identification of High Risk Pregnancy: Factors Associated with Increased Risk	304
The Fetus and the Newborn Infant	307
Conditions in Which Antenatal Diagnosis by Amniocentesis Has Been Made	308
The Role of the Nurse During Amniocentesis	308
Factors Implicated in the Etiology of Intrauterine Fetal Growth Retardation	315
Signs and Symptoms of Preeclampsia—Eclampsia	316
Treatment for Preeclampsia—Eclampsia	317
Interaction of Diabetes and Pregnancy	318
Cervical Dilatation	319
Normal Labor Graph	319
Labor Abnormalities	320
Mechanism of Labor-LOA	321
Fetal Monitoring	322
The Diagnosis of Acute Fetal Distress	325
The Treatment of Fetal Distress	325
Shock Hazards from Monitoring Equipment	326
Apgar Scoring	327
Emergency Childbirth	328
Postpartum	331
Disorders of Mothering	332
Estimation of Gestational Age	333
Common Variations in the Neonate	335
Danger Signs in the Newborn	338

References on Breast Feeding	338
Innovations in Maternity Care	341
Maternity Nursing Resources	345
Resources on Breast and Bottle Feeding	348

7. NURSING CARE OF CHILDREN — 369

Growth and Development	371
Essential Milestones	372
Summary of Normal Development in the First Three Years	373
Language Development	378
Typical Accidents Related to Developmental Level	380
Immunizations	381
Contraindications to Immunizations	382
Incubation Period and Duration of Infectivity of Common Infectious Diseases	382
Preventive Dental Practices for Children	383
Children in Hospitals	385
A Child's Letter	389
A Guide to the Development of Nursing Approach	390
Preferred Intramuscular Injection Sites for Older Children	392
Preferred Intramuscular Injection Sites for Premature and Newborn Infants	393
Factors Affecting Adjustment (to Hospitalization)	394
Signs Indicating Effects of Chronic Hospitalization	394
Pediatric Psychological Checklist for Surgery	395
Pediatric Resuscitation Kit	396
Observations of the Neonate	397
Reflexes of Neonates	397
Physical Observation and Appraisal of the Newborn	398
Significance of the Two Conditions	399
Equipment Required for Neonatal Intensive Care	400
Infant Suctioning Methods	400
Signs Indicative of Respiratory Distress in the Neonate	401
Signs and Symptoms of Cardiovascular Disorders in Infants	403
Parent-Parent Support in the Care of High-Risk Newborns	404
The Counseling of Families in the Professional Management of Sudden Infant Death Syndrome	409
The Management of SIDS	410

The Counseling Visit	412
Rule of Fives	413
Pediatric I.V.'s	413
Home Care for the Dying Child	414
Nursing Diagnoses and Interventions: The Disturbed Child's Family	414
The Nurse and the Abused Child	415
Further References on Child Abuse and Neglect	425
Resources in Pediatric Nursing	426
Growing Parents' Groups	429

8. GERONTOLOGICAL NURSING 458

Aging Changes	459
Innovations	460
Resources on Geriatrics	465
Schools Having Educational Programs in Geriatric Nursing	467

9. DEATH AND DYING 470

The Dying Person's Bill of Rights	470
Nurse Specialists for the Dying	471
Stages in the Acceptance of Death	472
Death—A Part of Living	472
Separation and Loss	473
Gramp	475
Resources on Death and Dying	478
Suggested References on Death and Dying	481
Audiovisual Materials on Death and Dying	484

10. MENTAL HEALTH AND PSYCHIATRIC NURSING 485

The Psychiatric Liaison Nurse in the General Hospital	486
The Private Practice of Psychotherapy in Psychiatric Nursing	493
Group Work Therapy and Practice	496
Self Acceptance	506
Erikson's Theory of Social Growth and Development	507
Ego Defense Mechanisms	508
Assessing Suicide Potential	509
The Professional Client	510
Sexual Myths and Facts to Refute Them	511

A Comparison of Approaches to Treating Sexual
   Dysfunction   513
Acceptance of the Client's Differences   515
Gay Rights in the Hospital   515
Comparison of Experimental and Dysfunctional Use
   of Drugs   516
Commonly Used Terms of the Drug User   518
Comprehensive Psychiatric Nursing   520
Resources in Mental Health and Psychiatric Nursing   521
Schools with Educational Programs for
   Psychiatric-Mental Health Nurse Practitioners   529

11. PUBLIC HEALTH NURSING   536
Extended Role of the Public-Health Nurse: A
   Statement of Policy   536
Specialization of Public Health Nurses   537
A Visiting Nurses Association's Affiliation with
   Group Physician Practices   539
Public-Health Nurse in Mental Health Follow-Up
   Care   541
Resources in Public Health   543

12. HOLISTIC HEALTH   545
Holistic Health   545
The Holistic Nurse   545
Therapeutic Touch in Practice   546
Mind-Body Relatedness   549
Resources in Holistic Health   551

13. PRIMARY NURSING   557
Definition of Primary Nursing   557
If You Are Instituting Primary Nursing   557
Resources in Primary Nursing   559
Nurse Faculty Fellowships   560

14. RESOURCES IN WOMEN'S HEALTH   561

15. RESOURCES IN MALE HEALTH CARE   567
The Men's Reproductive Health Clinic   567
Audiovisual Materials on Men and Male Health   568

16. FAMILY PLANNING AND INFERTILITY   569
Oral Contraceptives   569
Pill Side Effects: A Time Framework   571

CONTENTS

Pill Side Effects: Hormone Etiology	572
Contraindications to IUD Insertion	573
Resources in Family Planning and Infertility	574
17. RESOURCES IN SEXUALITY	**579**
National Sex Forum	579
18. NURSING RECORDS	**582**
What Is a Problem-Oriented Health Care Record?	582
S O A P	583
Resources on Nursing Records	584
19. NURSING INNOVATIONS	**585**
Audiovisual Materials on Nurses and Nursing	586
20. TRANSCULTURAL NURSING	**587**
Challenges of Cross-Cultural Encounters	587
Education in Transcultural Nursing	588
21. NURSING EDUCATION	**589**
Continuing Education	590
An Example of Continuing Education in Practice	590
Resources in Continuing Education	591
Publications on Continuing Education	592
Special Education Programs for Nurses: Career Mobility	593
Internship Programs	595
Doctoral Programs	596
Summer Program of Doctoral Study at U-T, Austin, Texas	596
Resources in Nursing Education	597
References on Scholarships and Grants for Nursing Education	598
22. NURSING RESEARCH	**599**
Regional Medical Libraries	599
Resources in Nursing Research	600
23. INDEPENDENT NURSING PRACTICE AND THE EXPANDED ROLE OF THE NURSE	**602**
Independent Nursing Practice	602
The Expanded Role of the Nurse	603
Audiovisual Materials on the Expanded Role of the Nurse	605

CONTENTS

24. NURSING AND THE LAW	606
Professional Liability Insurance Policy	607
Explanation of Admission Consent Form	607
An Innovative Approach to Protecting Patients' Rights	610
Selected References on Nursing and the Law	611
Audiovisual Materials on Nursing and the Law	612
25. MILITARY NURSING	613
Military Nursing Opportunities	613
26. JOB HUNTING	616
Practical Tips for Job Hunting	616
New Career Guide Now Available from NSNA	621
27. NURSING ABROAD	622
Sources of Information on Employment Opportunities in International Nursing	622
28. MISCELLANEOUS NURSING INFORMATION	623
Foreign Nurses Wishing to Work in the United States	623
Writing for Nursing Publications	624
Guide to Publishing Opportunities for Nurses	624
Fundraising	625
Grantsmanship: It Can Be Learned Part I	625
Grantsmanship: It Can Be Learned Part II	627
ANA Publishes Ethics Handbook	629
29. NURSING ORGANIZATIONS	630
Chronology of Nurse Associations	630
Nursing Organizations	631
30. SOURCES OF EQUIPMENT AND SUPPLIES OF USE TO NURSES AND THEIR CLIENTS	646
Stethoscopes	646
Sphygmomanometers	647
Sources for Patient Care Equipment and Supplies	648
Sources for Obstetrics Supplies and Equipment	661
Sources for Surgical Equipment and Supplies	663
Your Surgical Instruments & Their Care	667
Sources for Urological and Ostomy Supplies	669
Characteristics for Urostomy Appliances	671
Sources for Teaching Aids	672

Sources for Uniforms and Other Supplies for
Nurses   674
Nursing Uniforms Yesterday and Today   676

31. APPENDIX   678
Conversion of Pounds and Ounces to Grams   679
Average Height and Weight for Children   679
Head Circumference   680
Percentile Charts for Measurements of Infant Girls   681
Percentile Charts for Measurements of Girls   682
Percentile Charts for Measurements of Boys   683
Desirable Weights for Men Ages 25 and Over   684
Desirable Weights for Women Ages 25 and Over   684
Equivalents   685
Some Common Conversions to the Metric System of Measurement   687
State Boards of Nursing   688
Largest Poison Control Centers   692
State Departments of Vocational Rehabilitation   695
State Welfare Office Listings   698
Sources for Audiovisual Aids   701
Audiovisual Equipment   708
Index of Publishers   710
Abbreviations in Common Use   714

INDEX   723

1 Patients' Rights

The American Nurses' Association's "Code for Nurses"

1. The nurse provides services with respect for human dignity and the uniqueness of the client unrestricted by considerations of social or economic status, personal attributes, or the nature of health problems.

2. The nurse safeguards the client's right to privacy by judiciously protecting information of a confidential nature.

3. The nurse acts to safeguard the client and the public when health care and safety are affected by the incompetent, unethical, or illegal practice of any person.

4. The nurse assumes responsibility and accountability for individual nursing judgments and actions.

5. The nurse maintains competence in nursing.

6. The nurse exercises informed judgment and uses individual competence and qualifications as criteria in seeking consultation, accepting responsibilities, and delegating nursing activities to others.

7. The nurse participates in activities that contribute to the ongoing development of the profession's body of knowledge.

8. The nurse participates in the profession's efforts to implement and improve standards of nursing.

9. The nurse participates in the profession's efforts to establish and maintain conditions of employment conducive to high quality nursing care.

10. The nurse participates in the profession's effort to protect the public from misinformation and misrepresentation and to maintain the integrity of nursing.

11. The nurse collaborates with members of the health professions and other citizens in promoting community and national efforts to meet the health needs of the public.

Reprinted with permission of The American Nurses' Association. From *Code for Nurses with Interpretive Statements.* Copyright American Nurses Association.

2
A Patient's Bill of Rights

1. The patient has the right to considerate and respectful care.

2. The patient has the right to obtain from his physician complete, current information concerning his diagnosis, treatment and prognosis in terms the patient can be reasonably expected to understand. When it is not medically advisable to give such information to the patient, the information should be made available to an appropriate person in his behalf. He has the right to know, by name, the physician responsible for coordinating his care.

3. The patient has the right to receive from his physician information necessary to give informed consent prior to the start of any procedure and/or treatment. Except in emergencies, such information for informed consent should include but not necessarily be limited to the specific procedure and/or treatment, the medically significant risks involved and the probable duration of incapacitation. Where medically significant alternatives for care or treatment exist, or when the patient requests information concerning medical alternatives, the patient has the right to such information. The patient also has the right to know the name of the person responsible for the procedures and/or treatment.

4. The patient has the right to refuse treatment to the extent permitted by law and to be informed of the medical consequences of his action.

5. The patient has the right to every consideration of his privacy concerning his own medical care program. Care discussion, consultation, examination and treatment are confidential and should be conducted discreetly. Those not directly involved in his care must have the permission of the patient to be present.

6. The patient has the right to expect that all communications and records pertaining to his care should be treated as confidential.

7. The patient has the right to expect that within its capacity a hospital must make reasonable response to the request of a patient for services. The hospital must provide evaluation, service, and/or referral as indicated by the urgency of the case. When medically permissible, a patient may be transferred to

another facility only after he has received complete information and explanation concerning the needs for and alternatives to such a transfer. The institution to which the patient is to be transferred must first have accepted the patient for transfer.

8. The patient has the right to obtain information as to any relationship of his hospital to other health care and educational institutions insofar as his care is concerned. The patient has the right to obtain information as to the existence of any professional relationships among individuals, by name, who are treating him.

9. The patient has the right to be advised if the hospital proposes to engage in or perform human experimentation affecting his care or treatment. The patient has the right to refuse to participate in such research projects.

10. The patient has the right to expect reasonable continuity of care. He has the right to know in advance what appointment times and physicians are available and where. The patient has the right to expect that the hospital will provide a mechanism whereby he is informed by his physician or a delegate of the physician of the patient's continuing health care requirements following discharge.

11. The patient has the right to examine and receive an explanation of his bill regardless of source of payment.

12. The patient has the right to know what hospital rules and regulations apply to his conduct as a patient.

Reprinted with permission of the American Hospital Association.

Resources on Patients' Rights

The Rights of Hospital Patients, American Civil Liberties Union Handbook, by George Annas, Avon Books, 1975 (Price $1.75, Avon Books, 959 Eighth Ave., New York, N.Y. 10019).

Written for hospital patients and personnel to inform them of the legal rights of patients, this book discusses in detail the rights of patients in all areas. It is useful to nurses as a reminder that a hospital patient is a person first, with all the human rights that that entails. It is also useful to nurses in their role as patient advocates and as such is a good book to refer patients to for further knowledge of their rights.

2 Diagnostics and Physical Assessment

Nurses in many clinical settings are now required to take part in physical assessment of clients, including taking health histories, preparing patients for laboratory procedures, interpreting lab data, and assessing physical signs and symptoms. The material in this section includes guides to aid nurses in performing these functions.

I. **The Health History**

II. **Laboratory Values**
   Hematology
   Normal Chemistries
   Urine Chemistry
   Hematocrit and Hemoglobin
   Pediatric Laboratory Values

III. **Diagnostic Testing**
   Tests of Fetal Status
   Glucose Tolerance Test
   Urine Tests for Sugar
   Liver Function Tests
   Chromosomal Karyotypes

IV. **ABO Blood Typing System**

V. **Changes in Urine and Stool Caused by Drugs**

VI. **Some Components of the Physical Exam**
   Neurological Exam
   Assessment of Heart and Lungs
   Abdominal Palpation

VII. **More Diagnostic Procedures**
   Biopsies
   Radiologic Procedures
   Isotopic Procedures

VIII. **Differential Diagnoses**
   Shock
   Acid-base Imbalances
   Differential Diagnosis of High Fever
   Differential Diagnosis of Abdominal Pain
   Cardiac and Pulmonary Dyspnea

Cerebrovascular Accidents
Diabetes
Thrombophlebitis
Seizures
Breast Nodules
Cancer of the Cervix
Benign and Malignant Neoplasms
IX. **Recommended Resources on Physical Assessment**
Publications
Audiovisual Aids

Taking the Health History

"General Principles
1. The first step in caring for a patient and in soliciting his active cooperation is to gather a careful and complete history.
    a. In all patient concerns and problems, an accurate history is the foundation on which data collection and the process of assessment are based.
    b. The comprehensiveness of the history elicited will depend on the information available in the patient's record.
2. Time spent early in the nurse-patient relationship gathering detailed information about what the patient knows, thinks, and feels about his problems will prevent time-consuming errors and misunderstandings later.
3. Skill in interviewing will affect both the accuracy of information elicited and the quality of the relationship established with the patient. . . .
4. The purpose of the interview is to encourage an interchange of information between the patient and the nurse.
    a. The patient must feel that his words are understood and that his concerns are being listened to and dealt with sensitively.
    b. Some basic techniques for achieving these ends include the following:
        (1) Provide privacy for the patient in as quiet a place as possible and see that he is comfortable.
        (2) Begin the interview with a courteous greeting and an introduction. Explain who you are and why you are there.
        (3) Be sure that facial expressions, body movements,

and tone of voice are pleasant, unhurried, and nonevaluative, and that they convey the attitude of a sensitive listener, so that the patient will feel free to express his thoughts and feelings.
(4) Avoid reassuring the patient prematurely (before you have adequate information about the problem). This only serves to cut off discussion; the patient may then be unwilling to bring up a problem causing concern.
(5) At times a patient gives cues or suggests information, but does not tell enough. It may be necessary to probe for more information in order to obtain a thorough history; the patient must realize that this is done for his benefit.
(6) Guide the interview so that the necessary information is obtained, without cutting off discussion. Controlling the rambling patient is often difficult, but with practice it can be done skillfully, without jeopardizing the quality of the information gained."

Reprinted with permission from Brunner, L. S. and Suddarth, D. S., Eds.: *The Lippincott Manual of Nursing Practice*, 2nd Ed., p. 6. J. B. Lippincott, Philadelphia, 1978.

OUTLINE GUIDE FOR THE COLLECTION OF A HEALTH HISTORY

Date

I REASON FOR CONTACT

Reason for encounter with health personnel and facility.

II BIOGRAPHICAL DATA
A. Full name
B. Residence
C. Telephone Number
D. Age
E. Date of Birth
F. Place of Birth
G. Sex
H. Ethnic Group
I. Religion
J Primary Spoken Language
K. Marital Status
L. Education
M. Occupation
N. Health Insurance
O. Social Security Number
P. First Names of Parents; Mother's Maiden Name

III CURRENT HEALTH STATUS
A. *Details of Specific Complaint*
B. *Daily Habits and/or Activity Patterns*
 1. Diet
 2. Elimination
 3. Personal Hygiene
 4. Use of Tobacco and Drugs
 5. Recreation and Exercise/Play
 6. Sleep

IV PAST HEALTH HISTORY

A. *Developmental Data*
B. *Promotive and Preventive Practices*

1. Examinations
2. Counseling
3. Immunizations

C. *Restorative Interventions*

1. Past Illnesses, Injuries, and Surgery
2. Infectious Diseases

D. *Allergies*
E. *Foreign Travel*

V FAMILY HISTORY

A. *Composition of Family*

1. Relationship to Client
2. Age
3. Sex

B. *Health Status of Family Members*

1. General Description
2. Present Illnesses or Injuries
3. Other Major Stressors

C. *Familial Illnesses*
D. *Relationships Among Family Members*

1. Roles
2. Interactions

VI SOCIAL HISTORY

A. *Relationships*
B. *Occupation/School*

1. Type of Position
2. Length of Current Position
3. Conditions of Employment/School
    (a) Exposure to irritating or toxic agents
    (b) Unusual environmental conditions
    (c) Contact with various domestic or wild animals
    (d) Pressures

4. Relationships with Peers and Business Associates
5. Job or School Satisfaction
6. Financial Status
7. Past Employment/School
    (a) Types
    (b) Conditions
    (c) Dates or frequency of changes

C. *Environment*

1. Types of Living Conditions
2. Physical Facilities
3. Type of Community
4. Number of Persons in Household

VII REVIEW OF SYSTEMS

A. *General State of Health*

1. Recent Change in Weight and Height
2. Weakness
3. Fatigue
4. Malaise
5. Fever
6. Chills

B. *Integumentary System*

1. Skin
    (a) Texture
    (b) Excessive dryness or perspiration
    (c) Alteration in temperature
    (d) Unusual pigmentation
    (e) Pruritus
    (f) Lesions
    (g) Growths

2. Hair
    (a) Texture
    (b) Condition
    (c) Distribution
    (d) Abnormal growth or loss

3. Nails
    (a) Shape
    (b) Color
    (c) Condition

Continued on next page

C. *Head*
1. Pain
2. Trauma

D. *Eyes*
1. Itching
2. Redness
3. Edema
4. Pain
5. Diplopia
6. Blurring
7. Spots
8. Lacrimation
9. Visual Changes

E. *Ears*
1. Pain
2. Discharges
3. Hearing Changes
4. Vertigo
5. Tinnitus

F. *Nose and Sinuses*
1. Pain
2. Tenderness
3. Discharges
4. Obstruction
5. Sneezing
6. Olfactory Changes
7. Epistaxis

G. *Mouth and Throat*
1. Pain
2. Soreness
3. Lesions
4. Altered Taste
5. Difficulty in Chewing
6. Dysphagia
7. Bleeding
8. Voice Changes
9. Hoarseness
10. Condition of Teeth

H. *Neck*
1. Pain
2. Swelling
3. Enlargement
4. Limitation of Movement

I. *Breast*
1. Pain
2. Tenderness
3. Lumps
4. Dimples
5. Discharges
6. Changes in Nipples
7. Development
8. Lactation

J. *Respiratory System*
1. Pain
2. Dyspnea
3. Wheezing
4. Coughing
5. Sputum
6. Hemoptysis

K. *Cardiovascular System*
1. Pain
2. Dyspnea
3. Palpitations
4. Syncope
5. Edema

L. *Gastrointestinal System*
1. Pain
2. Pyrosis
3. Appetite Changes
4. Food Intolerance
5. Nausea
6. Emesis
7. Jaundice
8. Flatulence
9. Diarrhea
10. Constipation
11. Change in Bowel Habits

M. *Genitourinary System*

1. Urinary Tract
   (a) Dysuria
   (b) Burning
   (c) Urgency
   (d) Frequency
   (e) Hesitancy
   (f) Incontinence
   (g) Dribbling
   (h) Nocturia
   (i) Change in characteristics of urine
   (j) Retention
   (k) Oliguria
   (l) Polyuria

2. Genitalia
   (a) Pain
   (b) Burning
   (c) Lesions
   (d) Edema
   (e) Discharges
   (f) Secondary sex characteristics
   (g) Sexual drive/activity/ satisfaction
   (h) Contraceptive methods
   (i) Impotence/frigidity
   (j) Sterility

3. Menstrual/Menopausal
   (a) Age at onset
   (b) Date of last period
   (c) Amount of flow
   (d) Length of cycle
   (e) Duration
   (f) Amenorrhea
   (g) Menorrhagia
   (h) Metrorrhagia
   (i) Dysmenorrhea
   (j) Cessation of menses
   (k) Hot flashes

4. Obstetrical
   (a) Number of pregnancies
   (b) Deliveries; types
   (c) Stillbirths
   (d) Living children
   (e) Complications of pregnancy
   (f) Miscarriages
   (g) Abortions

N. *Musculoskeletal System*
1. Pain
2. Tenderness
3. Cramps
4. Swelling
5. Weakness
6. Deformities
7. Decreased Range of Motion
8. Atrophy

Continued on next page

O. *Neurological System*

1. General Status
   (a) Somnolence
   (b) Vertigo
   (c) Loss of consciousness
   (d) Convulsions
   (e) Weakness
2. Mental Status
   (a) Changes in disposition
   (b) Insomnia
   (c) Anxiety
   (d) Amnesia
   (e) Inability to meet responsibilities
   (f) Difficulty in interactions
   (g) Phobias
   (h) Hallucinations
   (i) Depression
3. Motor Status
   (a) Altered gait
   (b) Difficulty in coordination
   (c) Tremors
   (d) Paresis
   (e) Paralysis
4. Sensory Status
   (a) Pain
   (b) Paresthesia

P. *Hematopoietic System*

1. Bleeding Tendencies
2. Easy Bruisability
3. Lymph Node Enlargement
4. Exposure to Toxic Agents
5. Anemia
6. Blood Type

Q. *Endocrine System*

1. Change in Skin Texture
2. Excessive Dryness or Perspiration
3. Unusual Pigmentation
4. Abnormal Hair Distribution
5. Change in Weight and Height
6. Sensitivity to Temperature Variations
7. Change in Disposition
8. Abnormal Growth
9. Polydipsia
10. Polyphagia
11. Polyuria
12. Anorexia
13. Weakness
14. Drowsiness
15. Palpitations
16. Atrophy
17. Goiter

R. *Allergic and Immunological System*

1. Pruritus
2. Migraine
3. Dermatitis
4. Urticaria
5. Sneezing
6. Angioedema
7. Vasomotor Rhinitis
8. Conjunctivitis

Reprinted by permission of J. B. Lippincott Co. from Mahoney, E., Verdisco, L. and Shortridge, L.: *How to Collect and Record a Health History*, © 1976, J. B. Lippincott Company.

For further study see *American Journal of Nursing*, February, 1974, "Programmed Instruction on Taking a Patient's History."

Normal Values-Hematology

Determination	Normal Value	Clinical Significance
Bleeding time	30 sec.–6 min.	Prolonged in purpura hemorrhagica, in which platelets are reduced, and in chloroform and phosphorus poisoning.
Clotting time	5–10 min.	Prolonged in hemorrhagic disease and in various coagulation factor deficiencies.
Erythrocyte count	Males: 4,600,000–6,200,000 per cu. mm. Females: 4,200,000–5,400,000 per cu. mm.	Increased in severe diarrhea and dehydration, polycythemia, secondary polycythemia, acute poisoning, pulmonary fibrosis, and Ayerza disease. Decreased in all anemias, in leukemia, and after hemorrhage, when blood volume has been restored.
Reticulocytes	0.5–1.5% of red cells	Increased with any condition stimulating increase in bone marrow activity, i.e., infection, blood loss (acute and chronic); following iron therapy in iron deficiency anemia, polycythemia rubra vera. Decreased with any condition depressing bone marrow activity, acute leukemia, late stage of severe anemias.
Erythrocyte sedimentation rate	Males: 0–9 mm./hr. Females: 0–20 mm./hr.	Increased in tissue destruction, whether inflammatory or degenerative, and during menstruation, pregnancy, and in acute febrile diseases.
Leukocyte count Neutrophils Eosinophils Basophils Lymphocytes Monocytes	Total: 5,000–10,000 cu. mm. 60–70% 1–4% 0–0.5% 20–30% 2–6%	Elevated in acute infectious diseases—predominantly in the neutrophilic fraction with bacterial diseases, and in the lymphocytic and monocytic fractions in viral diseases. Eosinophils elevated in collagen diseases, allergy, intestinal parasitosis. Elevated in acute leukemia, following menstruation, and following surgery or trauma. Depressed in aplastic anemia, agranulocytosis and by toxic agents, such as chemotherapeutic agents used in treating malignancy.
Platelet Count	200,000–350,000 per cu. mm.	Increased with chronic granulocytic leukemia, hemoconcentration. Decreased in thrombocytopenic purpura, acute leukemia, aplastic anemia, and during cancer chemotherapy.

12

Normal Chemistries–Serum, Plasma, Whole Blood

Determination	Normal Adult Values	Clinical Significance (increased)	(decreased)

CO_2 content	Adults:
	  24–32 mEq/L.
	Infants:
	  18–24 mEq/L.
		Tetany
		Respiratory disease
		Intestinal obstruction
		Vomiting
			Acidosis
			Nephritis
			Eclampsia
			Diarrhea
			Anesthesia

Cholesterol	150–300 mg./100 ml.	Lipemia Obstructive jaundice Diabetes Hypothyroidism	Pernicious anemia Hemolytic anemia Hyperthyroidism Severe infection Terminal states of debilitating disease
Creatine	0.2–0.8 mg./100 ml.	Biliary obstruction Pregnancy Nephritis Renal destruction Trauma to muscle Pseudohypertrophic muscular dystrophy	

Creatine phosphokinase (CPK)	Males:
	  50–325 mU/ml
	Females:
	  50–250 mU/ml
		Myocardial infarction
		Skeletal muscle diseases
		Intramuscular injections
		Crush syndrome
		Hypothyroidism
		Delirium tremens
		Cerebrovascular diseases	

Creatinine	0.7–1.4 mg/100 ml	Nephritis Chronic renal diseases	
Creatinine clearance	100–150 mls of blood cleared of creatinine/min.		Kidney diseases

Determination	Normal Adult Values	Clinical Significance (increased)	(decreased)
Glucose	Fasting: 60–110 mg/100 ml Postprandial (2 hour): 65–140 mg/100 ml	Diabetes Nephritis Hyperthyroidism Early hyperpituitarism Cerebral lesions Infections Pregnancy Uremia	Hyperinsulinism Hypothyroidism Late hyperpituitarism Pernicious vomiting Addison's disease Extensive hepatic damage
Glucose tolerance (oral)	Features of a normal response: 1. Normal fasting between 60–125 mg/100 ml 2. No sugar in urine 3. The upper limits of normal are: fasting—125 1 hour—190 2 hours—140 3 hours—125	Hyperinsulinism Adrenal cortical insufficiency (Addison's disease) Anterior pituitary hypofunction Hypothyroidism Sprue and celiac disease	Diabetes Hyperthyroidism Primary adrenal cortical tumor or hyperplasia Severe anemia Certain central nervous system disorders
Icterus index	1–6 units	Biliary obstruction Hemolytic anemias	Secondary anemias
Iodine, protein-bound	4.0–8.0 micrograms/100 ml	Hyperthyroidism	Hypothyroidism
Iron	65–170 micrograms/100 ml	Pernicious anemia Aplastic anemia Hemolytic anemia Hepatitis Hemochromatosis	Iron deficiency anemia
Iron binding capacity	IBC: 150–235 micrograms/100 ml TIBC: 250–420 micrograms/100 ml % Saturation: 20–50	Iron deficiency anemia	Chronic infectious diseases
Lead (whole blood)	up to 40 micrograms/100 ml	Lead poisoning	
Lipids, total	400–1000 mg/100 ml	Hypothyroidism Diabetes Nephrosis Glomerulonephritis	Hyperthyroidism
Oxygen, saturation, arterial (whole blood)	96–100%	Polycythemia Anhydremia	Anemia Cardiac decompensation Chronic obstructive pulmonary disease

Continued on next page

14

Determination	Normal Adult Values	Clinical Significance (increased)	(decreased)
pCO₂ (whole blood) arterial	35–45 mm. Hg	Respiratory acidosis Metabolic alkalosis	Respiratory alkalosis Metabolic acidosis
pH (whole blood) arterial	7.35–7.45	Vomiting Hyperpnea Fever Intestinal obstruction	Uremia Diabetic acidosis Hemorrhage Nephritis
pO₂ (whole blood) arterial	95–100 mm. Hg	Directly related to oxygen saturation	
Phenylalanine	0–6 mg/100 ml first week 0.7–3.5 mg/100 ml thereafter	Phenylketonuria Oasthouse urine diease	
Potassium	3.5–5.0 mEq/L.	Addison's disease Oliguria Anuria Tissue breakdown or hemolysis	Diabetic acidosis Diarrhea Vomiting
Protein, total	6.0–8.0 gm/100 ml	Hemoconcentration Shock	Malnutrition Hemorrhage
Albumin	3.5–5.0 gm/100 ml	Multiple myeloma (globulin fraction)	Loss of plasma from burns
Globulin	1.5–3.0 gm/100 ml	Chronic infections (globulin fraction) Liver disease (globulin)	Proteinuria
Sodium	135–145 mEq/L.	Hemoconcentration Nephritis Pyloric obstruction	Alkali defecit Addison's disease Myxedema
T₃ Uptake	25–35%	Hyperthyroidism TBG deficiency Androgens and anabolic steroids	Hypothyroidism Pregnancy TBG excess Estrogens and anti-ovulatory drugs
T₃, Triiodothyronine (total circulating), by radioimmunoassay	75–200 nanograms/100 ml	Pregnancy Hyperthyroidism	Hypothyroidism

Determination	Normal Adult Values	Clinical Significance (increased)	(decreased)
T_4, Thyroxine by radioimmunoassay	4.5–11.5 micrograms/100 ml	Hyperthyroidism Thyroiditis Cases of elevated thyroxine-binding proteins caused by oral contraceptives Pregnancy	Primary and pituitary hypothyroidism Idiopathic involvement Cases of diminished thyroxine-binding proteins caused by androgenic and anabolic steroids Hypoproteinemia Nephrotic syndrome
T_4, Thyroxine, free	1.0–2.2 nanograms/100 ml	Euthyroid patients with normal free thyroxine levels may have abnormal T_3 and T_4 levels caused by drug preparations	
Urea nitrogen (BUN)	10–20 mg/100 ml	Acute glomerulonephritis Obstructive uropathy Mercury poisoning Nephrotic syndrome	Severe hepatic failure Pregnancy

Normal Values-Urine Chemistry

Determination	Normal Value	Clinical Significance (Increased)	(Decreased)
Acetone and acetoacetate	Zero	Uncontrolled diabetes Starvation	
Bence-Jones protein	None detected	Myeloma	
Creatine	0–200 mg/24 hr.	Muscular dystrophy Fever Carcinoma of liver Pregnancy Hyperthyroidism Myositis	

Continued on next page

16

Determination	Normal Value	Clinical Significance (Increased)	(Decreased)
Creatinine	0.8–2.0 gm/24 hr.	Typhoid fever Salmonella infections Tetanus	Muscular atrophy Anemia Advanced degeneration of kidneys Leukemia
Creatinine clearance	100–150 ml of blood cleared of creatinine/min.		Measures glomerular filtration rate Renal diseases
Estriol (placental)	Weeks of Pregnancy / mg/24 hr; 12 / less than 1 16 / 2–7 20 / 4–9 24 / 6–13 28 / 8–22 32 / 12–43 36 / 14–45 40 / 19–46		Decreased values occur with fetal distress of many conditions, including preeclampsia, placental insufficiency, and poorly controlled diabetes mellitus.
Glucose	Negative	Diabetes mellitus Pituitary disorders Intracranial pressure Lesion in floor of 4th ventricle	
Lead	Up to 150 micrograms/24 hr. Acetone and	Lead poisoning	
Phenolphthalein (PSP)	At least 25% excreted in 15 min., 40% by 30 min., and 60% by 120 min.	Primarily measures renal tubular function	Delayed in renal diseases Low in nephritis, cystitis, pyelonephritis, congestive heart failure
Urea nitrogen	9–16 gm/24 hr.	Excessive protein catabolism	Impaired kidney function
Uric acid	250–750 mg/24 hr.	Gout	Nephritis

Reprinted by permission of J. B. Lippincott Co. from Brunner, L. S., and Suddarth, D. S., Eds.: *The Lippincott Manual of Nursing Practice*, 2nd Ed., p. 1804ff. J. B. Lippincott, 1978.

Hematocrit

Normal range Expressed in millimeters per 100 millimeters (mm/100 mm) of column height, or as the percentage, which is the figure (that is, 50 mm/100 mm is the same as 50%).

Adults: Men: 40 to 50
Women: 35 to 45

Children: Newborn to 1 month: 42 to 54
1 month to 3 months: 29 to 54

Hemoglobin

Normal range Expressed in grams per 100 milliliters (gm/100 ml) of blood.

Adults: 12 to 18

Children: Newborn to 1 month: 14 to 19.5
10 months to 1 year: 11.2 to 14
1 year to 3 years: 11.2 to 12.5
3 years to 10 years: 12.5 to 13

From Solomon Garb, M.D., *Laboratory Tests in Common Use*, 6th ed., pp. 74–75. Copyright © 1976 by Springer Publishing Company, Inc., New York. Used by permission.

18
Some Pediatric Laboratory Values the Intensive Care Nurse Must Know

	Age	*Normal range*
Bilirubin (total)	Cord	under 2 mg./dl.
	0–1 day	under 6 mg./dl.
	3–5 days	under 12 mg./dl.
	after 5 days	under 1 mg./dl.
PO$_2$	Neonate	60–90 mm. Hg
pCO$_2$	(Venous)	40–50 mm. Hg
Fibrinogen	Newborn	150–300 mg./dl.
	after 1 month	200–400 mg./dl.
Fasting blood sugar	Premature	30–60 mg./dl.
	Newborn	30–80 mg./dl.
	Child	60–100 mg./dl.
	after	70–110 mg./dl.

Note: In newborn, under 30 mg. per cent means hypoglycemia. After 72 hours, under 40 mg. per cent means hypoglycemia.

Potassium	Premature cord	5.0–10.2 mEq./l.
	Premature 48 hours	3.0–6.0 mEq./l.
	Term newborn	5.0–7.7 mEq./l.
	Infant	4.1–5.3 mEq./l.
	Child	3.5–4.7 mEq./l.
	after	3.4–5.6 mEq./l.
Sodium	Premature 48 hours	128–148 mEq./l.
	Newborn	139–162 mEq./l.
	Infant	139–146 mEq./l.
	Child	138–145 mEq./l.
	Older	135–151 mEq./l.
BUN	0–infant	5–15 mg./dl.
	older	10–20 mg./dl.
pH	0–1 week	7.30–7.40
Chloride		95–110 mEq./l.
Calcium	Newborn	8.0–10.5 mg./100 ml.
Magnesium	Newborn	1–2 mg./100 ml.
Phosphorus	Newborn	3.5–8 mg./ml.

Reprinted by permission of W. B. Saunders Company from *Principles and Techniques in Pediatric Nursing*, 3rd edition, by Gloria Leifer, © Copyright 1977, W. B. Saunders Co.

HEMATOLOGIC VALUES DURING INFANCY AND CHILDHOOD

AGE	HEMOGLOBIN GM/DL % MEAN	RANGE	HEMATOCRIT % MEAN	RANGE	RETICULOCYTES % MEAN	WBC/MM.³ MEAN	RANGE	NEUTROPHILS % MEAN	RANGE	LYMPHOCYTES % MEAN (RELATIVELY WIDE RANGE)	EOSINOPHILS % MEAN	MONOCYTES % MEAN	NUCLEATED RED CELLS /100 WBC MEAN
Cord blood	16.8	13.7-20.1	55	45-65	5.0	18,000	(9-30,000)	61	(40-80)	31	2	6	7.0 (3-10)
2 weeks	16.5	13.0-20.0	50	42-66	1.0	12,000	(5-21,000)	40		48	3	9	0
3 months	12.0	9.5-14.5	36	31-41	1.0	12,000	(6-18,000)	30		63	2	5	0
6 mos.-6 yrs.	12.0	10.5-14.0	37	33-42	1.0	10,000	(6-15,000)	45		48	2	5	0
7-12 yrs.	13.0	11.0-16.0	38	34-40	1.0	8,000	(4500-13,500)	55		38	2	5	0
Adult Female	14	12.0-16.0	42	37-47	1.6	7,500	(5-10,000)	55	(35-70)	35	3	7	0
Male	16	14.0-18.0	47	42-52									

Reprinted by permission of W. B. Saunders, from *Nelson Textbook of Pediatrics*, 10th edition, by Vaughan and McKay, © Copyright 1975, W. B. Saunders Company.

20
Tests of Fetal Status

Urinary estriol—Assesses function of maternal-fetal-placement unit. Serial determinations done in later pregnancy, estriol rises progressively. Twenty-four hour urine samples should contain levels of 10 to 20 mg. estriol/24 hours. Low or decreasing values (40 percent less than the mean of three previous values) indicate fetal deterioration or impending death.

Ultrasonic determination of fetal biparietal diameter—Ultrasound B scan provides a two dimensional representation of the fetal skull, and the A scan produces unidirectional measurements for fetal cephalometry. This method of measurement does not have the hazards of x-ray examinations. A fetal biparietal diameter of 8.5 cm. indicates gestation of 36 weeks or more.

Lecithin/sphingomyelin ratio (L/S)—Lecithin is a major component of pulmonary surfactant, a substance which prevents collapse of alveoli with each breath. Comparison of the amount of lecithin present in amniotic fluid to the amount of sphingomyelin enables evaluation of fetal lung maturity. Mean concentrations of these do not differ until about the thirtieth week of gestation. An increase of lecithin at 35 weeks indicates pulmonary maturity. About 5 cc. of amniotic fluid is removed and chromatography performed in a laboratory requiring several hours. An L/S ratio equal to or more than 2:1 signifies fetal maturity with no respiratory distress syndrome likely upon delivery. A transitional ratio of 1.5 to 1.9:1 indicates the possibility of mild to moderate respiratory distress. A ratio of 1.0 to 1.4:1 usually means relatively immature lungs with respiratory distress a distinct possibility if the infant is delivered.

Snake test (rapid surfactant test)—A rapid test for surfactant in amniotic fluid can be performed outside a clinical laboratory. Amniotic fluid is withdrawn and diluted after centrifuging in two test tubes 1:1 and 1:2 with normal saline and ethanol. After vortexing, the tubes are set upright for 15 minutes. A complete ring of bubbles around the meniscus in both tubes indicates mature lungs; a complete ring in the 1:1 dilution only is intermediate; and no complete ring in either dilution indicates immaturity.

Amniotic fluid creatinine and bilirubin—Rising concentrations of creatinine in the amniotic fluid are correlated with gestational age, with concentrations of less than 1.8 mg./dl. prior to the thirty-sixth week and greater than this value after the thirty-sixth week. After 37 weeks, creatinine concentration is 2 to 4 mg./dl. Bilirubin in amniotic fluid decreases as term approaches (only used for nonisoimmunized patients) by spectrophotometric analysis. Levels above 0.01 occur in gestations less than 35 weeks; 0.0 levels at 36 weeks.

Oxytocin challenge test—Decelerations in fetal heart rate with uterine contractions usually indicate fetal hypoxia. Weekly challenge tests during late pregnancy allow an index of fetal condition. Using an external fetal monitor and tocohynamometer for uterine contractions, a baseline is first obtained of FHT and uterine activity. Then intravenous oxytocin is given at gradually increasing doses until there are three contractions per 10 minutes. With no late decelerations for 30 minutes, the test is negative. Positive tests are combined with other data to make decisions about terminating the pregnancy.

Reproduced by permission of J. B. Lippincott Co. from *Health Care of Women* by Leonide L. Martin, © Copyright 1978, J. B. Lippincott Company.

ORAL GLUCOSE TOLERANCE TEST (GTT)

An appropriate prior diet of $\geq$ 250 gm of carbohydrate daily and no alcohol for 3 days before the test should be prescribed. Patient should be fasting for 10–12 hours before test, with no smoking or drinking of coffee. Do not test in presence of fever or infection.

For older persons without elevated fasting levels, without glycosuria (alone or during oral GTT), without positive family history of diabetes, limits of normal at 1 and 2 hours should be increased 10 mg/100 ml at age 50 and an additional 10 mg for each subsequent decade (e.g., 30 mg/100 ml at age 70).

To detect early diabetes in pregnancy, upper limits of normal are 165 at 1 hour, 145 at 2 hours, 125 at 3 hours. If results are equivocal test should be repeated in 3 months or IV GTT should be done. If suggestive diagnosis of diabetes is not definite during pregnancy, additional workup should be done after delivery.

U.S. Public Health Service criteria for diagnosis of diabetes: Assign 1 point each to elevated fasting and 3-hour levels, and ½ point each to the 1- and 2-hour levels. Total of two points or more is considered diagnostic.

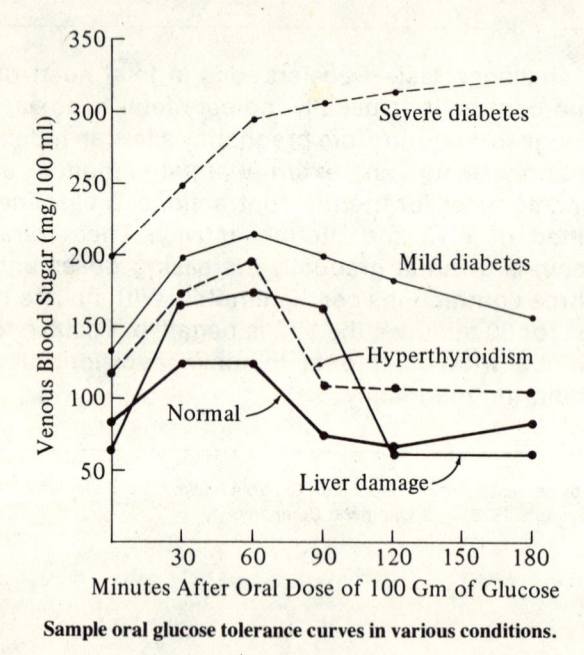

Sample oral glucose tolerance curves in various conditions.

Reprinted by permission of Little, Brown and Company from *Interpretation of Diagnostic Tests, A Handbook Synopsis of Laboratory Medicine*, 3rd edition, by Jacques Wallach, M.D., © Copyright 1978, Little, Brown and Company.

METHODS OF URINE TESTING FOR SUGAR

	Chemical Reduction Method	Enzyme Method
Basis of Test	Substances used for testing contain metallic ions (e.g., copper and bismuth). When urine containing glucose is heated, the ions are reduced. Due to ion reduction, precipitation occurs, and the urine changes color, depending upon the amount of glucose present.	Substances used for testing contain an enzyme called glucose oxidase. When urine containing glucose contacts glucose oxidase, a color change occurs which varies with the amount of glucose present.
Types of Tests	(a) Benedict's test (used only in laboratories today). (b) Clinitest tablets (Ames Company).	(a) Test Tape (Eli Lilly and Company). (b) Clinistix (Ames Company).
Procedure	Clinitest: (a) Place in test tube 5 drops urine, 10 drops water, and 1 Clinitest tablet. (b) Allow solution to boil. (c) When boiling stops, wait 10 seconds and compare color of urine to color chart accompanying set-up. (d) *Blue color indicates negative result*, *yellow moderately positive for sugar*, and *orange highly positive for sugar*.	(a) Dip a tape (Tes Tape) or enzyme strip (Clinistix) into the urine. (b) Wait one minute. (c) Compare tape or strip with color chart accompanying set-up to evaluate if acetone or glucose is present.
Specificity of method	Reaction not specific to glucose alone; test also detects galactose, lactose, fructose, maltose, salicylates.	Reaction occurs *only* in the presence of glucose.
Advantages	Inexpensive; reasonably reliable; colors of urine easily differentiated.	Extremely simple to use; easy to transport tape or tablets when traveling; reacts positively only to glucose.
Disadvantages	More difficult to use than enzyme methods; equipment somewhat cumbersome; positive reactions can occur in presence of substances other than glucose.	Expensive; less reliable than Clinitest; positive reactions occur in presence of even tiny amounts of glucose; difficult to differentiate colors.
Sources of Error	Tablets become inactive if exposed to air; keep bottle tightly closed. Administration of vitamin C may cause a false-positive reaction.	Tes-Tape deteriorates in 4 months, Clinistix strips within a few months. Use only fresh testing materials. Administration of vitamin C and the diuretic Mercuhydrin may cause a false-negative reaction.

Reprinted by permission of W. B. Saunders Co. from *Medical-Surgical Nursing: A Psychophysiological Approach* by Joan Luckmann and Karen Sorenson, © 1974, W. B. Saunders Co.

24

Liver Function Tests

	Test	Normal Values	Hepatocellular Disease	Obstructive Disease
Excretion	Bilirubin, serum			
	Direct	0.1-0.4 mg/100 ml	Increased	Increased
	Indirect	0.2-0.7 mg/100 ml	Increased	Increased
	Bilirubin, urinary	Absent	Present	Present
	Urobilinogen Urinary	0-4 mg/24 hours	Increased	Absent or variable
	Fecal	40-280 mg/24 hours	Decreased	Absent or variable
	Bromsulphalein® 5 mg/kg	0-5% retention in 45 min.	Increased retention	Increased retention until obstruction relieved
Synthesis	Protein, serum*			
	Albumin	4.5-5.5 gm/100 ml	Decreased	Normal or decreased
	Globulin	1.5-3.0 gm/100 ml	Increased	Normal or decreased
	Total	6.0-8.0 gm/100 ml	Decreased or normal	Normal or decreased
	Thymol turbidity, serum	0-5 units	Increased	Normal
	Zinc turbidity, serum	0-12 units	Increased	Normal
	Cephalin flocculation, serum	0-1+ in 48 hours	Positive	Negative
	Prothrombin, plasma			
	Before vitamin K	70-130% of normal control	Decreased	Decreased
	After vitamin K	15% increase in 48 hours	Poor or no response	Rapid response
	Cholesterol, Esterified	60-75% of total	Greatly decreased	Normal
	serum Total	150-240 mg/100 ml	Slightly decreased	Increased
Enzymatic	Phosphatase, alkaline serum	2-4.5 Bodansky units 5-13 King-Armstrong units	Slightly increased	Greatly increased
	Transaminase, serum			
	SGOT	5-40 units	Increased	Normal or slightly increased
	SGPT	5-35 units		

*Normal protein fractions as determined by electrophoresis as % of total protein are albumin 52-68, α_1 globulin 2.4-4.4, α_2 globulin 6.1-10.1, β globulin 8.5-14.5, and γ globulin 10-21.

Reprinted by permission of Jones Medical Publications, from *Handbook of Medical Treatment*, 15th edition, by Milton J. Chatton, M.D., © Copyright, 1977, Jones Medical Publications.

Chromosome Number and Karyotype in Various Clinical Conditions

Clinical Condition	Chromosome Number and Karyotype	Incidence
Normal male	46 XY	
Normal female	46 XX	
Turner's syndrome	45 XO	1 in 3,000 live female births
	46 XX	Rare
	Mosaics	Infrequent
Klinefelter's syndrome	47 XXY	1 in 600 live male births
	48 XXXY	
	48 XXYY	Rare
	49 XXXXY	
	49 XXXYY	
	Mosaics	Infrequent
Superfemale	47 XXX	1 in 1–2,000 live female births
	48 XXXX	
	49 XXXXX	Rare
	Mosaics	
Supermale	47 XYY	1 in 1,000 live male births
	48 XYYY	Rare
	Mosaics	Rare
Down's syndrome (mongolism; trisomy 21)	47 XX, G+ or 47 XY, G+	1 in 700 live births (2% are 46 count due to translocation and have 10% risk of Down's syndrome in subsequent pregnancies; 2% are 46/47 mosaics)
D_1 trisomy	47 XX, D+ or 47 XY, D+	1 in 5,000 live births
	Translocations	Rare
	Mosaics	Rare
E_{18} trisomy	47 XX, E+ or 47 XY, E+	1 in 3,000 live births
	Translocations	Rare
	Mosaics	Rare
Cri du chat syndrome	46 with partial B deletion	1 in 30,000 live births

Reprinted by permission of Little, Brown and Company from *Interpretation of Diagnostic Tests, A Handbook Synopsis of Laboratory Medicine*, 3rd edition, by Jacques Wallach, M.D., © Copyright 1978, Little, Brown and Company.

26
ABO System of Antigens and Antibodies for Determining Blood Compatibility

			Compatibility	
Blood group	Antigen	Antibody	Can be donor to type	Can receive from type
A	A	Anti-B	A or AB	A or O
B	B	Anti-A	B or AB	B or O
AB	A and B	No antibodies	AB	A, B, AB, or O
O	No antigen	Anti-A and Anti-B	A, B, AB, or O	O

Reprinted by permission of McGraw-Hill Book Company, from *Comprehensive Pediatric Nursing* by Gladys Scipien, et al., © Copyright McGraw-Hill Book Company, 1975.

DRUGS THAT MAY CAUSE COLOR CHANGES IN STOOL

Drug	*Resulting Color*
Alkaline antacids and aluminum salts	White discoloration or speckling
Anticoagulants (excess)	Due to bleeding
Anthraquinones	Brown staining
Bismuth salts	Black
Charcoal	Black
Dithiazine	Green to blue
Indomethacin	Green (due to biliverdin)
Iron salts	Black
Mercurous chloride	Green
Phenazopyridine	Orange-red
Phenolphthalein	Red
Phenylbutazone and oxyphenbutazone	Black (due to bleeding)
Pyrvinium pamoate	Red
Rhubarb	Yellow
Salicylates	Due to bleeding
Santonin	Yellow
Senna	Yellow to brown
Tetracyclines in syrup (due to glucosamine)	Red

Reprinted by permission of Little, Brown and Company from *Interpretation of Diagnostic Tests, A Handbook Synopsis of Laboratory Medicine*, 3rd edition, by Jacques Wallach, M.D., © Copyright 1978, Little, Brown and Company.

DRUGS THAT MAY ALTER URINE COLOR

Urine coloration due to drugs may mask other abnormal colors (e.g., due to blood, bile, porphyrins) as well as interfere with various chemical determinations (fluorometric, colorimetric, photometric)

Drug	Resulting Color
Acetophenetidin	Hematuria or pink-red due to metabolite
Aminosalicylic acid (PAS)	Discoloration abnormal but not distinctive
Amitriptyline	Blue-green
Anisindione (indandione)	Orange (alkaline urine), pink-red-brown (acid urine)
Anthraquinones	Pink to brown
Anticoagulants	Pink to red to brown (due to bleeding)
Cascara	Brown (acid urine), yellow-pink (alkaline urine), black on standing
Chloroquine	Brown
Chlorzoxazone (metabolite)	Purple, red, pink, rust
Cinchophen	Red-brown
Dihydroxyanthraquinone	Pink to orange (alkaline urine)
Emodin	Pink to red to red-brown (alkaline urine)
Ethoxazene	Orange, red, pink, rust
Furazolidone	Brown
Indomethacin	Green (due to biliverdin)
Iron sorbitol	Brown
Methocarbamol	Dark brown, black, blue or green on standing

Drug	Resulting Color
Methyldopa	Red darkens on standing, pink or brown
Methylene blue	Greenish-yellow to blue
Metronidazole (metabolite)	Dark brown
Nitrofurantoin and derivatives	Brown, yellow
Pamaquine	Brown
Phenacetin	Dark brown
Phenazopyridine	Orange to red
Phenindione	Red-orange in alkaline urine
Phenolphthalein	Pink to red to magenta (alkaline urine), orange, rust (acid)
Phenothiazines	Pink, red, purple, orange, rust
Phensuximide	Pink, red, purple, orange, rust
Phenytoin sodium	Pink, red, red-brown
Primaquine	Rust yellow to brown
Quinacrine (mepacrine)	Deep yellow on acidification
Quinine and derivatives	Brown to black
Rhubarb	Yellow-brown (acid), yellow-pink (alkaline). darkens
Riboflavin	Yellow
Rifampin	Red-orange
Salicylates	Pink to red to brown (due to bleeding)
Salicylazosulfapyridine	Pink, red, purple, orange, rust
Senna	Red (alkaline urine), yellow-brown (acid urine)
Sulfonamides	Rust, yellow, or brown
Thiazolsulfone	Pink, red, purple, orange, rust
Tolonium	Blue, green
Triamterene	Green, blue with blue fluorescence

Reprinted by permission of Little, Brown and Company from *Interpretation of Diagnostic Tests, A Handbook Synopsis of Laboratory Medicine*, 3rd edition, by Jacques Wallach, M.D., © Copyright 1978, Little, Brown and Company.

Summary of Basic Components of Neurological Examination

FUNCTION OR STRUCTURE TESTED	AREA OF OBSERVATION	TYPE OF TEST
Cerebral Function	Behavior, emotional status, intellectual performance and thought content, level of consciousness	Observation of appearance Observation of physical and emotional behavior Response to questions and to mental tasks (e.g., repeating number series)
	Cortical function: sensory interpretation, motor integration	Recognition of objects by sight, sound, feel Carrying out of motor acts
	Language	Communication in and response to spoken and written language
Cranial Nerve Function	I Olfactory nerve	Recognition of familiar odors
	II Optic nerve	Visual acuity Ophthalmoscopic examination of fundus Visual fields
	III Oculomotor nerve IV Trochlear nerve VI Abducens nerve } these three nerves are generally tested together	Observation of pupil size, shape, equality, reaction to light Range and direction of ocular motion
	V Trigeminal nerve	Facial sensation-touch, warmth, cold Equality of sensation on both sides of face Maxillary reflex Corneal reflex
	VII Facial nerve	Facial muscle symmetry: at rest, in motion Ability to taste sweet and salt

Cranial Nerve Function (*continued*)	VIII Acoustic nerve: cochlear part	Hearing (watch tick)
	: vestibular part (not routinely tested)	Lateralization of sound (tuning fork)
		Air and bone conduction
	IX Glossopharyngeal nerve ⎫ tested together	Pharyngeal gag reflex; palatal reflex
	X Vagus nerve ⎭	Ability to swallow
		Symmetrical movement of vocal cords
		Clarity of speech
	XI Accessory nerve	Strength and size of sternocleidomastoid and trapezius muscles
	XII Hypoglossal nerve	Lateral deviation, atrophy, or tremor of tongue
Cerebellar Function	Balance and coordination	Touch finger to nose, to examiner's finger (eyes open and closed)
		Rapidly alternating movements (e.g., pat knees)
		Make figure-of-eight movement with foot
		Standing and walking balance (eyes open and closed)
Motor Function	Muscle size, tone, strength	Measurement of muscle size
	Abnormal movements	Inspection for abnormal movements
		Joint flexion and extension: without and against resistance
Sensory Function	Tactile sense	Sensitivity to light touch (wisp of cotton)
	Temperature sensitivity	Response to hot and cold objects
	Vibration sensitivity	Ability to feel vibration (tuning fork)
	Superficial pain	Response to pinprick
	Deep pressure pain	Response to squeezing forearm and calf muscles and Achilles tendon
	Position and motion	Identification of position of passively moved fingers and toes (eyes closed)

Continued on next page

FUNCTION OR STRUCTURE TESTED	AREA OF OBSERVATION		TYPE OF TEST
	Discriminatory sense	: two point	Two-point touch: varying distances apart : different parts of body
		: single point	Single point touch to various parts of body
		: extinction	Recognition of two points of touch on opposite sides of body
		: texture	Recognition of material by feel
		: stereognostic	Recognition of familiar objects by feel
Reflexes	Superficial reflexes	: upper and lower abdominal : cremasteric : plantar : gluteal	Response to stroking skin in specified area with a moderately sharp object
	Deep reflexes	: biceps : brachioradialis : triceps : patellar : Achilles	Contraction response to tapping a tendon or bony prominence, sudden muscle stretching
	Pathologic Babinski: pyramidal tract pathology (Chaddock, Oppenheim, and Gordon reflexes elicit same response)		Stroke lateral aspect of sole of foot: big toe dorsiflexes, toes fan out
	Hoffman: muscular hypertonia		Flick distal phalanx of middle finger: thumb flexes

* For details of the neurologic examination, the reader is referred to a neurology textbook or to Francis A. Vazuka: "Essentials of the Neurological Examination," Smith, Kline and French Laboratories, Philadelphia, 1962.

Reprinted by permission of McGraw-Hill Company from *Nursing Care of the Patient With Medical-Surgical Disorders*, 2nd edition, by Harriett Moidel, Elizabeth Giblin, and Berniece Wagner, © 1976, McGraw-Hill Book Company.

Neurologic Examination for Testing Cranial Nerves

Nerve	Equipment	Clinical Examination
1. Olfactory	Four small bottles of volatile oils, such as (1) turpentine, (2) oil of cloves, (3) oil of wintergreen, (4) vanilla	Instruct the patient to sniff and to identify the odors. Each nostril is tested separately. The patient is asked if he perceives the smell and if he can identify it.
2. Optic	Ophthalmoscope	In darkened room the patient is asked to look straight ahead at a distant object while the examiner looks for choked disc, optic atrophy, and retinal and vascular lesions. Special equipment is used for examination of visual fields. Eye chart is used to check visual acuity.
3. Oculomotor 4. Trochlear 5. Abducens	Flashlight	Because of close association, these nerves are examined collectively. They innervate pupil and upper eyelid and are responsible for extraocular muscle movements.
6. Trigeminal	Test tube of hot water Test tube of ice water Cotton wisp from cotton applicator stick	*Sensory branch*—Vertex to chin tested for sensations of pain, touch, and temperature. This includes reflex reaction of cornea to wisp of cotton.
	Pin	*Motor branch*—Ability to bite is tested.

* See material which follows for detailed description of testing cranial nerve function.

Continued on next page

Nerve	Equipment	Clinical Examination
7. Facial	Four small bottles with solutions which are salty, sweet, sour, and bitter (Four wet cotton applicators)	Observe symmetry of face and ability to contract facial muscles. Instruct patient to taste and to identify substance used. He should rinse his mouth well between each drop of solution. This is a test for the anterior ⅔ of tongue.
8. Acoustic	Tuning fork	Tests for hearing, air and bone conduction.
9. Glossopharyngeal	Cotton applicator stick	Test posterior ⅓ of tongue for taste and also check for gag reflex.
10. Vagus	Tongue depressor	Checking voice sounds, observing symmetry of soft palate will give suggestion of function of vagus.
11. Spinal Accessory		Since this innervates the sternocleidomastoid and the trapezius muscles, the patient will be instructed to turn and to move his head and to elevate shoulders with and without resistance.
12. Hypoglossal		Observe tongue movements.

Reprinted by permission of J. B. Lippincott Co. from *The Lippincott Manual of Nursing Practice*, 2nd edition, Lillian Brunner, and Doris Suddarth, © 1978, J. B. Lippincott Co.

Deep Tendon Reflexes

Reflexes	Elicitation of Reflex	Normal Response
Biceps reflex	The arm is half-flexed at the elbow with the elbow resting in the examiner's hand. The examiner places his thumb over the biceps tendon and taps the tendon with a reflex hammer.	Flexion of the forearm and contraction of the biceps muscle.
Triceps reflex	The arm is flexed at the elbow and held across the chest or rested on the examiner's hand. The triceps tendon is struck above the olecranon process.	Contraction of the triceps muscle with extension of the forearm.
Brachiordialis reflex	The forearm is semiflexed and semipronated with the hand supported by the examiner's hand. The styloid process of the radius is tapped.	Flexion of the forearm and supination of the forearm.
Patellar reflex (quadriceps reflex, "knee jerk")	*Sitting position*: The legs hang freely over the bed or an examining table. The patellar tendon is struck just below the knee. The examiner should place one hand over the quadriceps femoris muscle as he strikes the patellar tendon with the other in order to feel the contraction of the muscle. *Lying position*: The person's knee is flexed slightly by placing the hand under the knee and raising the knee off the bed. The patellar tendon is tapped.	Extension of the leg at the knee and contraction of the quadriceps femoris muscle.
Achilles reflex ("ankle jerk" or triceps surae reflex)	*Sitting position*: The legs should dangle freely over the bed or table. The patient's foot is grasped and pressure exerted upward on the ball of the foot to a position of moderate dorsiflexion. The Achilles tendon is tapped on the posterior surface of the calcaneous. *Lying position*: The thigh and leg are rotated slightly outward and the knee is flexed. The examiner places his hand under the foot and exerts pressure upward to produce dorsiflexion. The Achilles tendon is tapped.	Contraction of the gastrocnemius, soleus, and plantaris muscles which produce plantar flexion of the foot.

Reproduced by permission of J. B. Lippincott Company from *Advanced Concepts in Clinical Nursing,* 2nd edition, edited by Kay Corman Kintzel, © Copyright 1977, J. B. Lippincott Co.

Pathological Reflexes

Pathological Reflex	Site of Stimulus	Response to Stimulus
Babinski—One of the most important tests for neurologic disease. Indicative of pyramidal tract involvement and occurs most frequently in pyramidal tract disease.	The lateral (outer) aspect of the sole of the foot is stroked with a blunt point from the midpoint of the heel up to the ball of the foot and then across the ball of the foot.	Dorsiflexion of the great toe and fanning of the small toes. Dorsiflexion of the foot and flexion of the knee occur concomitantly.
Chaddock's sign—Appears in pyramidal tract disease.	The lateral aspect of the foot under the external malleolus is stimulated.	Dorsiflexion of the great toe.
Gordon's sign—Pyramidal tract response.	Deep pressure is applied to the calf muscles by squeezing or pressing firmly.	Dorsiflexion of the great toe.
Oppenheim's sign—Pyramidal tract response.	The examiner strokes downward on the anteromedial tibial surface toward the ankles with the thumb and index finger or with the knuckles of the fingers.	Dorsiflexion of the great toe.
Hoffman's sign—Pathological hand reflex seen in pyramidal tract involvement.	Flicking or snapping the nail of the middle finger.	Flexion of the index finger. Flexion and adduction of the thumb.
Clonus—A continuous contraction of muscle which has been stimulated through stretch. Present in pyramidal tract disease.	*Finger clonus*—The patient's fingers are held and the hand is quickly dorsiflexed at the wrist.	Alternating flexion and extension at the wrist.

Quadriceps (patellar) clonus—With the leg in extension and lying flat, the knee is held with the thumb and index finger and pushed down toward the feet.

Rhythmical movements of the patella.

Ankle clonus—With the knee flexed, relaxed and supported, the foot is held with the free hand and quickly dorsiflexed.

Alternate flexion and extension of the foot due to repeated contractions of triceps surae muscle.

Reproduced by permission of J. B. Lippincott Co. from *Advanced Concepts in Clinical Nursing*, 2nd edition, edited by Kay Corman Kintzel, © Copyright 1977, J. B. Lippincott Co.

AVERAGE PULSE RATES AT REST

AGE	LOWER LIMITS OF NORMAL		AVERAGE		UPPER LIMITS OF NORMAL	
	Girls	*Boys*	*Girls*	*Boys*	*Girls*	*Boys*
Newborn	70	70	120	120	170	170
1-11 months		80		120		160
2 years		80		110		130
4 years		80		100		120
6 years		75		100		115
8 years		70		90		110
10 years		70		90		110
12 years	70	65	90	85	110	105
14 years	65	60	85	80	105	100
16 years	60	55	80	75	100	95
18 years	55	50	75	70	95	90

Reprinted by permission of W. B. Saunders Co. from *Nelson Textbook of Pediatrics*, 10th edition, by Vaughan and McKay, Copyright © 1975, W. B. Saunders Co.

Approximate Respiratory Rates At Various Ages

Age	Rate per minute
Newborn	30–50
2 years	24–32
6 years	22–28
10 years	20–26
12 years	18–24
Adult	16–22

Reprinted by permission of W. B. Saunders Co. from *Principles and Techniques in Pediatric Nursing*, 3rd edition, by Gloria Leifer, Copyright © 1977, W. B. Saunders Co.

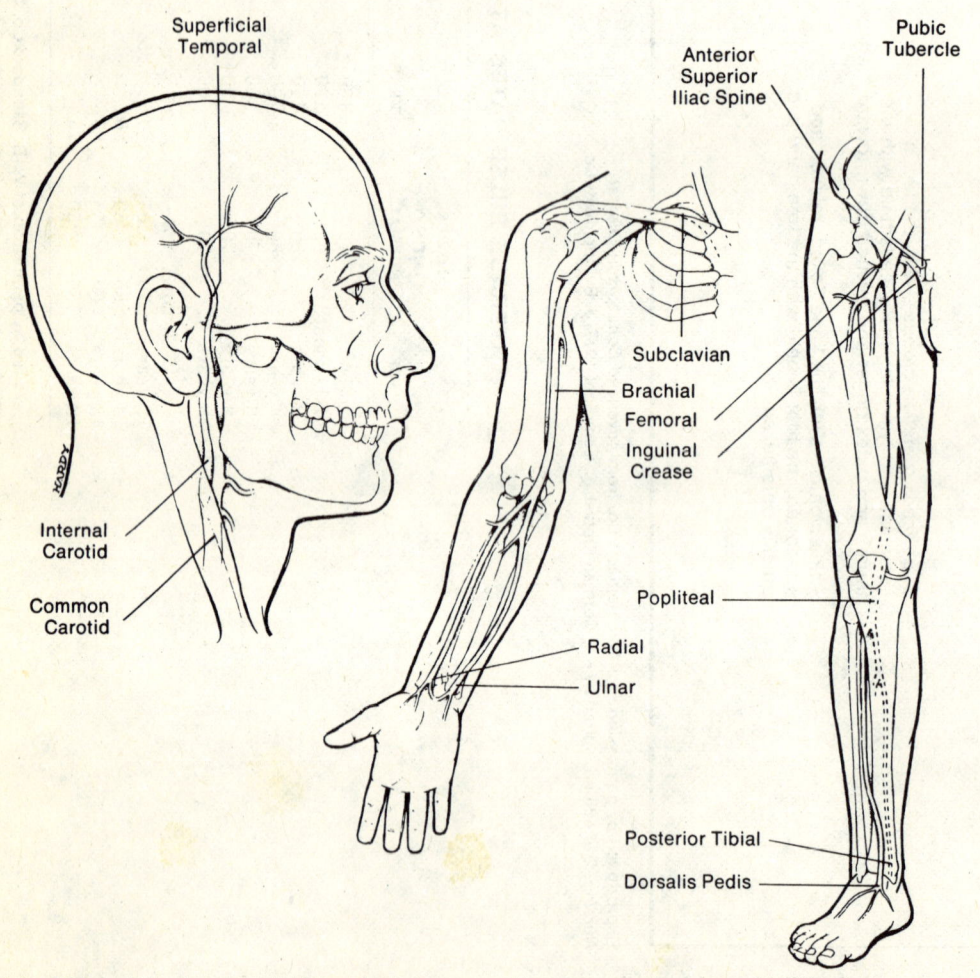

Pulse Points. The drawings indicate the points on major arteries of the head, neck and extremities where a pulse can most easily be palpated.

Reprinted by permission from J. B. Lippincott Co. from *The Practice of Emergency Nursing*, James Cosgriff and Diann Anderson, © 1975, J. B. Lippincott Co.

Sequence of auscultating heart sounds*

Auscultatory site	Chest location	Characteristics of heart sounds
Aortic area	Second right intercostal space close to sternum	S_2 heard louder than S_1; Aortic closure heard loudest
Pulmonic area	Second left intercostal space close to sternum	Splitting of S_2 heard best, normally widens on inspiration; pulmonic closure heard best
Erb's point	Second and third left intercostal space close to sternum	Frequent site of innocent murmurs and those of aortic or pulmonic origin
Tricuspid area	Fifth right and left intercostal space close to sternum	S_1 heard as louder sound preceding S_2 (S_1 synchronous with carotid pulse)

Mitral or apical area	Fifth intercostal space, left midclavicular line (third to fourth intercostal space and lateral to left midclavicular line in infants)	S_1 heard loudest; splitting of S_1 may be audible because mitral closure is louder than tricuspid closure
		
		S_3 heard best at beginning of expiration with child in recumbent or left side-lying position, occurs immediately after S_2, sounds like word "Ken-tuc-ky"
		    S_1 S_2 S_3
		
		S_4 heard best during expiration with child in recumbent position (left side-lying position decreases sound), occurs immediately before S_1, sounds like word "Ten-nes-see"
		  S_4 S_1 S_2

*Use both diaphragm and bell chestpieces when auscultating heart sounds. Bell chestpiece is necessary for low-pitched sounds of murmurs, S_3 and S_4.

Reprinted by permission of The C. V. Mosby Co. from *Nursing Care of Infants and Children,* by Lucille Whaley and Donna Wong. © 1979, The C. V. Mosby Co., St. Louis.

38

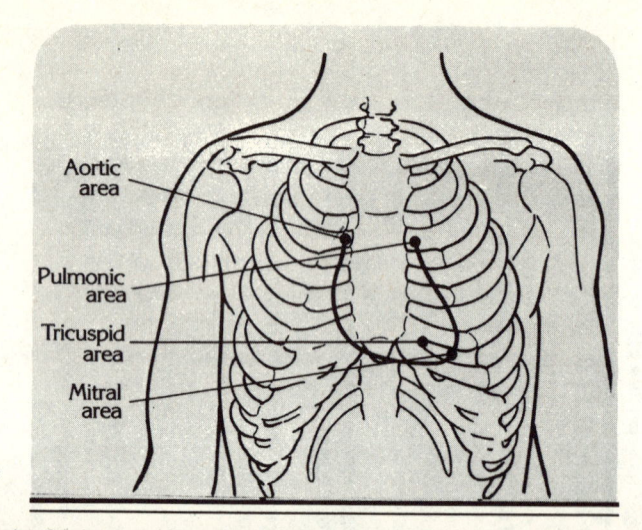

Aortic area
Pulmonic area
Tricuspid area
Mitral area

The placement of the bell of the stethoscope to hear heart sounds.

Reprinted from *Fundamentals of Nursing Concepts and Procedures*, by Barbara Kozier and Glenora Lea Erb, © Copyright Addison-Wesley Publishing Company, Menlo Park, California, 1979.

The Electrocardiograph Leads

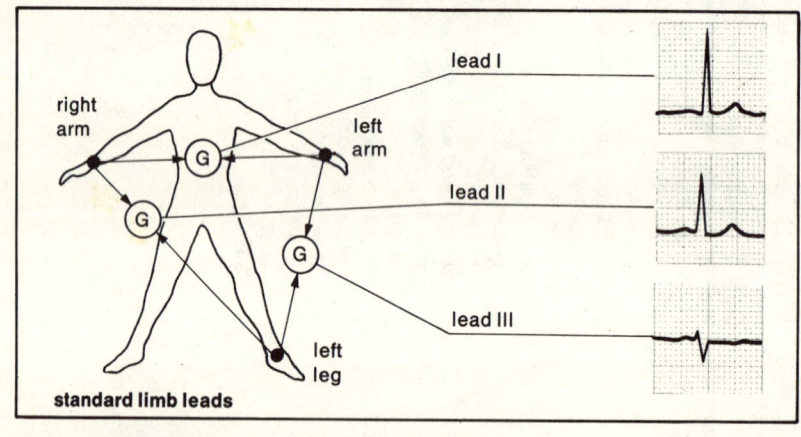

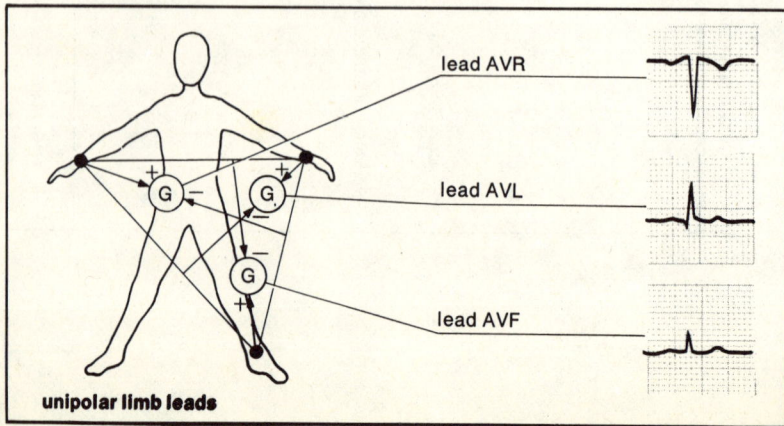

right arm
left arm
left leg
lead I
lead II
lead III

standard limb leads

lead AVR
lead AVL
lead AVF

unipolar limb leads

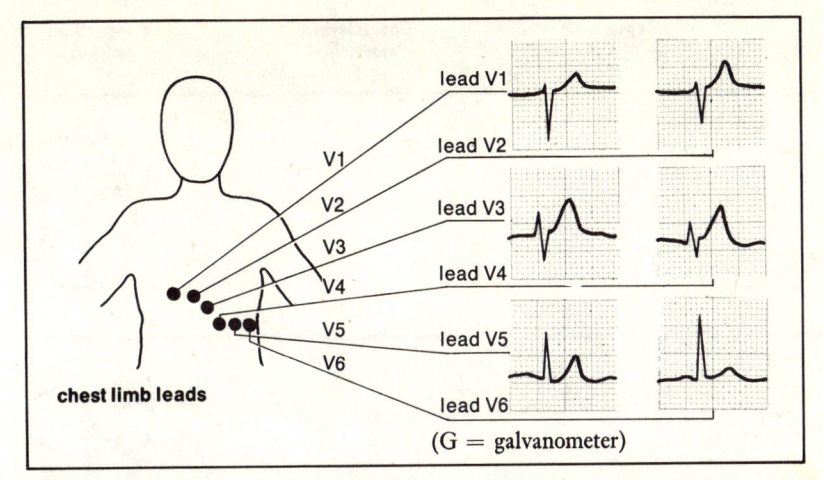

[Figure: Chest limb leads V1–V6 placement with corresponding ECG tracings (G = galvanometer)]

Reprinted by permission of Churchill Livingstone from *Penguin Library of Nursing, The Cardiovascular System* by P. P. Turner, © Copyright 1976, Churchill Livingstone, Longman Group, Ltd.

Summary of basic arrhythmias

Type of arrhythmia	Appearance of ECG	Characteristic abnormality	Conduction pathway
Normal rhythm			
Sinus arrhythmia		Irregular rhythm	
Sinus tachycardia		Rate 100-150	
Sinus bradycardia		Rate below 60	
PACs		Premature P; normal QRS	
PAT		Rate 140-250	
Atrial flutter		Saw-toothed flutter waves	

Continued on next page

Type of arrhythmia	Appearance of ECG	Characteristic abnormality	Conduction pathway
Atrial fibrillation		No clearly defined P; irregular rhythm	
Junctional rhythm		Inverted or hidden P	
JPCs		Premature beat; inverted or hidden P; normal QRS	
PVCs		Premature beat; no P; wide, distorted QRS	
Ventricular tachycardia		Series of PVCs; rate 150-200	
Ventricular fibrillation		No well-defined complexes	
First degree heart block		PR greater than 0.20; constant PR	
Second degree Mobitz I (Wenckebach)		Progressively longer PR until dropped beat; cyclic pattern	
Second degree Mobitz II		Some nonconducted Ps (2:1, 3:1, or occasional); constant PR	
Third degree complete heart block		No relationship between P and QRS	

Reprinted by permission of Medical Economics Company, from *How To Read An ECG*, Revised edition, by Blowers and Smith, Copyright © 1977 by Medical Economics Company, a division of Litton Industries, Inc. All rights reserved.

Effect of drugs and electrolytes on the ECG. Changes in the shape of the ECG complex may result from presence or absence of certain substances that influence myocardial tissue. Here are the most common, showing their ECG effect.

Agent	Effect on myocardium	ECG change	Example
Hypokalemia (low serum potassium)	Increases irritability (ectopic beats)	Decreases height of T wave; produces U wave	
Hyperkalemia (high serum potassium)	Depresses automaticity (standstill)	Creates tall, peaked T waves; prolongs PR interval	
Hypocalcemia (low serum calcium)	Decreases threshold for stimulation	Prolongs Q-T interval	
Hypercalcemia (high serum calcium)	Increases threshold for stimulation	Shortens Q-T interval	
Digitalis	Depresses conduction; increases automaticity (predisposes to many arrhythmias)	Produces downward deflection of S-T segment; prolongs PR interval	
Quinidine	Depresses conduction and automaticity	Widens QRS; prolongs PR interval	

Reprinted by permission of Medical Economics Co., from *How To Read An ECG*, Revised Edition, by Blowers and Smith, Copyright © 1977 by Medical Economics Company, a division of Litton Industries, Inc. All rights reserved.

Guidelines for Adult Coronary Risk Assessment and Health Maintenance

Risk Factor or Indicator	Assessments of Increased Risk	Health Maintenance
Age and Sex	Men over 35; peak incidence age 50-60	No immediate referral unless other risks are present
	Women over 50; peak incidence age 60-70	Same as for men (regular health care indicated for high risk groups)
Heredity	Family history of premature heart attack (before 65), stroke, or diabetes	Regular health evaluation
Hypertension*	Assess systolic and diastolic pressures separately	Annual blood pressure measurements for all adults
	All adults with: Diastolic 120 mm Hg or higher**	Immediate Medical Evaluation+
	Systolic 160 mm Hg or higher Diastolic 95 - Hg or higher	Confirm elevation within one month+
	Adults under 50 with: Systolic 140 - 160 mm Hg Diastolic 90 - 95 mm Hg	Blood pressure check within 2-3 months+
	Adults over 50 with: Systolic 140 - 160 mm Hg Diastolic 90 - 95 mm Hg	Check within 6-9 months+
Elevated Cholesterol	High saturated fat diet	Minimum yearly tests for high risk patients Serum cholesterol and dietary education
	Family history of hyperlipidemia, premature coronary or peripheral vascular disease	Regular health evaluation

	Presence of xanthoma (flat slightly elevated soft round plaque or nodule usually on the eyelids, palmar creases, or tendinous surfaces)	Medical evaluation
	Presence of arcus senilis (opaque white ring around the corneal periphery due to fat granules) under age 40	Medical evaluation
Cigarette Smoking	Risk increases with the amount smoked	Recommend that patient stop smoking and inform of resources for assistance to quit
Obesity	Estimate overweight (mild, moderate, or severe)	Based on degree of obesity and presence of other risk factors
Left Ventricular Hypertrophy (LVH)	ECG criteria: (not valid for persons under 25) The R wave in Lead I *plus* the S wave in Lead III exceeds 26 mm or The S wave in V_1 *plus* the R wave in V_5 or V_6 (whichever is taller) total more than 36 mm	If other risks are negative and ECG and patient status non-acute, no immediate treatment needed Establish a primary source for further evaluation of cardiovascular status Indicative of hypertensive heart disease when blood pressure is elevated
Glucose Intolerance‡	Criteria: Presence of diabetes	Regulate diabetes
	Trace or more of sugar in the urine	Further assessment in ED or referral to primary care source
	A non-fasting whole blood glucose level of 120 mg% or greater	Further evaluation

*The American Heart Association recommends that diastolic pressure be recorded at the point when the Korotkoff sound disappears (fifth phase) rather than at the muffling of sound (fourth phase).
**Many physicians recommend treatment at the lower levels of diastolic elevations (90 mm Hg) for all persons.
+Prompt referral to a primary source for followup.
‡Possible medication-induced hyperglycemia due to caffeine, catecholamines, chlorpromazine, corticosteroids, phenytoin, ethacrynic acid, furosemide, indomethacin, marijuana, nicotine, oral contraceptives, and thiazides.

Reprinted by permission of *JEN* from "Assessment of Coronary Risk Factors" by Beverly A. Krogseng in JEN: JOURNAL of EMERGENCY NURSING, March/April, 1979, Vol. 5, No. 3, © 1979, Emergency Department Nurses Association.

ABNORMALITIES IN RATE AND RHYTHM OF BREATHING

NORMAL

Inspiration *Expiration*

Time

Volume of air

The respiratory rate is about 16 to 20 per minute in adults and up to 44 per minute in infants.

TACHYPNEA

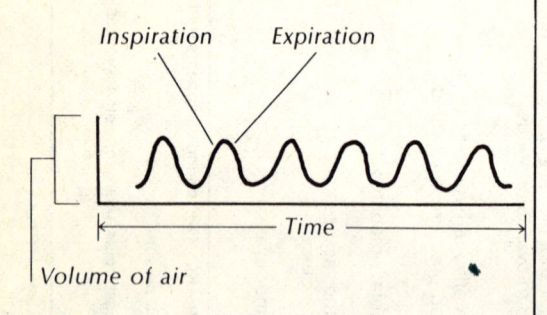

Breathing is faster than normal and usually more shallow.

HYPERPNEA OR HYPERVENTILATION

Breathing is increased in both rate and depth.

CHEYNE-STOKES BREATHING

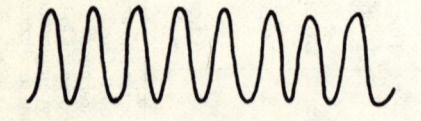

Hyperpnea *Apnea*

Periods of hyperpnea alternate with periods of apnea (cessation of breathing). Overly brief inspection will miss this important sign. Stay alert to the patient's breathing pattern over several minutes.

SIGHING RESPIRATION

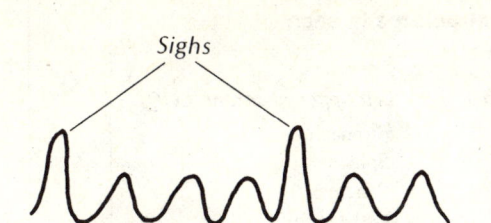

Sighs

OBSTRUCTIVE BREATHING

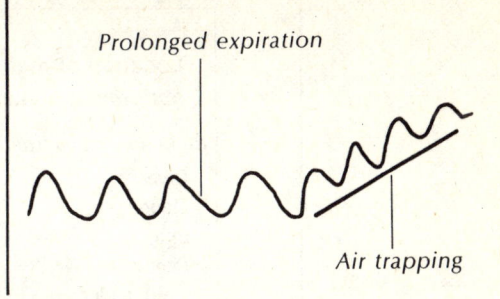

Prolonged expiration

Air trapping

Reprinted by permission of J. B. Lippincott Company, from *A Guide to Physical Examination* by Barbara Bates, M.D., Copyright © 1974, J. B. Lippincott Company.

Adventitious Sounds in the Chest Examination

RALES

RHONCHI AND WHEEZES

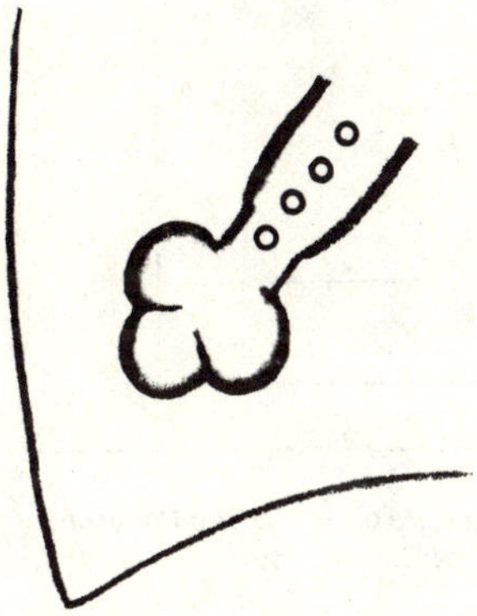

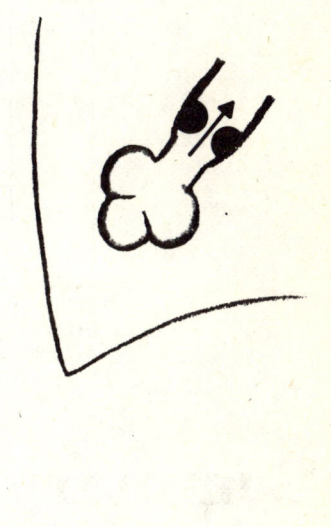

PLEURAL FRICTION RUBS

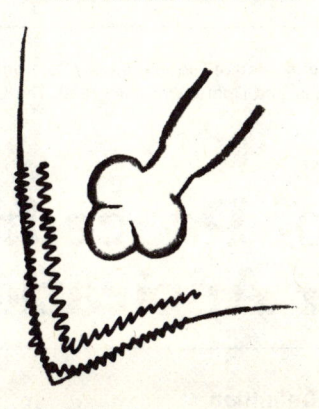

Reprinted by permission of J. B. Lippincott Company, from *A Guide to Physical Examination* by Barbara Bates, M.D., Copyright © 1974, J. B. Lippincott Company.

Location of major structures in each abdominal quadrant

Right upper quadrant (RUQ)
 Liver*
 Duodenum
 Pylorus
 Pancreas
 Gallbladder
 Hepatic flexure of colon
 Part of transverse and ascending colon

Left upper quadrant (LUQ)
 Stomach
 Spleen*
 Pancreas
 Left kidney
 Splenic flexure of colon
 Part of transverse and descending colon

Right lower quadrant (RLQ)
 Cecum
 Appendix
 Part of ascending colon
 Right overy and fallopian tube
 Right femoral pulse*

Left lower quadrant (LLQ)
 Sigmoid colon
 Part of descending colon
 Left ovary and fallopian tubes
 Left femoral pulse*

Midline
 Umbilicus*
 Aorta*
 Bladder
 Rectum
 Uterus

*Organs that are usually palpable.

Reprinted by permission of The C. V. Mosby Co. from *Nursing Care of Infants and Children*, by Lucille Whaley and Donna Wong, © 1979, The C. V. Mosby Co., St. Louis.

Summary of Procedures of Biopsy or Aspiration

Name of Procedure	Definition	Special Care or Observations
Abdominal paracentesis	Puncture through abdominal wall and aspiration of fluid from peritoneum	Observe pulse and respirations during and following procedure. Observe for abdominal

Name of Procedure	Definition	Special Care or Observations
		tenderness, fever, or rigidity indicating peritonitis
Thoracentesis	Puncture through chest wall and aspiration of pleural fluid	Observe for shock during procedure. Observe for pain on breathing, dyspnea, fever indicating pneumothorax, hemothorax, or infection
Lumbar puncture	Puncture made into subarachnoid space between lumbar vertebrae and aspiration of cerebrospinal fluid	Observe for symptoms and signs of collapse during the procedure. Headache may follow
Bone-marrow biopsy	Aspiration of marrow from sternum, usually anterior or posterior iliac crest	Should cause little discomfort. Sterile dressing applied to puncture site. Bleeding is uncommon
Liver biopsy	Needle aspiration of liver tissue with intercostal approach or epigastric	Observe pulse and respirations during procedure. Patient remains in bed for 12 h with BP and pulse q 30 min. Observe site for hemorrhage. Signs of hemorrhage are usually seen within 4 h—increasing restlessness, hypotension, tachycardia, sweating. Observe for abdominal pain, rigidity, indicating peritonitis (possible bile leakage into peritoneum)

Reprinted by permission of McGraw-Hill Book Company from *Nursing Care of the Patient With Medical-Surgical Disorders,* 2nd edition, by Harriet Moidel, Elizabeth Giblin, and Berniece Wagner, © 1976, McGraw-Hill Book Company.

48

Summary of Common Radiological Procedures

System	Structure	Procedure	Medium	Nursing Considerations
Nervous Brain	Ventricles	Ventriculogram	Air: injected directly into ventricles	Patient will have had head shaved and burr holes made in skull; headache may follow; patient to lie flat.
	Ventricles and meningeal spaces	Pneumoencephalogram	Air: injected into subarachnoid space	Headache may follow; patient to lie flat
	Subarachnoid spaces and ventricles	Encephalogram	Air: introduced by lumbar puncture	Headache may follow; patient to lie flat. Observe for signs of increased intracranial pressure or convulsion
	Cerebral vessels	Cerebral angiogram	Dye: injected into carotid or vertebral arteries	Observe neck for obstruction from swelling. Check movement of extremities and facial mobility

Spine	Spinal sub-arachnoid space	Myelogram	Air or dye: introduced by lumbar puncture	Observe for signs of meningeal irritation
If air used, position patient flat for several hours
If dye used and not removed, elevate head to prevent flow of dye to brain
Gastrointestinal
Upper	Esophagus
Stomach
Duodenum	Barium swallow	Barium sulfate: taken by mouth	Patient fasted for procedure
Stools may be light in color for following few days
Note absence of stool, abdominal discomfort indicating constipation following procedure
Lower	Colon
Rectum	Barium enema	Barium sulfate: given by enema	Before examination: bowel cleared by enemas
After examination: retained barium can cause constipation and impaction; cathartics and/or
	Polypoid masses	Double contrast	Air: injected into colon after expulsion of barium	

Continued on next page

System	Structure	Procedure	Medium	Nursing Considerations
				enemas may be required; encourage intake of natural laxative foods and fluids to promote elimination
Biliary	Gallbladder	Cholecystogram	Dye: by mouth or intravenously Fatty meal (e.g., cream) following first x-ray series	Before examination: cathartics and enemas to empty gastrointestinal tract for better visualization : fats withheld at evening meal : patient fasted for procedure Dye tablets (given preceding evening) may cause mild diarrhea
	Cystic, hepatic, common ducts	Cholangiogram	Dye: injected directly into biliary tree, or intravenously (less frequent)	Rarely, bile peritonitis may result from leakage into peritoneal cavity via needle tract

Renal	Kidney Renal pelves Ureters Bladder	Intravenous pyelogram Retrograde pyelogram	Dye: injected intravenously or by ureteral cathether	Patient fasted Gastrointestinal tract may be cleared by enemas During and after procedure: observe for any signs of reaction to intravenously administered dye (skin flushing, nausea, abdominal cramps)
Cardiovascular	Heart and great vessels	Cardio-angiogram	Dye: injected into heart by cardiac catheter	Patient will require postoperative cardiac catheterization care
		Angio-cardiogram	Dye: injected intravenously	
	Arteries and veins	Venogram Arteriogram Aortogram	Dye: injected into desired area of vascular system	
Respiratory	Lungs	Bronchogram	Dye: instilled into bronchi intratracheally	After procedure: patient placed on postural drainage for removal of oily dye substance

Reprinted by permission of McGraw-Hill Book Company from *Nursing Care of the Patient With Medical-Surgical Disorders,* 2nd edition, by Harriet Moidel, Elizabeth Giblin, and Berniece Wagner, © 1976, McGraw-Hill Book Company.

52

Summary of Common Isotopic Procedures

Organ or Function Tested	Isotopes Used and Administration Route	Measurement Type and Time After Tracer Dose	Comments
Thyroid gland iodine uptake	^{131}I, oral or IV	Urine, blood, over thyroid 6 and 24 h	24-h uptake normally 10–40%. Need not fast. Tracer uptake bears constant relationship to amount of inorganic iodide accumulated by thyroid. Many substances can affect test (e.g., iodide administration, radio-opaque dyes, etc.)
Protein-bound iodine	^{131}I, oral	Blood—48 or 72 h	Measures organically bound ^{131}I in circulation at a specified time interval after tracer dose. Takes into account hormone synthesis and release by thyroid gland. Normal—usually 4.0–8.0 μg/ml
Thyroid scan	^{131}I, oral	Detector over gland, 24 h	Thyroid normally has butterfly appearance. Test determines morphology—size, shape, nodules, tumors

Brain scan	^{131}I albumin ^{197}Hg Chlormerodrin ^{99m}Tc injected	24 h (detector) 3–5 h (detector) ½ h (detector)	Used to detect tumors, cerebrovascular disease, head trauma, skull lesions, intracranial infections, congenital defects
Lung function	^{133}Xe, inhaled	Detector over lungs, immediately	Measures regional ventilation. Patient takes single breath to total lung capacity and distribution of radioactivity is measured
	^{133}Xe, injected	Detector over lungs, immediately	Measures distribution of regional blood flow. Tracer injected through superior vena cava catheter, patient holds breath, Xe moves into alveolar space and distribution of radioactivity measured
Lung scan	^{131}I albumin microaggregated, IV	Detector over lungs, immediately	Tracer is trapped in pulmonary arteriolar-capillary bed. Detects pulmonary embolus, tuberculosis, bronchogenic cancer, chronic obstructive pulmonary disease

Continued on next page

Organ or Function Tested	Isotopes Used and Administration Route	Measurement Type and Time After Tracer Dose	Comments
Gastrointestinal tract	^{51}Cr-labeled red blood cells, IV	Blood sample at start and end (72 h) 72-h stool sample	Detects gastrointestinal blood loss
Liver function	Rose Bengal Sodium ^{131}I, IV	Detector against lateral aspect of head and midabdomen. Counts taken at each site for 30 min.	Patient must be in fasting state. Rate at which substance is removed from blood assesses functional capacity of liver cells, liver blood flow, and biliary tract patency
Liver scan	Rose Bengal Sodium ^{131}I Gold 198, IV	Detector over liver, 30 min 5 min	Helpful in diagnosing hepatomegaly, atrophy, lesions, displacement of the liver, trauma, abscesses, cysts, tumors
Kidney renogram	Iodohippurate ^{131}I, IV	Detectors over kidneys immediately, for 15 min or longer	Patient is normally hydrated. Detects decreased kidney function and blood supply
Bone scan	Strontium 85 Strontium 87m Fluorine 18	1 h (detector) 30 min (detector) 2 h (detector)	Patient should void prior to scan and have laxative and enema preparation evening before. Indications for bone

scan are bone pain, suspected cancer metastases, tumors

Reprinted by permission of McGraw-Hill Book Company from *Nursing Care of the Patient With Medical-Surgical Disorders,* 2nd edition, by Harriet Moidel, Elizabeth Giblin, and Berniece Wagner, © 1976, McGraw-Hill Book Company.

Summary of Signs and Symptoms of Shock

	Early	Late
Blood pressure	Normal	Less than 90 mm Hg systolic
Pulse	Increase in rate	Increase in rate; weak
Skin color	Normal	Pale
Skin temperature	Cool, moist	Cold
Sensorium	Anxious	Coma
Respiration	Increase in rate and depth	Increase in rate, shallow

Reprinted by permission of The C. V. Mosby Co. from *First Aid in Emergency Care,* Guy S. Parcel, © 1977, The C. V. Mosby Company.

Diseases Associated with Unusual Odors

DISEASE	ENZYME DEFECT	ODOR	CLINICAL FEATURES	TREATMENT
Diabetes mellitus	Lack of insulin or insulin activity	Acetone on breath	Polyuria, polyphagia, polydipsia, weight loss, acidosis, coma	Insulin administration
Phenylketonuria	Phenylalanine hydroxylase	Musty, "mousy," "horsey"	Progressive mental retardation, eczema, decreased pigmentation, seizures, spasticity	Diet low in phenylalanine
Maple syrup urine disease	Branched chain decarboxylase	Maple syrup	Marked acidosis, seizures, coma leading to death in first year or two of life or mental subnormality without acidosis or intermittent acidosis without mental retardation	Diet low in branched chain amino acids; protein restriction and/or thiamine in large doses
Oasthouse urine disease	Defective transport of methionine, branched chain amino acids, tyrosine, and phenylalanine	Yeast-like Dried-celery-like	Mental retardation, spasticity, hyperpnea, fever, edema	Restrict methionine in diet
Odor of sweaty feet, Syndrome I	Isovaleryl CoA dehydrogenase	Sweaty feet	Recurrent bouts of acidosis, vomiting, dehydration, coma, aversion to protein foods	Restrict leucine in diet
Odor of sweaty feet, Syndrome II	Green acyldehydrogenase	Sweaty feet	Onset of symptoms in first week of life with acidosis, dehydration, seizures, and death	High CHO diet(?) Low fat diet(?)
Odor of cats syndrome	Beta-methyl-crotonyl-CoA carboxylase	Cat's urine	Neurologic disorder resembling Werdnig-Hoffmann disease, ketoacidosis, failure to thrive	Leucine restriction(?) Biotin administration

Fish odor syndrome	Unknown	Like dead fish	Stigmata of Turner's syndrome, neutropenia, recurrent infections, anemia, splenomegaly	Unknown
Fish odor syndrome	Trimethylamine oxidase	Like dead fish	Unusual odor of sweat, skin and urine. Normal development	Elimination of fish from the diet
Odor of rancid butter syndrome	Unknown	Rancid butter	Poor feeding, irritability, progressive neurologic deterioration with seizures and death; hepatic dysfunction; possibly same as acute tyrosinosis	Response to decreased phenylalanine and tyrosine intake(?)

Reprinted by permission of W. B. Saunders Co. from *The Whole Pediatrician Catalog* by McMillan, Nieburg and Oski, © 1977, W. B. Saunders Co.

Summary of Assessment of Acid-Base Imbalance

Acid-base imbalance		Blood gases*							
Type	Common causes	Arterial blood pH	BE and HCO_3^-	Pa_{CO_2}	Respirations	Urine pH†	Neurological signs	Electrolytes (K^+)	Effects on cardiac function
Metabolic acidosis	Diabetic ketoacidosis Shock Lactic acidosis Renal failure (retained H^+, loss of base)	<7.40 Lungs may partially correct	Lowered HCO_3^- base excess (BE) −2 or <	Lowered during compensation	Rapid, deep	< 6.0	Apathy Confusion Disorientation Stupor Coma	Hyperkalemia during acidosis →	Widening pulse pressure due to falling diastole Severe arrhythmias Cardiac arrest

Continued on next page

Acid-base imbalance		Blood gases*							
Type	Common causes	Arterial blood pH	BE and HCO_3^-	Pa_{CO_2}	Respirations	Urine pH†	Neurological signs	Electrolytes (K^+)	Effects on cardiac function
Metabolic alkalosis	Diarrhea (loss of base) K^+ depletion (diuretics, tap-water enemas, laxatives) Vomiting or GI suctioning Excessive intake of antacids	≥ 7.45 Lungs may partially correct	Elevated HCO_3^- BE +2 or >	Elevated during compensation	Shallow, slow periods of apnea	> 7.0	Belligerence Irritability Disorientation Lethargy Tetany Convulsions	Hypokalemia during correction, may fall to 1.7 meq/liter Hypokalemia	Irregular and/or slow pulse Cardiac arrest Irregular and/or slow pulse
Respiratory acidosis	Chronic obstructive lung disease Surgery, abdominal or chest	Normal, if kidneys compensating; otherwise < 7.40	Elevated, if kidneys compensating	Elevated	Hypoventilation Respiratory arrest	< 6.0	Confusion Disorientation Lethargy Stupor Coma	Normal	—
Respiratory alkalosis	Mechanical ventilation with volume-cycled ventilator	Normal, if kidneys compensating; otherwise > 7.45	Lowered, if kidneys compensating	Lowered	Hyperventilation (aggravates loss of CO_2)	> 7.0	Hyperreflexia Muscle twitching Convulsions	Normal	—

*Normal values for the parameters measured in blood gases are blood pH = 7.35–7.45; BE = ±2; HCO_3^- = 24 meq/liter; Pa_{CO_2} = 40 mmHg. †Normal urine pH is 4.8–7.5.

Reprinted by permission of McGraw Hill from *The Nurses Guide to Fluid and Electrolyte Balance* by Audrey Burgess, 2nd edition, © 1979, McGraw Hill Book Company.

Differential Diagnosis of High Fever

Disease (Illness)	Onset of Illness	Symptoms	Physical Findings
Upper respiratory tract infection Lobar pneumonia	Sudden onset. History of chills. Onset acute	Stuffy nose, coryza, general malaise, cough Coughing, chest pain, rust-colored sputum	Congested throat. Nasal secretions present. Moist rales may be heard; sound of breathing diminishes, speech accelerated.
Lung abscess and bronchiectasis	History of respiratory tract infections	Chest pain, coughing, purulent sputum, which shows 3-layer separation inside container.	Moist rales possibly heard; fingers clubby if disease of long duration.
Tuberculosis	Onset insidious, though sudden in small children	Coughing, recurrent afternoon fever which drops to below 37°C in the morning, hidrosis weight loss, poor appetite, insomnia.	Fine rales possibly heard in tuberculosis cases; percussion pain over kidney region in renal tuberculosis.
Rheumatism	History of tonsillitis and skin infections	Large joints red, swollen, hot and painful (of migrating nature); sweating, palpation, circular red patches, small subcutaneous nodes.	Increased heart rate, lowered heart sounds or murmurs heard in region of heart valves.
Urinary tract infections		Urinary frequency, dysuria, chills	Percussion pain over kidney region, pressure pain over suprapubic region.
Measles	History of measles epidemics usually occurring during winter-spring	Coughing, running nose and tearing	Red buccal membrane showing spots, exanthem first appearing as maculopapular rash, starting from neck, then spreading to face, body, and extremities. After fever has subsided, skin desquamation takes place.
Scarlet fever	Onset acute and history of contact; occurring mostly during winter-spring.	Sore throat	Congested throat exanthem scarlet red, small maculopapular rash that blanch upon pressure. Pale lips, strawberry tongue, skin peeling in large patches.

Continued on next page

Epidemic meningitis	Likely to occur during winter-spring	Headache, projectile vomiting, coma	Dull red petchiae, neck rigidity, Kernig's sign positive, sole scratch test positive.
Epidemic Japanese B encephalitis	Likely to occur during summer-fall	Headache, vomiting, sleepiness, delirium	Neck resistance present; possibly positive Kernig's sign and sole [foot] scratch test.
Typhoid	Onset slow, history of contact	Gradual temperature rise, continuous high fever 1 week later; nausea and vomiting possibly present; expression dull and listless.	Hepatosplenomegaly, roseola, relatively slow pulse.
Infectious hepatitis	History of contact	Poor appetite, nausea and vomiting, weakness, upper abdominal discomfort, appearance of jaundice upon temperature drop in some cases.	Hepatomegaly, pressure pain felt over liver region, urine dark tea-colored and foamy, the foam also dark.
Leptospirosis	Likely to occur in summer-fall, history of contact with infected water.	Chills and muscular aches throughout body, particularly pronounced in the gastrocnemius muscle of the leg; sometimes bleeding and jaundice.	Pressure pain obvious over the gastrocnemius; possibly hepatosplenomegaly.
Acute schistosomiasis	History of contact with infected	Fever over long duration, coughing, diarrhea.	Hepatomegaly, pressure pain, spleen possibly palpable.
Malaria	History of mosquito bites	Course of rigors, fever, sweating and temperature drop in tertian or quartan pattern	Possibly splenomegaly and anemia
Septicemia	History of infection	Headache, chills, frequently accompanied by nausea, vomiting and diarrhea.	Subcutaneous bleeding points, hepatosplenomegaly, pressure pain, slight jaundice
Various malignant tumors		Fever over a long period of time, ineffective antibiotic therapy, rapid loss of weight	Lymphadenopathy and hepatosplenomegaly possible, anemia.
Acute mastitis	Mostly in primiparas	Painful breasts, chills	Cracked nipples, local redness, swelling, burning and pain.
Puerperal fever	3–5 days postpartum	Chills, unpleasant odor to lochia	Pressure pain over and alongside uterus

From *A Barefoot Doctor's Manual: The American Translation of the Official Chinese Paramedical Manual.* Copyright © 1977 Running Press. Reprinted courtesy of Running Press, 38 South 19th St., Philadelphia, Pa. 19103. (This is an excellent resource for nurses wishing to know more about Chinese medical practices. It is also a good source for diagnostic and treatment information in this country as well since much of the information is applicable here. The book includes a large section on Chinese medicinal herbs as well. This paperback edition is a bargain at $6.95.)

Differential Diagnosis of Abdominal Pain

Disease	Disease Onset and History	Site of Abdominal Pain	Nature of Abdominal Pain	Abdominal Symptoms	Other Symptoms
Acute appendicitis	Gradual onset	Beginning in upper abdomen or around umbilicus, shifting gradually to lower right quadrant	Continuous pain accompanied by slight increase in paroxysmal pain	Localization of tenderness and pain in right lower quadrant, muscular tension present	Slight rise in body temperature, accompanied by nausea and vomiting
Acute cholecystitis and cholelithiasis	Onset frequently sudden, usually on evenings after a diet of greasy foods	Middle or right epigastrium	Continual or periodic colicky pain radiating toward the right shoulder	Tactile tenderness over right epigastrium, muscles tense, percussion pain frequently present over liver, gallbladder sometimes palpable.	High fever accompanied by chills, nausea, and vomiting, and possibly jaundice
Bile duct ascariasis	Onset sudden. Has history of taking an anthelmentic recently	Right lower part of the xiphoid of the sternum	Recurring acute colicky pain, a "drilled-through-the-top" feeling	Slight degree of tenderness and rebound tenderness felt under the xiphoid on the lower right	No fever in early stage. Chills, high fever, nausea and vomiting (sometimes vomiting up ascaris) accompanying infections of the bile ducts.
Acute perforation of peptic and duodenal ulcer	Sudden onset, frequently after a full meal. History of ulcers.	Upper and midabdomen rapidly involving the whole abdomen	Continual stabbing pain	Considerable tactile tenderness abdominal muscles tense, liver hard and murmurs over boundary of liver dissipated	Body temperature drops during state of shock, showing obvious rise 6–2 hours later, accompanied by nausea and vomiting.

Continued on next page

Disease	Disease Onset and History	Site of Abdominal Pain	Nature of Abdominal Pain	Abdominal Symptoms	Other Symptoms
Acute intestinal obstruction	Onset sudden, history of surgery and extraperitoneal hernia possible	Arising usually from midabdomen	Intermittent colicky pain	Tenderness and distension present, sometimes intestinal type, peristaltic rushes strong, bubbly and metallic sound present	No fever in early stage, though bile and fecal fluid may be vomited. No bowel movements, no flatus expelled via anus.
Acute pancreatitis	Sudden, usually following gluttonous consumption of food and drink, sometimes accompanied by shock	Upper abdomen	Continuous acute pain, usually radiating toward back	Horizontal tenderness, slight muscular rigidity, abdominal distension in severe cases	Fever occurring 2–3 days later, with nausea and vomiting
Renal colic	Sudden. Past history of hematuria	Upper abdomen or sides [at waistline]	Intermittent acute colicky pain, usually radiating toward external genitals along medical aspect of thigh, accompanied by painful micturition	Slight tenderness, though percussion pain over kidneys definite	Chills and fever, nausea and vomiting accompanying infection
Intestinal parasites	Gradual. History of ascaris expulsion positive in many cases	Peri-umbilical area	Intermittent colicky pain	Tenderness not felt over definite area, no noticeable abdominal distension, sometimes knotted beltlike mass caused by ascaris felt.	Nausea and vomiting possible
Acute gastroenteritis	Sudden onset, usually with history of ingesting food less than clean	Whole abdomen	Intermittent colicky pain	Tenderness not localized, rigidity usually lacking.	Chills and fever usually seen, vomiting occurring before onset of abdominal pain, the severity

			of abdominal pain lessened after stools have been passed. Chills, high fever
Lobar pneumonia	Sudden, accompanied by symptoms of respiratory infection	Upper abdomen	Continual pain, accompanied possibly by chest and shoulder pain that is heightened by deep breathing	Tenderness over epigastrium
Acute salpingitis	Onset gradual, accompanied often by increased leukorrhea. Usually occurring during or after menstrual periods.	Lower abdomen	Continual pain, frequently accompanied by low back pain.	Site of tenderness somewhat lower, but frequently symmetrical	Chill and fever
Rupture of ectopic gestation	Onset sudden, frequently accompanied by shock. History of menstrual period overdue. Also history of sterility for many years.	First on one side of lower abdomen, developing to generalized abdomen pain later on	Continuous pain, frequently radiating toward shoulder	Marked tenderness over one side of lower abdomen, but muscular rigidity slight. Shifting dullness sometimes present

From *A Barefoot Doctor's Manual: The American Translation of the Official Chinese Paramedical Manual.* Copyright © 1977 Running Press. Reprinted courtesy of Running Press, 38 South 19th St., Philadelphia, Pa. 19103.

Differential Diagnosis of Cardiac and Pulmonary Dyspnea

	Cardiac	Pulmonary
History	Exertional dyspnea; orthopnea; true paroxysmal nocturnal dyspnea; ankle swelling; angina pectoris	Usually exertional dyspnea only; chronic cough; long history of being "bronchial"; frequent URIs or pneumonias
Electrocardiogram	Definite abnormalities or completely normal; notched P waves may be seen; evidence of old myocardial infarction	Right axis deviation; peaked P waves or completely normal
Physical examination	Heart sounds prominent; atrial or ventricular gallops present; systolic murmurs present	Heart sounds frequently obscured; sounds best heard below xiphoid
	Good diaphragmatic excursion and normal transmission of breath sounds; basilar, coarse or crepitant rales	Poor diaphragmatic excursion and poorly transmitted breath sounds; wheezing on forced expiration or at rest
Chest x-ray	Cardiac enlargement; pulmonary congestion	Normal or small heart; overinflated lungs
Pulmonary function test	Vital capacity and maximum breathing capacity moderately reduced in parallel fashion; normal expiratory flow rates	Maximum breathing capacity and expiratory flow rates markedly reduced; vital capacity may be normal or slightly reduced
Response to diuretic	Decrease in dyspnea and amelioration of rales, loss of weight > 3 pounds	No effect
Response to nebulized bronchodilator	No definite effect	Improvement

If several positive findings are present from both columns, the patient probably has both heart and lung disease.

From Ayres, Giannelli and Mueller. Care of the Critically Ill, 2nd edition, 1974. Courtesy of Appleton-Century-Crofts, Publishing Division of Prentice-Hall, Inc.

What to expect in seven types of cerebrovascular accidents

	INTRACEREBRAL HEMORRHAGE	SUBARACHNOID HEMORRHAGE
ONSET	rapid: minutes to 1 or 2 hrs	sudden; varied progression
DURATION	permanent if lesion is large; small lesions are potentially reversible	variable: complete clearing may occur in days or weeks
RELATION TO ACTIVITY	usually occurs during activity	most commonly related to head trauma
CONTRIBUTING OR ASSOCIATED FACTORS	hypertensive cardiovascular disease; coagulation defects	intracerebral arterial aneurysm; trauma; tumor; vascular malformations
SENSORIUM	coma common	coma common
NUCHAL (NECK) RIGIDITY	frequently present	present
LOCATION OF CEREBRAL DEFICIT	focal: arterial syndrome not common	diffuse: aneurysm may give focal sign before and after
CONVULSIONS	common	common
CEREBROSPINAL FLUID	bloody unless hemorrhage entirely intracerebral	grossly bloody; increased pressure
SKULL X-RAYS	pineal shift edema, hemorrhage, or hematoma	normal or calcified aneurysm
RECURRENCE IN SURVIVORS	common	common

Continued on next page

SUBDURAL HEMORRHAGE	EXTRADURAL HEMORRHAGE	FOCAL CEREBRAL ISCHEMIA	CEREBRAL THROMBOSIS	CEREBRAL EMBOLISM
insidious; occasionally acute	rapid: minutes to hours	rapid: seconds to minutes	minutes to hours	sudden
hours to months	initially fluctuating, then steadily progressive	seconds to minutes	permanent if lesion is large; potentially reversible if lesion is small	rapid improvement may occur depending on collateral flow
usually related to head trauma	almost always related to head trauma	occurs during activity if related to decreased cardiac output	usually occurs at rest	unrelated to activity
chronic alcoholism	any condition that predisposes to trauma	peripheral and coronary atherosclerosis; hypertension	peripheral and coronary atherosclerosis; hypertension	atrial fibrillation; aortic and mitral valve disease; myocardial infarct; atherosclerotic plague
generally clouded	rapidly advancing coma	usually conscious	usually conscious	usually conscious
rare	rare	absent	absent	absent
frontal lobe signs, ipsilateral pupil may dilate	temporal lobe signs, ipsilateral pupil may dilate, high intracranial pressure	focal; or arterial syndrome	focal; or arterial syndrome	focal; or arterial syndrome
infrequent	common	rare	rare	rare
normal to slightly elevated protein	increased pressure; color and cells usually normal	usually normal	usually normal	usually normal
frequent contralateral shift of pineal	frequently fracture across middle meningeal artery groove	may show calcification of intracranial arteries	possible arterial calcification and pineal shift from edema	usually normal
can recur after surgery	none with adequate initial treatment	common	common	common

Reprinted with permission from *RN Magazine*, January, 1979, pages 68 and 69, © 1979 by Litton Industries, Inc.

A Comparison of Juvenile Diabetes and Adult-Onset Diabetes

A COMPARISON OF JUVENILE DIABETES AND ADULT-ONSET DIABETES

Factors	Juvenile Diabetes	Adult-Onset Diabetes
Age at onset	May occur at any age; usually appears before age 15	Usually occurs in obese persons over age 40
Synonyms	Growth-onset diabetes, labile diabetes, brittle diabetes, insulin-dependent diabetes	Maturity-onset diabetes, senile diabetes, mild diabetes
Possible etiology	*Absolute* deficiency of insulin caused by deficiency of pancreatic islets	*Relative* insulin deficiency possibly cuased by insulin antibodies, by insulin antagonists, or by excessive demands for insulin due to obesity, persistent stress, etc.
Severity	Very severe; little or no circulating insulin may be present	Usually mild; some circulating insulin almost always present
Therapeutic control	Insulin injections and careful planning of diet essential	Insulin injections often unnecessary; condition controlled by diet and oral hypoglycemic agents
Sequelae	Vascular and neural damage inevitably develops	Same

Reprinted by permission of W. B. Saunders Co. from *Medical-Surgical Nursing: A Psychophysiological Approach* by Joan Luckmann and Karen Sorenson, © 1974, W. B. Saunders Co.

68

Comparison of Clinical Features of Insulin Reactions and Diabetic Coma

Clinical Feature	Insulin Reaction	Diabetic Coma
Onset	Sudden or gradual (minutes to hours)	Slow (days)
Causes	Delayed mealtime Omission of meal Excessive exercise Insulin overdosage	Neglect of treatment Intercurrent disease
Symptoms	Nervousness Weakness Sweating Hunger Blurred or double vision Abnormal behavior Unconsciousness Convulsions	Thirst Headache Nausea Vomiting Abdominal pain Dim vision Constipation Drowsiness Shortness of breath
Signs	Pallor Shallow respiration Sweating Pulse normal Eyeballs normal	Florid face Air hunger Loud, labored breathing Dry skin Rapid pulse Soft eyeballs Acetone breath Loss of consciousness
Urinalysis:		
Sugar	Usually absent, especially in second voided specimen	Positive
Acetone	Negative	Positive
Diacetic acid	Negative	Positive
Response to Treatment	Rapid; occasionally delayed	Slow

From Rosenthal, H., and Rosenthal, J.: *Diabetic Care in Pictures*. 3rd ed. Philadelphia, J. B. Lippincott Company, 1960, p. 141, as reprinted by Luckmann & Sorensen in *Medical-Surgical Nursing, A Psychophysiologic Approach,* © 1974, W. B. Saunders Co. Reproduced by permission of J. B. Lippincott Co.

Clinical Appraisal of Thrombophlebitis

Veins	Causative Factors	Signs and Symptoms	Edema	Pulmonary Embolism	Venous Insufficiency
Superficial Veins: saphenous, median cephalic, median basilic	Varicose veins; I.V. injections; Buerger's disease; blood dyscrasias; cancer	Tender, indurated, red, visible palpable cord along vein; ovoid nodules in skin	Rare	Rare	Rare
Deep Small Veins: femoral, tibial, popliteal, pelvic	Postoperative; postpartum; prolonged bed rest; congestive heart failure; blood dyscrasias; cancer; oral contraceptives; fractures and dislocations	Increased muscle turgor over tenderness on affected vein; minimal or no venous distention; deep muscle tenderness; limb may be warmer than opposite limb; dorsiflexion of foot may cause calf pain (Homans' sign); occasionally fever—rarely exceeds 101°F.	Occasional edema may be masked and revealed by measuring circumference of extremities	Always a possibility	Rare
Major Deep Veins: femoral, ileal, axillary, subclavian, superior and inferior vena cava		No superficial signs of inflammation; cyanosis of extremity; venous distention of limbs	Usually	Always a possibility	Frequent

Reprinted by permission of W. B. Saunders Co. from *Medical-Surgical Nursing: A Psychophysiological Approach*, by Joan Luckmann and Karen Sorenson, © 1974, W. B. Saunders Co.

Categories of Seizure Types

Seizure	Behavior
Grand mal	Seizure may be preceded by an aura or prodromal twitching, localized spasm, irritability, headache, digestive disturbance, or mental dullness.
	Seizure itself involves generalized convulsion with tonic and clonic phases of muscular spasms as well as involuntary urination and/or defecation from contraction of abdominal muscles.
	The convulsion is followed by sleep.
Petit mal	Seizures consist of transient loss of consciousness. Motor manifestations include upward rolling of eyes, moving of lids, dropping or rhythmic nodding of head, quivering of trunk and limb muscles.
	Clinical evidence of petit mal rarely appears before age 3 and frequently disappears by puberty.
	Intellectual development is rarely impaired.
Psychomotor seizures	This is the most difficult type to recognize and control.
	A slight aura may manifest itself in a shrill cry or an attempt to run for help.
	The seizure itself consist of purposeful but inappropriate motor acts which are repetitive and often complicated, characterized by gradual loss of postural tone.
	After 1 to 5 minutes of unconsciousness, normal activity may resume or sleep may ensue.
Status epilepticus	Seizure involves successive major convulsions without intervening recovery of consciousness.
	The most frequent cause is sudden withdrawal of anticonvulsant medication: an attack may occur 2 to 4 days after phenobarbital is withdrawn, 7 to 12 days after withdrawal of Dilantin.
	Seizure may be precipitated by an acute respiratory infection or the administration of chlorpromazine.
	An attack constitutes medical emergency requiring vigorous treatment.

Reprinted by permission of McGraw-Hill Book Co., from *Comprehensive Psychiatric Nursing*, by Haber, Leach, Schudy, and Sideleau, © Copyright 1978, McGraw-Hill Book Company.

Differentiation of Common Breast Nodules

Despite the classic differences listed below, definitive diagnosis usually depends on aspiration of cysts or surgical biopsy. Differentiation is most difficult in cases where it is most desirable—the early small nodule.

PATHOLOGY	CYSTIC DISEASE Single or Multiple Cysts	ADENOFIBROMA A Benign Neoplasm	CANCER A Malignant Neoplasm
Findings by palpation (The illustrations do not imply visibility to inspection.)			
Usual age	30–55, regresses after menopause	Puberty and young adulthood, up to 55	30–80, most common in middle-aged and elderly
Number	Single or multiple	Usually single, may be multiple	Usually single although may coexist with other nodular lesions
Shape	Round	Round, discoid or lobular	Irregular or stellate
Consistency	Soft to firm, usually elastic	May be soft, usually firm	Firm or hard
Delimitation	Well delineated	Well delineated	Not clearly delineated from surrounding tissues
Mobility	Mobile	Very mobile	May be fixed to skin or underlying tissues
Tenderness	Often tender	Usually non-tender	Usually non-tender
Retraction signs	Absent	Absent	Often present

Reprinted by permission of J. B. Lippincott Company from *A Guide to Physical Examination* by Barbara Bates, M.D., Copyright © J. B. Lippincott Company.

International Classification of Cancer of the Cervix

Stage	Description
Stage 0	Carcinoma in situ
Stage I	Carcinoma confined to the cervix
Stage IA1	Early stromal invasion
Stage IA2	Occult cancer
Stage IB	All other cancers limited to the uterus
Stage II	Cancer involves the vagina, but not the lower third, or infiltrates the parametrium, but not out to the sidewall
Stage IIA	Cancer involves the vagina, but there is no evidence of parametrial involvement
Stage IIB	Infiltration of the parametria, but not out to the sidewall
Stage III	Cancer involves the lower third of the vagina or extends to the pelvic sidewall
Stage IIIA	Cancer involves the lower third of the vagina, but is not out to the pelvic sidewall if the parametria are involved
Stage IIIB	Involvement of one or both parametria out to the sidewall
Stage III (urinary)	Obstruction of one or both ureters on intravenous pyelogram without other criteria for Stage III disease
Stage IV	Cancer extends outside the reproductive tract
Stage IVA	Involvement of the bladder or rectum
Stage IVB	Distant metastasis or disease outside the true pelvis

Reproduced by permission of J. B. Lippincott Co. from *Health Care of Women* by Leonide L. Martin, © Copyright 1978, J. B. Lippincott Company.

A Comparison of the Characteristics of Benign and Malignant Neoplasms

Characteristic	Benign Neoplasm	Malignant Neoplasm
Speed of growth	Grows slowly usually continues to grow throughout life unless surgically removed; may have periods of remission during which growth stops for a time	Grows usually rapidly, tends to grow relentlessly throughout life; rarely, neoplasm may *regress spontaneously*
Mode of growth	Grows by enlarging and expanding; always remains localized; never infiltrates surrounding tissues	Grows by infiltrating surrounding tissues; may remain localized (in situ) but usually spreads out to infiltrate other tissues
Presence of capsule	Almost always contained and confined within a fibrous capsule; capsule does not prevent expansion of neoplasm but does prevent growth by infiltration; capsule advantageous because it and enclosed tumor cells can be easily removed surgically	Never contained and confined within a capsule; absence of capsule allows neoplastic cells to invade surrounding tissues; absence of capsule makes surgical removal of tumor more difficult
Characteristics of cells composing tumor	Usually well differentiated; mitotic figures absent or scanty; cells appear adult; anaplastic cells absent; cells function poorly in comparison with normal cells from which they arise; if neoplasm arises in glandular tissue, cells may be capable of secreting hormones	Usually poorly differentiated; large numbers of normal and abnormal mitotic figures present; cells tend to be anaplastic, i.e., young, embryonic type cells; cells too abnormal to perform any physiologic functions; occasionally a malignant tumor arising in glandular tissue may secrete hormones
Recurrence	Recurrence extremely unusual when surgically removed	Recurrence common following surgery because of spread of tumor cells into surrounding tissues
Metastasis or spread of tumor from original site to other organs of body	Metastases never occur	Metastases very common; most dangerous and deadly aspect of neoplastic disease (see discussion below)

Continued on next page

Effect of neoplasm on tissues and body as a whole	Not harmful to host unless neoplasm located in area where it causes compression of tissues or obstruction of vital organs; does not produce *cachexia* (weight loss, debilitation, anemia, weakness, wasting); neoplasm located in glandular tissue may secrete the hormone normally produced, resulting in excess of hormone in blood	Always harmful to the host; will result in death unless removed surgically or destroyed by radiation or chemotherapy; causes disfigurement of the body, disrupted organ functions, and nutritional imbalances; may result in ulcerations, sepsis, perforations, hemorrhage, and tissue slough; almost always produces cachexia, which leaves patient prone to pneumonia, anemia, etc.; infrequently malignant tumors secrete hormones, causing a hormonal imbalance; usually cells too poorly differentiated to produce normal body secretions
Prognosis	Very good; tumor generally removed surgically	Depends upon speed with which cancer diagnosed; poor prognosis indicated if cells are poorly differentiated and evidence exists of metastatic spread; good prognosis indicated if cells still resemble normal and there is no evidence of metastasis

Reprinted by permission of W. B. Saunders Co. from *Medical-Surgical Nursing: A Psychophysiological Approach* by Joan Luckmann and Karen Sorenson, © 1974, W. B. Saunders Co.

Recommended Sources on Physical Assessment for Nurses

Bates, Barbara, *A Guide to Physical Examination,* J. B. Lippincott, Philadelphia, 1974.

De Gowin, Elmer and Richard De Gowin, *Diagnostic Examination,* The MacMillan Co., London, 1969.

De Gowin, Elmer and Richard De Gowin, *Bedside Diagnostic Examination,* 3rd edition, The MacMillan Co., 1976.

Fowkes, William, and Virginia Hunn, *Clinical Assessment for the Nurse Practitioner,* The C. V. Mosby Co., St. Louis, 1973.

Hochstein, Elliot and Albert Rubin, *Physical Diagnosis,* McGraw-Hill Book Co., New York, 1964.

Judge, Richard, and George Zuidema, eds., *Physical Diagnosis: a Physiologic Approach to the Clinical Examination,* 2nd ed., Little Brown and Co; Boston, 1968.

Lehmann, Janet, "Auscultation of the Heart Sounds" in *AJN,* July, 1972, p. 1242–46.

Littman, D. "Stethoscopes and Auscultation" in *AJN,* July, 1972, p. 1239–41.

Lynsugh, Joan and Barbara Bates, "Physical Diagnosis: A Skill for All Nurses?" in *AJN,* January, 1974, p. 58–59.

Mechner, F. and G. Brown, "Patient Assessment: Auscultation of the Heart, Part II" in *AJN,* February, 1977, p. 275–298.

Morgan, William and George Enghe, *The Clinical Approach to the Patient,* W. B. Saunders Co., Philadelphia, 1969.

Nursing Skillbook, *Assessing Vital Functions Accurately,* Intermed Communications, Inc., Horsham, Pa. 1977.

Prior, John, et al., *Physical Diagnosis: The History and Examination of the Patient,* 3rd edition, The C. V. Mosby Co., St. Louis, 1969.

Slesson, G., "Auscultation of the Chest—a clinical nursing skill" in *Canadian Nurse,* April, 1973, p. 40–43.

Traver, Gayle A., "Assessment of Thorax and Lungs" in *AJN,* March, 1973, p. 466–71.

A series of brochures on differential diagnosis of *Abdominal Pain* is available from Roche Laboratories.

A "Patient Assessment Series," consisting of 18 units on various aspects of physical assessment is available from the American Journal Of Nursing Company.

Audiovisual Materials on Physical Assessment

A set of six cassettes on cardiac auscultation is available from Merck, Sharp and Dohme.

"Physiological And Clinical Aspects Of Cardiac Auscultation," a series of 18 modules including booklets, films, audiocassettes, and slides, on normal and abnormal findings in cardiac auscultation, is available from Lippincott's Audiovisual Media.

"Stethoscopic Heart Records" and "Heart Recordings" are two records on auscultation of the heart, from Columbia Special Products.

ACCEL, the American College Of Cardiology Extended Learning, produces several audiovisual aids in cardiology including auscultation of the heart and detailed programs on cardiovascular disease.

"A Simplified Introduction to Lung Sounds," an audiocassette and booklet, is available from Stethophonics.

"Physical Assessment: Eye And Ear" and "Physical Assessment: Heart And Lungs" are filmstrip series with sound cassettes from Concept Media.

"Essentials Of The Neurological Examination" is a film from Association-Sterling Films.

"Physical Examination Films" is a series of 12 films based on the book, *A Guide To Physical Examination,* by Dr. Barbara Bates. From Lippincott's Audiovisual Media.

An excellent series of 15 films on physical diagnosis is available to educational institutions for rental or purchase from Wayne State University. The series is produced by the University in conjunction with CIBA Pharmaceutical Co.

3 Pharmacology

Nurses in all fields of practice are involved with medications in some way. If not directly involved with administering medications, they may need a knowledge of the medications a patient is taking and their effects and interactions. This section contains general information on the administration of drugs, including basic mathematical formulas for nurses and injection sites, and information on specific drug categories, followed by resource information.

I. **Computing Drug Dosages**
II. **Calculating Drops per Minute**
III. **Injection Sites**
   A. Intramuscular—Adults
   B. Intramuscular—Pediatric
   C. Subcutaneous
IV. **Meals and Drug Administration**
V. **Antidotes for Toxic Agents**
VI. **Drug Incompatibilities with 5% Glucose I.V.**
VII. **Drug Interactions**
VIII. **Specific Drug Categories**
   A. Analgesics
   B. Anesthetics
   C. Antianemics
   D. Antihypertensives
   E. Antipsychotic Agents
   F. Barbiturates
   G. Cardiac Glycosides
   H. Cardiac Emergency Drugs
   I. Chemotherapeutic Agents
   J. Diuretics
   K. Gonorrhea Therapy
   L. Insulins
   M. Radioisotopes
   N. Penicillins
IX. **Drugs Causing Blood Dyscrasias**
X. **Drug Effects on Sexual Behavior**
XI. **Abused Drugs**
XII. **Resources in Pharmacology**

Formulas Used for Computation of Correct Dosage for Administration

I. $$\frac{D \text{ (dose required)}}{X \text{ (units to be administered)}} = \frac{H \text{ (dose available)}}{\text{(no. units containing dose available)}}$$

Example: The physician orders 16 mg of elixir of phenobarbital. The dose on hand is 4 mg/4 ml. How many millimeters should be administered?

(1) $\quad\quad\quad\quad\quad\quad\quad\quad\quad\quad \dfrac{16}{X} = \dfrac{4}{4}$

(2) $\quad\quad\quad\quad\quad\quad\quad\quad\quad\quad 4X = 64$

(3) $\quad\quad\quad\quad\quad\quad\quad\quad\quad\quad X = 16 \quad\quad\quad\quad$ Ans. 16 ml

Example: The physician orders prednisone 20 mg. The tablets on hand are 5 mg each. How many tablets should be administered?

(1) $\quad\quad\quad\quad\quad\quad\quad\quad\quad\quad \dfrac{20}{X} = \dfrac{5}{1}$

(2) $\quad\quad\quad\quad\quad\quad\quad\quad\quad\quad 5X = 20$

(3) $\quad\quad\quad\quad\quad\quad\quad\quad\quad\quad X = 4 \quad\quad\quad\quad$ Ans. 4 tablets

II. *Clark's rule* used for computation of pediatric dosage:

$$\frac{\text{Weight in pounds} \times \text{adult dose}}{150} = \text{safe dosage range for individual child}$$

III. *Fried's rule* used for computation of pediatric dosage for infant or child up to 2 years of age:

$$\frac{\text{Child's age in months} \times \text{adult dose}}{150} = \text{safe dosage for individual infant or child}$$

IV. *Young's rule* used for computation of pediatric dosage for child over 2 years of age:

$$\frac{\text{Age in years} \times \text{adult dose}}{\text{Age in years} + 12} = \text{safe dosage for child}$$

V. Formula using *Surface Area of Child* for computation of pediatric dosage for child:

$$\frac{\text{Surface area of child (in square meters)} \times \text{adult dose}}{1.7} = \text{safe dosage for individual child}$$

VI. Formula based upon *Recommended Pediatric Dosage per Kilogram of Body Weight:*

Milligrams × kilograms of child's body weight = safe dosage for 24 hr

Example: John weighs 88 lb. The recommended pediatric dosage for chlortrimeton is 2 mg/kg/24 hr. What would be a safe dose for John for the total 24 hours?

88 lb/2.2 lb/kg = 40 kg
40 kg × 2 mg/kg = 80 mg = safe dosage for 24 hr for John

Note: Safe dosage for adrenal steroids, digitalis, and antineoplastics are not computed by mg/kg/24 hr since these drugs have a wide dosage range and specialized usage.

Total doses for 24 hours are to be divided and administered at appropriate intervals as indicated by the physician.

Reprinted by permission of John Wiley and Sons, Inc., from *The Nurse's Drug Handbook* by Loebl, Spratto, Wit and Heckheimer, Copyright © 1977, John Wiley and Sons, Inc.

Calculating Drops per Minute

Rate of flow in drops per minute is determined by the number of cc the patient must receive in a given period of time. Infusions may be calculated using the following general formula:

$$\frac{(\text{Total amount of solution in cc})\left(\frac{gtt}{cc}\right)}{(\text{Number of hours to infuse})\left(\frac{60 \text{ minutes}}{1 \text{ hour}}\right)} = X \text{ gtt/minute}$$

Example: If 1000 cc must be infused in 12 hours using Abbott equipment (15 gtt/cc), what will be the rate of flow in drops per minute?

$$\frac{(\cancel{1000}^{500} \text{ cc})\left(\frac{\cancel{15}^{1} \text{ gtt}}{cc}\right)}{(\cancel{12}_{6} \text{ hours})\left(\frac{\cancel{60}^{4} \text{ minutes}}{1 \text{ hour}}\right)} = X \text{ gtt/minute}$$

$$\frac{(\cancel{500})^{125}(1)}{(6)(\cancel{4}_{1})} = X \text{ gtt/minute}$$

$$\frac{125}{6} = X \text{ gtt/minute}$$

$$X = 20.8, \text{ or } 21 \text{ gtt/minute}$$

The rate of flow will be 21 gtt/minute.

Continued on next page

Flow rates may also be calculated in steps using ratios and proportion. The first step determines the number of cc per hour; the second converts cc per hour to cc per minute; the third converts cc per minute to drops per minute.

Example: If 1000 cc must be infused in 12 hours with Abbott equipment (15 gtt/cc), what will be the rate of flow in drops per minute using ratios and proportion?

(1) Determine the number of cc per hour.

$$\frac{\text{Total number of cc to be infused}}{\text{Number of hours to infuse}} = \frac{X \text{ cc}}{1 \text{ hour}} \qquad \frac{1000 \text{ cc}}{12 \text{ hours}} = \frac{X \text{ cc}}{1 \text{ hour}}$$

$$(12)(X \text{ cc}) = (1000)(1)$$

$$X \text{ cc} = \frac{1000}{12}$$

$$X = 83.3, \text{ or } 83 \text{ cc/hour}$$

(2) Convert cc per hour to cc per minute.

$$\frac{\text{Number of cc/hour}}{60 \text{ minutes}} = \frac{X \text{ cc}}{1 \text{ minute}} \qquad \frac{83 \text{ cc}}{60 \text{ minutes}} = \frac{X \text{ cc}}{1 \text{ minute}}$$

$$(60)(X \text{ cc}) = (83)(1)$$

$$X \text{ cc} = \frac{(83)(1)}{60}$$

$$X = 1.38, \text{ or } 1.4 \text{ cc/minute}$$

(3) Convert cc per minute to drops per minute.

$$\frac{\text{Number of gtt}}{1 \text{ cc}} = \frac{X \text{ gtt/minute}}{\text{Number of cc/minute}}$$

$$\frac{15 \text{ gtt}}{1 \text{ cc}} = \frac{X \text{ gtt/minute}}{1.4 \text{ cc/minute}}$$

$$(1)(X \text{ gtt}) = (15)(1.4)$$

$$X = 21 \text{ gtt/minute}$$

The rate of flow will be 21 gtt per minute.

If you were using Cutter or Travenol equipment, 20 gtt/cc or 10 gtt/cc would have been plugged into Step 3. If you were using McGaw (15 gtt/cc), Step 3 would be identical to the above.

Reprinted by permission of the Medical Economics Co., from *How to Calculate Drug Dosages: A Ready Reference and Textbook*, by Angela R. Pecherer and Suzanne L. Vertuno, Copyright © 1978, The Medical Economics Co.

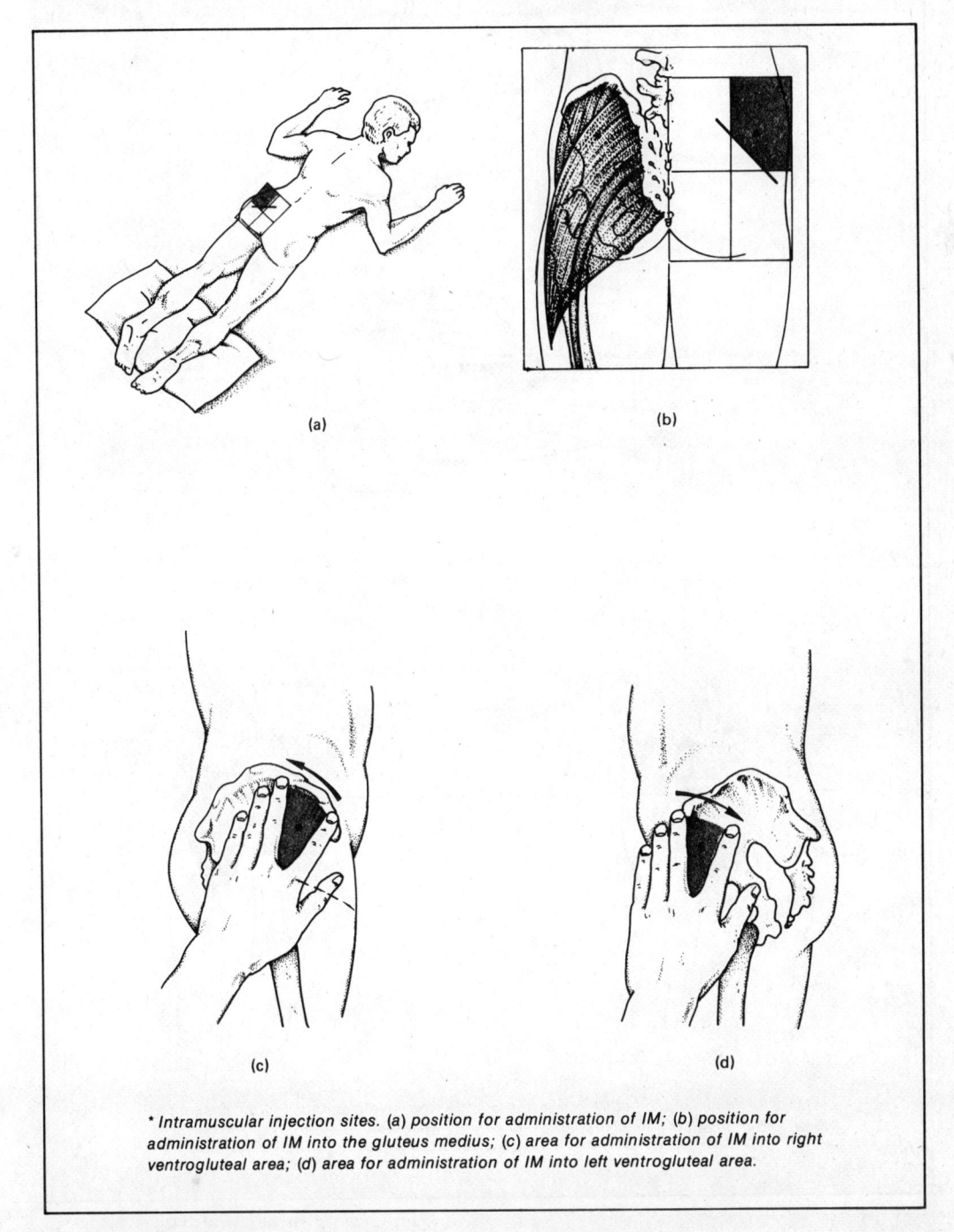

Intramuscular Injection Sites

(a)

(b)

(c)

(d)

* Intramuscular injection sites. (a) position for administration of IM; (b) position for administration of IM into the gluteus medius; (c) area for administration of IM into right ventrogluteal area; (d) area for administration of IM into left ventrogluteal area.

Continued on next page

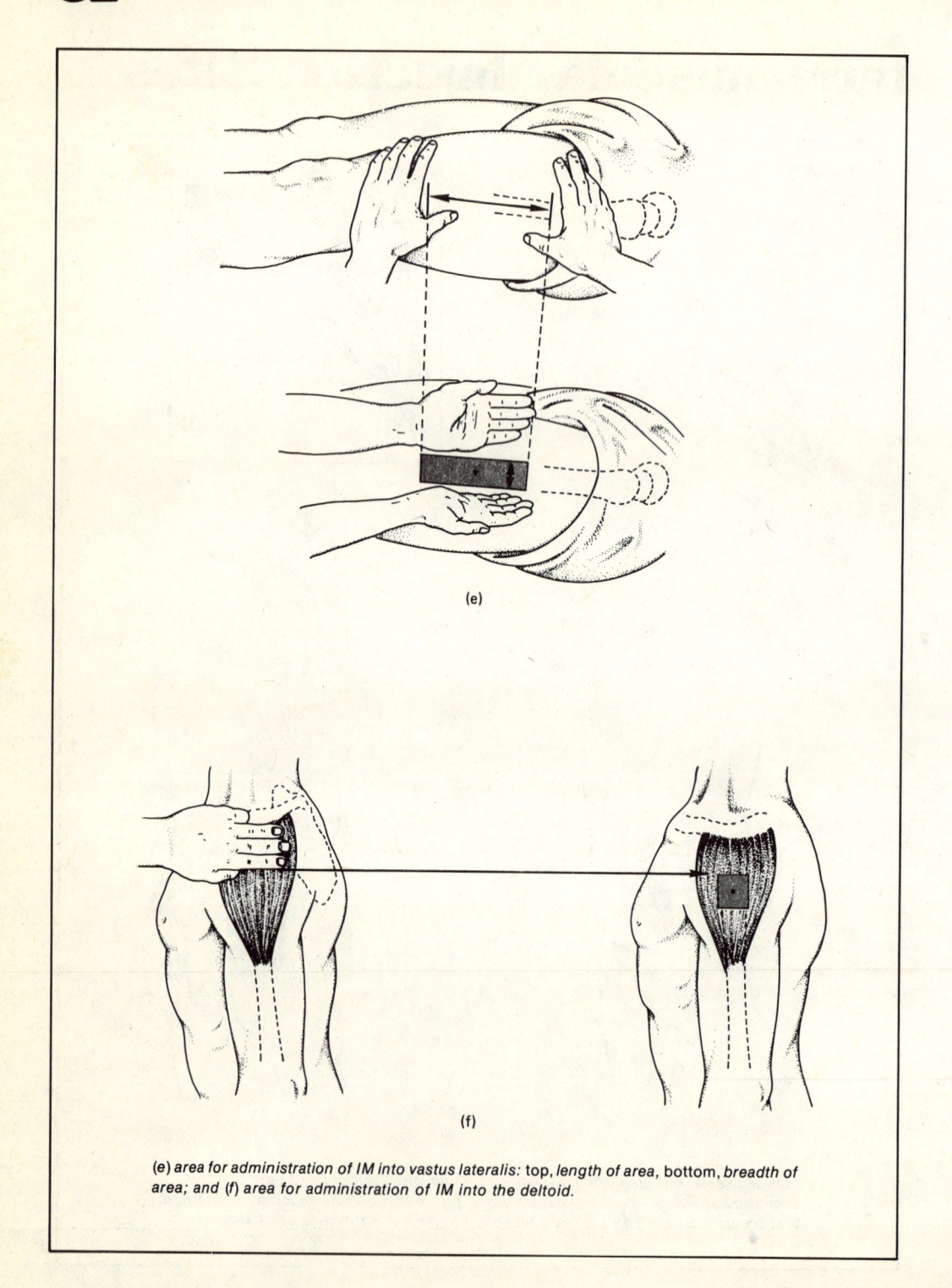

(e) area for administration of IM into vastus lateralis: top, length of area, bottom, breadth of area; and (f) area for administration of IM into the deltoid.

Continued on next page

Pediatric intramuscular injection sites. (a) *deltoid;* (b) *anterior surface of midlateral thigh;* and (c) *anterolateral surface of upper thigh.*

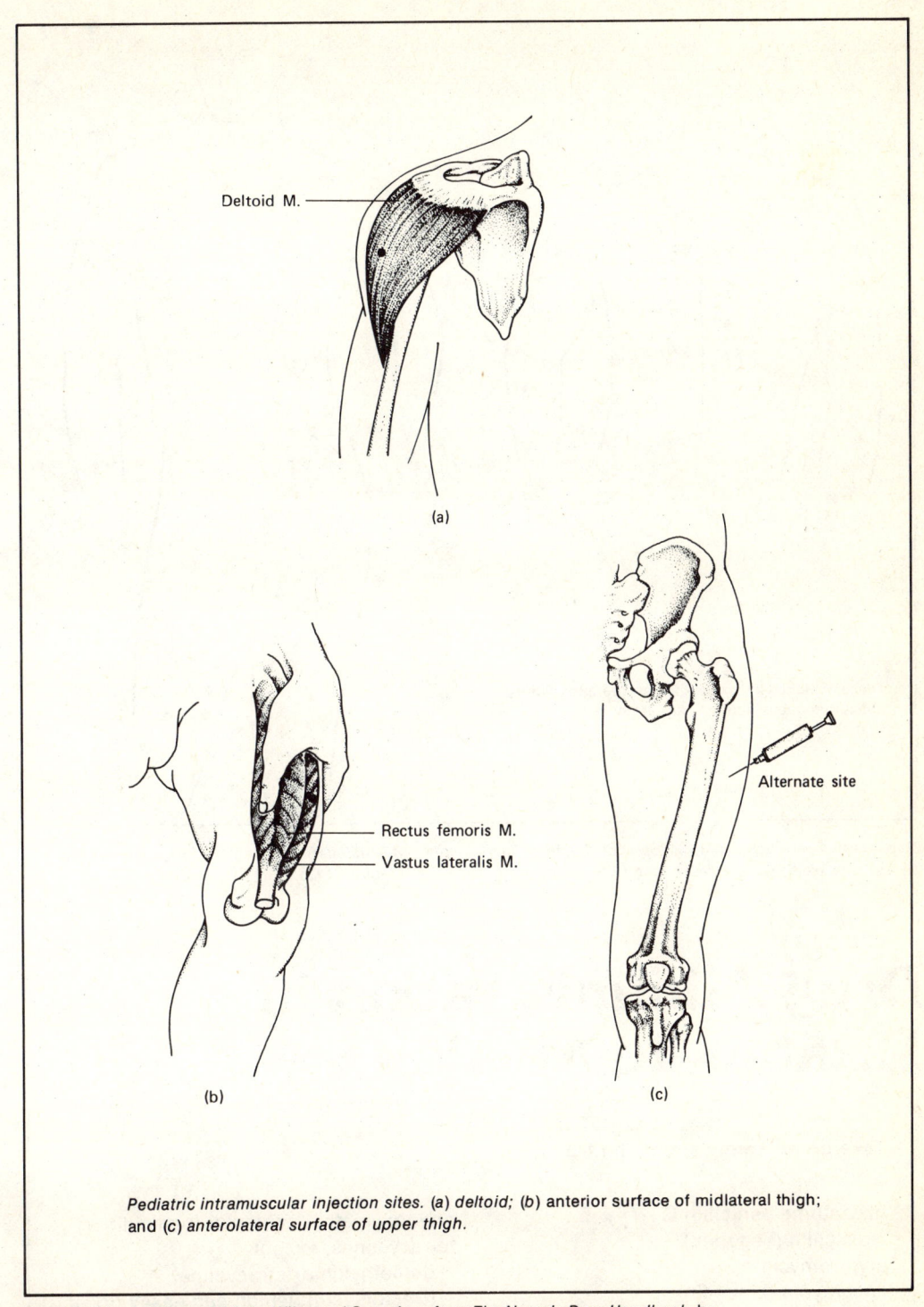

Reprinted by permission of John Wiley and Sons, Inc., from *The Nurse's Drug Handbook*, by Suzanne Loebl, George Spratto, Andrew Wit, and Estelle Heckheimer, Copyright © 1977, John Wiley and Sons.

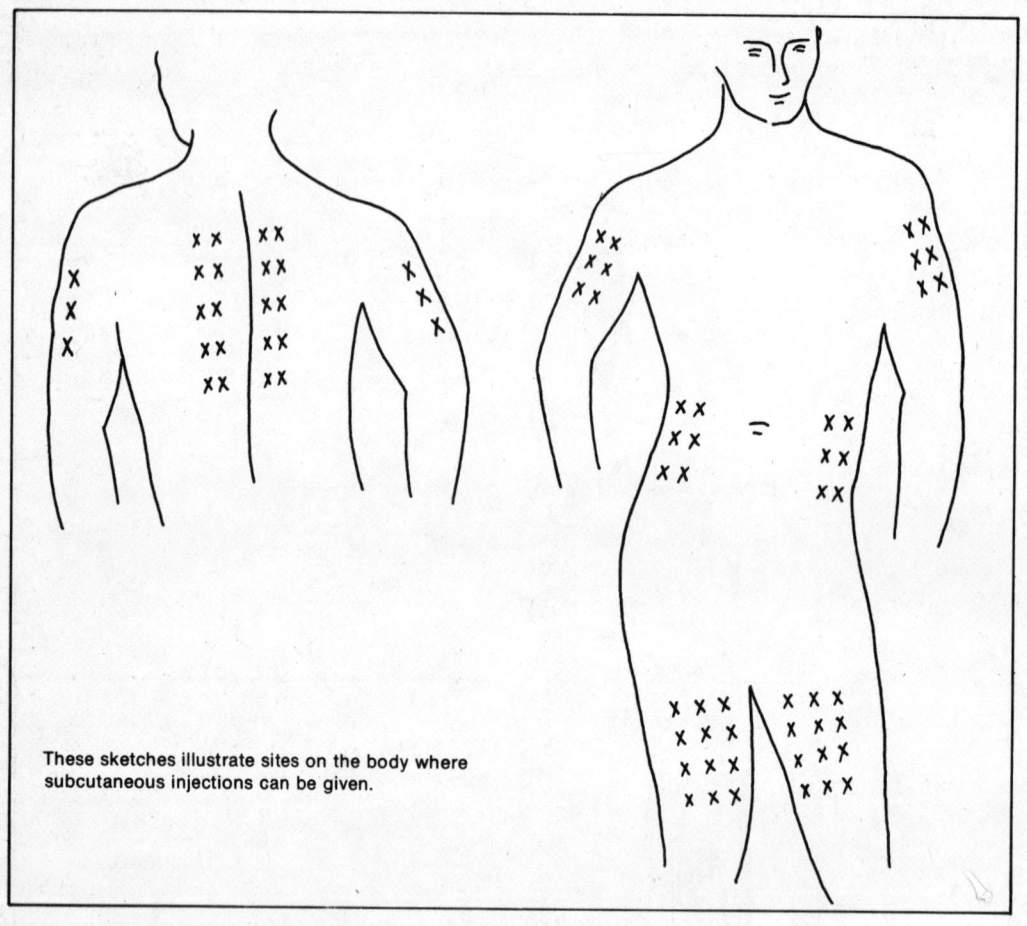

These sketches illustrate sites on the body where subcutaneous injections can be given.

Reprinted by permission of J.B. Lippincott Co. from *Fundamentals of Nursing*, 6th edition, by LuVerne Wolff, Marlele Weitzel, and Elinor Fuerst, © 1979, J.B. Lippincott Co.

Drug Administration in Relation to Meals

Take on an empty stomach (2–3 hours a.c.):

benzathine penicillin G
cloxacillin (Tegopen)
erythromycin
lincomycin (Lincocin)
methacycline (Rondomycin)
phenoxymethyl penicillin (penicillin V)
tetracyclines, except demethylchlortetracycline (Declomycin), which can easily upset the stomach

Continued on next page

Take ½ hour before meals:
belladonna and its alkaloids
chlordiazepoxide hydrochloride
 (Librax)
hyoscyamine sulfate (Donnatal)
methylphenidate (Ritalin)
phenmetrazine hydrochloride
 (Preludin)
phenazopyridine (Pyridium)
propantheline bromide (Pro-banthine)

Take with meals or food:
aminophylline
antidiabetics
APC (acetylsalicylic acid, phenacetin,
 caffeine)
chlorothiazide, (Diuril) (Hydrodiuril)
diphenylhydantoin (Dilantin)
mefenamic acid (Ponstel)
metronidazole (Flagyl)
nitrofurantoin (Furadantin)
 (Macrodantin)
prednisolone
prednisone
rauwolfia and its alkaloids
reserpine (Serpasil)
triamterene (Dyrenium)
trihexyphenidyl hydrochloride (Artane)
trimeprazine tartrate (Temaril)

Do not take with milk:
bisacodyl (Dulcolax)
potassium chloride
potassium iodide
tetracyclines except doxycycline
 (Vibramycin)

Do not take with fruit juices:
ampicillin
benzathine penicillin G
cloxacillin (Tegopen)
erythromycin

Do not drink alcohol while taking:
acetohexamide (Dymelor)
antihistamines
chlorpropamide (Diabinese)
chlordiazepoxide (Librium)
chloral hydrate
diphenoxylate hydrochloride (Lomotil)
MAO inhibitors
meclizine hydrochloride (Antivert)
methaqualone (Quaalude)
metronidazole (Flagyl)
narcotics
phenformin hydrochloride (DBI)
tolbutamide (Orinase)

Lambert, Martin L., Jr. Copyright 1975, American Journal of Nursing Company. Reproduced with permission from the *American Journal of Nursing*, March, Vol. 75, No. 3.

Specific Antidotes for Toxic Agents

TABLE 12–1 SPECIFIC ANTIDOTES FOR TOXIC AGENTS

Toxic agent	Antidote
(1) Opiates	Naloxone hydrochloride (Narcan)
(2) (Insulin)	(Glucose)
(3) Cholinesterase inhibitors	Atropine and pralidoxime chloride
(4) Methanol	Ethanol
(5) Iron	Sodium ferrocyanide and deferoxamine mesylate

Continued on next page

(6) Atropine or scopolamine	Cholinesterase inhibitors (physostigmine)
(7) Warfarin	Vitamin K
(8) Arsenic or mercury	Dimercaprol (BAL)
(9) Lead	Ethylenediaminetetraacetic acid (EDTA)
(10) Cyanide	Nitrites and sodium thiosulfate
(11) Carbon monoxide	Oxygen or hyperbaric oxygen

Reprinted by permission of J. B. Lippincott Co. from *The Practice of Emergency Nursing* by James Cosgriff and Diann Anderson, Copyright © 1975, J. B. Lippincott Co.

Selected Drug Incompatibilities with Intravenous 5 Per Cent Glucose

When using 5 per cent glucose intravenous solution:

When this drug is added:	**Do not mix with these drugs:**
Aminophylline	Vitamin B complex with vitamin C
	Tetracycline HCl
	Methicillin
	Chloramphenicol
Ampicillin	Vitamin B complex with vitamin C
	Tetracycline HCl
	Sodium phenobarbital
	Epinephrine chloride
	Chloramphenicol
	Atropine
Chloramphenicol or sodium succinate	Vitamin B complex with vitamin C
	Tetracycline
	Hydrocortisone phosphate
	Erythromycin
	Epinephrine

Continued on next page

	Digitoxin
	Ampicillin
	Aminophylline
Kanamycin	Sodium bicarbonate
	Phenobarbital
	Methicillin
	Hydrocortisone
	Heparin
	Calcium gluconate
Methicillin	Vitamin B complex with vitamin C
	Tetracycline
	Sodium bicarbonate
	Potassium chloride
	Kanamycin
	Hydrocortisone
	Epinephrine
	Calcium chloride
	Atropine
	Aminophylline
Penicillin G potassium	Vitamin B complex with vitamin C
	Tetracycline
	Heparin
	Epinephrine
	Dilantin
Potassium chloride	Novobiocin
	Methicillin
Sodium bicarbonate	Vitamin B complex with vitamin C
	Tetracycline
	Phenobarbital
	Methicillin
	Kanamycin
	Hydrocortisone
	Calcium gluconate
	Calcium chloride
	Atropine

Reprinted by permission of W. B. Saunders Co. from *Principles and Techniques in Pediatric Nursing*, by Gloria Leifer, 3rd edition, Copyright © 1977, W. B. Saunders Company.

Summary of Drug Interactions

	Drugs	Effects of Combination
Alcohol Antidiabetic drugs	C.N.S. depressants	The effects of central depressant drugs, are increased by alcohol, and may cause respiratory depression. Antidiabetic drugs may cause hypoglycaemia
Anticoagulants (excluding heparin)	Chloral, Gluthethimide Griseofulvin Phenobarbitone	Phenobarbitone and some other drugs, increases the production of drug-metabolising enzymes by the liver, and this activity may require the administration of larger doses of anticoagulants. Withdrawal of the sedative may result in a rise in the anticoagulant response, with possible haemorrhage.
	Clofibrate, phenylbutazone, phenytoin, salicylates	These drugs increase the effects of anticoagulants on the clotting time of the blood by the displacement of the anticoagulant that is bound to the plasma protein.
	Rifampicin	Rifamycin decreases the activity of oral anticoagulants, and combined therapy requires adjustment of dose.
Barbiturates	Alcohol and other C.N.S. depressants (q.v.) Anticoagulants (q.v.) Griseofulvin Phenytoin	Phenytoin is given with phenobarbitone in the treatment of epilepsy, but the increased production of drug-metabolising enzymes induced by phenobarbitone may reduce the duration of action of the phenytoin. Phenobarbitone can also reduce the blood level of griseofulvin.
Chloral	Anticoagulants (q.v.)	
Chlorpromazine and related drugs	Alcohol and other C.N.S. depressants (q.v.) Hypotensive agents (q.v.)	
Clofibrate	Anticoagulants (q.v.) Oral antidiabetic agents (q.v.)	
Digitalis	Thiazide diuretics (q.v.)	
Griseofulvin	Anticoagulants (q.v.)	
Hypotensive agents	Monoamine Oxidase inhibitors (q.v.) Thiazide diuretics (q.v.) Antidepressants Pressor drugs	Tricyclic antidepressants may antagonise the action of guanethidine and other antihypertensive drugs. Sympathomimetic drugs, by their pressor action, have a similar effect.
Monoamine oxidase inhibitors	Alcohol Antihistamines Amphetamines and other pressor drugs Benzhexol and other drugs used in parkinsonism	The monoamine oxidase inhibitors may increase or modify the action of a wide range of unrelated substances. The action of any C.N.S. stimulant will be increased, and the effects of narcotic analgesics, tricyclic antidepressants, hypotensive drugs and thiazide diu-

Continued on next page

Drugs		Effects of Combination
	Hypotensive drugs (q.v.) Insulin Levodopa Narcotic analgesics Oral antidiabetic drugs Thiazide diuretics (q.v.) Tricyclic antidepressants	retics may also be potentiated. Monoamine oxidase inhibitors increase hepatic glycolysis and potentiate the action of oral antidiabetic drugs. The pressor effects of tyramine, present in foods such as cheese, broad beans, yeast extracts and chianti will also be increased by the monoamine oxidase inhibitors.
Morphine pethidine and similar narcotics	Monoamine oxidase inhibitors (q.v.)	
Oral antidiabetic drugs	Barbiturates (q.v.) Beta blocking Clofibrate (q.v.) Phenylbutazone Salicylates Sulphonamides Monoamine oxidase inhibitors (q.v.)	The action of oral antidiabetic drugs may be increased by displacement from plasma binding, or by increasing the activity of liver enzymes.
Penicillin	Chloramphenicol and tetracyclines	Chloramphenicol and the tetracyclines are bacteriostatic in action, whereas penicillin is bactericidal. Mixtures of bacteriostatic and bactericidal antibiotics may have an antagonistic action.
Phenylbutazone and related compounds	Anticoagulants (q.v.) Long acting sulphonamides	These sulphonamides can be displaced from plasma bindings by other drugs, such as phenylbutazone. Such displacement modifies both duration of action and tissue concentration of the sulphonamide.
Phenytoin	Anticoagulants (q.v.)	
Propranolol and related beta-blocking agents	Anaesthetics Antidiabetic agents	Hypotensive effects potentiated. Loss of reflex tachycardia. May be unwise to use propranolol in diabetics with hypertension.
Salicylates	Anticoagulants (q.v.) Oral antidiabetic drugs (q.v.) Insulin Methotrexate	Salicylates increase the uptake and use of glucose by the tissues, and increase the effects of antidiabetic agents. Salicylates displace methotrexate from binding sites.
Thiazide diuretics	Digitalis Hypotensive drugs (q.v.) Monoamine oxidase inhibitors (q.v.)	The loss of potassium caused by the thiazide diuretics may increase the sensitivity of the heart to digitalis.
Tubocurarine and other muscle relaxants	Neomycin and related antibiotics Neostigmine and similar anticholinesterase	These antibiotics also have some curare-like properties, and may extend the relaxant action of tubocurarine. Neostigmine inhibits the breakdown of acetylcholine at nerve endings and reverses the action of curareform muscle relaxants. This effect is used to promote prompt return of muscle function after operation. (Suxamethonium is not reversible by neostigmine.)

Reprinted by permission of Churchill Livingstone Publishers from *Drugs and Pharmacology For Nurses*, 7th edition, S. J. Hopkins, Copyright 1979, Churchill Livingstone, Edinburgh, London and New York.

Analgesics

Generic Name	Trade Name	How Supplied	Routes	Usual Dose	Comments
Morphine sulfate		Tablets 8 mg., 10 mg., 15 mg., 30 mg., 60 mg. Various strengths for parenteral use.	P.O. I.M. I.V. Sc.	8–15 mg. q. 3h. p.r.n.	Included within the jurisdiction of Control Substances Act (CSA)
Codeine sulfate		Tablets 15, 30, 60 mg. Various strengths for parenteral use.	P.O. I.M. Sc.	15–60 mg. q. 3h. p.r.n.	Included within the jurisdiction of CSA.
Meperidine hydrochloride	Demerol	Tablets 50 mg., 100 mg. Elixir 50 mg./tsp. Vials 30 cc., 50 mg./cc., 20 cc., 100 mg./cc. Ampuls 0.5 cc., 1 cc., 1.5 cc., 2 cc., 50 mg./cc., 1 cc., 100 mg./cc. Disposable syringe 50 mg./cc., 75 mg./cc., 100 mg./cc.	P.O. I.M. I.V. Sc.	25–100 mg. q. 3h. p.r.n.	Included within the jurisdication of the CSA. Disposable syringes may contain an additional cc. volume to enable mixing with other drugs.
Pentazocine	Talwin	Tablets 50 mg. Multiple dose vials 10 cc., 30 mg./cc.	P.O. Sc. I.M.	1–2 tablets q. 3–4h. p.r.n. 30 mg. I.V., I.M. and S.C.	Total daily dosage not to exceed 600 mg. orally, 360 mg. parenterally. Aspirin

90

		Ampuls 1 cc., 30 mg./cc. I.V. 2 cc., 30 mg./cc.	q. 3–4h. p.r.n.	may be administered concomitantly. Not recommended for children under twelve. Doses over 30 mg. I.V. or 60 mg. I.M. or S.C. not recommended.
Methotrimeprazine	Levoprome	Ampuls 1 cc., 20 mg./cc. Vials 10 cc., 20 mg./cc.	I.M.	10–20 mg. I.M. q. 4–6h.	May be mixed in a syringe with atropine sulfate or scopolamine hydrobromide only. When multiple injections are used, rotation of the injection site is advisable. Not to be confused with Levophed or levodopa.
Acetylsalicylic acid	A.S.A.	Capsules, tablets, suppositories (commonly 5 gr. tablets)	P.O. rectal	0.3–0.6 gm. q. 3–4h. p.r.n.	Not to exceed 3 gm. in 24 hours.
Acetaminophen	Tylenol	Tablets 325 mg. Chewable tablets 120 mg.	P.O.	1–2 tablets t.i.d. or q.i.d. p.r.n. children's dosage ad-	Not to be confused with Talwin. The elixir must not be

Continued on next page

Generic Name	Trade Name	How Supplied	Route	Usual Dose	Comments
		Elixir 120 mg./5 cc. Drops 60 mg./0.6 cc.		justed according to age.	confused with the drops, which are much more concentrated.
Opium camphorated tincture	Paregoric	Bottles of various sizes.	P.O.	2–10 cc. p.r.n.	Included within the jurisdiction of C.S.A.
Diphenoxylate hydrochloride with atropine sulfate	Lomotil	Tablets 2.5 mg. diphenoxylate and 0.025 mg. atropine sulfate Liquid 2.5 mg. diphenoxylate and 0.025 mg. atropine sulfate/teaspoon	P.O.	2 tablets q.i.d. 2 teaspoons q.i.d.	Dosage may be decreased as desired response is reached. Used with caution in children. Do not use tablets for children under twelve. Contraindicated for children under two.
Methysergide maleate	Sansert	Tablets 2 mg.	P.O.	4–8 mg. q.d. with meals.	There must be a three-to-four week interval free of medication after each six-month course of treatment.

Reprinted by permission of J. B. Lippincott from *Review and Application of Clinical Pharmacology* by Susan E. Ralston and Marion F. Hale, Copyright 1977, J. B. Lippincott.

Agents Used in Anesthesia Administration

Agent	Administration	Induction	Advantages	Disadvantages	Nursing precautions
Halothane (Fluothane)	Inhalation	Rapid and smooth	Nonflammable Pleasant odor Nonirritating Little excitement Rapid emergence Seldom causes nausea or vomiting	Requires special vaporizer Narrow margin of safety May depress cardiovascular system Limited relaxation Expensive May cause liver damage	Watch for bradycardia and hypotension Use of epinephrine, with this agent, may cause cardiac arrhythmias, including ventricular fibrillation
Nitrous oxide	Inhalation	Rapid	Rapid induction and recovery Nonflammable Few aftereffects	Poor relaxation May produce hypoxia Except for short procedures, must be used with other agents	When used with other agents, follow those precautions
Vinyl ether (Vinethene)	Open drop Inhalation	Rapid	Good for short procedures Good relaxation Small incidence of excitement	May cause kidney and liver damage Great danger of overdose Irritating Flammable and explosive Irritating to skin	Protect skin and eyes Practice explosion safeguards
Penthrane	Inhalation	Slow	Nonflammable and nonexplosive Excellent muscle relaxation Seldom causes nausea or vomiting	Requires special vaporizer and skillful administration May cause kidney or liver damage	Long postoperative depressant action Patient requires close observation
Enflurane (Ethrane)	Inhalation	Rapid and smooth	Nonflammable Nonirritating to respiratory tract Good muscle relaxant Eliminated rapidly	Not compatible with epinephrine Requires special vaporizer	Administration with epinephrine may cause ventricular fibrillation Body temperature may fall and patient may shiver following prolonged use Watch for hypotension, respiratory depression, arrhythmias, nausea, and vomiting

Continued on next page

Agent	Administration	Induction	Advantages	Disadvantages	Nursing precautions
Isoflurane (Forane)	Inhalation	Rapid	Nonflammable Rapid recovery Cardiac output remains stable Good muscle relaxant No evidence of renal or hepatic damage	Requires special vaporizer May be irritating to respiratory tract during induction	Watch for nausea, vomiting, excitement, and shivering
Ether	Open drop Inhalation	Slow	Good relaxation and wide margin of safety Inexpensive Nontoxic	Long recovery (elimination may take 8 hours) Unpleasant odor Irritating to skin, mucous membranes, lungs, and kidneys Causes nausea and vomiting, urinary retention, and acidosis Explosive and flammable	Protect skin and eyes Expect nausea and vomiting Prevent aspiration Practice explosion safeguards
Cyclopropane	Inhalation	Rapid and pleasant	Rapid induction and emergence Wide margin of safety Good relaxation Well tolerated	Explosive May cause cardiac arrhythmias, shock, bronchospasm, and acidosis	Use explosion safeguards Observe blood pressure
Ketamine (Ketalar)	Intravenous Intramuscular	Rapid	Short action Excellent for diagnostic and short, topical surgical procedures May be used to supplement weaker agents such as nitrous oxide	Too rapid administration causes respiratory depression Induces blood pressure rise May produce dreams or hallucinations Patients may act irrationally when emerging from anesthesia	Avoid stimulation of patient by touching or talking Resuscitative equipment must be available
Thiopental sodium (Pentothal Sodium)	Intravenous Rectal	Rapid and pleasant	Rapid, pleasant induction and recovery (patient has no recollection of mask) Nonirritating; nonflammable Easy administration Good for short procedures and hypnosis during regional anesthesia	Large doses cause respiratory-circulatory depression Wide variation in tolerance Poor relaxation	Watch for respiratory and circulatory depression Be prepared for possible laryngospasm

Agent	Administration	Induction	Advantages	Disadvantages	Nursing precautions
Innovar (combination of inapsine and sublimaze)	Intramuscular Intravenous	Rapid	Produces a state of quiescence with decreased motor activity and decreased responsiveness to painful stimuli Patient is unresponsive to auditory stimuli but does not lose consciousness Good premedication for anesthesia	Should not be given in combination with hypnotics or strong analgesics May cause respiratory depression, apnea, laryngospasm, bronchospasm, and hallucinations	Observe for respiratory depression, cardiac arrhythmias
Fentanyl (Sublimaze)	Intramuscular Intravenous	Rapid	Rapid induction 80 to 100 times more potent than morphine Duration of action shorter than morphine or meperidine	Degree of respiratory depression may be greater than morphine May cause respiratory depression, nausea, vomiting, bradycardia, muscular rigidity	Observe for muscular rigidity and respiratory depression Doses of narcotics should be reduced by ¼ to ⅓ of usual dose
Lidocaine hydrochloride (Xylocaine)	Infiltration Topical Block or spinal	Rapid	Action is more rapid, more intense, and longer acting than procaine Is a local vasodilator Used to treat arrhythmias during heart surgery or general anesthesia; suppresses laryngeal or pharyngeal reflexes	Few; well tolerated Untoward effects may occur from allergy, overdose, or faulty injection	Initial effect of overdose is depression rather than excitement Watch for drowsiness, respiratory arrest, cardiovascular collapse, and cardiac arrest
Procaine hydrochloride (Novocaine; Ethocaine)	Subcutaneous Intramuscular Intravenous Spinal	Rapid	Low toxicity Good duration of action Inexpensive	Possible idiosyncrasy Slow action	May involve central nervous and cardiovascular systems; watch for reaction; hypotension, bradycardia, thready pulse, shock
Cocaine	Topical	Rapid	Rapid action Patient is conscious	Abolishes throat reflexes when applied in this area High toxicity May be fatal if injected	Watch for cocaine reaction: excitement, restlessness, confusion, hypertension, tachycardia, rapid shallow respirations

Reprinted by permission of The C. V. Mosby Co. from *The Surgical Patient*, 2nd edition, by Barbara J. Gruendemann, Shirley B. Casterton, Sandra C. Hesterly, Barbara B. Minckley, and Mary G. Shetler, Copyright © 1979, The C. V. Mosby Co., St. Louis.

Antianemics

DRUG	MAIN USE	DOSAGE	REMARKS
Ferrocholinate (Chel-iron, Ferrolip, Kelex)	Microcytic, hypochromic anemias due to iron deficiency	Liquid, syrup and tablets: **PO**: 330 mg (equivalent to 40 mg elemental iron) t.i.d. **Infants and children less than 6 yr:** 104 mg daily	Better tolerated than ferrous gluconate or ferrous sulfate
Ferrous fumarate (Eldofe, Feostat, Fumasorb, Fumerin, Ircon, Laud-Iron, Palmiron, Span-FF, Toleron)	Microcytic, hypochromic anemias due to iron deficiency	Tablets, chewable tablets, extended release: **PO, adults:** 600–800 mg (equivalent to daily 200–260 mg elemental iron) daily in 3 to 4 divided doses. **Children under 5 yr and infants:** 100–300 mg (equivalent to 33–99 mg elemental iron) daily in 3 to 4 divided doses	Better tolerated than ferrous gluconate or sulfate
Ferrous gluconate (Fergon, Ferralet)	Microcytic, hypochromic anemias due to iron deficiency	Capsules, Elixir, Tablets: **PO:** 320–640 mg (equivalent to 40–80 mg elemental iron) t.i.d. **Infants and children less than 6 yr:** 120–300 mg daily. **Children 6–12 yr:** 100–300 mg t.i.d.	Particularly indicated for patients who cannot tolerate ferrous sulfate because of gastric irritation
Ferrous sulfate (Fero-Gradumet, Mol-Iron) Dried ferrous sulfate (Feosol, Fer-In-Sol)	Microcytic, hypochromic anemia due to iron deficiency (drug of choice)	**PO:** 300–1200 mg (equivalent to 60–240 mg elemental iron) daily in divided doses. **Children less than 6 yr:** 1–3 ml (equivalent to 25–75 mg elemental iron) of the pediatric preparation. **Children 6–12 yr:** 120–600 mg (equivalent to 24–120 mg elemental	Least expensive, most effective iron salt for oral therapy

		iron) daily in divided doses. Prophylaxis for premature or poorly developed infants: 3–6 mg/kg daily. **Pregnancy:** 300–600 mg daily (equivalent to 60–120 mg elemental iron)	
Iron dextran injection (Imferon) (See also special drug entry in text, p. 195)	Microcytic, hypochromic anemias due to iron deficiency	Dosage formula: **IM, adults** (over 50 kg), 50 mg first day and up to 250 mg every other day or twice weekly until the total calculated dose is given. **Adults and children** (9–50 kg), no more than 100 mg daily. **Infants** (3.5–9 kg), no more than 50 mg daily. **Infants** (under 3.5 kg), no more than 25 mg daily. **IV, adults,** 15–30 mg to start, increase by 10 mg daily until hemoglobin levels return to normal (maximal daily dose, 50–65 mg).	Used mainly for patients intolerant to oral iron. See drug entry
Iron sorbitex (Jectofer) (See also special drug entry in text, p. 196)	Microcytic, hypochromic anemias due to iron deficiency	**IM:** 1.5 mg/kg body weight, or 100 mg for patient weighing 60 kg or more, daily. Higher doses, 200 mg daily are used occasionally	Used mainly for patients intolerant to oral iron

Reprinted by permission of John Wiley and Sons, Inc., from *The Nurse's Drug Handbook* by Loebl, Spratto, Wit and Heckheimer, Copyright © 1977, John Wiley and Sons, Inc.

Antihypertensive Agents

Generic Name	Trade Name	How Supplied	Routes	Usual Dose	Comments
Methyldopa Methyldopate hydrochloride	Aldomet	Tablets 125 mg., 250 mg., 500 mg. Ampuls 5 cc. 250 mg./5 cc.	P.O. I.V.	500 mg.–2.0 gm. 250–500 mg. q. 6 hr.	Not recommended for use in pregnant patients. Parenteral form is used to control acute hypertensive crisis.
Hydralazine hydrochloride	Apresoline	Tablets 10 mg., 25 mg., 50 mg., 100 mg. Ampuls 1 cc. 20 mg./cc.	P.O. I.V. I.M.	50 mg. P.O. q.i.d. 20–40 mg. repeat p.r.n.	Initial doses are small, then dosage is increased until desired effect is reached.
Reserpine	Serpasil	Tablets 1 mg., 0.25 mg., 0.1 mg. Elixir 0.2 mg./tsp. (4 cc.) Multiple dose vials 10 cc., 2.5 mg./cc. Ampuls 2 cc. 2.5 mg./cc.	P.O. I.M.	Maintenance dose 0.1 mg.–0.25 mg. q.d. Initial dose 0.5 mg. to 1 mg. I.M., followed by 2–4 mg. at three hour intervals until blood pressure reaches the desired levels.	Should be given after meals to lessen gastrointestinal discomfort.
Phentolamine	Regitine	Tablets 50 mg. Ampuls I cc., 5 mg./cc.	P.O. I.V. I.M.	50 mg. P.O. q.i.d. 5 mg. I.V.	Regitine blocking test may be used for diagnosis of pheochromocytoma. Also used to prevent dermal necrosis following I.V. administration or extravasation of norepinephrine.

Reprinted by permission of J. B. Lippincott Co. from *Review and Application of Clinical Pharmacology* by Susan E. Ralston and Marion F. Hale, Copyright 1977, J. B. Lippincott Co.

Commonly Used Antipsychotic Agents

	Usual Oral Dosages (3-4 Times Daily)	Comment
Phenothiazines		
Chlorpromazine (Thorazine®)	25-50 mg	The standard drug of its class. In hospitalized psychotics, total daily dose may exceed 800 mg/day. Available for 25-100 mg I.M. or I.V. injection.
Thioridazine (Mellaril®)	10-25 mg	Increased incidence of pigmentary retinopathy.
Promazine (Sparine®)	50-200 mg	Higher incidence of agranulocytosis and hypotension.
Trifluoperazine* (Stelazine®)	1-5 mg	Larger doses (up to 40 mg/day) may be considered in some cases. Extrapyramidal effects frequent.
Perphenazine* (Trilafon®)	2-8 mg	Larger doses (up to 40 mg/day) may be considered in some cases. Extrapyramidal effects frequent.
Fluphenazine* (Permitil®, Prolixin®)	1-2.5 mg	Prolixin Enanthate®, 25 mg subcut. or I.M. every 2 weeks, for uncooperative patients.
Prochlorperazine (Compazine®)	5-30 mg	
Mesoridazine (Serentil®)	10-100 mg	
Nonphenothiazines		
Chlorprothixene (Taractan®)	25-100 mg	Hypotension common. Fewer extrapyramidal reactions. Anti-emetic action.
Thiothixene* (Navane®)	2-10 mg	Extrapyramidal effects frequent.
Haloperidol* (Haldol®)	0.5-2 mg	Extrapyramidal effects frequent.
Hydroxyzine (Atarax®, Vistaril®)	25-100 mg	Also has an antihistaminic effect.

*"Stimulant tranquilizers" causing less somnolence but more extrapyramidal effects.

Reprinted by permission of Jones Medical Publications from *Handbook of Medical Treatment*, 15th edition, by Milton J. Chatton, M. D., Copyright © 1977, Jones Medical Publications.

Barbiturates

DRUG	USE	DOSAGE	REMARKS
Amobarbital (Amytal) Amobarbital sodium (Amytal sodium)	Sedation, hypnotic, acute convulsive disorders	Amobarbital is given **PO** only. Sedation: 30–50 mg 2–3 times daily. Hypnotic: 100–200 mg. Amobarbital sodium: **PO, IM** and **rectally**: dose highly individualized, essentially the same regardless of route of administration	Intermediate acting. *Administration:* When dissolving dry-packed ampules with accompanying sterile water for parenteral use, rotate ampule for mixing. Solutions that are not clear after 5 min should be discarded. Not more than 30 min should elapse between opening of ampule and usage. IM: Inject deeply in large muscle, no more than 5 ml at one site. IV: Inject slowly at rates not exceeding 1 ml/min. Patients requiring IV administration should be closely monitored
Aprobarbital (Alurate)	Daytime sedation, hypnotic	**PO** Sedation: 40 mg t.i.d. Hypnotic: 80–160 mg. The preparation is supplied as red or green elixir. One teaspoon (5 ml) contains 40 mg	Intermediate-acting barbiturate
Barbital Barbital sodium	Mild, prolonged sedation	**PO** Sedation: 65–130 mg 2–3 times daily. Hypnotic: 300–600 mg 1 to 2 hr before sleep desired. Preparation available as capsules or tablets	Long-acting barbiturate. Not metabolized by liver.
Butabarbital sodium (BBS, Butacaps, Butisol Sodium)	Hypnotic, mild sedation for anxiety	**PO** or **IM** Sedation: 15–30 mg 3–4 times daily. Hypnotic: 50–100 mg. **Pediatric:** Sedation: 8–30 mg in divided doses daily. Available as tablets, capsules, elixir, and release tablets.	Intermediate-acting barbiturate. Used more as a sedative than as a hypnotic
Hexobarbital (Sombulex)	Hypnotic, preanesthetic, preoperative or postoperative sedation	Hypnotic: 250–500 mg. Pediatric dosage has not been established	Short-acting barbiturate

DRUG	USE	DOSAGE	REMARKS
Mephobarbital (Mebaral, Menta-Bal)	Sedation and as anticonvulsant as required in epilepsy (grand mal and focal seizures, not for petit mal or psychomotor), tension, anxiety, neurasthenia, hysteria, mild psychosis, alcoholism, delirium tremens, and restlessness. As adjunct in cardiovascular disease and allergies	Sedation: 32–100 mg 3–4 times daily. *Delirium tremens*: 200 mg 3 times daily. *Epilepsy*: 400–600 mg daily. **Pediatric:** Up to age 5: 16–32 mg 3–4 times daily; over age 5: 32–64 mg 3–4 times daily. Administer at bedtime if seizures are likely to occur at night. Increase dosage gradually until optimum is reached	Long-acting barbiturate with anticonvulsant activity. The hypnotic effects are mild and compound causes little drowsiness or lassitude. For epilepsy, mephobarbital is often administered concurrently with diphenylhydantoin. Drug has specific antiepileptic action because it is broken down in body to phenobarbital
Metharbital (Gemonil)	Anticonvulsant, suitable for treatment of petit mal, grand mal, myoclonic epilepsy and mixed types of seizures (not agent of first choice, however)	Individualized. Usual **adult:** 100 mg 1–3 times daily, to be increased gradually until control is established. **Pediatric:** 5–15 mg/kg daily	Long-acting barbiturate, anticonvulsant with specific antiepileptic action
Methohexital sodium (Brevital sodium)	General anesthetic for brief procedures (oral surgery, gynecologic, and genitourinary examinations, reduction of fractures, prior to electroshock therapy)	**Induction:** 50–120 mg. **Maintenance:** Administer 20–40 mg as required usually q 4–7 min (as a 1% solution) or by continuous drip (0.2% solution—1 drop/min)	Ultrashort acting; duration of anesthesia 5–8 min
Pentobarbital sodium (Nebralin, Nembutal Sodium)	Sedative, hypnotic, adjunct in diagnostic procedures, emergency use in convulsive states	Drug can be given **PO, IM, rectally,** and even by cautious **IV** administration. Dosage is essentially the same regardless of route. Sedation: 20–40 mg 3–4 times daily up to maximum of 120 mg daily. Hypnotic: 100 mg. **Pediatric** (Hypnotic): Children under 6 yr:	Short-acting barbiturate. *Administration:* Since pentobarbital is a potent CNS depressant that may cause adverse respiratory and circulatory response, the IV dose is given in fractions. Adults receive 100 mg initially; children and debilitated persons 50 mg. Subsequent fractions are administered after 1-min observation periods

Continued on next page

DRUG	USE	DOSAGE	REMARKS
		30–60 mg; older children: 60–120 mg. **IV** (*control of acute convulsions*): 200–500 mg depending on response of patient (see Remarks)	Overdosage or too rapid administration may cause spasms of larynx or pharynx, or both. Pentobarbital solutions are highly alkaline. *Administration:* (1) Administer no more than 5 ml at one site IM because of possible tissue irritation (pain, necrosis, gangrene). (2) Observe for pain, delayed onset of hypnosis, pallor, cyanosis, and patchy discoloration of skin, signs of intraarterial injection. (3) Stop IV injection if there is any pain in limb
Phenobarbital (Eskabarb, Hypnette, Luminal, Pheno-Squar, Solfoton) Phenobarbital sodium (Luminal sodium)	Sedative, anticonvulsant, antiepileptic (grand mal and focal cortical epilepsy only, can exacerbate psychomotor and petit mal)	Phenobarbital is given **PO**. Phenobarbital sodium is given **PO, IM, IV, SC and rectally.** Sedation: 16–32 mg 2–4 times daily. Hypnotic: **PO** 100–300 mg. Anticonvulsant: Individualized. Aim at minimum effective dose. Usual **PO:** 120–200 mg daily. **IM:** 200–320 mg. Total adult daily dose should not exceed 650 mg. IV dose should not exceed 300 mg. **Pediatric** (Sedative) **PO:** 6 mg/kg. Anticonvulsant: 1–6 mg/kg daily. **Parenteral** (*epilepsy*): 3–5 mg/kg daily.	**Additional Nursing Implications** Observe closely for respiratory depression, which is the first sign of overdosage Long-acting barbiturate. A drug of choice for grand mal epilepsy. Give major fraction of anticonvulsant dosage according to when seizures are likely to occur. On arising for daytime seizures, at bedtime when seizures occur at night. In most cases, when used for epilepsy, drug must be taken regularly to avoid seizures—even when no seizures are imminent. For epilepsy, may be given with amphetamine to overcome sedation. Aqueous solution for injection must be freshly prepared. Some ready-dissolved solutions for injection are available. The vehicle is propylene glycol, water, and alcohol. These solutions are stable. IM administration is preferred. *IV Administration:* Inject very slowly at rate of 50 mg/min

Secobarbital (Seconal) Secobarbital sodium (Seconal Sodium)	Mild sedation, hypnotic, acute convulsive disorders, dentistry, minor surgery, obstetrics	**PO, IM, and rectally:** Same dosage regardless of route. Sedation: 30–50 mg t.i.d. Hypnotic: 100–200 mg. **Pediatric** (hypnotic) (up to 6 mo): 15–50 mg; (6 mo–3 yr): 60–65 mg; (older children): 50–100 mg. Preoperative sedation: 200–300 mg 1 to 2 hr before surgery	Short-acting barbiturate. Not effective for epilepsy. *Administration:* (1) Aqueous solutions for injection must be freshly prepared from dry-packed ampules. (2) Stable aqueous-polyethylene glycol solutions are available. These should be stored below 10°C. Aqueous solution preferred to polyethylene glycol—which may be irritating to kidneys, especially in patients with signs of renal insufficiency
Talbutal (Lotusate)	Mild sedation, hypnotic	PO (Hypnotic): 120 mg	Intermediate-acting barbiturate
Thiamylal sodium (Surital Sodium)	Anesthesia	**IV:** 3–4 ml of a freshly prepared 2.5% solution. Maximum dose: 1 gm (or 40 ml of 2.5% solution) **Rectal (adult and pediatric)** for *diagnostic procedures:* 800–1000 mg/22.5 kg. Maximum dose: 3 gm. Two-thirds of calculated dose may be sufficient for obstetric cases	Ultrashort-acting barbiturate. *Administration:* (1) Solution should be administered slowly: 1 ml every 5 sec. Can also be administered by IV drip as 0.2 or 0.3% solution. (2) Rectal: Administer through small catheter. Effect is maximal after 30 min and lasts 1 hr. Use 5% solution **Additional Nursing Implications** Do not use soap suds enemas if this drug is to be administered rectally. Soap interferes with drug **Additional Contraindications** Porphyria
Thiopental sodium (Pentothal Sodium)	Preanesthetic or general anesthesia only	**IV** only. Dosage determined by anesthesiologist to fit needs of situation	Ultrashort-acting barbiturate. Administer cautiously to avoid severe respiratory depression

Reprinted by permission of John Wiley and Sons, Inc. from *The Nurse's Drug Handbook* by Loebl, Spratto, Wit and Heckheimer, Copyright © 1977, John Wiley and Sons, Inc.

Cardiac Glycosides

DRUG	DIGITALIZING DOSE (DD) AND MAINTENANCE (MD)	ONSET (ON) AND DURATION (DR)	REMARKS	ADDITIONAL NURSING IMPLICATIONS
Acetyldigitoxin (Acylanid)	DD: **PO** 1.6–2.2 mg in 1–4 doses **IV** 0.6 mg MD: 0.1–0.2 mg daily	ON: (**PO**) 1–2 hr DR: 1–3 days	More rapid onset and more quickly eliminated from the body than digitoxin. It is not completely absorbed from the GI tract	
Deslanoside (Cedilanid-D)	DD: **IM** or **IV** 1.2–1.6 mg in 1–2 equal doses **Pediatric IM** or **IV**: 22 μg/kg body weight MD: **IV** 0.4 mg daily	ON: 10–30 min DR: 3–6 days	Used for rapid digitalization in emergency situations (acute cardiac failure with pulmonary edema, atrial arrhythmias). Injection vehicle contains ethyl alcohol and glycerin. Protect from light	
Digitalis, glycosides mixture (Digiglusin)	DD: **PO** 10–15 U.S.P. units; **IV** 4 U.S.P. units MD: 0.8–1.6 units **PO** daily	ON: 25 min–2 hr Maximum effect: 4–12 hr DR: 2–3 weeks		
Digitalis leaf, powdered (Digifortis, Pil-Digis)	DD: **PO** 50–150 mg 3–4 times daily for 3–4 days to a maximum of 1 gm. MD: 100 mg daily	ON: 25 min–2 hr Maximum effect: 4–12 hr DR: 2–3 weeks	This preparation contains standardized amount of dried leaves of *Digitalis purpurea* plant for PO use	
Digitoxin (Crystodigin, Digitaline Nativelle,	DD: **PO, IM, IV** 1.0–1.5 mg. Give 30%–50% of dose initially, followed by ⅛–⅓ of	ON: 25 min–2 hr Maximum effect: 4–12 hr DR: 2–3 weeks	Most potent of digitalis glycosides. Its slow onset of action makes it unsuitable for emergency use.	*Administration:* Inject deeply into gluteal muscle

Purodigin	total dose q 3–6 hr. Or: 200 µg b.i.d. for 4 days **Pediatric:** 33 µg/kg MD: 0.05–0.3 mg daily		Drug of choice for maintenance. 1 mg digitoxin is therapeutically equivalent to 1 gm digitalis leaf. Is almost completely absorbed from GI tract	*Storage:* Incompatible with acids and alkali. Protect from light
Digoxin (Lanoxin)	DD: **PO, IM** 2.0–3.0 mg over a 24-hr period. Give ¼–½ of total dose initially, and the remainder in ¼ doses at 6-hr intervals. **IV** 1–1.5 mg. Give 0.5–1.0 mg every 2–4 hr as required. **Pediatric:** 44–88 µg/kg **PO** MD: 0.25–0.75 mg daily	ON: 5–30 min Maximum effect: 2–5 hr DR: 2–6 days	Action more prompt and shorter than digitoxin. Injection vehicle contains propylene glycol, sodium phosphate, and citric acid. May be drug of choice for congestive heart failure because of (a) rapid onset, (b) relatively short duration, (c) can be administered PO, IM, IV	Give full DD only if patient has not received digoxin during previous week; if patient has received an even more slowly excreted cardiac glycoside, full DD should be withheld for 2 weeks *Administration:* Inject deeply into muscle and follow by vigorous massage. Rotate IM injection site. *Storage:* Incompatible with acids and alkali. Protect from light
Gitalin (Gitaligin)	DD: **PO** 4.0–8.0 mg over a 3–4 day period. Give 2.5 mg initially, 0.75 mg q 6 hr thereafter MD: 0.25–1 mg daily **Pediatric:** 100 µg/kg in 3 doses	ON: 10–20 min DR: 10–12 days	Oral only. Give only to patients who have not received digitalis therapy during previous 2 weeks	*Storage:* Protect from light

Continued on next page

DRUG	DIGITALIZING DOSE (DD) AND MAINTENANCE (MD)	ONSET (ON) AND DURATION (DR)	REMARKS	ADDITIONAL NURSING IMPLICATIONS
Lanatoside C (Cedilanid)	DD: **PO** 8–10 mg. Give 3.5 mg on day 1, 2.5 mg on day 2, 2.0 mg on day 3, 2.0 mg daily thereafter MD: 0.5–1.5 mg daily	DR: 16 hr–3 days	Oral only. Only give to patients who have not received digitalis during previous 2 weeks. Rarely given due to poor absorption from GI tract	*Storage:* Protect from light
Ouabain (G-Strophanthin)	DD: **IV** 1 mg. Initiate with 0.25 mg followed by 0.1–0.25 mg at 30–60 min intervals	ON: 3–10 min Peak effect: 30–60 min DR: 1–3 days	Most potent of the pure cardiac glycosides. IV only. Used only for rapid digitalization for emergency treatment of acute congestive heart failure; paroxysmal, atrial, or nodal tachycardia; or atrial flutter. Only given to patients who have not received digitalis therapy during previous 3 weeks	*Storage:* Protect from light

Reprinted by permission of John Wiley and Sons, Inc., from *The Nurse's Drug Handbook* by Loebl, Spratto, Wit and Heckheimer, Copyright © 1977, John Wiley and Sons, Inc.

Drugs Used in Cardiac Emergencies

Drug	Suggested dose and route of administration	Remarks
(1) Sodium bicarbonate	I.V. bolus or continuous infusion. Initial dose, 1 mEq./kg. Repeat, then monitor according to blood gases.	Repeat dose following blood pH results if base deficit.
(2) Calcium chloride (10%)	I.V. bolus, 2.5–5 cc. every 10 minutes.	If digitalized, watch carefully following administration. Check calcium blood levels frequently, as high levels are detrimental. Don't mix with sodium bicarbonate.
(3) Epinephrine (Adrenalin)	I.V. bolus, 0.5 cc. of 1:1,000 solution diluted to 10 cc.	Note dilution. (Dilution for child is 1:10,000.)
(4) Lidocaine (Xylocaine)	I.V. bolus, 50–100 mg., may repeat. I.V. drip, 1–3 mg./minute. Mix I.V. bottle 500 mg./500 cc. D5W (yields 1 mg./cc.).	Do not exceed 100 mg./hour in children or 4 mg./minute in adults.
(5) Atropine	I.V. bolus, 0.5 mg. Repeat every 5 minutes until pulse is greater than 60.	Adult: Total dose not to exceed 2 mg. (except in 3rd-degree block).
(6) Levarterenol (Levophed)	I.V. bolus, 2–5 mg. every 5–10 minutes. I.V. drip, 0.4 mg./ml. in D5W.	Don't use in endotoxic shock or renal shutdown. Titrate for desired blood pressure.
(7) Metaraminol (Aramine)	I.V. drip, 0.5 mg. in 500 cc. D5W.	Titrate for desired blood pressure.
(8) Isoproterenol (Isuprel)	I.V. drip, 1 mg. in 500 cc. D5W.	Titrate for desired effect.

Reprinted by permission of J. B. Lippincott Co. from *The Practice of Emergency Nursing*, by James Cosgriff and Diann Anderson, © 1975, J. B. Lippincott Co.

Major Drugs (Used in Chemotherapy)

Drug	Usual doses	Indications	Toxicity Manifestations	Toxicity Management
Antimetabolites 5 FU (5 Fluorouracil; Efudex, Fluoroplex ointment)	500 to 100 mg/wk orally or IV	Gastrointestinal Breast	1. Stomatitis 2. Diarrhea 3. Nausea 4. Bone marrow suppression (stops when drug discontinued)	1. Good oral hygiene 2. Do not use laxatives; determine previous bowel habits for baseline, and chart amount. 3. Nausea after small frequent meals—carbonated beverage, tea, antiemetics, prochlorperazine maleate (Compazine), or chlorpromazine hydrochloride (Thorazine) 4. Check CBC
MTX (methotrexate)	2.5 mg/24 hr orally 25 mg/wk IV	Alone or in combination (MOPP) Metastatic trophoblastic disease, leukemia, lymphosarcoma, advanced unresponsive psoriasis	1. Stomatitis 2. Diarrhea 3. Dermatitis 4. Pancytopenia — resistance to infection 5. Hepatic toxicity 6. Renal failure 7. Cystitis 8. Menstrual dysfunction 9. Alopecia 10. Headache and blurred	Management same as 5FU NOTE: Observe for adequate renal function. Drug must be stopped immediately or if renal function deteriorates. Obtain SMA-12s, and check creatinine. Drug accumulates in tissues, especially liver, leading to higher serum levels in higher doses. Drug inter-

			Toxicity	
Drug	**Usual doses**	**Indications**	**Manifestations**	**Management**
			vision	acts with sulfonomides, diphenylhydantoin, antibacterials, folic-acid—containing vitamins.
6 MP (6-mercaptopurine; Purinethol)	50 to 150 mg/24 hr orally	Leukemia	1. Oral and gastrointestinal tract ulceration 2. Bone marrow depression 3. Leukopenia 4. Thrombocytopenia	1. Oral care and frequent antacids 2. Check CBC
Ara C (cytosine arabinoside, cytarabine, Cytosar)	1 to 3 mg/kg/24 hr orally	Leukemia	1. Bone marrow depression 2. Nausea and vomiting 3. Megaloblastosis 4. Leukopenia 5. Thrombocytopenia	1. Check CBC 2. Antiemetics
Hydroxyurea (Hydrea)	20 to 30 mg/kg/24 hr orally	Leukemia	1. Nausea 2. Bone marrow depression	1. Antiemetics 2. Check RBC
Miotitic inhibitors Vincristine (Oncovin) Vinblastine (Velban)	1 to 2 mg/wk IV 5 to 10 mg/wk IV	Combination therapy Combination therapy	1. Neuropathy 2. Paresthesia 3. Bone marrow suppression 4. Neurotoxicity	1. Watch tendon reflexes 2. Watch for constipation
Antibiotics Adriamycin (doxorubicin)	0.4 to 0.6 mg/kg/wk 60 mg/M² every 3 weeks	Breast cancer Combination therapy	1. Stomatitis 2. Pancytopenia 3. Cardiac abnormalities 4. Alopecia— 5. Urine may be red	1. As with 5FU 2. As with 5FU 3. Electrocardiogram and CPK should be monitored 4. Advise patient that alopecia will surely occur

Continued on next page

| | | | Toxicity | |
Drug	Usual doses	Indications	Manifestations	Management
Dactinomycin (actinomycin D; Cosmegen)	0.5 to 1 mg/wk IV Also given in more intensive courses	Miscellaneous cancers, and in combination with other drugs	1. Stomatitis 2. Pancytopenia 3. Alopecia 4. Acne in males	As with adriamycin Advise patient that alopecia will probably occur
Mithramycin (Mithricin)	0.5 mg/kg IV q.o.d. and 4 doses	Cancer of testis	1. Hypocalcemia 2. Thrombocytopenia 3. Phlebitis 4. Epistaxis — may be first sign of toxicity	Fatal sx have occurred suddenly
Bleomycin (Blenoxane)	15 to 30 mg 2 or 3x/wk IV	Cancer of testis Cancer of larynx, head, and neck Lymphomas	1. Pulmonary fibrosis 2. Fever 3. Dermatitis	1. Chest x-ray films
Streptozotocin	12.5 mg/kg/wk	Pancreatic islet cell tumors	1. Nausea 2. Vomiting	Still under investigational use
Hormones Corticosteroids, Cortisone-acetate Prednisone-dexamethasone	25 to 37.5 mg/24 hr orally 0.75 to 16 mg/24 hr orally	Cancer of prostate Brain tumors	1. Cushing's syndrome 2. Fluid retention 3. Hypertension 4. Osteoporosis 5. Susceptibility to infection	1. Check electrolytes 2. Check BP
Estrogens Premarin, DES, TACE	1 to 5 mg/24 hr (males) 5 to 15 mg/24 hr (elderly females)	Cancer of prostate Metastatic cancer of breast	1. Fluid retention 2. Cardiac failure 3. Feminization	1. Check electrolytes 2. ECG
Androgens— fluoxymesterone (Halotestin), calusterone (Methosarb), testalactone Teslac	100 mg 3x/wk 30 mg/24 hr 200 mg/24 hr	Metastatic cancer of breast	1. Masculinization 2. Nausea 3. Fluid retention 4. Jaundice	1. Check electrolytes

			Toxicity	
Drug	Usual doses	Indications	Manifestations	Management
Progestins— medroxy- progesterone acetate (Provera, Depo- Provera) hydroxy- progesterone caproate (Delalutin)	2500 to 5000 mg/wk	Cancer of endometrium Cancer of kidney	1. Susceptibility to infection 2. Euphoria or depression 3. Cushing's syndrome 4. Peptic ulcers 5. Osteoporosis 6. Myopathy 7. Hyperglycemia 8. Virilization 9. Thromboembolism	1. Avoid contact with infectious organisms 2. Assess mental and emotional status 4. Bland diet 6. Assess muscle weakness
Alkylating agents Cyclophospha- mide (Cytoxan)	50 to 150 mg/24 hr orally 500 to 1000 mg/wk IV	Lymphosarcoma Leukemia Cystadenocarcinoma of ovary Breast cancer Lung cancer	1. Hemorrhagic cystitis 2. Nausea and vomiting 3. Alopecia	1. Encourage 2 to 3 quarts of fluid per 24 hours; early with breakfast 2. Management same as 5FU
Thio-Tepa	30 to 60 mg IV — can be given by intrapleural or intraperitoneal route	1. Cystadenocarcinoma of ovary 2. Lymphoma 3. Breast cancer	1. Pancytopenia	1. Check blood counts frequently and adjust dosage accordingly
Mechloretha- mine hydrochlo- ride (nitrogen mustard; Mustargen)	Initially 0.4 mg/kg IV or as daily doses of 0.1 mg/kg for 2 to 4 days IV, or a single intracavitary dose	Pleural effusions	1. Nausea and vomiting 2. Irritating to tissues 3. Permanent bone marrow depression	1. Give Thorazine or Compazine 30 to 50 minutes before administration 2. Prevent extravasation or drug coming into contact with skin 3. Watch blood counts carefully
Melphalan (L- phenylala- nine mus-	2 to 4 mg tablets orally per	Breast cancer	1. Nausea after leukopenia and throm-	1. Check course frequently

Continued on next page

Drug	Usual doses	Indications	Toxicity Manifestations	Toxicity Management
tard, L-PAM; Alkeran)	24 hours for 5 days repeated every 6 weeks		bocytopenia	
Procarbazine (Matulane, Natulan)	50 mg/24 hr orally	Combination therapy MOPP Hodgkin's disease	1. Nausea and vomiting 2. Neurotoxicity	1. Antiemetics
Busulfan (Myleran)	4.8 mg/24 hr orally	Chronic leukemia	1. Bone marrow depression	1. Check RBC
Miscellaneous drugs Nitrosoureas, CCNU, BCNU	100 to 200 mg/M² every 4 to 6 weeks	Glioblastomas	1. Nausea and vomiting 2. Bone marrow depression	1. Antiemetics 2. Check RBC
Quinacrine (Atabrine) Chloquine (Aralen)	500 to 1000 mg into affected pleural cavity	Pleural effusion	1. Fever 2. Malaise 3. Severe vomiting	1. Check temperature 3. Antimetics
BCG vaccine *	1 ml intralesionally, orally, or intradermally by scarification	Peripheral tumors, malignant melanoma	1. Fever 2. Nausea and vomiting	1. Check temperature 2. Antiemetics
DTIC (dimethyltriazenomicarboxamide dacarbazine)	IV push Alone 4.5 mg/kg over 10-day period	Combination therapy Alone for malignant melanoma	1. Same as for BCG with flulike syndrome	1. Same as for BCG 2. Burns during injection. Avoid extravasation

Reprinted by permission of The C. V. Mosby Co. from Mantz, Cynthia Allison, and Hill, George J., II: Role of the nurse in antineoplastic drug research. In: Peterson, Barbara Holz, and Kellogg, Carolyn Jo, editors: *Current Practice in Oncologic Nursing*, vol. I, St. Louis, 1976, The C. V. Mosby Co.

Diuretics

Generic Name	Trade Name	How Supplied	Route	Usual Dose	Comments
Mercaptomerin sodium	Thiomerin	Ampuls 1 cc., 2 cc. Vials 10 ml., 30 ml., 125 mg./ml.	Sc. I.M. (deep) I.V.	0.2–2 ml. daily	I.M. injections are painful; massage of the site often helps to relieve the pain.
Spironolactone	Aldactone	Tablets 25 mg.	P.O.	25 mg. q.i.d.	Children's daily dose is 1.5 mg./lb. of body weight.
Acetazolamide	Diamox	Tablets 125 mg., 250 mg. Capsules 500 mg. (sustained release) Vials 500 mg.	P.O. I.V.	250 mg. q.d. or q.o.d.	
Urea	Ureaphil	Vials 150 cc. 40 gm./vial	I.V.	1 gm./kg. of body weight or 8–20 gm. several times a day. Not to exceed 1.5 gm./kg.	Given in 30% solution; rate not to exceed 60 gtts/minute. Dose should not exceed 120 gm. daily. Should be freshly prepared each dose.
Benzthiazide	Aquatag	Tablets 25 mg., 50 mg.	P.O.	50 mg. b.i.d.	Larger doses may be necessary until "dry weight" is obtained.

Continued on next page

Generic Name	Trade Name	How Supplied	Route	Usual Dose	Comments
Furosemide	Lasix	Tablets 20 mg., 40 mg.	P.O.	40–80 mg. P.O. q.d.	Exposure of the drug to light may cause discoloration, which does not alter its potency. This drug is contraindicated in women of childbearing potential. I.V. doses should be given slowly.
		Ampuls 2 cc., 10 mg./cc. 10 cc., 10 mg./cc.	I.M. I.V.	20–40 mg. I.M. or I.V.	
Ethacrynic acid	Edecrin	Tablets 25 mg., 50 mg.	P.O.	50–200 mg. P.O. q.d.	Edecrin should not be given intramuscularly or subcutaneously. When some 5% dextrose solutions are used to reconstitute the dry material, the solution may appear hazy. I.V. use of these solutions is not recommended. Discard unused solution after 24 hours. Edecrin is not recommended for pregnant women or nursing mothers.
Sodium ethacrynate	Sodium Edecrin	Vials 50 cc., 1 mg./cc.	I.V.	50 mg. I.V., or 0.5–1 mg. per kg. of body weight.	

Reprinted by permission of J. B. Lippincott from *Review and Application of Clinical Pharmacology* by Susan E. Ralston and Marion F. Hale, Copyright 1977, J. B. Lippincott.

Antibiotic Therapy in Gonorrhea

Drug	Dosage Adolescents	Dosage Children	Method	Administration
Procaine penicillin G	4.8 million U	75,000 U/kg	IM	Administered at two sites during single visit
Probenecid	1 g	25 mg/kg	PO	Administered simultaneously or 20-30 minutes prior to IM penicillin as initial dose to delay excretion of penicillin by kidneys
	500 mg	10 mg/kg	PO	Given every 6 hours for 24 hours
Ampicillin	3.5 g	100 mg/kg	PO	Single dose preceded 30 minutes earlier by probenecid
Amoxicillin	Same as ampicillin	—	PO	Can be given without probenecid
Spectinomycin dihydrochloride (Trobicin)	2 g	—	IM	For patients allergic to penicillin. Single-dose drug, therefore useful only in treatment of uncomplicated disease. Not used in children who weigh less than 50 kg (110 pounds)
Tetracycline	1.5 g	25 mg/kg	PO	Initial dose
	500 mg	10-15 mg/kg		Given 4 times per day for total dosage of 9.5 g (adolescents). Given every 6 hours for 5 days (children)

Reprinted by permission of The C. V. Mosby Co. from *Nursing Care of Infants and Children,* by Lucille Whaley and Donna Wong, © 1979, the C. V. Mosby Co., St. Louis.

Insulins

	TRADE NAME	APPEARANCE	DOSAGE**	ONSET	PEAK (Hours)	DURATION	COMPATIBLE WITH:
Fast Acting							
Insulin injection	Regular Insulin Regular Iletin	Clear	Individualized 5–100 U.S.P. units 1 to 4 times daily	½–1	2–3	5–8	All preparations
Prompt insulin zinc suspension	Semilente Iletin Semilente Insulin*	Cloudy suspension	Individualized 10–80 U.S.P. units	½–1	3–9	12–16	All preparations
Intermediate Acting							
Globin zinc insulin suspension		Clear	Individualized 10–80 U.S.P. units	1–4	6–16	16–24	All preparations
Insulin zinc suspension	Lente Iletin Lente Insulin*	Cloudy suspension	Individualized 10–80 U.S.P. units	1–4	7–12	24–30	All preparations
Isophane insulin suspension	NPH Iletin NPH Insulin	Cloudy suspension	Individualized 10–80 U.S.P. units	1–2	7–12	24–30	All preparations
Long Acting							
Extended zinc insulin suspension	Ultralente Iletin Ultralente Insulin*	Cloudy suspension	Individualized	4–8	10–18	30–36	All preparations
Protamine zinc insulin suspension	PZI Protamine, Zinc, and Iletin	Cloudy suspension	Individualized 10–80 U.S.P. units	4–8	12–24	30–36	All preparations

*Contains only beef insulin.
** Number of times drug is given is highly individualized.
Remark: These preparations are derived from cattle and/or hogs.

Reprinted by permission of John Wiley and Sons, Inc. from *The Nurse's Drug Handbook*, by Suzanne Loebl, George Spratto, Andrew Wit, and Estelle Heckheimer, Copyright © 1977, John Wiley and Sons, Inc.

Radioisotopes and Their Therapeutic Uses

Radioisotope and symbol	Kind of internal radiotherapy	Uses	Half-life	Emissions Alpha	Emissions Beta	Emissions Gamma
Cobalt 60 (^{60}Co)	Interstitial (beads)	Buccal mucosa carcinoma	5 years			X
Iodine 131 (^{131}I)	Systemic (p.o. or IV)	Primary and metastatic thyroid carcinoma (papillary and follicular carcinoma), hyperthyroidism	8 days		X	X
Phosphorus 32 (^{32}P)	Systemic (IV), intracavitary (instillation)	Polycythemia vera, palliative treatment for CML and CLL, metastatic breast and prostate carcinoma, bone cancer, malignant pleural effusions	14 days		X	
Radon 222 (^{222}Rn)	Interstitial (seeds)	Cancers of the tongue, neck, etc.	4 days			X
Radium 226 (^{226}Ra)	Interstitial (needles)	Oral Cancers	1600 years			X
	Intracavitary (applicator)	Cervical/uterine cancers	1600 years			X
Iridium 192 (^{192}Ir)	Interstitial (seed, wire)	Head and neck cancers	75 days			X
Gold 198 (^{198}Au)	Intracavitary (instillation)	Palliative management of malignant ascites and pleural effusions, bladder cancers	3 days		X	X
Cesium 137 (^{137}Cs)	Interstitial, intracavitary	Cervical/uterine and head and neck cancers	30 years			X

Reprinted by permission of McGraw-Hill Book Co. from *Dynamics of Oncology Nursing* by Pamela Burkhalter and Diana Donley, Copyright © 1978, McGraw-Hill Book Co.

The Penicillins

Approved name	Other name	Resistant to gastric acid	Resistant to penicillinase	Antibacterial spectrum	Remarks
Natural penicillins Benzylpenicillin (penicillin G)	Penicillin G	No	No	High activity against gram-positive bacteria Low activity against gram-negative bacteria	Only one-third oral dose absorbed, so oral dose must be three to five times that given parenterally For maximum absorption give oral dose 1 hour before or 2 to 3 hours after meal
Semisynthetic penicillins Penicillin V (phenoxymethyl penicillin: Compocillin V)	Pen-Vee	Yes	No	Like penicillin G but less potent	Yields a serum peak level two to five times greater than penicillin G Can be given orally
Phenethicillin	Syncillin Chemipen Darcil	Yes	No	Like penicillin G but slightly less active against gram-positive cocci More active against penicillinase-producing *Staphylococcus aureus*	Give between meals since food delays absorption
Methicillin	Staphcillin	No	Yes	Like penicillin G but with lower activity; only 1/150 as potent	Use only for penicillinase-producing staphylococci Intramuscular injections quite painful

Oxacillin	Prostaphlin Resistopen	Yes	Yes	Less active than penicillin G, more active than methicillin	Give between meals since food delays absorption
Cloxacillin	Tegopen	Yes	Yes	Effective against staphylococci resistant to penicillin G Like methicillin	Yields a serum peak level two times that of oxacillin Available only for oral use
Dicloxacillin	Dynapen Pathocil Veracillin	Yes	Yes	More active against penicillinase-producing *Staphylococcus aureus* than oxacillin or cloxacillin	Yields a serum peak level four times that of oxacillin
Nafcillin	Unipen	—	Yes	Staphylococci, pneumococci, group A beta-hemolytic streptococci More active than methicillin	Irregular absorption when given orally
Ampicillin	Polycillin Penbriten	Yes	No	Like penicillin G but more active against gram-negative bacteria; broad spectrum	Produces higher blood levels of antibiotic than ampicillin
Amoxicillin		—	No	Like ampicillin	
Carbenicillin		No	—	Like ampicillin High activity against some *Proteus* species Moderate activity against *Pseudomonas aeruginosa*	Not absorbed when given orally Under clinical investigation

Reprinted by permission of The C. V. Mosby Co. from *Pharmacology in Nursing*, 14th edition, by Betty S. Bergerson, Copyright © 1979, The C. V. Mosby Co., St. Louis

Examples of Drugs Known to Cause Blood Dyscrasias, by Disorder

Disorder	Generic drug name	Trade drug name
(1) Agranulocytosis (Granulocytopenia or Leukopenia)	Methyldopa Acetylsalicylic acid Phenylbutazone Chloramphenicol Prochlorperazine Chlorothiazide Thioridazine Tolbutamide Benzylpenicillin sodium Propylthiouracil Tripelennamine Quinidine sulfate Streptomycin Sulfonamides Tetracycline Imipramine HCl	Aldomet (Aspirin) Butazolidin Chloromycetin Compazine Diuril Mellaril Orinase (Penicillin) Pyribenzamine (Quinidine) Tofranil
(2) Aplastic Anemia	Methyldopa Acetylsalicylic acid Barbiturates Phenylbutazone Chloramphenicol Chlorpropamide Acetazolamide Chlorothiazide Sulfisoxazole Sulfamethoxypyridazine Tolbutamide Benzylpenicillin sodium Quinidine sulfate Streptomycin Trimethadione	Aldomet (Aspirin) Butazolidin Chloromycetin Diabinese Diamox Diuril Gantrisin Kynex Orinase (Penicillin) (Quinidine) Tridione
(3) Hemolytic Anemia	Acetylsalicylic acid Probenecid Chloramphenicol Nitrofurantoin Isonicotinic Hydrazide Para-aminosalicylic acid Benzylpenicillin sodium Quinidine sulfate Sulfonamides	(Aspirin) Benemid Chloromycetin Furadantin I.N.H. (P.A.S.) (Penicillin) (Quinidine)

Continued on next page

	Tetracycline Chlorpromazine Vitamin K	Thorazine
(4) Megaloblastic Anemia	Anticonvulsants Barbiturates Diphenylhydantoin sodium	Dilantin
(5) Pancytopenia	Methyldopa Acetylsalicylic acid Barbiturates Phenylbutazone Chloramphenicol Chlorpropamide Acetazolamide Chlorothiazide Meprobamate Sulfisoxazole Sulfamethoxypyridazine Tolbutamide Benzylpenicillin sodium Quinidine sulfate Streptomycin Tetracycline	Aldomet (Aspirin) Butazolidin Chloromycetin Diabinese Diamox Diuril Equanil Gantrisin Kynex Orinase (Penicillin) (Quinidine)
(6) Thrombocytopenia	All of the above.	All of the above.

Reprinted by permission of J. B. Lippincott Co. from *The Practice of Emergency Nursing*, by James Cosgriff and Diann Anderson, © 1975, J. B. Lippincott Co.

Drug Effects on Human Sexual Behavior

Drug or drug category	Effect	Probable mechanism of action
Oral contraceptives	Positive	Permits separation of sexual activity from concern about conception

Antihypertensives
  Guanethidine (Ismelin)
  Mecamylamine (Inversine)
  Reserpine (Serpasil)
  Spironolactone (Aldactone)
  Trimethaphan (Arfonad)
	Negative	Peripheral blockade of nervous innervation of sex glands

Antidepressants
  Amitriptyline (Elavil)
  Desipramine (Norpramin, Pertofrane)
	Negative	Central depression; peripheral blockade of nervous innervation of sex glands

Continued on next page

Imipramine (Tofranil)		
Nortriptyline (Aventyl)		
Pargyline (Eutonyl)		
Phenelzine sulfate (Nardil)		
Protriptyline (Vivactil)		
Tranylcypromine sulfate (Parnate)		
Antihistamines	Negative	Blockade of parasympathetic nervous innervation of sex glands
Chlorpheniramine (Chlor-Trimeton)		
Diphenhydramine (Benadryl)		
Promethazine (Phenergan)		
Antispasmodics	Negative	Ganglionic blockage of nervous innervation of sex glands
Glycopyrrolate methobromide (Robinul)		
Hexocyclium (Tral)		
Methantheline (Banthine)		
Poldine (Nacton)		
Sedatives and tranquilizers	Negative and positive	Central sedation; blockade of autonomic innervation of sex glands; suppression of hypothalamic and pituitary function
Benperidol		
Chlordiazepoxide (Librium)		
Chlorpromazine (Thorazine, Megaphen)		
Chlorprothixene (Taractan)		
Diazepam (Valium)		Tranquilization and relaxation
Mesoridazine (Serentil)		
Phenoxybenzamine (Dibenzyline)		
Prochlorperazine (Compazine)		
Thioridazine (Mellaril)		
Ethyl alcohol	Negative	Central depression; suppression of motor activity; diuresis
	Transiently positive	Release of inhibitions; relaxation
Barbiturates	Negative	Central depression; suppression of motor activity; hypnosis
Sex hormone preparations	Negative	Antiandrogenic effects on sexual function; loss of libido; decreased potency
Cyproterone acetate		
Methandrostenolone (Dianabol)		
Nandrolane phenpropionate (Durabolin)		
Norethandrolone (Nilevar)		
Methadone	Negative	Suppresses secondary sex organ function in male
Potassium nitrate (saltpeter)	Questionable	Diuresis
Cantharis (Spanish fly)	Negative	Irritation and inflammation of genitourinary tract, systemic poisoning
Yohimbine	Questionable	Stimulation of lower spinal nerve centers
Strychnine	Questionable	Stimulation of neuraxis; priapism

Continued on next page

Narcotics and psychoactive drugs
  Amphetamines
  Cocaine
	Negative	Central depression; decreased libido and impaired potency

Heroin
  LSD
  Marihuana
  Morphine
	Transiently positive	Release of inhibitions; increased suggestibility; relaxation

L-Dopa and *p*-chlorophenylalanine (PCPA)	Questionable	Improvement of well-being
Amyl nitrite	Questionable	Vasodilation of genitourinary tract; smooth muscle relaxation
Caffeine	Questionable	Central nervous system stimulant
Vitamin E	Questionable	Supports fertility in laboratory animals
Selenium	Questionable	Supports fertility in laboratory animals

Reprinted by permission of The C. V. Mosby Co. from *Human Sexuality in Health and Illness*, 2nd edition, by Nancy Fugate Woods, Copyright 1979, The C. V. Mosby Co.

Characteristics of Abused Drugs and Their Acute Reactions in Adolescents

CLASS	EXAMPLE	ROUTE	BEHAVIORAL SIGNS	PHYSICAL SIGNS	MEDICAL COMPLICATIONS
Opiates	Heroin, methadone morphine	Subcutaneous, intranasal, intravenous	Euphoria, lethargy to coma	Constricted pupils, respiratory depression, cyanosis, rales	Injection site infection, hepatitis, bacterial endocarditis, amenorrhea, peptic ulcer, pulmonary edema, tetanus
Hypnotic-sedatives	Barbiturates, glutethimide	Oral, intravenous	Slurred speech, ataxia, short attention span, drowsiness, combative, violent	Constricted pupils (barbiturates), dilated pupils (glutethimide), needle marks	Injection site infection, hepatitis, endocarditis
	Alcohol	Oral	As above		Gastritis, CNS depression
Stimulants	Amphetamines	Oral, subcutaneous, intravenous	Hyperactive, insomnia, anorexic paranoia, personality change, irritability	Hypertension, weight loss, dilated pupils	Injection site infections, hepatitis, endocarditis, psychosis, depression
	Cocaine	Intravenous, intranasal	Restless, hyperactive, occ. depression or paranoia	Hypertension, tachycardia	Nausea, vomiting, inflammation or perforation of nasal septum
Hallucinogens	LSD, THC, PCP, STP (DOM), mescaline, DMT*	Oral	Euphoria, dysphoria, hallucinations, confusion, paranoia	Dilated pupils, occ. hypertension, hyperthermia, piloerection	Primarily psychiatric with high risk to individuals with unrecognized or previous psychiatric disorder
Hydrocarbons, fluorocarbons	Glue (toluene)	Inhalant	Euphoria, confusion, general intoxication	Nonspecific	Secondary trauma, asphyxiation from plastic bag used to inhale fumes

	Cleaning fluid (trichloroethylene)	Inhalant	Euphoria, confusion, general intoxication, vomiting, abdominal pain	Oliguria, jaundice	Hepatitis, renal injury
	Aerosol sprays (freon)	Inhalant	Euphoria, dysphoria, slurred speech, hallucinations	Nonspecific	Psychiatric
Cannabis	Marihuana, hashish, THC	Smoke, oral	Mild intoxication and simple euphoria to hallucination (dose-related)	Occ. tachycardia, delayed response time, poor coordination	Occ. psychiatric, with depressive or anxiety reactions

Reprinted by permission of W. B. Saunders Co. from *Nelson Textbook of Pediatrics*, 10th edition, by Vaughan and McKay, Copyright © 1975, W. B. Saunders Co.

Publications on Pharmacology

Brief Guide To Major Hypnotic Drug Interactions And Their Management, a booklet, is available from Roche Laboratories, Nutley, N.J. 07110.

A wide variety of publications on drug information is available from the American Society Of Hospital Pharmacists, 4630 Montgomery Avenue, Washington, D.C., 20014. These include the *American Journal Of Hospital Pharmacy* and *American Hospital Formulary Service.* Write for complete list.

Imferon IM/IV (iron dextran injection, U.S.P.), a pamphlet on the use of Imferon, is available from Merrell-National Laboratories, Cincinnati, Ohio 45215.

PDR—Physician's Desk Reference (revised yearly). This source of information on thousands of drugs (the book is over 2000 pages) is available from Medical Economics Co., Box 58, Oradell, New Jersey 07649. Price: $13 each, bulk rates available.

Periodicals

The Medical Letter, 56 Harrison St. New Rochelle, N.Y. 10801. *The Medical Letter* is a newsletter for physicians published every two weeks. It contains up-to-date information on drugs and drug research. (Cost: $19.50/year. $9.75 for students.)

This material is adapted from *Medical Self-Care,* Number Six, Fall, 1979, review by Joe Graedon.

The *Nurses' Drug Alert* (Nurses' Drug Alert, Inc., 12 East 63rd St., New York, New York 10021) contains up-to-date information on drugs. It includes abstracts from other journals and the latest studies on drugs. It is published semimonthly in March, June, September and December, and monthly all other months. Cost: $14 per year in the U.S. and Canada and $17 in all other countries.

Audiovisual Materials on Pharmacology

"Drugs: Action And Interaction" and "Drugs: Autonomic And Somatic Nervous Systems," filmstrips plus cassette tapes or records, are available from Concept Media.

"Current Drug Therapy: Nursing Focus, Volume 1" is a series of six audiocassettes and study guides, from American Journal Of Nursing Co.

4 Medical-Surgical Nursing

Medical-Surgical Nursing is a specialty with many subspecialties, including emergency care, chronic and acute disease care, critical and coronary care, orthopedics, surgical nursing, rehabilitation, and many others. Included in this section are reference guides from each of these areas to aid the practicing nurse.

Patient teaching is a component of all nursing and is particularly important in the medical-surgical field in helping clients adjust to illness and in teaching health promotion. Methods of patient teaching are included here as a reminder of the importance of this nursing function. The resource section at the end of this chapter is a further aid to nurses in this area, since it includes valuable information on services and educational aids available to patients. This information can be incorporated into patient teaching.

The resource section is further intended as a reminder to consider the "whole" patient. The more we know of the resources available to patients, the better we can anticipate their needs and make appropriate referrals. In doing this we come closer to being "the caring link" described so eloquently in the following pages by the authors of *Leadership for Change: A Guide for the Frustrated Nurse* and by Lore Kruger and Karen Jasper. Their words are fitting reminders of the need to develop our caring, human skills, as we gain in technical expertise.

I. Nurses—The Caring Link
II. A Mother's Letter
III. Methods of Patient Teaching
IV. First Aid
    Cardiopulmonary Resuscitation
    The Heimlich Maneuver
    Red Cross Recommendations
    Equipment for an Emergency Cart for Cardiopulmonary Resuscitation
V. Body Water Balance

- VI. **Operation and Examination Positions**
  Assessment, Intervention and Evaluation
  Superficial Veins
  Prevention and Assessment of Complications
- VII. **Range of Motion Exercises**
- VIII. **Wound Healing**
- IX. **Hot and Cold Applications**
- X. **Oxygen Administration**
- XI. **I.V. Therapy**
- VII. **Range of Motion Exercises**
- XII. **Intravascular Monitoring Techniques**
- XIII. **Hemolytic Transfusion Reactions**
- XIV. **Peritoneal Dialysis**
- XV. **Urinary Catheterization**
- XVI. **Assessment and Treatment of Acute Head Injury**
- XVII. **Chemotherapy Treatment**
- XVIII. **Burn Care**
  "Rule of Nines"
  Chemical Burns
  Methods of Burn Care
  Educational Programs in Burn Care
- XIX. **Hypertension**
- XX. **Orthopedics**
  Cast Care
  Complications from Fractures
- XXI. **Spinal Cord Injury**
  A Message to Helping Professionals
  Functional Goals and Potential Equipment
- XXII. **Plan of a Coronary Care Unit**
- XXIII. **Radiation**
- XXIV. **Effects of Industrial Agents on the Worker**
- XXV. **Preoperative Assessment Guidelines**
- XXVI. **Clinical Nurse Specialist for Intraoperative Care**
- XXVII. **Medical-Surgical Resources**
  General Medical-Surgical Resources
  Resources on Burns and Burn Care
  Resources on Cancer
  Resources on Communicable Diseases
  Resources on Diabetes
  Resources on Environmental and Occupational Health
  Resources on the Handicapped
  Resources on Self-Help and Consumer Oriented Health Care
  Resources on Smoking
  Resources on Speech and Hearing Disorders
  Resources on Vision and Blindness

Nurses-The Caring Link

"As technology has provided medicine with newer, more complicated and more sophisticated methods of diagnosing and treating illness, we (nurses) remain the caring link between the hardware of that technology and the human needs of the client and his family. We remain the health care providers who relate not just to the person's lungs, liver, heart and housing, but to all of him physically and emotionally, and to all of him in the context of his social environment."

Reprinted with permission of J. B. Lippincott Co., from *Leadership For Change: A Guide For the Frustrated Nurse,* by Dorothy Brooten, Laura Hayman and Mary Naylor, © J. B. Lippincott Co., 1978.

A Mother's Letter

The following letter from a bereaved mother serves as a reminder to all of us of the need for compassion and caring along with technical expertise in the nursing care we give.

> Despite my deep and crushing pain, I feel a dire need to share a tragic and dehumanizing, absolutely shattering experience.
>
> Our daughter was taken to a hospital following an automobile accident of August 6. She had left home only a few hours earlier to spend the evening with friends. The next moment she was dead. Our big-little girl had been taken to a hospital's emergency room. We were called there. Doctors were on duty and in charge. Theirs was the voice that pronounced our Lore's end. We had every right to expect awareness of our overwhelming grief, tenderness toward our massive loss, calm to assist us through those first moments of shock.
>
> Instead the doctor greeted us with, "Your daughter didn't make it." He insisted on immediate identification and immediate signature on the autopsy report. He insisted we wait for the police. And the nurse said, "Don't worry about it. We see this every day."
>
> Whether by instinct, character or training, these "helpers" hurt two distraught parents. We needed human help. They insisted on bureaucratic protocol. We needed a moment to hold our hearts. They insisted on immediate action. We needed to retreat to our home to grasp our grief. They insisted we await the uniformed authorities.
>
> Months have passed since then. We are learning to deal with our agonies and grief, but those words continue to ring in my ears and haunt my very silence. We were bowed in dismayed grief. Impersonal pronouncements perhaps protected doctoral pain. They added considerably to ours.

Continued on next page

> Doctors, please search yourselves for resources to deal helpfully with others like us. Seek ways to make the few moments available for deeply troubled persons times of healing rather than destruction. Plan ways of staffing your facilities with, or have immediately available to them, someone who is full of heart and wise in the administration of compassion. We need caring, so desperately.
>
> Lore Kruger

Reprinted with permission of *The Washington Post*, from a letter to the Editor by Lore Kruger in *The Washington Post*, March 3, 1977, © *The Washington Post*, 1977.

Methods of Patient Teaching

A prime function of nursing in all areas of practice is patient teaching. The following table lists various teaching methods and their particular uses for patient teaching.

Some Techniques for Producing Desired Behavioral Outcomes

RATIONALE	TEACHING METHODS
If you wish to:	*Use:*
impart *generalizations* about experience.	lecture, symposium, panel, reading, audiovisual aids, a book- or pamphlet-based discussion.
apply information to experience through insight and *understanding*.	feedback devices, problem-solving discussions, laboratory experimentation, group participation, case problems.
build *skills*.	role playing, drill, coaching, demonstration, and return demonstration.
create new *attitudes*. (Attitudes are learned through repeated reinforcement of a response to a stimulus. If a response different from the original one is given and reinforced over a period of time, a change in attitude occurs, evidenced by a change in behavior in a particular set of circumstances [21]. Eventually the attitude may become a value.)	reverse role playing, experience-sharing discussion, counseling-consultation, environmental support, games designed to produce certain attitudes, and nonverbal exercises which draw out certain attitudes through gestures, posture, and facial expression, positive and negative reinforcement.
change *values* through the rearrangement of the priority of beliefs.	speakers who have adjusted satisfactorily to a certain condition now facing the patient, biographical or autobiographical reading, drama, philosophical or direct-value-placement discussion with provision for reflection.
promote new *interests*.	field trips, audiovisual aids, reading, creative experiences.

Reprinted by permission of Prentice-Hall, Inc. from *Nursing Concepts for Health Promotion*, 2nd edition, by Ruth Beckmann Murray and Judith Proctor Zentner, © 1979, Prentice-Hall, Inc.

First Aid in Cardiopulmonary Resuscitation

In the event of an accident or sudden illness that causes the cessation of breathing or the interruption of normal circulation, the first aider should be prepared to properly administer cardiopulmonary resuscitation. The following ABCD steps of cardiopulmonary resuscitation should be followed by the first aider:

*A*irway opened
    Place in supine position
    Tilt head back
    Extend neck
    Clear and remove obstructions
*B*reathing restored
    Pinch nose
    Form seal with mouth
    Inflate lungs
    Check circulation
*C*irculation restored
    Locate lower half of sternum
    Compress sternum
    Alternate with ventilation
*D*efinitive therapy
    Get medical help

Reprinted by permission of the C. V. Mosby Co. from *First Aid in Emergency Care* by Guy S. Parcel, © 1977, The C. V. Mosby Company.

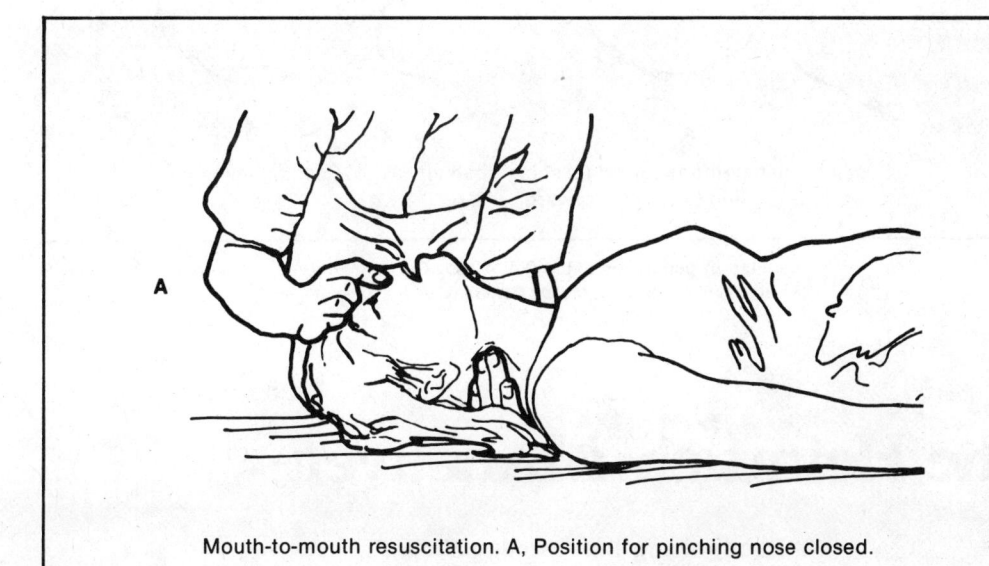

Mouth-to-mouth resuscitation. A, Position for pinching nose closed.

Continued on next page

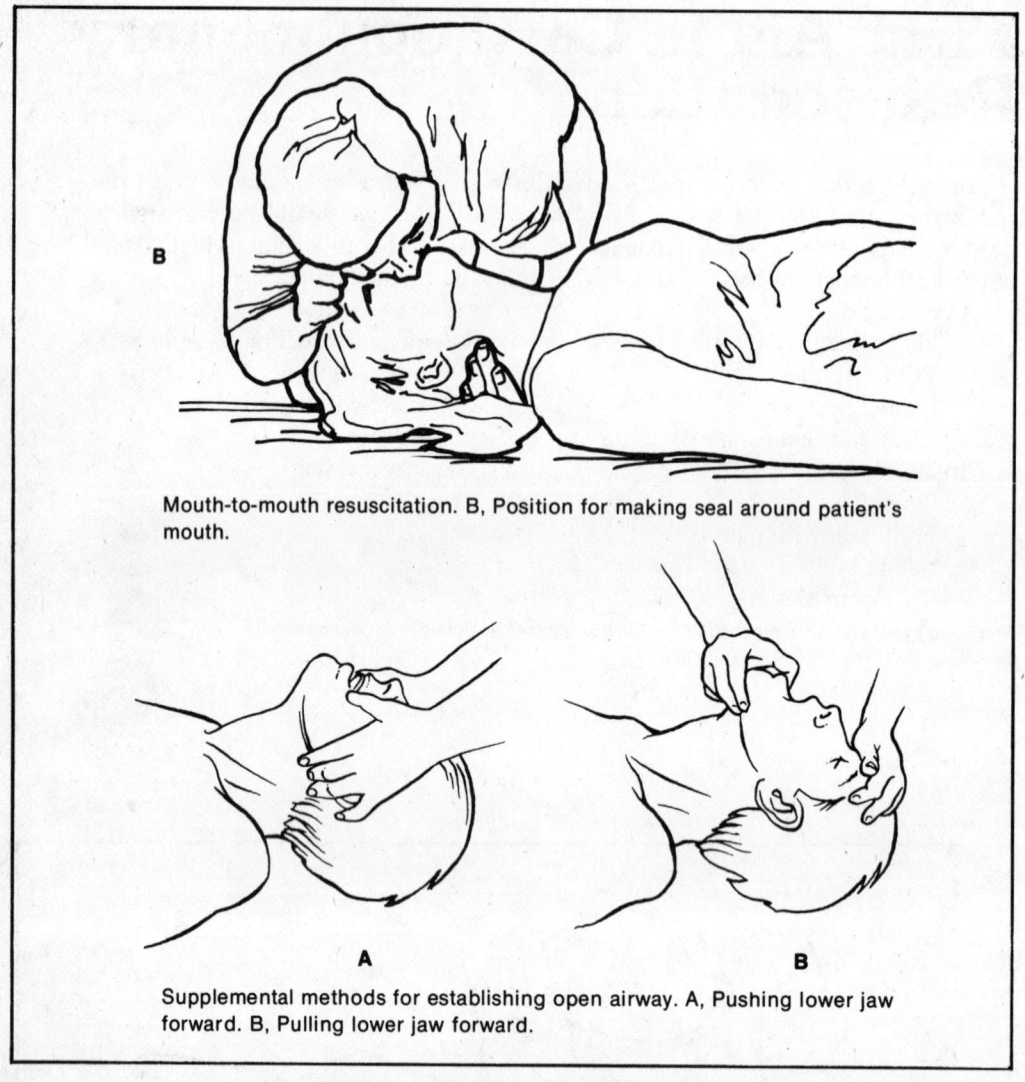

Mouth-to-mouth resuscitation. B, Position for making seal around patient's mouth.

Supplemental methods for establishing open airway. A, Pushing lower jaw forward. B, Pulling lower jaw forward.

Reprinted by permission of the C. V. Mosby Co. from *First Aid in Emergency Care*, Guy S. Parcel, © 1977, The C. V. Mosby Company.

The Heimlich Maneuver

I. Recognizing the Choking Victim

A. Heimlich sign: Victim may bring hand to throat (Heimlich sign) to indicate choking. Rescuer should ask "Are you choking?" Victim will be unable to speak but may nod his assent.

B. Symptoms. When sign is not given or goes unrecognized, the following indicate choking:
 1. Victim cannot speak or breathe.
 2. He rapidly becomes pale and then increasingly cyanotic.
 3. He loses consciousness and collapses.

II. Heimlich Maneuver—Victim Standing

 1. Rescuer stands behind victim and wraps his arms around victim's waist.
 2. Rescuer makes a fist with one hand and places the thumb side of the fist against the victim's abdomen, slightly above the navel and below the rib cage.
 3. Rescuer grasps fist with other hand and presses into victim's abdomen with a quick upward thrust.
 4. Thrust is repeated several times if necessary.

III. Heimlich Maneuver—Victim Seated

Same technique as for standing victim. Back of chair acts as a support and enhances effectiveness of Maneuver.

IV. Heimlich Maneuver—Victim Supine

Victim on back with face up. Facing victim, rescuer kneels astride victim's hips. Rescuer then places his hands one on top of the other with the heel of the bottom hand on victim's abdomen, slightly above the navel and below the rib cage. He presses into abdomen with a quick upward thrust. Thrust repeated several times if necessary.

V. Heimlich Maneuver—Self-Save Technique

A. Standard Heimlich technique. Victim positions his own hands slightly above the navel and below the rib cage, and presses his fist into his abdomen with a quick upward thrust. Thrust is repeated several times if necessary.
B. Alternative technique. Victim positions himself over edge of fixed horizontal object such as a chair back, railing or table edge, and presses abdomen into edge with a quick movement. Movement repeated if necessary.

VI. Heimlich Maneuver—Infant Victim

Infant is either held in rescuer's lap or placed face up on a firm surface with the rescuer at his feet. Rescuer places index and middle fingers of both hands on child's abdomen, slightly above navel and well below the rib cage, and presses into abdomen

FIRST AID FOR CHOKING

UNIVERSAL CHOKING SIGN

If victim can cough, speak, breathe → Do not interfere

If victim cannot cough speak breathe →

TAKE ACTION: FOR CONSCIOUS VICTIM

Have someone call for help. Telephone: _____ (Number)

with a quick upward thrust. Several thrusts may be necessary to expel the object.

Reprinted by permission of CIBA Pharmaceutical Company from *Clinical Symposia*, Volume 31, Number 3, by Henry J. Heimlich M.D., and Milton Uhley M.D., illustrated by Frank Netter M.D., Copyright 1979, CIBA Pharmaceutical Company, Division of CIBA-GEIGY Corporation.

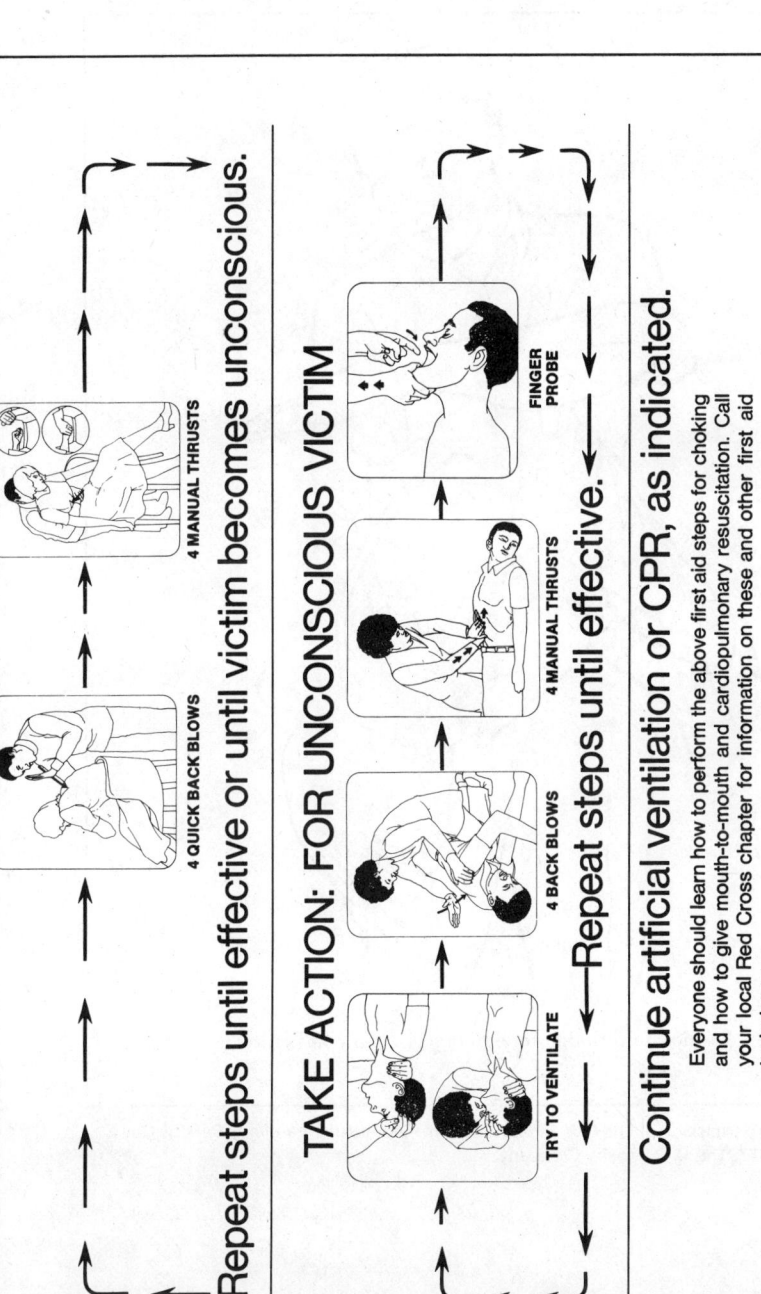

Repeat steps until effective or until victim becomes unconscious.

4 QUICK BACK BLOWS

4 MANUAL THRUSTS

TAKE ACTION: FOR UNCONSCIOUS VICTIM

TRY TO VENTILATE

4 BACK BLOWS

4 MANUAL THRUSTS

FINGER PROBE

Repeat steps until effective.

Continue artificial ventilation or CPR, as indicated.

Everyone should learn how to perform the above first aid steps for choking and how to give mouth-to-mouth and cardiopulmonary resuscitation. Call your local Red Cross chapter for information on these and other first aid techniques.

Caution: Abdominal thrusts may cause injury. Do not practice on people.

American Red Cross Poster 1030, (5–76), prepared by the American National Red Cross, showing the Red Cross' recommendations for dealing with choking victims. Copies of the poster for public education may be obtained from the National Office of the Red Cross or your local chapter.

Instructional materials on the Heimlich Maneuver, including posters, flyers and wallet cards, a cassette tape and slides, and T-shirts with illustrations of the Heimlich Maneuver, can all be obtained from Edumed, Inc., P.O. Box 52, Cincinnati, Ohio. These materials are approved for use by Dr. Henry Heimlich.

136
Position to Dislodge Foreign Object from Child's Airway

Position to dislodge foreign object from child's airway.

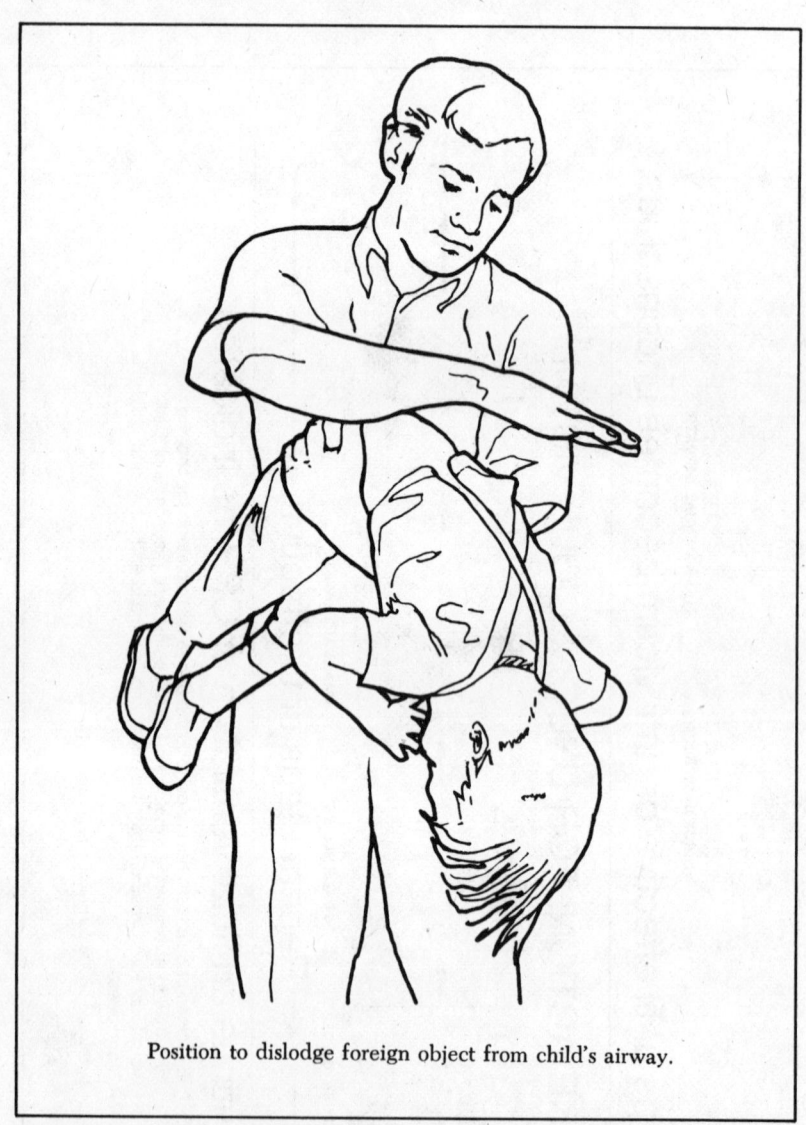

Reprinted by permission of The C. V. Mosby Co. from *First Aid in Emergency Care* by Guy S. Parcel, © 1977, The C. V. Mosby Company.

Equipment for an Emergency Cart for Cardiopulmonary Resuscitation

The equipment should include the following items:

Emergency thoracotomy kit

1 Scalpel handle no. 4 with blade no. 20
1 Rib retractor, wedge retractor, or notched tube
  or
1 Finochietto or Harken self-retaining retractor

Ventilation and resuscitation equipment

Resuscitubes
Ambu resuscitator (air shields type), anesthesia machine, or Kreiselmann resuscitator
Airways
Endotracheal tubes
Laryngoscope
Suctioning apparatus

Syringes (Luer control-type) and needles
(each hospital committee determines sizes needed)

5 Syringes, 2 ml.
1 Syringe, 10 ml.
2 Syringes, 20 ml.
1 Syringe, 50 ml.
5 Needles, 25-gauge, $\frac{5}{8}$ in.
5 Needles, 20-gauge, $1\frac{1}{2}$ in.
5 Needles, 18-gauge, $1\frac{1}{2}$ in.

Emergency drugs

Sodium bicarbonate
Isoproterenol (Isuprel)
Calcium chloride or calcium gluconate
Epinephrine
Lanatoside C (Cedilanid)
Caffeine and sodium benzoate
Aminophylline
Procaine hydrochloride
Potassium hydrochloride
Procaine amide (Pronestyl)
Levarterenol (Levophed)

Infusion equipment

Fluids for intravenous injection
Phleboclysis set
Infusion tubing sets
Blood
Cutdown set and intracatheters

Cardiac support equipment

Defibrillator (pacemaker)
Cardiac monitoring equipment (electroencephalograph and electrocardiograph)

THORACOTOMY SETUP

The items included are the following:

Cutting instruments

1 Scapel handle no. 4 with blade no. 20
1 Mayo scissors, straight
1 Suture scissors

Holding instruments

2 Tissue forceps, 1 and 2 teeth, $5\frac{1}{2}$ in.
1 Tissue forceps, 1 and 2 teeth, 8 in.
1 Foerster sponge forceps, 10 in.
4 Backhaus towel clamps, 5 in.
1 Rib approximator

Clamping instruments

6 Halsted hemostats, straight, $5\frac{1}{2}$ in.
6 Crile hemostats, curved, $6\frac{1}{4}$ in.
2 Rochester-Ochsner hemostats, straight, 1 and 2 teeth, 8 in.

Exposing instruments

1 Pair Volkmann retractors, blunt, 4-pronged, $8\frac{1}{2}$ in.

Reprinted by permission of The C. V. Mosby Co. from *Alexander's Care of the Patient in Surgery*, 6th edition, by Marie J. Rhodes, Barbara J. Gruendemann, and Walter F. Ballinger, © 1978, The C. V. Mosby Co.

Continued on next page

Suturing instruments

    2 Mayo-Hegar needle holders, medium, 6 in.
    3 Ferguson needles, medium
Prepackaged no. 3-0 silk on straight milliner needles

Accessory instruments

1 Suction tubing and tube
1 Plastic chest drainage catheter
1 Rubber drainage tube, large, no. 28 or 32 Fr.

Instructions for cardiac arrest

The instructions for cardiac arrest should be printed on a laminated board and posted in a designated area in each room. Instructions may read as follows:

Respiratory measures

1. Establish an airway.
2. Connect the airway to an oxygen supply.
3. Practice artificial ventilation.
4. Lower the patient's head.

Cardiac measures

1. Apply closed chest massage.
2. Apply open heart massage, as follows:
    a. Enter the left side of the chest through an incision extended from the sternal margin to the midaxillary line.
    b. Insert a rib wedge or chest retractor.
    c. Massage the heart to produce a palpable peripheral pulse at a rate of 60 to 70 beats per minute.

The instructions must be carried out by a physician.

Reprinted by permission of The C. V. Mosby Co. from *Alexander's Care of the Patient in Surgery*, by Marie J. Rhodes, Barbara J. Gruendemann, and Walter F. Ballinger, © 1978, The C. V. Mosby Co.

Body Water Balance in the Adult over a 24-hour Period

Intake	ml.	Output	ml.	
Oral fluids	1200	Urine from kidneys	1500	
"Hidden" water from foods	1100	Water vapor from lungs	400	insensible water loss
Metabolic sources	300	Sweat from the skin	600	

(Water of oxidation):
  Protein = 40 ml./100 Gm.
  Fat = 100 ml./100 Gm.
  CHO = 100 ml./100 Gm.
		Feces from the bowel	100	

	2,600		2600	

Reprinted by permission of W. B. Saunders Co. from *Medical-Surgical Nursing: A Psychophysiological Approach*, by Joan Luckmann and Karen Sorenson, © 1974, W. B. Saunders Co.

Operation and Exam Positions

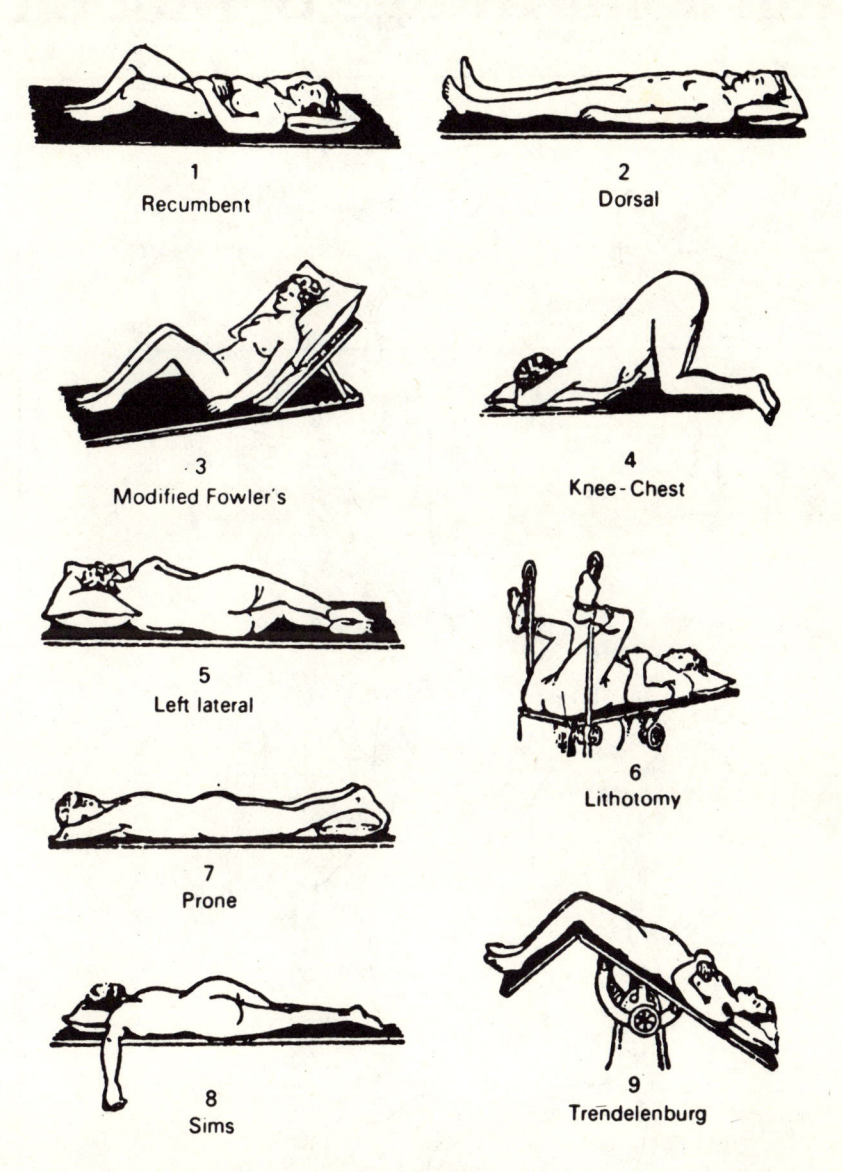

1 Recumbent

2 Dorsal

3 Modified Fowler's

4 Knee-Chest

5 Left lateral

6 Lithotomy

7 Prone

8 Sims

9 Trendelenburg

Operation positions

Reprinted by permission from *New American Pocket Medical Dictionary*, by Nancy Roper, adapted by Jane Clark Jackson, © 1978, Churchill Livingstone.

140
Examples of Exercises to Help Maintain Joint Range of Motion

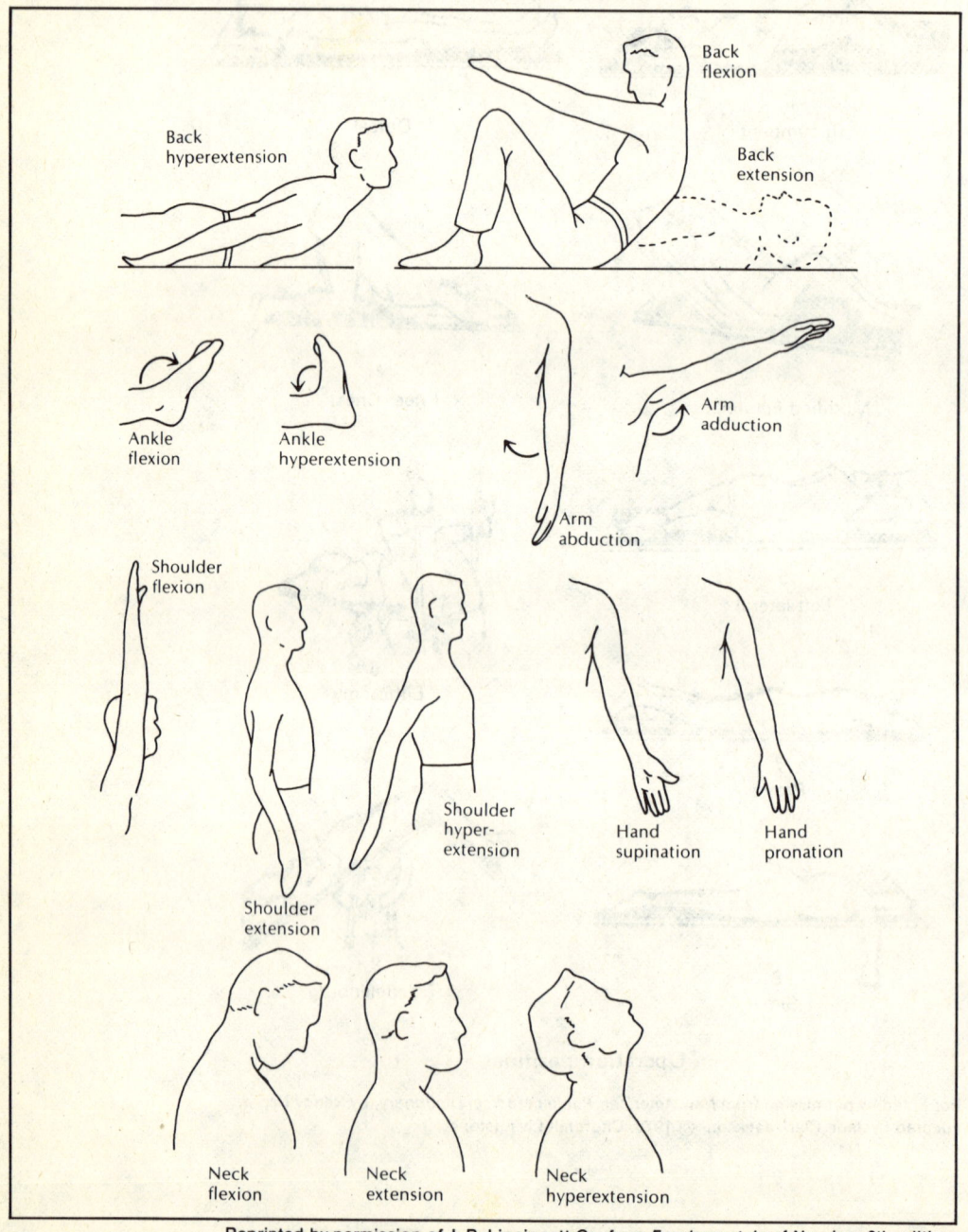

Reprinted by permission of J. B. Lippincott Co. from *Fundamentals of Nursing*, 6th edition, by LuVerne Wolff, Marlene Weitzel, and Elinor Fuerst, © 1979, J. B. Lippincott Co.

Which wounds to watch

CATEGORY	DESCRIPTION	EXAMPLES	RISK OF INFECTION
Clean	Procedures in which the surgeon enters a sterile body cavity and exits through the same cavity, makes no contact with areas having bacterial populations (such as the gastrointestinal and upper respiratory tracts), encounters no inflammation or pus, and experiences no break in sterile technique.	Open heart surgery, herniorrhaphy, mastectomy.	1-2%
Clean/ Contaminated	Surgery, during which no major break in sterile technique occurs, performed on organs or areas with a bacterial population but no inflammation or pus, or on sterile organs or cavities connected with areas containing bacteria. This includes procedures in which the surgeon enters a sterile body cavity and exits through another cavity with a bacterial population.	Appendectomy, gastric and small bowel resections, abdominal hysterectomy, cesarean section (sterile uterus connects to bacterially contaminated vagina), open fractures less than eight to 10 hours old.	Approximately 5%
Contaminated infected	Surgery performed on areas where there's acute inflammation and/or pus and on wounds containing foreign matter; procedures during which drainage spills from one organ or body cavity to another, or a significant break in sterile technique occurs.	Appendectomy with perforation; colon, rectal, and vaginal surgery; bowel resection with peritonitis or perforation; lacerations and open fractures more than eight to 10 hours old; oral surgery; incision and drainage of abscesses, boils, and infected pilonidal cysts.	30% or greater

Continued on next page

How wounds heal

The wound healing process includes eight basic stages:

1. Red blood cells and other blood elements form a clot, which fills the wound and begins to knot its edges together with shreds of fibrin.

2. Dried proteins form a scab that seals off the wound, to prevent fluid loss and bacterial invasion.

3. White blood cells remove bacteria and foreign material from the wound by phagocytosis. Inflammation and edema can occur.

4. Epithelial cells migrate into the wound from the edges, closing the surface under the scab.

5. Fibroblasts synthesize collagen, to form new connective tissue and aid in scar formation.

6. Granulation tissue, containing new capillary buds, forms from existing capillaries and further promotes scar formation.

7. Collagen fibers realign along the stress line, to form the final thickness of the scar.

8. Scar tissue shrinks and contracts.

Although all wounds go through the same basic healing process, they don't all heal in an identical manner. Depending on the amount of tissue loss or damage, they'll heal by first intention or second intention. The major differences between these two types of healing lie in the time required for each stage in the healing process, and the amount of scar formation involved.

Clean incised (closed surgical) wounds and other wounds involving a minimal amount of tissue destruction usually heal by first intention (primary healing), since their edges can be approximated. Shreds of fibrin connect the approximated edges of the wound, epithelialization and collagen formation occur, and a small amount of granulation tissue fills in the area. There is little suppuration or inflammation, and minimal scarring.

Second intention healing occurs in wounds where the edges can't be approximated because of extensive tissue damage or loss. These include open or infected surgical (and traumatic) wounds—for example, excision of cysts and tumors and excision and drainage of abscesses. Second intention healing is also known as healing by granulation, or indirect union. A large amount of granulation tissue forms to fill the gap between the edges of the wound and to allow epithelial cells to migrate across the wound surface from the edges. (Epithelialization is essential to proper collagen formation within the wound.) Second intention healing takes longer than first intention healing and usually produces greater scarring, which can lead to severe contraction of the skin and deformity or malfunction of affected body parts.

Reprinted by permission from "Post-Op Wound Dressings" by Cecelia Meshelany in *RN Magazine*, May 1979, Copyright 1979, Litton Industries.

Pain

Patients' Responses When Asked What Nurses and Doctors Could Do About Pain

"Slow down, don't hurry so, you can't hurry pain."

"What is more important than talking to patients about pain?"

"Be prompt. Try to understand. Make more of an effort."

"Stop telling people they don't have pain when they actually do. Don't try to feel for people when you can't know if they hurt or not."

"Don't make judgments when you don't know and haven't hurt."

"Don't ignore patients in pain and give them the brushoff—we aren't a bunch of neurotics."

"Have confidence you can help the pain—if you had more confidence we would, too."

"Be realistic about pain. Don't be too casual or flip."

"Don't assume the shot or pill helps."

"If you had hurt just once, you wouldn't hand out this 'It won't hurt a bit' routine."

"I'd like one doctor and one nurse each shift. There isn't enough energy to describe the pain over and over again."

"See patients as individuals and not textbook pictures."

"Don't be callous. You treat patients like a garage repairman but we aren't automobiles."

"Prescribe fewer pain pills and shots and get down to the cause."

Reprinted from "The Spectrum of Suffering by Laurel Copp in the *American Journal of Nursing,* March, 1974, p. 493.

Comparative Uses of Hot and Cold Applications

Hot Applications

Dilate local superficial blood vessels.
Increase blood flow (perhaps more than doubling the flow).
Increase capillary pressure, thus causing more transudation of fluid through capillary walls with increased lymph formation and accelerated lymph flow.
Reduce local inflammatory swellings, reduce tissue pressure, and reduce pain from pressure.
Reduce painful muscle spasm by causing muscle to relax.
Increase peristaltic movement in intestines if the abdominal wall is heated. (This is important in treating painful abdominal distention caused by paralytic ileus of the bowel.)

Cold Applications

Constrict local superficial blood vessels.
Decrease blood flow.
Produce temporary reduction of inflammatory swelling which, in turn, reduces pain.
Reduce pain sensitivity since marked chilling acts as a local anesthetic.
Decrease peristaltic movement in intestines if the abdominal wall is cooled. (This is important in the treatment of inflammatory disorders in the peritoneal cavity since intestinal immobilization slows down spread of infection.)

Reprinted by permission of W. B. Saunders Co. from *Medical-Surgical Nursing: A Psychophysiological Approach* by Joan Luckmann and Karen Sorenson, © 1974, W. B. Saunders Co.

Methods of Oxygen Administration

METHOD	L/MIN	CONCENTRATION PERCENTAGE	ADVANTAGES, DISADVANTAGES, GENERAL COMMENTS
Nasal catheter	6-8	30-50	Causes little restriction of movement. Mouth breathing prevents an adequate concentration. If inserted too deeply can cause gastric distention from swallowing air. Some nasal irritation usually occurs.
Nasal cannula	4-6	30-40	The general comments above pertain. Cannulas can cause severe irritation.
Mask—without bag —bag	6-8 10-12	35-55 55-65	Can be removed easily by patient. It is hard to fit. May allow CO_2 retention at lower liter flows. Some patients complain of moisture around face.
Tent	10-15	21-50	Provides cool environment and relative freedom of movement for patient who needs bed rest. Expensive. Some patients complain of coolness and moisture accumulations. Patient may feel claustrophobic.
IPPB units pressure-controlled	0-15	0-100	Depends on cooperation of conscious patient. Helps overcome pulmonary resistance. Medications may be nebulized and instilled with air.
Volume-controlled respirators	0-25	0-100	Best method in respiratory insufficiency. Size and noise of machine may bother conscious patient if used long-term. Patient is immobilized while it is in use.

Reprinted with permission of J. B. Lippincott Company from *Advanced Concepts in Clinical Nursing,* 2nd edition, edited by Kay Corman Kintzel, © Copyright J. B. Lippincott, 1977.

General Nursing Assessment, Intervention, and Evaluation During IV Therapy

Parameter	Assessment	Intervention	Evaluation

Renal function	Prior to starting infusion:
	1. Obtain base-line measurements for urine sugar and sp gr.
	
	2. If sp gr is ≤ 1.010, obtain sp gr q 4 h.
	
	3. a. Obtain base-line body weight.
	   b. Observe hourly urine output if patient is intensively ill, diabetic, aged, comatose, postsurgery or has head injury, pulmonary infection, or pulmonary cancer.
		1. Measure and record urine output q 8 h unless otherwise indicated.
		
		2. a. If base-line specific gravity ≤ 1.010, measure and record urine output q 1 h.
		   b. If base-line measurement indicates glycosuria, report to doctor. If infusion is glucose, watch for changes in levels of consciousness, diuresis.
		   c. If patient is diabetic and infusion is glucose, check with doctor for insulin coverage.
		
		3. a. Insert Foley catheter, measure urine output q 1 h.
		   b. Weigh daily, using bed scale if necessary.
		   c. Report weight change of 5%/24 h, gain or loss, to doctor.
			1. Urine output during IV therapy should
			   a. Range from 30–60 ml/h to amount infused over last 1–3 h.
			   b. Be less during the night than during the day (i.e., normal diurnal rhythm).
			   c. Be less during first 24–48 h after surgery.
			   d. Be reported immediately if it increases beyond infusion per hour or decreases below 30–60 ml/h.
			
			2. Urine specific gravity during IV therapy:
			   a. Normal for the specific patient, i.e., similar to base-line sp gr, or rising if patient is dehydrated or postsurgery. Falling sp gr indicates too-rapid IV flow rate, renal failure, or ↑ ADH. Decrease flow rate, observe sp gr and output, and notify doctor.
			   b. Urine sugar during dextrose infusion should be negative. Glycosuria indicates IV flow rate is too rapid or kidney is failing. If output is also greatly increased, osmotic diuresis is occurring. Decrease flow rate. If glycosuria and increased output continue, notify doctor.
			
			3. a. If weight gain > 5%/24 h, observe for mania, inattention, staring, sudden convulsions, anorexia, nausea, vomiting, and water intoxication symptoms. Stop infusion. Call doctor.

Continued on next page

Parameter	Assessment	Intervention	Evaluation
Cardiac function	At beginning of infusion:		
	1. Obtain base-line BP, noting pulse pressure (i.e., systolic − diastolic (normal pulse pressure = 30 mmHg).	1. a. Unless orders indicate otherwise, start IV at recommended flow rate for tonicity. (See ranges in Table 10-12.) (1) Hypertonic, 100 ml/h (2) Hypotonic, 200 ml/h (3) Isotonic, 400 ml/h b. Obtain precise order for flow rate, requesting a minimal-maximal range.	1. Narrowing pulse pressure indicates decreased cardiac output. Increase IV flow rate. Notify doctor.
	2. Observe neck veins for distention.	2. If patient has pulse pressure < 30 mmHg, distended neck veins, rapid or slow pulse, and/or, history of a cardiac or pulmonary problem a. Obtain order for central venous pressure monitering. b. If there is no order for a flow rate range, start IV at minimal flow rate for tonicity and obtain physician's order for a flow rate range, i.e., a minimal-maximal range over which IV may be adjusted relative to changes in BP, pulse, or central venous pressure.	2. Distended neck veins indicate failing heart and circulatory overload. Decrease IV flow rate. Notify doctor.
	3. Check pulse for rate and rhythm.		3. Increasing pulse rate indicates heart is attempting to compensate for decreased cardiac output. Increase flow rate. Notify doctor.
	4. Check history for cardiac or pulmonary problems.		4. Rising CVP indicates possible onset of cardiac failure and overload. Decrease flow rate and notify doctor. Falling CVP indicates poor venous return and possible onset of shock. Increase flow rate and notify doctor.

5. Auscultate lungs for moist-breath sounds.

5. Dyspnea rates indicate circulatory overload and pulmonary edema. Decrease flow rate. Notify doctor.

Central nervous system function

At start of infusion:
1. Obtain and record base-line observations of
   a. Level of consciousness.
   b. Activity (e.g., restlessness).
   c. Neuromuscular irritability (e.g., twitching muscles, jerking foot).
   d. Mental state (e.g., irritability, confusion, disorientation).
2. Note if patient had narcotic or anesthesia.
3. Before making judgments concerning aged and intensively ill patients
   a. Listen carefully to conversation to be certain before labeling patient confused.
   b. Check environment for misleading cues, i.e., paging system, lights on 24 h day, monitor alarms.
   c. Check environment for lack of cues to date or time, i.e., no radio, television, newspaper, clock, or calendar.

1. Maintain hypotonic fluid at flow rate appropriate to tonicity. Use slower rate for aged, postsurgical, neurological, and neurosurgical patients and for those with pulmonary infections or pulmonary cancer (patients with poor circulation or increased ADH secretion).
2. Have periodic, scheduled check of the patient's central nervous system function. That is, when urine output is being checked, check level of consciousness, mental status, etc.
3. Provide for rest, comfort, and relief of pain. Also provide sensory stimuli and control sensory overload in order to create environment in which responses elicited from the patient will be more reflective of response to therapy.

1. Stop infusion if there are any sudden behavioral changes (e.g., violence, mania, irritability, confusion) during hypotonic infusion. Notify doctor.
2. Call the doctor if there is a change in level of consciousness with any tonicity infusion.
3. Increased temperature and increased serum sodium with behavioral and/or level of consciousness changes may indicate onset of hyperosmolar coma. Notify doctor. If IV is saline, use minimal to midrange flow rate. If IV is 5% D/W, use very slow flow rate. If given too rapidly, extracellular fluid will be diluted too rapidly and fluid will shift into brain. (See symptoms of water intoxication.)

Reprinted with permission of McGraw-Hill Book Company from *The Nurse's Guide to Fluid and Electrolyte Balance*, by Audrey Burgess, © Copyright 1979 McGraw-Hill.

Superficial Veins, Dorsal Aspect of Hand.

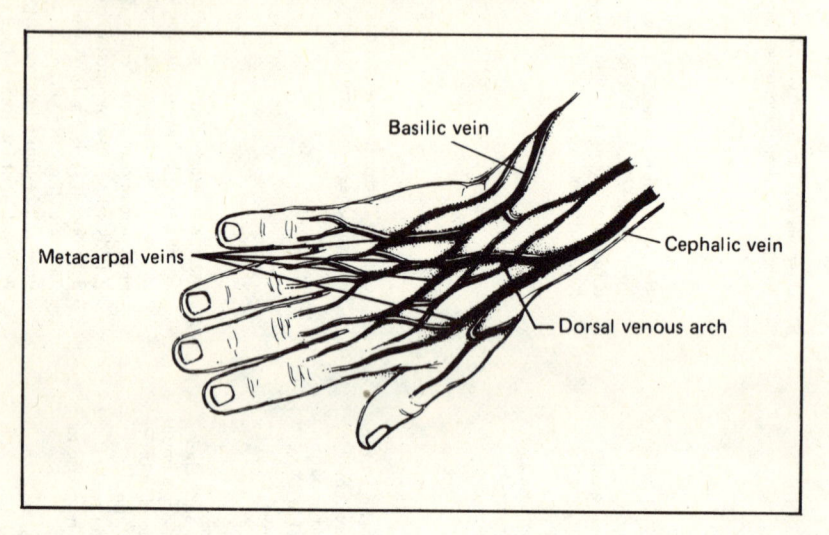

- Basilic vein
- Metacarpal veins
- Cephalic vein
- Dorsal venous arch

Superficial Veins, Forearm.

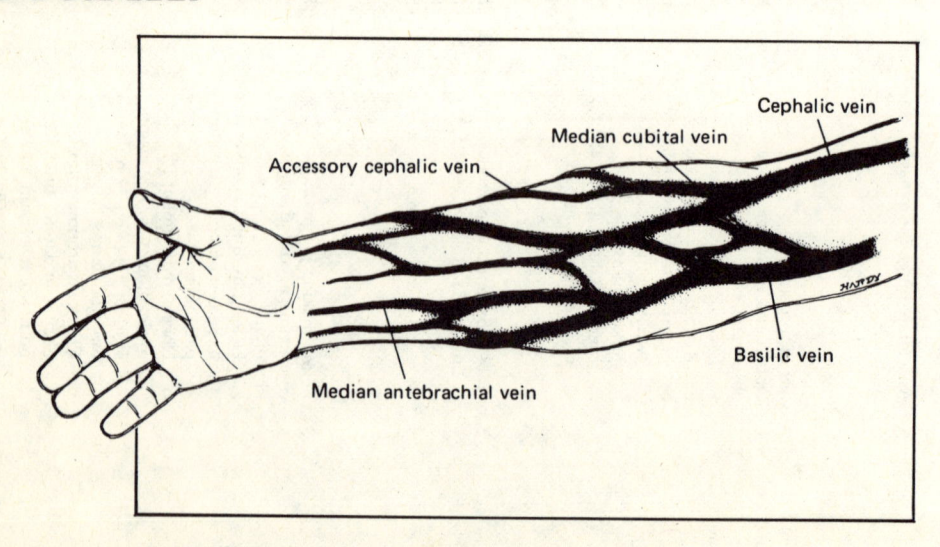

- Accessory cephalic vein
- Median cubital vein
- Cephalic vein
- Median antebrachial vein
- Basilic vein

Reprinted by permission of J. B. Lippincott Co. from *The Lippincott Manual of Nursing Practice*, 2nd edition, by Lillian Brunner and Doris Suddarth, © 1978, J. B. Lippincott Co.

Prevention, Assessment, and Intervention Methods for Complications of IV Therapy

Complication	Prevention	Assessment	Intervention
Infiltration	Stabilize IV site well.	Edema Hardness of skin at IV site Pain Sloughing with Levophed or calcium solutions	1. Stop infusion. 2. Apply warm soaks to site. 3. If Levophed, get order to inject the IV site with Regitine (phentolamine) 5–10 mg/10–15 ml 0.9% saline. 4. Restart IV in new site.

Pyrogenic reaction	Don't give solutions which are:
	  Cloudy.
	  In an open bottle.
	  In a cracked bottle.
		During first hour of IV:
		Fever
		Chills
		Flushed face
		Tingling sensations and sudden change in pulse rate (↑)
			1. Stop infusion.
			2. Notify doctor.
			3. Record name of solution, lot number, manufacturer, added medications.
			4. Save solution for laboratory analysis.

Thrombophlebitis	1. Don't milk IV tubing vigorously. 2. Adjust needle carefully in vein.	Pain Redness of vein Swelling of site Keflin (cephalothin), penicillin, $NaHCO_3$ 3–5% or NH_4Cl 2.14% all predispose to development of thrombi.	1. Stop infusion. 2. Restart in another extremity. 3. Do not massage limb or site. 4. First apply cold compresses, then warm.

Continued on next page

150

Complication	Prevention	Assessment	Intervention

Speed shock	1. Know and use safe flow rate for tonicity of fluid.
	2. If drugs are added to fluid, consider age and cardiac and renal status of patient.
	3. May result from patient's position during sleep.
	   a. Normal ↓ urine formation at night ↓ rate of fluid removal from blood during sleep.
	   b. Position change can increase flow rate.
		Pounding headache
		Chills
		Apprehension
		Fainting
		Dyspnea
		Back pain
			1. Stop infusion.
			2. Notify doctor.

Air embolism	1. Nonrigid containers reduce risk of air embolism. 2. Run IV fluid through tubing before starting IV. 3. Discontinue IV before it runs dry. Clamp off empty bottle in a tandem set, or air will be drawn into vein. 4. Don't elevate extremity being infused above level of heart. 5. Occurs most commonly with subclavian catheter administration. 6. Some electric pumps may pump air into veins when bottle is empty.	Cyanosis Falling BP Tachycardia Falling CVP Loss of consciousness	1. Stop infusion. 2. Give oxygen. 3. Place on left side in Trendelenburg position. 4. Notify doctor.

Reprinted with permission of McGraw-Hill Book Company from *The Nurse's Guide to Fluid and Electrolyte Balance* by Audrey Burgess, © Copyright 1979, McGraw-Hill Book Company.

Summary of Bedside Intravascular Monitoring Techniques in Critically Ill Patients

Procedure	Needle or catheter used	Site	Technique	Complications
Single arterial blood sampling	20-gauge with heparinized syringe	Brachial, femoral radial arteries	Percutaneous	Local hematoma, occlusion
Multiple arterial blood samples	20-gauge, 1.5-inch Longdwell catheter-needles (Becton, Dickson & Co, Rutherford, NJ)	Radial artery	Percutaneous	Local hematoma, occlusion
	18-gauge Cournand needle with stylet (Becton, Dickinson & Co, Rutherford, NJ)	Brachial artery	Percutaneous	Local hematoma, occlusion
	18-gauge Longdwell catheter needle with stylet (Becton, Dickinson & Co, Rutherford, NJ)	Brachial artery	Percutaneous	Local hematoma, occlusion
Monitoring intraarterial pressure	16-gauge Deseret radiopaque catheter, 24 inches (Deseret Pharmaceutical Co, Sandy, Utah)	Radial artery advanced to subclavian artery, brachial artery	Arteriotomy	Local occlusion, embolism
	No. 7 French Gensini percutaneous catheter, 100 cm (U.S. Catheter and Instrument Corp, Glens Falls, NY)	Femoral artery	Percutaneous by Seldinger technique (18-gauge Cournand needle and 125-cm 0.035-inch spring guide)	Local hematoma and occlusion, embolism

Continued on next page

Procedure	Needle or catheter used	Site	Technique	Complications
Monitoring left ventricular pressure	No. 5.5F precurved Kifa radiopaque polyethylene catheter, 100 cm (U.S. Catheter & Instrument Corp, Glens Falls, NY)	Femoral artery	Percutaneous by Seldinger technique; blind passage or fluoroscopic control across the aortic valve	Local occlusion embolism; ventricular arrhythmia, myocardial perforation
Monitoring central venous pressure	16-gauge Deseret radiopaque catheter, 24 inches (Deseret Pharmaceutical Co, Sandy, Utah)	Median basilic vein Subclavian vein	Percutaneous or cutdown Percutaneous	Phlebitis Pneumothorax, air embolism; hemothorax
		Deep brachial, cephalic, or external jugular vein	Cutdown	Phlebitis
Monitoring pulmonary artery and wedge pressures	No. 5 French Swan-Ganz flow-directed right heart catheter—No. 7 French Swan-Ganz thermodilution flow-guided catheter used for thermodilution technique of measuring cardial output (Edwards Laboratories, Santa Ana, Calif)	Median basilic or deep brachial vein most commonly used Femoral vein	Cutdown Percutaneous via Deseret catheter introducer system (USCI)	Ventricular inability, VPCs V fibrillation
Monitoring coronary sinus lactate and coronary blood flow	No. 7 French Goodale-Lubin Dacron, standard wall 125-cm catheter (U.S. Catheter & Instrument Corp, Glens Falls, NY)	Left median basilic or deep brachial vein	Cutdown	Occlusion, perforation of coronary sinus

Reprinted from Ayres, Gianelli and Mueller. *Care of the Critically Ill*, 2nd Ed., 1974. Courtesy of Appleton-Century-Crofts, Publishing Division of Prentice-Hall, Inc.

Hemolytic Transfusion Reaction

Care in Hemolytic Transfusion Reaction

Drugs and Treatments Used to Counteract Reaction

1. Intravenous infusions of dextrose in water to counteract shock and promote diuresis.
2. Oxygen and epinephrine to treat dyspnea and wheezing.
3. Sedation to counteract restlessness and apprehension.
4. Indwelling catheter to accurately evaluate urine output.
5. Mannitol (an osmotic diuretic) to counteract oliguria. (See Chapter 26.)
6. Blood transfusion (with properly matched blood) to control shock.
7. Vasopressor drugs in event of severe shock (Chap. 26).

Nursing Actions

1. Discontinue blood immediately.
2. Notify physician and laboratory.
3. Return blood and sample of patient's blood to laboratory for another type and crossmatch.
4. Connect bottle of dextrose in water as ordered to blood or I.V. tubing to keep I.V. open.
5. Administer oxygen and other drugs as ordered.
6. Take vital signs every 15 to 30 minutes; observe for hypotension and shock.
7. Start intake and output record; observe for oliguria or anuria.
8. Insert Foley catheter and measure urine hourly.
9. Allay patient's anxiety.
10. Observe for effects of vasopressor drugs (Chap. 26).

Care in Bacterial Transfusion Reaction

Drugs and Treatments Used to Counteract Reaction

1. Intravenous infusions of dextrose in water to counteract shock and promote diuresis.
2. Vasopressor drugs to maintain systolic blood pressure above 100 mm. mercury.
3. Corticosteroids to abate inflammatory reaction.
4. Broad spectrum antibiotics in high dosages.

Nursing Actions

1. Discontinue blood and notify physician.
2. Return blood and sample of patient's blood to laboratory for culture and sensitivity tests.
3. Take vital signs every 15 to 30 minutes despite patient's "rosy" coloring; observe for hypotension and shock.

Continued on next page

5. Indwelling catheter to properly evaluate urine output.
6. Blood (properly retested for contaminants) to counteract shock.

Care in Allergic Transfusion Reaction

*Drugs and Treatments Used
to Counteract Reactions*

Nursing Actions

1. *Mild reactions*: antihistamines and antipyretics given directly to patient and *not* into the blood transfusion.
2. *Severe reactions*: epinephrine, vasopressors and corticosteroids.
3. Appropriate respiratory therapy.

1. *Slow* blood if *mild* reaction; *stop* blood if *severe* reaction and connect intravenous fluids.
2. Notify physician.
3. Give medications to patient as ordered.
4. Allay anxiety.

Care in Circulatory Overload

*Drugs and Treatments Used
to Counteract Reactions*

Nursing Actions

1. Digitalis to counteract congestive heart failure.
2. Venesection or rotating tourniquets to remove excess fluid from the general circulation. (See Unit X.)

1. Stop transfusion and notify physician.
2. Give digitalis as ordered.
3. Set up for venesection or rotating tourniquets.

(Continued from previous column)

4. Start I.V. fluids; give medications as ordered.
5. Insert Foley catheter; record intake and output.
6. Take temperature every hour; start cooling measures (alcohol rubs, cool sponge) if temperature is elevated above 101°F.

Reprinted by permission of W. B. Saunders Co. from *Medical-Surgical Nursing: A Psychophysiological Approach*, by Joan Luckmann and Karen Sorenson, © 1974, W. B. Saunders Co.

Nursing Assessment, Intervention, and Evaluation During Peritoneal Dialysis

Time	Assessment	Intervention	Evaluation

Serial determinations prior, during, and after dialysis	Body weight
	Serum electrolytes and albumin
	Blood gases
	Blood glucose
	Urine sugars
	Vital signs
		1. Always weigh patient at same point in the cycle, i.e., with fluid in or out of peritoneal cavity.
		2. Preparation of dialysate
		  a. Warm to body temperature to promote diffusion and conserve body heat.
		  b. Add all medications to 1 liter of the dialysate to help prevent infection.
		  c. Use aseptic technique.
		3. Run fluid through administration tubing to remove air.
		4. Heparin is added to dialysate to prevent clot formation and promote drainage.
		5. Change administration tubing once every 24 h.
			1. "Wet" weight serves as a baseline to determine rapidity of fluid removal.
			2. 2.2 lb weight loss or gain indicates 1 liter of fluid removed or retained.
			3. If high serum Na^+, observe for signs of hypernatremia, e.g., drowsiness.
			4. If high HCO_3^-, observe for signs of increasing alkalosis (e.g., drowsiness, hypoventilation).
			5. ↑blood sugar, and/or glycosuria Report to physician, who may order insulin or a reduction in concentration of dialysate.
			6. Watch for hypotension, a sign of too rapid fluid removal.
			7. Do not heat dialysate above body temperature.
			8. Air in peritoneal cavity will cause pain and/or poor returns.

Inflow period	Respirations Pulse Abdominal discomfort and pain	1. Position patient at 45° angle. 2. Slow inflow rate to alleviate discomfort, pain, or mild dyspnea. 3. Optimum inflow period time is 5–10 min. 4. Record amount of dialysate infused, unusual thirst,	1. Acute dyspnea, tachycardia, rales, rapid respirations, and orthopnea may indicate acute pulmonary edema. Stop inflow and call doctor. 2. Acute pain may indicate bowel perforation. *Continued on next page*

	hypotension, and/or glycosuria.	
	5. Hypoventilation and drowsiness should be reported to the physician.	
Equilibration period	Respirations Level of consciousness Blood pressure Thirst Comfort Urine sugar q 6 h	1. Shorter equilibration may be ordered to increase rate of K^+ removal. 2. Longer equilibration, if ordered, indicates need to observe urine more frequently for sugar. Dextrose may be absorbed into blood. Also observe for hypoventilation, changes in levels of consciousness. Increased HCO_3^- in blood → compensatory hypoventilation, retention of CO_2.
	1. Change position of patient frequently to promote diffusion and control hypoventilation. 2. Give hygienic care during this period. 3. Optimum equilibration period time is 20–30 min.	

Outflow period	Dialysate returns
	Body weight
		1. Returns should be clear.
		  a. Mucous, shreds, pus or cloudy returns indicate infection.
		  b. Fecal matter indicates bowel perforation.
		  c. Blood-tinged after first few cycles indicates possible bowel perforation.
		2. If less dialysate is returned than infused, patient is retaining fluid. Desired result is a loss of fluid, that is, more fluid returned than fluid infused.
		3. "Dry" weight serves as a guide to the patient for weight change between dialysis treatments. Expected gain is no more than 1 lb/day.

	1. Collect specimen of returns for each cycle. Mark cycle 1, 2, etc., and tape to head of bed. Optimum outflow period is 20 min. 2. Position patient to obtain maximum outflow. 3. Record amount of dialysate returned. 4. If amount returned is less than that infused, the difference is recorded in the "plus" column, since the patient gained fluid. 5. If amount returned is greater than that infused, the difference is recorded in the "minus" column, since the patient lost fluid. 6. Weigh at end of dialysis.	

Reprinted with permission of McGraw-Hill Book Company from *The Nurse's Guide to Fluid and Electrolyte Balance* by Audrey Burgess, © Copyright 1979, McGraw-Hill Book Company.

Bladder Elimination

I. Catheterization

A Equipment
1 Two or more sterile catheters
2 Sterile towels
3 Sterile collecting basin for urine
4 Sterile basin with sterile antiseptic solution
5 Sterile swabs
6 Sterile lubricant
7 Sterile gloves
8 Sterile specimen bottle
9 Standing lamp with flexible neck

B Method of Preparation
1 Equipment
 a Place lamp so that light is directed to perineal area
 b Unwrap sterile equipment and supplies and place conveniently on a flat surface

2 Patient
 a Female patient lying flat on back with knees flexed and feet spread wide; male patient flat on back
 b Drape each leg and body of patient so that only perineal area of female or penis of male is exposed

C Method of Procedure
1 Put on sterile gloves or surgically scrub hands
2 Place sterile towels over pubes and under perineal area of female or under penis of male

Continued on next page

3 Lubricate catheter
4 Female
  a With thumb and index finger, spread labia and expose meatus of urethra
  b Cleanse meatus with sterile swabs dipped in antiseptic solution and discard swab
  c Gently insert catheter into meatus
  d After initial contraction of meatus, insert catheter 3 to 4 cm (1½ to 2 inches)
5 Male
  a Retract foreskin of penis
  b Cleanse tip of penis with antiseptic solution
  c Insert catheter 8 to 10 cm (4 to 5 inches)
6 Place open end of catheter into sterile collecting basin
7 When urine ceases to flow, remove catheter and dry perineum with sterile towel
8 Remove equipment and cover patient
9 Measure quantity of urine and record on chart

D Special Considerations
1 The danger of bladder infection is so great that catheterization should not be done *unless absolutely necessary and other methods of encouraging voiding fail*
2 Sterile technique must be used
3 Catheter should not be inserted in female until you are positive you see the meatus of urethra; if catheter touches other than meatus, it is contaminated
4 If specimen is desired, collect specimen in a sterile specimen container before placing end of catheter in collecting basin

II. Retention Catheterization

A Equipment
The same as for a catheterization, except catheters have inflatable bags around tip (Foley catheters) and three additional parts are needed:
1 Sterile connecting tip
2 Sterile rubber or plastic tubing
3 Sterile collecting bag or bottle

B Method of Preparation
  1 Equipment
    a Same as for catheterization
    b Check balloon in retention catheter
  2 Patient. Same as for catheterization

C Method of Procedure
  1 Catheterize patient as directed
  2 Leave catheter in place and inflate bag at tip
  3 Connect catheter, tubing, and drainage bottle, using sterile technique
  4 Remove remaining equipment
  5 Cover patient
  6 Suspend collecting bottle from bedframe at side of bed
  7 Pin tubing to bottom sheet, leaving some slack to allow patient to move

D Special Considerations
  1 Indwelling catheters carry a high risk of bladder infection; every effort should be made to help the patient void normally
  2 If the catheter must be irrigated, sterile technique must be used
  3 Patients with indwelling catheters usually require extra fluids by mouth

Reprinted by permission of John Wiley and Sons, Inc., from *Handbook of Fundamental Nursing Techniques*, by Mildred Montag and Alice Rines, © 1976, by John Wiley and Sons, Inc.

Acute head injury: A plan

FIRST PRIORITY: The abc's of trauma

AIRWAY
Determine patency of airway immediately; do not leave unconscious patient unattended; have oral suction ready for use.

BREATHING
Note rate, rhythm, and depth of respirations; observe patient's color for signs of inadequate O₂ exchange.

CIRCULATION
Check rate of pulse, and quality; look for signs of hemorrhaging.

PERTINENT HISTORY

Determine:
- Circumstances of injury
  —acceleration-deceleration
  —direct blow
- Time lapsed since injury
- Clinical course since injury
- Treatment prior to arrival
- Period of unconsciousness
- Patient's memory of accident
  —events before
  —events after
- History of illness (e.g., diabetes, heart disease, glaucoma), and medications being taken

VITAL SIGNS

(With increased intracranial pressure (ICP), changes in vital signs are opposite to hypovolemic shock.)
- Rectal temperatures q2h (Hyperthermia is a later sign of ICP.)
- Pulse (rate, rhythm, quality) q15min until stable
- Respirations (rate rhythm, depth) q30min (Also assess breath sound initially, and observe for ataxic breathing, hyperventilation, and Cheyne-Stokes respiration.)
- Blood pressure q15min (Widening pulse pressure indicates ICP.)

PHYSICAL EXAM

- Rule out possible spinal injury
- Describe injury to other organ systems.
- Note location and size of abrasions, lacerations, hematomas, ecchymoses.
- Observe for clinical signs of basal skull fracture:
  Hemotympanum (blood behind eardrum)
  CSF rhinorrhea, or otorrhea
  Periorbital ecchymosis (without history of eye injury)
  Battle's sign (mastoid ecchymosis)

TREATMENT

Maintain airway
- Oral airway
- Cuffed ET tube
- Assisted/mechanical ventilation
- Oral suction
- Mechanical hyperventilation (By decreasing pCO₂, the intravascular blood volume of the brain also drops, thereby decreasing ICP.)

Maintain adequate circulation and perfusion
- Control hemorrhage
- Pulse and blood pressure q15min until stable

Basic first aid
- Immobilize until spinal injury is ruled out.
- Cleanse abrasions and lacerations; apply sterile dressing.
- Apply ice to hematomas.
- Splint obvious fractures.

Diagnostic tests
- Skull X-rays
- Lateral cervical spine X-ray
- CT scan
- Angiography
- Echoencephalography
- Laboratory values (CBC, UA, ABG, glucose, and serum chemistry)

REMEMBER:

- If a head trauma patient is semi-comatose on arrival in the ED, it's essential to observe if the patient's level of consciousness is stable or improving (sign suggests concussion), or if the patient regained consciousness after impact and is now deteriorating (sign suggests cerebral edema or intracranial hematoma).

- Skull fractures without associated intracranial hemorrhage or cerebral edema will not necessarily cause coma or clinical deterioration.

- Acute head injury alone does not cause signs of shock; look for other causative factors.

- Head trauma may cause damage at the point of injury as well as point directly opposite the injury (contracoup).

- Because of their small total blood volume, infants and small children may lose blood volume from scalp lacerations sufficient to cause hypovolemia.

- In a brightly lit room, pupils may show minimal or no response

for assessment

NEUROLOGICAL EXAM

Check level of consciousness:
- Alert
- Lethargic
- Stuporous
- Semi-comatose
- Comatose

Assess orientation:
- Time
- Place
- Person

(Disorientation occurs first to time, last to person.)

Assess pupil size and consensual reactivity.

Note slurred speech or aphasia.

Note restless, combative, or irrational behavior (may indicate rising ICP).

Assess motor function:
- Spontaneous motor activity (note symmetry, purposefulness)
- Response to pain
  purposeful (withdraws from or pushes stimulus away)
  stereotyped
  —*decerebrate (marked extension of all extremities)*
  —*decorticate (flexion of arms at elbows, extension of legs)*
- Cranial nerve function (frown, grimace, whistle, stick out tongue, raise eyebrows)
- Spinal nerve function (deep tendon reflexes are graded on a sliding scale where +1 = diminished; +2 = normal; +3 = brisker than normal; and +4 = hyperactive)
- Gag reflex
- Corneal reflex

- Babinski sign (abnormal—great toe extends, other toes fan)
- Oculocephalic eye movements (abnormal—eyeball of unresponsive patient remains in midposition when head is turned from right to left)
- Arm raise (have patient close eyes and extend arms horizontally for 30 seconds. If one arm drifts down without patient's realizing it, motor impairment is indicated.)
- Leg raise (Have patient raise legs alternately off the bed. Difficulty or inability to perform this may indicate motor impairment.)
- Gait
  —*normal*
  —*ataxic (uncoordinated, staggering)*
  —*Parkinsonian (shuffling, stooped)*
- Seizure activity (if present, describe)
- Bowel and bladder control

Monitor for rising ICP
- Vital signs q15min until stable, then q2h
- Neuro checks q15min initially, then q1h
- Report variations in pulse, respirations, or blood pressure; and irregular respirations

Supportive treatment
- IV fluids at "keep open" rate
- Nasogastric tube
- Urinary catheter (monitor urine output)

Medications
- Mannitol (20%) 1.5 gm/kg IV over 30-60 min
- Decadron 10 mg IV initially, then maintenance dosage

Definitive treatment
- Surgery to evacuate intracranial hematomas, or to debride and align depressed skull fractures

---

to light because they are already constricted. Dim room lights to evaluate patient's reactivity to light.

- The corneal reflex test may produce an opposite side response, or a diminished response on the compression side. For example: with fifth nerve compression, you'll get a diminished direct response on the stroked side, and a consensual response on the other side.

- Pupil dilation occurs on the same side as the brain injury. It is important for you to remember that a common cause of pupil dilation, however, is direct eye injury.

- Motor deficit occurs on the side opposite the injury.

- As intracranial pressure rises, it can exceed the systemic arterial pressure resulting in decreased cerebral blood flow and hypoxia. To compensate for this, the systolic blood pressure rises in an attempt to increase cerebral blood flow, thus causing a widened pulse pressure. As arterial pressure rises, the heart rate slows as a result of stimulation to receptors in the carotid sinus.

Reprinted by permission from *RN Magazine*, May, 1979, by Terri Poehland, R.N., Copyright 1979, Litton Industries.

Nursing Interventions for Patients on Chemotherapy

Symptom	Cause	Nursing Intervention
Gastrointestinal toxicity Anorexia, nausea, emesis.	5-FU, Cytoxan, nitrogen mustard, bleomycin, 6-MP, Imidazole carboxamide, Alkeran, Leukeran, Thio-TEPA, Cytosar, mithramycin, Actinomycin D, androgens, estrogens, progesterones, Thioguanine.	Provide good mouth care, encourage fluids, give appetizing meals. Foods should be bland, not highly spiced. Antiemetics such as Atarax, Vistaril, or Tigan may be given, though these drugs should be used with caution in patients who have liver disease or obstruction. IVs may be necessary.
Stomatitis (oral or stoma), GI ulcerations.	5-FU, Cytoxan, Imidazole carboxamide, nitrogen mustard. Cytosar, 6-MP, Thioguanine, Daunomycin, mithramycin, adriamycin, prednisone.	Provide good mouth care using swabs instead of toothbrushes. Give soft, bland foods. Drugs will be stopped. Mineral oil or Vaseline may be used to soothe the lips. Mouthwashes will only be irritating; may be 1/2 H_2O 1/2 H_2O_2, followed by water rinse. If severe pain exists, Xylocaine viscous may be used before meals, or Chlorseptic mouthwash.
Diarrhea.	5-FU, Cytoxan, nitrogen mustard, Actinomycin D, Imidazole carboxamide, methotrexate, estrogens. May also be caused by some antacids.	Usually drugs will be stopped if there are more than three diarrhea stools a day. Encourage fluids. Kaopectate, Lomotil, or antispasmodics may be given. (Patient should be checked for impaction if he or she has been constipated prior to receiving chemotherapy.) IVs may be needed to replace fluid loss.
Dehydration, electrolyte imbalance.	Any of the above drugs, especially those leading to diarrhea.	Give serum electrolytes, IVs, electrolyte replacement therapy. Patients with dehydration are much more susceptible to hemorrhagic cystitis if on Cytoxan. They are also more likely to get obstructive uropathy if their uric acid level is high.
Gastric ulcers.	Prednisone.	Antacids must be given with steroids and continued for at least 1 week after discontinuance of the drug.
Constipation	Vincristine, vinblastine.	Stop drugs. Laxatives and stool softeners are used as preventatives when patients are placed on these drugs.
Bone marrow depression Leukopenia.	Nitrogen mustard, 5-FU, methotrexate, Cytoxan, Imidazole carboxamide, Actinomycin D, vincristine, vinblastine, Alkeran, 6-MP, Cytosar, Thioguanine, Myleran, Leukeran, Daunomycin.	Reduce exposure to infection: give IV care, care for skin lesions, keep infected people away from the patient. If any signs of infection appear, stop chemotherapy drugs, begin antibiotics. May need reverse isolation.

Symptom	Cause	Nursing Intervention
Thrombo-cytopenia.	Same drugs that cause leukopenia.	Take bleeding precautions: patient should shave with an electric razor. Care must be taken with IV or IM injections, and pressure must be held over an injection site for 3–5 min. Requisitions for blood work should have "Bleeding Precautions" written on them. Aspirin in any form should never be given to any chemotherapy patient. If bleeding occurs and is not controlled by pressure dressings Collodian may be applied with a few fibers of cotton and then pressure dressing applied. Platelet transfusions may be given.
Anemia	Same drugs that cause leukopenia. Hemorrhage due to hemorrhagic cystitis or due to mithramycin. Hemorrhage may also be due to GI ulceration from any of the drugs under GI ulcerations.	If there is active bleeding, cause must be found and eliminated. If drug-induced, stop drug and give transfusions while awaiting repopulation of the bone marrow. If due to GI bleeding, surgical intervention may be necessary.
Alopecia	Mithramycin, Cytoxan, nitrogen mustard, 5-FU, vincristine, vinblastine, Actinomycin D, Daunomycin, Adriamycin, prednisone.	Hair loss is usually temporary, and hair will grow again when the drug is discontinued. With some drugs, hair is lost initially but begins to grow again as therapy continues. There is no way to prevent hair loss, but keeping hair clean and neat will help the patient's morale. The patient may wear a hairnet to prevent it from falling all over the bed or floor. Wigs or caps may boost the patient's morale.
Skin sensitivities		
Increased pigmentation, acne, itching, urticaria, nail changes.	5-FU, methotrexate, Myleran, Actinomycin D, Daunomycin, prednisone, bleomycin, androgens.	If urticaria or itching is severe enough, drug may be stopped. Soothing lotions such as Alpha Keri or Caladryl may be used.
Genitourinary toxicity		
Hemorrhagic cystitis.	Cytoxan.	Stop drug immediately. This symptom is caused by high concentrations of drug in the urine due to dehydration. Encourage fluids, give IVs, insert Foley to watch the progress of the bleeding and to get an accurate output. Care must be taken to prevent fluid overload, especially in patients who have preexisting coronary disease. Transfusions may be needed if patient becomes anemic.
Pulmonary toxicity		
Pulmonary fibrosis, cough, hemoptysis.	Bleomycin (fibrosis and hemoptysis), Myleran (cough). Irritation of bronchus by tumor.	Drugs must be stopped. Fibrosis is irreversible, and steroids may be given to suppress symptoms. Cough may be controlled by codeine.
Cardiac toxicity		
Congestive heart failure (peripheral edema, lethargy,	Adriamycin, Daunomycin.	Stop drugs immediately, and it will be reversible if caught in time. To be treated as is failure caused by any other disease.

Continued on next page

Symptom	Cause	Nursing Intervention
drowsiness, etc.)		
Neurotoxicity		
Tingling of fingers and toes. Loss of deep tendon reflexes.	Vincristine, vinblastine. May also be caused by tumor infiltration into area, e.g., in leukemia.	Stop drugs. If caught early enough, may be reversible. If not caught in time, may progress to irreversibility.
Hepatic toxicity		
Jaundice, lethargy, weakness, pruritis, coma.	Cytosar, 6-MP, methotrexate, mithramycin.	Drugs must be stopped. Give IVs, antibiotics as indicated, supportive care.
Blood chemistry changes		
Hypocalcemia.	Mithramycin.	Stop drug. Give calcium gluconate IV.
Hypercalcemia.	Increased bone destruction from any metastatic disease. Adrenal cancer.	Give Mithramycin in low doses. May also use x-ray therapy to the bone lesions to destroy the cancer and promote healing.
Hyperuricemia.	Increased cell death, whether due to tumor destruction or to normal tissue destruction.	Give Zyloprim (blocks the formation of uric acid). Force fluids or patient can go into renal shutdown from uric acid crystals.
Endocrine toxicity		
Diabetes.	Prednisone.	Drug must be stopped. Condition is then reversible. Control of preexisting diabetes is made much more difficult when prednisone is given.
Additional toxicity		
Constipation.	Vincristine, vinblastine.	Stop drugs. Laxatives and stool softeners are used as preventatives when patients are placed on these drugs.
Psychological changes		
Dizziness, headache, confusion, lethargy, euphoria, depression, psychosis.	Nitrogen mustard, Thio-TEPA, Imidazole carboxamide, vinblastine, Actinomycin D, prednisone, estrogens.	Dosage must be adjusted or drug may be stopped.
Fever	Cytosar, Imidazole carboxamide, bleomycin, Daunomycin. Infection. CNS leukemia.	If drug-induced, may give Tylenol or steroids to suppress the symptoms. If patient is on chemotherapy and develops any fever, he or she may be placed on appropriate antibiotics as a precautionary measure after cultures are done. If fever is caused by CNS leukemia, the disease may be controlled by methotrexate given intrathecally.

Reprinted with permission of McGraw-Hill Book Company from *Dynamics of Oncology Nursing* by Pamela Burkhalter and Diana Donley, © Copyright 1978, McGraw-Hill Book Company.

Burn Care

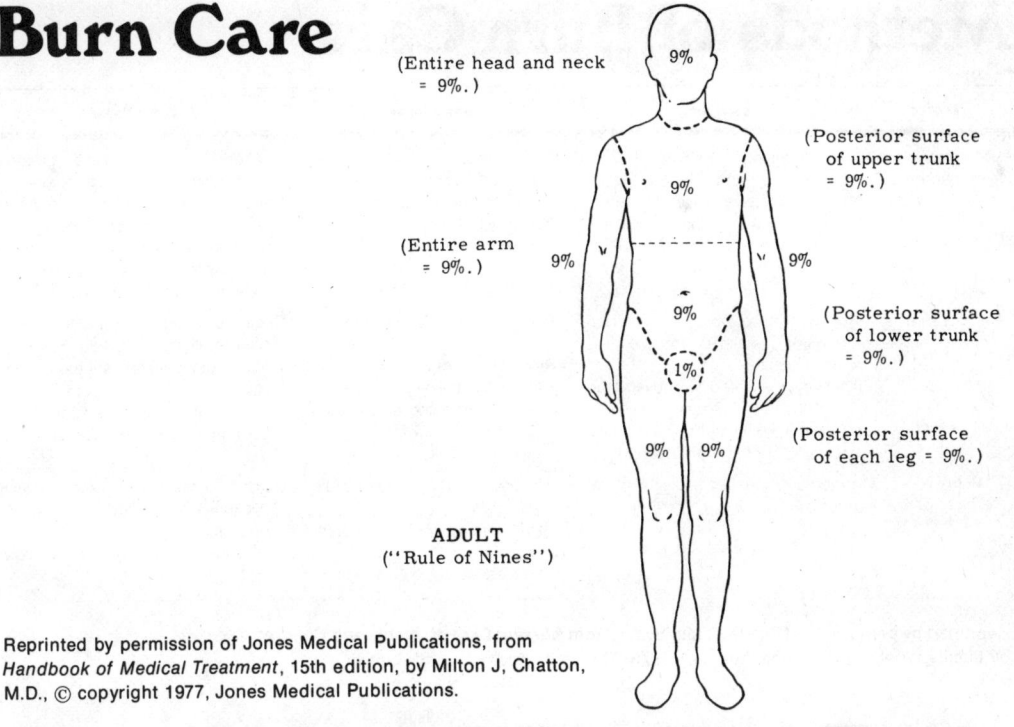

(Entire head and neck = 9%.)

(Posterior surface of upper trunk = 9%.)

(Entire arm = 9%.)

9% 9% 9%
9%
1%
9% 9%

(Posterior surface of lower trunk = 9%.)

(Posterior surface of each leg = 9%.)

ADULT
("Rule of Nines")

Reprinted by permission of Jones Medical Publications, from *Handbook of Medical Treatment*, 15th edition, by Milton J, Chatton, M.D., © copyright 1977, Jones Medical Publications.

Management of Chemical Burns

Agent	Cleansing	Neutralization	Débridement

Acid Burns
  Sulfuric
  Nitric
  Hydrochloric
  Trichloracetic
	Water	Sodium bicarbonate solution	Débride loose, nonviable tissue

Phenol	Ethyl alcohol	Sodium bicarbonate solution	Débride loose, nonviable tissue.
Hydrofluoric	Water	Same as other acids plus magnesium oxide, glycerin paste, local injection, calcium gluconate	Débride loose, nonviable tissue

Alkali Burns
  Potassium hydroxide
  Sodium hydroxide
  Ammonia
	Water	0.5–5.0% acetic acid or 5.0% ammonium chloride	Débride loose, nonviable tissue

Lime	Brush off powder	0.5–5.0% acetic acid or 5.0% ammonium chloride	Débride loose, nonviable tissue
Phosphorus	Water	Copper sulfate soaks	Débride and remove particles of phosphorus
Mustard gas	Water	M-5 ointment	Aspirate; then excise blebs during flushing with water
Tear gas	Water	Sodium bicarbonate solution	Débride loose tissue

Reprinted with permission of J. B. Lippincott Company, from *Advanced Concepts in Clinical Nursing*, 2nd edition, edited by Kay Corman Kintzel, © Copyright 1977, J. B. Lippincott.

Methods of Burn Care

Method	Description	Advantages	Disadvantages
Exposure therapy	After cleansing, wound remains exposed to air and allowed to dry. Natural protective barrier formed by hard coagulum from exudate of partial-thickness burns and dry eschar of full-thickness burns	Patient not immobilized with bulky dressings. Allows frequent inspection. Dry crust is poor culture medium. Fluid loss less in initial phases. Less odor	Risk of cross contamination greater. Requires strict isolation technique. Requires maintenance of optimal environmental temperature. Often requires restraints on extremities to prevent picking at crust. Presents unsightly appearance
Occlusive dressings	Wound surface covered with non-adherent, water-permeable fine-mesh gauze. Inner layer covered with even layer of absorptive, resilient fluffed gauze held in place by nonconstricting stretch gauze bandages	Protection from cross contamination. Protection from injury. Better immobilization, if desired. Aids in positioning and putting injured part at rest. Less pain initially	Requires skilled nursing care. Higher incidence of hyperpyrexia. Warm, moist environment more conducive to bacterial growth. Often requires pain medication for uncomfortable dressing changes
Primary excision	Immediate surgical excision of devitalized tissue and grafting	Immediate removal of necrotic eschar. Permanent coverage of damaged skin. Reduces exposure to infection	Difficult to distinguish between full-thickness and deep partial-thickness injury. Associated with significant blood loss

Reprinted by permission of The C. V. Mosby Co. from *Nursing Care of Infants and Children,* by Lucille Whaley and Donna Wong, © 1979, The C. V. Mosby Co., St. Louis.

Educational Programs and Materials in Burn Care Research

Published by: American Burn Association Department of Surgery
Cornell Medical Center—New York Hospital
525 East 68th Street
New York, New York 10021

This catalog (approximately 90 pages, revised yearly) lists and describes training programs for burn nurses in California, Connecticut, Illinois, Indiana, Michigan, Missouri, New York, Ohio, Oklahoma, Pennsylvania, Texas, Virginia, Washington, and Wisconsin. The programs range from short-term for continuing education, to long-term graduate programs.

There is also a listing of burn training programs for M.D.s, physical and occupational therapists, and listings of research programs in burn treatment.

Information is included on sources of materials for educating the public to prevention of burn injuries.

For the nurse working in burn care, there is information on how to obtain manuals on clinical care from various burn centers as well as an extensive guide to publications on burn nursing including independent study guides and educational modules. Sources are given for movies, videotapes, newsletters, slide sets and posters.

For any nurse working in the direct care of burn patients or for those involved in public education on burn prevention, this resource catalog will be most useful.

Phases of Hypertension

Phase	Characteristics	Therapy
Prehypertensive	Blood pressure mildly elevated: systolic pressure below 200 mm. Hg, diastolic pressure below 100 mm. Hg; symptoms of anxiety may be present: headache, insomnia, irritability, forgetfulness	No specific therapy; occasionally tranquilizers or sleeping medication
Mild benign	Systolic pressure remains below 200 mm. Hg, diastolic pressure above 100 mm. Hg; vague symptoms of anxiety: headache, fatigue, palpitations	Weight reduction; Na⁻-restricted diet; mild antihypertensive drugs; diuretics with K⁻ replacements
Moderately severe benign	Systolic blood pressure above 200 mm. Hg, diastolic pressure above 110 mm. Hg; no evidence of vascular damage	Weight reduction; Na⁻-restricted diet; more potent drugs: Aldomet, Apresoline, Eutonyl
Severe benign	Systolic blood pressure up to 250 mm. Hg or higher, diastolic blood pressure persistently above 120 mm. Hg; abnormal neurologic signs: severe occipital headaches, anginal pain	Postganglionic blocking agents, e.g., Ismelin; ganglionic blocking agents if postganglionic blocking agents fail to control BP, e.g., Ansolysen
Malignant	Sudden sharp elevation in blood pressure: diastolic pressure above 130 mm. Hg; papilledema; rapidly progressive renal failure with albuminuria, proteinuria, decreased specific gravity, increased blood urea nitrogen; severe epigastric pain; left ventricular failure; mortality 100% in 2 years if not treated	Most potent antihypertensive drugs available, e.g., Ismelin, administered concomitantly with thiazides and reserpine; hospitalize promptly
Acute	Greatly elevated diastolic blood pressure (above 140 mm. Hg); rapid development of following conditions: Hypertensive encephalopathy, severe headache, mental confusion, nausea, vomiting, convulsions, coma, papilledema, retinal hemorrhages; intracranial hemorrhage; acute congestive heart failure with pulmonary edema	Medical emergency requiring immediate treatment; diastolic blood pressure must be reduced rapidly; chemotherapy with reserpine I.M. or I.V., Aldomet I.V., ganglionic blocking agents subcut. or I.V., Arfonad I.V. diluted in dextrose; have patient in sitting position; monitor BP continuously while patient is receiving parenteral medications; when BP controlled, Ismelin or ganglionic blocking agents and reserpine may be given orally

Reprinted by permission of W. B. Saunders Co. from *Medical-Surgical Nursing: A Psychophysiological Approach* by Joan Luckmann and Karen Sorenson, © 1974, W. B. Saunders Co.

Orthopedics

Tips in Caring for Your Cast

- ... If it becomes soiled, clean with a cloth dampened with dry cleanser. If still soiled, use white shoe polish, but *sparingly;* too much may saturate and soften cast.
- ... Avoid getting water on or in your cast. If it becomes damp, use a hair dryer to dry area.
- ... Plastic bags are good covering in wet weather.
- ... If cast becomes rough on edges, cover rough area with tape.

Caring For Your Skin While Wearing Your Cast

- ... Wash skin area around cast taking care not to saturate cast in the process.
- ... Rub the areas around the cast frequently with alcohol. Lotion has a tendency to build up on the inside of the cast and becomes sticky, so it should never be used around the cast or under it.
- ... If edges are causing irritation to the skin, pad with some soft materials such as cotton or foam. Be sure the padding is well anchored to the cast, as loose material slipping into the cast, will cause even more irritation.

Important Things to Watch For and Do While You Are Wearing Your Cast

Twice a day check your fingers, if the cast is on your arm; and toes, if the cast is on your leg.

- ... Are they pink in color? Squeeze the nail till white; when released, they should have an immediate return to their pink color. If return is slow, call your doctor.
- ... Do not be alarmed if your foot appears darker when it is down. This is normal.
- ... Watch for swelling. Compare it to the other hand or foot. Are they about the same?
- ... Move fingers or toes, NOT JUST WIGGLE, but fully extend the fingers or toes. If any loss of motion or any increased pain, call your doctor.
- ... Make sure there is feeling on all surfaces of the hand and fingers, or foot and toes. If *any* numbness, tingling, or pinprick pain develops, call your doctor.
- ... Check around cast for any odors other than those that may be from something spilled on or around the cast. Ordinarily, casts won't smell. Be especially conscious of odors if there

are stitches under the cast. If any smell is noticed, don't delay, call your doctor. Also watch for any staining of, or discharge from, the cast.

... If swelling is noted after activity, elevate the extremity, the higher the better.

... Arm casts are most comfortable with a sling support.

If Your Doctor Permits—Then—

... To keep shoulder from becoming stiff, EACH DAY, four times a day, remove the sling and exercise the arm by putting it through its full range of motion. In other words, move it the way it normally goes.

... For the leg in a cast, if possible, work at "setting," that is, tightening, then relaxing the thigh muscles, doing this frequently, or every two hours while awake. You should discuss this with your doctor FIRST, but some exercise is essential.

... If skin under the cast begins to itch, DO NOT try to stick anything inside the cast to scratch, especially if there is an area with stitches. Parents, especially be alert to children sticking forks, sticks, or other ingenious objects inside the cast.

Remember:
Cast Care Must Continue As Long As Your Cast Is On.

When a patient undergoes a cast change, the whole process of observation and care begins anew.

Possible Complications from Fractures

Complication	Early Clinical Features	Recommended Nursing Action	Most Common Fracture Type—Location
Pulmonary Embolism (may occur *without* clinical symptoms)	1. *Sub-sternal pain* 2. Dyspnea 3. Rapid weak pulse	Administer oxygen. Notify physician immediately— as to pain and vital signs.	Lower extremities
Fat Embolism	1. *Mental confusion,* apprehension, restlessness *due to hypoxia*	It is advisable to have a standing order to draw blood gases at first sign	Lower extremities and/or multiple fractures

Continued on next page

Complication	Early Clinical Features	Recommended Nursing Action	Most Common Fracture Type—Location
	2. Followed by fever, tachycardia, tachypnea, dyspnea	of mental confusion. Notify physician immediately. Administer oxygen.	
Gas Gangrene	1. *Mental aberration* followed by signs of infection	Notify physician immediately of mental status, vital signs and appearance of wound.	Compound (esp. with small open area)
Tetanus	*May be none* until: patient has tonic twitchings and difficulty opening mouth	Notify physician immediately. Check to see if patient is getting compazine.*	Compound

*One of the side effects of the normal therapeutic dose of compazine *is* hypertonia

Reprinted with permission of J. B. Lippincott Company from *Illustrated Guide to Orthopedic Nursing* by Jane Farrell, © 1977, J. B. Lippincott Company.

Spinal Cord Injury Rehabilitation: A Message to Helping Professionals

by Karen Jasper

Too often, it seems to me, we in the helping professions focus upon a medical-vocational model of rehabilitation, even when it is clear to us that the major issues are not exclusively medical and/or vocational, but emotional, interpersonal, and functional. To a spinal cord injured person who must learn to **trust** again—in essence, to **live** again—we do a great disservice when we assume that he/she can or should handle these major life issues alone; too often we fail to provide the encouragement, the faith, and the means which will assist him/her in "making it." It is with ironic reversal, I think, that it becomes **we** who are overwhelmed by the countless and multi-leveled needs and demands of a spinal cord injury, and it is often **we** who lose faith or give up in the full rehabilitation process. Because the obstacles appear so overwhelming, we translate a message of hopelessness to a person who perhaps, with support and opportunity, **could** become "properly" rehabilitated.

I know I am not alone in sometimes wondering if we truly know what we are doing at this point in the rehabilitation of spinal cord injured people. For example, there may be psychological effects that are delayed one, five, and ten years after an injury, and an individual's "readiness" for the massive reconstitution process required may vary unpredictably over so large a number of years. Perhaps a person's long period of withdrawal, depression, and/or lack of interest may simply be due to an unrecognized attempt to gather the psychic energy needed to tackle such a reconstitution. At this point in time, due especially to a major lack of long-term research in the psychological processes of spinal cord injured persons, we simply do not know enough about our part in the rehabilitation of people who become traumatically disabled.

I once heard Dr. Tom Stuart, then a psychiatrist at the West Roxbury V.A. Hospital, say that the learning of technical skills, although obviously important, is not a substitute for learning to live in a different way; and learning a new life means thinking a new way. The magnitude of such a life task can demand months, years, of working through and of non-judgementally coming to terms with who one is. In a period of five or ten years, we **all** change in major ways as we face life's major issues—a severe physical disability even further complicates this process through the multiplicity of crises inherent in such an injury.

The goal of rehabilitation never changes—its direction is always toward the promotion of self-worth and ego integrity of accepting and valuing who one is. Our aim is to assist a disabled person in **reformulating a self that approves of continuing to be:** simply, a self that is predicted on worth, not on deficiency; a self that recognizes that despite its physical characteristics, it has worth and meaning. The most valuable contribution we helping professionals can make to an individual's rehabilitation is, I submit, a willingness to concretely share the burden of this reformulating process—to accept at times a part of the heavy burden of learning to live again. Perhaps we as separate human beings must be willing to share not only the **issues** of discomfort and dependence and disease, but also the **experiences** of each: counseling someone toward a re-involvement in social activities, for example, is not the same as supporting and sharing those activities with him. And telling a client that life can be OK again or that she/he is not "motivated" to live independently, is not as helpful as respecting the despair behind the inactivity while actively participating and encouraging the process of making life OK again.

It is not an easy road—the process of becoming "whole" once again. We must understand this. And, yet, it is not an impossible road either. Caring, knowledgeable people can have a profound effect on how a traumatically disabled person will view the world, as well as his or her place in that world.

Peer Counseling

In recent years, Peer Counseling has become a very effective means of dealing with and supporting the multi-faceted problems of physical disability. It has shown to be an effective way for the disabled person, as well as their family and friends, in coping with, and understanding severe physical disability. Peer Counseling can be a formal program or service, or it can simply be contact and assistance from another disabled person, family member, or friend.

Reprinted from *National Resource Directory*, published by the National Spinal Cord Injury Foundation, 1979.

Functional Goals and Potential Equipment in Spinal Cord Lesions

It is often through the use of assistive devices that independent function become possible.

The following list of equipment is to serve as a guideline only in the determination of equipment needs of individuals with various levels of injury. Most individuals will not need all of the items listed. On the other hand, the individual may have specific needs not accounted for here. This represents only a summary of equipment considered reasonable for respective levels of injury.

Functional Spinal Cord Level	Muscle Function	Functional Goals	Potential Equipment
C4	Neck control Scapular elevators	Manipulate electric wheelchair with devices Mouth-stick (communication) Use environmental controls	Electric wheelchair with appropriate controls Light-weight travel wheelchair Collapsible commode chair or bowel training wheelchair Electric hospital bed Over-bed table Reading stand Environmental controls Patient lifter: car/home Self-aid devices: mouth-stick Foot-board
C5	Partial shoulder control Partial elbow flexion	Independent in light hygiene and feeding activities with devices Propel wheelchair with assistive devices Swivel bar transfer Adapted sports: swimming, archery, bowling	Wheelchair with modifications as needed — possible power Shower/bowel training wheelchair Hospital bed — regular or electric, with trapeze, swinging davit, straps Patient lifter: car/home (if swivel bar transfer not possible) Self-aid devices: Pushing gloves

Continued on next page

Functional Spinal Cord Level	Muscle Function	Functional Goals	Potential Equipment
C6	Shoulder control Elbow flexion Wrist extension Supinators	Independent in dressing activities Independent in transfer activities car and bed Driving with adapted equipment Adapted sports: track and field table tennis	Dressing gloves Hand splints Aids for feeding Mobile arm support Over-bed table Wheelchair with modifications as needed Shower/bowel training wheelchair Hospital bed — trapeze, davit, straps Transfer board or stool for car transfers Self-aid devices: Functional splints Dressing gloves Leg-bag straps & clamp
C7 and C8	Shoulder depression Elbow extension Some hand function	Independent in eating with adapted devices Independent in application of condom drainage Independent transfers car, bed, commode chair and/or tub stool Assisted bowel care (C8)	Wheelchair with modifications as needed Shower wheelchair Hospital bed Raised toilet seat Tub seat Car transfer stool or board Standing frame Self-aid devices: Leg-bag straps Bathroom grab-bars

Continued on next page

Level	Function	Activities	Equipment
T1–5	Normal upper extremity muscle function	Total wheelchair independence Independent transfer wheelchair to tub Move from wheelchair to floor and back Assisted standing activities All wheelchair sports	Wheelchair Shower wheelchair Raised toilet seat Standing frame Bathroom grab-bars
T6–10	Partial trunk stability	Exercise ambulation with bilateral long leg braces and crutches	Same as T1–5 Long leg braces/standing frame Bathroom grab-bars
T11–L1	Trunk stability	Possible household ambulation	Wheelchair Shower wheelchair Raised toilet seat Bracing for ambulation Bathroom grab-bars
L2	Hip flexors	Household ambulation	Same as T11–L1
L3–4	Abductors, quadriceps	Community ambulation with long or short leg braces and crutches or cane	Wheelchair Bracing for ambulation Shower chair Bathroom grab-bars
L5–S2	Hip extensors, abductors Knee flexors Ankle control	No equipment needed if plantar flexion is enough for push-off and there is no foot-drop	Ambulation aids

* Obtained from the West Roxbury VA Hospital, W. Roxbury, Massachusetts.

Reprinted from *National Resource Directory*, published by the National Spinal Cord Injury Foundation, 1979.

Plan of a Coronary Care Unit

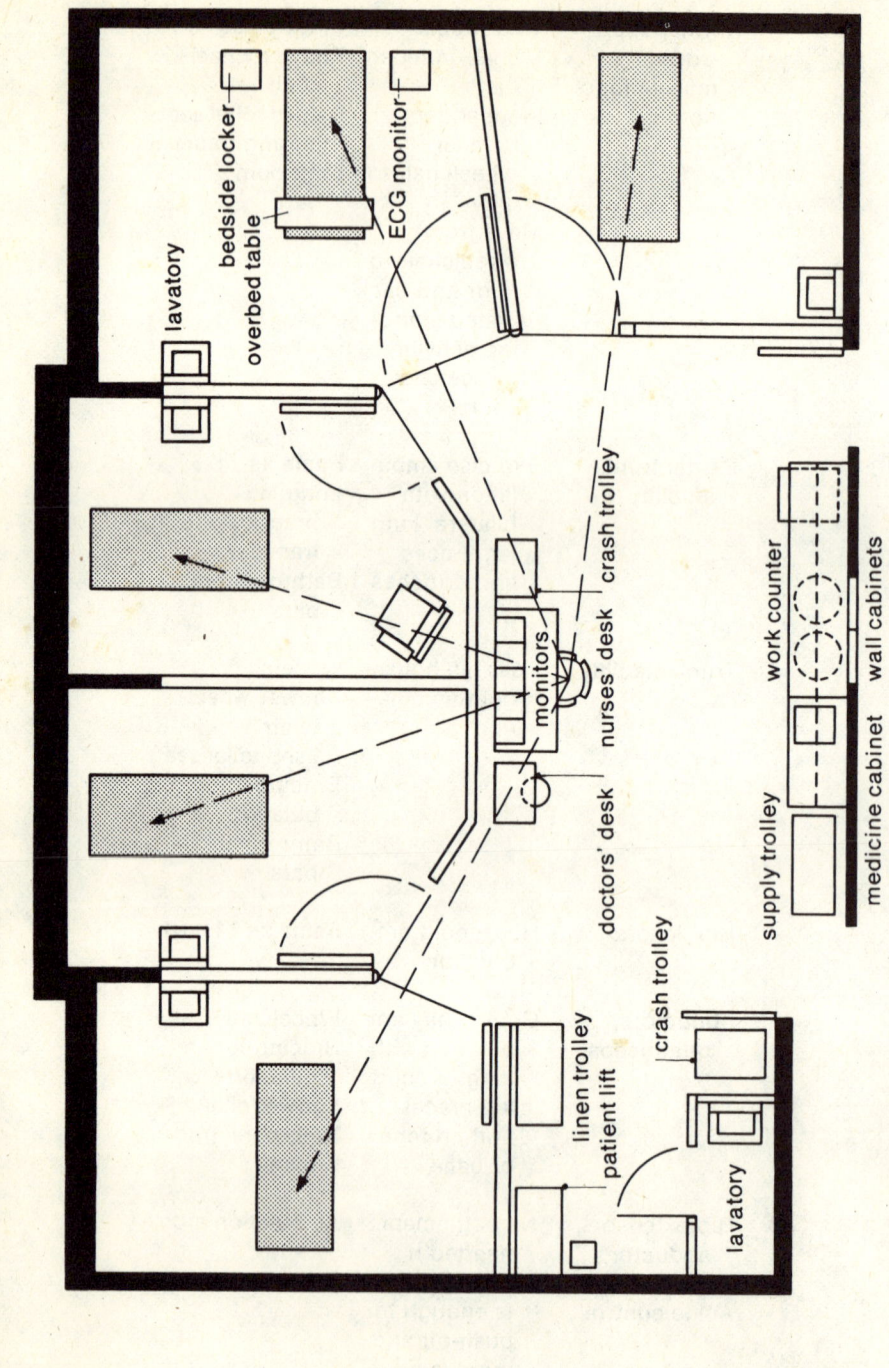

The ABGs of radiation

Radioactivity: The process of spontaneous disintegration of an atom's nucleus, resulting in the emission of radiation in the form of alpha, beta, and gamma rays. Alpha rays are positively charged, beta rays negatively charged. Gamma rays, more penetrating than either of the others, are emitted in electromagnetic radiation (like X-rays), and in nuclear accidents.

X-ray: A form of energy produced when high-speed electrons collide abruptly with an object.

Roentgen: A unit of X-ray exposure in air.

Rad: The standard unit of "radiation absorbed dose." (Equivalent to the rem, for gamma rays and electrons.)

Millirad: One thousandth of a rad.

Rem (Roentgen equivalent man): A unit of measurement of the biologic effectiveness of a given radiation dose. (Equivalent to the rad for gamma rays and electrons.)

Average exposure (in rems) in one year: Estimated to be about 100-200 millirems, from sources including the sun, cosmic rays, television sets, and diagnostic X-rays. One chest X-ray, depending on the equipment and technique used, yields 30-60 rems exposure.

Permissible levels of exposure (as established by the National Council on Radiation Protection and Measurement):
General population—500 millirems per year;
Nuclear plant workers—up to 5,000 millirems (5 rems) per year;
Hospital personnel working with radionuclides—3,000 millirems (3 rems) per 13 weeks. Maximum permissible lifetime rem exposure, however, is determined by using the formula 5(N-18), where N is the age of the individual. For example, a 30-year-old nurse could receive 5(30-18) rems—a total of 60 rems—during her lifetime, including the average number of rems received from non-work related sources. The radiation safety officer in each hospital's nuclear medicine department should keep records of each employee's exposure, to insure that the maximum permissible limit is not exceeded.

Reprinted by permission from RN Magazine, June, 1979, page 71, Copyright 1979, Litton Industries.

"In the event of radiation exposure..."

The following protocol for handling victims of radiation contamination and poisoning is based on the emergency plan of New York's Mount Sinai Hospital.

It is the responsibility of the senior Emergency Department staff member on duty, on receipt of notification of the momentary arrival of a case involving radiation exposure or contamination, to:

1. Notify the responsible staff physician or radiation safety officer (trained health physicist or trained technician from the Nuclear Medicine or X-ray Department). When the responsible person is not on duty, the administrator should be notified so he can contact the responsible person.

2. Obtain an appropriate survey meter from the Radiation Safety Office; if the office is closed, Security has keys to it. When a meter is removed from the office, a note must be left indicating who has it and where it can be found. If no survey meter can be procured in the hospital, notify the administrator or radiation safety officer, so that equipment can be obtained from the Police Department.

WHEN THE PATIENT ARRIVES AT THE HOSPITAL:

3. Check the patient for contamination while he is on the stretcher (preferably as the stretcher is being removed from the ambulance), and perform a survey of his clothing, and the ambulance, before undertaking any other activity or bringing the patient inside the hospital.

4. If clothing is contaminated, place in a special container marked "Radioactive: Do Not Discard." Handle contaminated patient and objects as in surgical procedures, using gown, gloves, cap, mask, etc.

5. Notify the hospital administrator so he may seek expert professional consultation for technical management of the case.

6. Prepare a separate examining room or outside hallway immediately adjacent to the entrance to the Emergency Department. Cover the floor—in an area adequate for the stretcher-cart, disposal hampers, and working space—with absorbent paper. Mark and close off this area. If dust is involved, be prepared to shut off air circulation system, to prevent spread of contamination.

WHEN THE PATIENT IS BROUGHT INTO THE EXAMINATION/ TREATMENT AREA:

7. If seriously injured, give emergency lifesaving assistance immediately.

8. If possible external contamination is involved save all clothing, bedding from ambulance, blood, urine, stool, vomitus, and other objects (jewelry, belt buckles, dental plates, etc.). Label with patient's name, body location, time, and date. Save in containers marked "Radioactive: Do Not Discard."

9. Begin decontamination, if medical status permits, with cleansing and scrubbing of the areas highest in contamination first. If an extremity alone is involved, clothing may serve as an effective barrier; the affected limb should still be scrubbed. Initial cleansing should be done with soap and hot water. If the body as a whole is involved or clothing generally permeated, showering and scrubbing will be necessary. Pay special attention to hair, body orifices, and body folds. Remeasure with survey meter and record measurement after each washing or showering.

10. If a wound is involved, prepare and cover it with self-adhering disposable surgical drape. Cleanse neighboring skin surfaces. Seal off cleansed areas with self-adhering disposable surgical drapes. Remove wound covering and irrigate wound with sterile water, catching the irrigating fluid in a basin or can to be marked as above. Each step in the decontamination process should be preceded and followed by monitoring and recording of the location and extent of contamination.

11. Save physicians', nurses', and attendants' scrub or protective clothing as described for patients. Staff must follow the same monitoring and decontamination procedures as the patients.

12. If confronted with a grossly contaminated wound (dirt particles and crushed tissue), the physician in attendance should be prepared to do a preliminary simple wet debridement. Further measurements may necessitate use of sophisticated wound counting detection instruments supplied by the consultant, who will advise further definitive debridement when necessary.

STANDING ORDERS:
When the accident has occurred at a plant, university, or medical unit regularly working with nuclear material, the health physicist or supervisor, a co-worker, or the patient should be able to inform the rescue squad of the nature of the accident, type of radiation exposure or radioactive contamination involved, and possible body areas that may be affected.

Reprinted with permission of *RN* Magazine from *RN*, June 1979, page 73, © *RN* Magazine.

Effects of Some Common Industrial Agents Upon the Worker

TABLE 9-1
Effects of Some Common Industrial Agents Upon The Worker

AGENT	TYPE OF INDUSTRY OR OCCUPATION	BODY AREA AFFECTED
Acetaldelhyde	Chemical, Paint	All body cells, especially brain and respiratory tract.
Acetic anhydride	Textile	Exposed tissue damage, especially eye and respiratory tract.
Acetylene	Welding, Plastic, Dry Cleaning	Respiratory tract asphyxiant. Explosive, especially when combined with certain substances.
Acrolein	Chemical	Skin, eye, respiratory tract.
Allyl Chloride	Plastic	Skin, respiratory tract, kidney.
Ammonia	Chemical, Leather, Wool, Farmers, Refrigeration Workers	Eyes, skin, respiratory tract.
Aniline	Paint, Rubber	Skin, hematopoietic system.
Arsenic	Mine, Smelter, Leather, Chemical, Oil Refinery, Insecticide Makers and Sprayers	Skin, lung, liver (cancer). Nervous system damage.
Asbestos	Mine, Textile, Insulation, Shipyard Workers, Construction	Respiratory and gastrointestinal tract (cancer) as well as asbestosis (lung scarring). More harmful to people who smoke.
Benzene	Rubber, Chemical, Explosives, Paint, Shoemakers, Dye Users	Skin, liver, brain, hematopoietic system (cancer, leukemia).
Berylluim	Foundry, Metallurgical, Aerospace, Nuclear, Household appliance production	Skin and eye (inflammation, ulcers), respiratory tract (acute inflammation and berylliosis—chronic lung infection), systemic effects on heart, liver, spleen, kidneys.
Butyl Alcohol	Lacquer, Paint	Eye, skin, respiratory tract.
Carbon Disulfide	Rubber, Viscose Rayon	Gastrointestinal, heart, liver, kidney, brain.
Carbon Tetrachloride	Solvent, Dry Cleaning	Skin, gastrointestinal, liver, kidney, brain.
Chlorine	Industrial Bleaching	Eye, respiratory tract.
Chloroform	Chemical, Plastic	Heart degeneration, liver, kidney.

Chromium	Chrome Plating, Chemical, Industrial Bleaching, Glass and Pottery, Linoleum Makers, Battery Makers	Irritating to all body cells. Skin, eye, respiratory tract, (cancer) liver, kidney.
Coal Combustion Products (Soot, Tar)	Gashouse Workers, Asphalt, Coal Tar, or Pitch Workers, Mine, Coke Oven Workers	Skin, respiratory tract, scrotum, urinary bladder (carcinogenic to all areas).
Cotton, Flax, Hemp Lint	Textile	Respiratory tract (byssinosis-chest tightness, dyspnea, cough, wheezing; chronic bronchitis). Cigarette smokers especially affected.
Creosol	Chemical, Oil Refining	Denatures and precipitates all cellular protein. Skin, eye, respiratory tract, liver, kidney, brain.
Dichloroethyl Ether	Insecticide, Oil Refining	Respiratory tract.
Dimethyl Sulfate	Chemical, Pharmaceutical	Eye, respiratory tract, liver, kidney, brain.
Fungus, Parasites	Food, Animal, Outdoor Workers	Skin, respiratory tract.
Iron Oxide	Mine, Iron Foundry, Metal Polishers and Finishers	Respiratory tract (cancer).
Lead	Auto, Smelter, Plumbing, Paint, Metallurgical, Battery Making, Exposure in 120 different industries	Hematopoietic, liver, kidney, brain, muscles, bone, gastrointestinal tract. Causes fetal damage during first trimester of pregnancy.
Leather	Leather, Shoe	Nasal cavity and sinuses, urinary bladder (carcinogenic for each).
Manganese	Mine, Metallurgical	Respiratory tract, liver, brain.
Mercury	Electrical, Laboratory Workers, Exposure in 80 different types of industries	Toxic to all cells. Respiratory tract, liver, brain. Exposure of pregnant woman causes congenital defects and retardation.
Mica	Rubber, Insulation	Respiratory tract.
Nickel	Metallurgical, Smelter, Electrolysis Workers	Skin, respiratory tract (cancer).
Nitrobenzene	Synthetic dyes	Skin, hematopoietic system, brain.
Nitrogen Dioxide	Chemical, Metal	Eye, respiratory tract, hematopoietic system.
Petroleum Products	Rubber, Textile, Aerospace, Workers in contact with fuel oil, coke, paraffin, lubricants	Skin, respiratory tract, scrotum (carcinogenic to each).
Phenol	Plastics	Corrosive to all tissue. Liver, kidney, brain.

Continued on next page

AGENT	TYPE OF INDUSTRY OR OCCUPATION	BODY AREA AFFECTED
Rubber Dust	Rubber	Respiratory tract (chronic disease).
Silica	Mine, Foundry, Ceramic or glass production	Respiratory tract (silicosis).
Talc Dust	Mine	Respiratory tract (cancer), calcification of pericardium.
Tetraethyl Lead	Chemical	Hematopoietic system, brain.
Thallium	Pesticide, Fireworks or Explosives	Skin, respiratory and gastrointestinal tract, kidney, brain.
Toluene	Rubber, Paint	Skin, respiratory tract, liver, hematopoietic system, brain.
Trichloroethylene	Chemical, Metal Degreasing	Skin, liver, kidney, brain.
Vinyl Chloride	Plastic, Rubber, Insulation, Organic-Chemical Synthesizers, Polyvinyl Resin Makers	Skin, respiratory tract, (asthma), cancer in the liver, kidney, spleen and brain. Exposure of pregnant woman to polyvinyl chloride causes defective fetus.

Reprinted by permission of Prentice-Hall, Inc. from *Nursing Concepts for Health Promotion*, 2nd Ed., by Ruth Beckmann Murray and Judith Proctor Zentner, © 1979, Prentice-Hall, Inc.

Preoperative assessment guidelines

Date _____ ORN note:
Problem: Surgical intervention

S—Subjective: Patient responses to
  What do you understand the doctor is going to do tomorrow?
  How do you feel about having this particular surgery?
  Who will be here tomorrow? (Tell them where to wait)
  Have you ever had surgery before? What do you recall about it?
  Do you have any problem areas that we should know about? (back trouble? trick knee? meds from home? etc)
  Is there anything you are especially concerned about at this time?
  Do you have any other questions?

O—Objective: Observed facts of patient or chart
  Physical appearance: obese, slender, short (< 5 ft), tall (> 6 ft), age, pulses
  Physical impairments: hearing, sight, speech, motor ability, skeletal position limitations, pain, bleeding, drainage, bowel or bladder dysfunction

Skin: Intact, breaks, scars, dry, moist, reddened, bruises, rash, flushed, pale, jaundiced, edematous, ulcers, or sores, etc
Mental/emotional state: level of consciousness, responds to name, crying tremor, muscular tenseness, anger, talkative, composed, calm, sad, etc
Therapeutic devices/measures: oxygen, transfusions, drains, catheters, trach, levine, cast, traction, colostomy, laryngectomy, etc

A—Analysis of subjective and objective
  Oriented to time and place
  Knowledge of illness
  Emotional summary: availability of support from wife, husband, children, family, religion
  Concerns: finances, loneliness, outcome of surgery, change of body image, fear of unknown

P—Plan of nursing care
  Identify patient
  Called "＿＿＿＿＿＿＿＿＿＿" at home
  Position with precautions
  Blood and x-ray availability
  Allergy precautions (tape, iodine, meds) with alternative
  Operative permit signed
  Referrals
  Suggestion for instrumentation
  Special considerations

Hints: Don't say, "Everything will be all right"; instead, say, "We will be there when you need us."

Tell patient about:
  1. shave
  2. removal of water pitcher
  3. changing into hospital gown and removing all valuables
  4. preop meds and what they may do (Note: Not all pt get meds)
  5. nurse aide will transport
  6. then to OR suite
  7. may go to holding room area
  8. describe some sounds within the OR (suction, for example)
  9. anesthesia will be at your head
  10. OR lights—size and mirror give distorted image
  11. arms tucked into sides
  12. awake in recovery room, which will be large ward and cold
  13. transfer when fully awake

Tell family:
  1. where to wait
  2. that operation starting time is often an hour after they last see patient
  3. physician and recovery room nurse will talk with them postoperation

Reprinted from "SOAPing the Preoperative Interview" by Susan Kleinbeck in *AORN Journal,* December, 1978. Reprinted by permission of *AORN Journal.*

Innovation in Surgical Nursing
Clinical Nurse Specialist For Intraoperative Care

Daniel Freeman Hospital
Inglewood, California

BACKGROUND: Although most patients are given sedative medication prior to arrival in surgery, many patients arrive with less than optimal sedative effect. The literature reports postoperative patients recall their sedated conscious experiences in the operating room and operating room corridor. Often, operating room personnel are preoccupied with tasks and overlook the patients. Patients' need for support, comfort, and information about the operating room experience has been documented.

PURPOSE: The role of the clinical nurse specialist in intraoperative care is to link the preoperative and postoperative phases of care with the intraoperative period, including direct care, teaching of staff and patients, and research.

NURSING ROLE: The clinical nurse specialist in intraoperative care coordinates, teaches, and assists operating room nurses in teaching a basic operating room nursing program in the hospital. Her direct-care activities include preoperative assessment and teaching of selected surgical patients and their families. She communicates to operating room nurses any problems that have relevance for nursing care in the operating room and provides assessment and intervention during the immediate preoperative period when the patient is in the surgery corridor or in the operating room, but is not yet undergoing surgery. She serves as a communication link between the operating room and the families of patients in the operating room and assists with and directs care given by the nurses in the operating room and evaluates the results of interventions provided.

The clinical nurse specialist participates in research, such as a project to determine the effectiveness of puppet therapy as a preoperative teaching modality for pediatric surgical patients and an intraoperative quality-care research project using a process audit method. Ultimately, she develops patient outcome criteria for the intraoperative period of care. She is a resource for staff, a facilitator and problem solver, a liaison with various areas of the hospital and community, and a clinical supervisor and contact person for graduate students in medical-surgical nursing from a university program.

EVALUATION: Although no systematic evaluation has been conducted, there is evidence that this role is valued by the patients and staff and that care for surgical patients is improving.

CONTACT FOR FURTHER INFORMATION:
   Mary Gill Nolan, RN, MN
   Clinical Nurse Specialist for Surgical Patients
   Daniel Freeman Hospital
   333 North Prairie Avenue
   Inglewood, California 90301
   (213) 672-0112

Reprinted from *Analysis and Planning for Improved Distribution of Nursing Personnel and Services,* Sheila Kodadek, Editor, 1976, Division of Nursing, Health Resources Administration, U.S. Department of H.E.W.

General Medical-Surgical Resources

American Association of Blood Banks
Suite 608
1828 L Street, N.W.
Washington, D.C. 20036

This is a national organization which promotes improvement in blood bank services and voluntary blood donations. Several publications are available from the Association on transfusion and other topics related to blood donation and distribution.

American College Health Association (ACHA)
2807 Central Street
Evanston, Ill. 60201

ACHA is a national organization for institutions and individuals concerned with providing health care in colleges and universities. Publications include the *Journal Of The American College Health Association,* published six times a year; "Recommended Standards And Practices For A College Health Program," "Functions, Standards And Qualifications For College Nurses In

Student Health Services," and other publications of interest to nurses working in a college health program.

American Heart Association
44 East 23rd Street
New York, N.Y. 10010

This is the national organization for research and education on heart disease. Services available through local chapters include cardiopulmonary resuscitation courses, support and educational groups for heart patients and their families, materials for strep disease screening programs, smoking clinics, and symposia and workshops for professionals (the services provided by local affiliates vary—contact your local Heart Association for information on its services). Publications include a variety of educational materials on all aspects of heart disease and *Cardio-Vascular Nursing,* a monthly publication for nurses, available from the local affiliates.

American Hospital Association
840 N. Lake Shore Drive
Chicago, Ill. 60611

The American Hospital Association is composed of hospitals and related institutions. It makes available many publications of interest to nurses, including: information on the Association and its functions, materials on hospital careers, hospital administration, continuing education, manuals for training hospital staff, infection control, hospital law, hospital safety, record keeping, and many other topics. Periodicals include *Hospital Week,* a weekly newsmagazine, *Hospitals, Journal Of The American Hospital Association,* published twice monthly. Write for free resource catalog.

American National Red Cross
National Headquarters
Washington, D.C. 20006

The Red Cross is a national volunteer-directed organization for preventing emergencies and helping people cope with them when they do occur. The Red Cross provides blood services, disaster preparedness and relief programs, and conducts training programs in first aid, preparation for childbirth and parenthood, water safety, home nursing and health care. Among the publications available are: booklets on disaster services, the blood program and use of blood, safety and first aid materials, and the textbook, *Family Health and Home Nursing,* © 1979, American National Red Cross, an excellent health teaching resource and a useful reference for all homes.

The Arthritis Foundation
3400 Peachtree Road, N.E.
Atlanta, Ga. 30326

The Foundation provides patient services and education on arthritis. It includes an Allied Health Professions Section for professionals working with people with rheumatic disease.

Association For The Advancement
Of Health Education
American Alliance For Health,
Physical Education, Recreation
1201 16th Street, N.W.
Washington, D.C. 20036

This is an organization for all professionals involved in health education. It provides services, educational materials and resource information on health education for professionals and lay people. It also promotes research and legislation on health education. Publications include *Health Education,* a magazine published six times yearly; a newsletter published three times a year; publications on school health and school nursing and patient education, and many other aspects of health education. The membership fee is $25 a year.

Asthma And Allergy Foundation Of America
National Office
801 Second Avenue
New York, N.Y. 10017

This Foundation is a national non-profit organization which supports research into the allergic diseases, provides information and educational materials to the public on these diseases, and supports the education of professionals to work in immunology. Publications include the pamphlets, "Questions And Answers About Asthma and Allergic Diseases," "Handbook For The Asthmatic," "Allergy in Children," and related topics.

Epilepsy Foundation Of America
1828 L Street., N.W.
Washington, D.C. 20036

The Epilepsy Foundation is a non-profit organization which promotes the needs and concerns of people with epilepsy. Local chapters provide referrals, education, and many other services. Many books, pamphlets, reprints, cassettes and slides, and films on epilepsy for lay people and professionals are available. "Nurses Talk About Epilepsy" is a film of particular interest to nurses as it considers the nurse's role in working with people with epilepsy.

International Association For Enterostomal Therapy, Inc.
2506 Gross Point Road
Evanston, Ill. 60201

A specialty organization for nurse Enterostomal Therapists, IAET accredits professional educational programs in enterostomal therapy and provides literature for patient education. Publications include *Enterostomal Therapy Journal*. Write for list of accredited schools for training nurse Enterostomal Therapists.

Medic Alert Foundation International
P.O. Box 1009
Turlock, Calif. 95380

Medic Alert is a non-profit organization providing emergency medical identification for people with "hidden medical problems." Necklaces and bracelets with information on the person's medical problem (e.g., "allergic to penicillin") and a phone number to call in an emergency, are available from Medic Alert (cost: $10 stainless steel, $17.50 sterling silver, and $28 gold filled). Wallet-sized I.D. cards with emergency medical information are also available. Literature available includes "Suggestions For Registered Nurses" and "Suggestions for Emergency Department Nurses." Nurses should inform clients who have need of this service of its availability and help to educate other health professionals to look for the Medic Alert emblem.

National Association of Patients on Hemodialysis and Transplantation (NAPHI)
505 Northern Blvd.
Great Neck, N.Y. 11021

NAPHT is an organization which promotes the well-being of kidney patients. It provides professionals and lay people with education on kidney disease and treatment.

The organization is made up largely of kidney patients and serves as their voice. There are several local chapters. Activities include patient support, providing lists of dialysis centers, and promoting organ donation. Publications include *NAPHT News,* a quarterly magazine for kidney patients ($8.50/year, available in Spanish); *Dialysis Worldwide for the Traveling Patient* ($1.00 each); pamphlets such as "Living With Renal Failure," "Renal Failure and Diabetes," and "Transplant Kidneys—Don't Bury Them;" a "Na-K Counter" for patients which details the sodium and potassium content of several foods; and a "Kidney Patient Identification Card."

The National Asthma Center At Denver
1999 Julian Street
Denver, Colo. 80204

This is a center for research and treatment for asthma and related disorders. Patients are accepted from all 50 states and foreign countries if they have chronic illness which does not respond to local treatment. Literature available (free of charge) includes booklets on asthma, allergy and immunology.

National Foundation for Ileitis and Colitis, Inc.
295 Madison Avenue
New York, N.Y. 10017

This is a national voluntary agency for research into ileitis and ulcerative colitis. It provides literature on these diseases to health professionals and the general public. Publications include a quarterly newsletter and educational brochures.

National Kidney Foundation
116 East 27th Street
New York, N.Y. 10016

This is the national voluntary agency concerned with the prevention and treatment of kidney diseases. The Foundation sponsors research, a national program of organ donors, education, and patient services, through local affiliates. Publications include booklets on kidney functioning and kidney disease and on the organ donor program.

National Multiple Sclerosis Society
205 East 42nd Street
New York, N.Y. 10017

This is the national voluntary agency concerned with research into the causes and prevention of multiple sclerosis and educational programs on the disease. Local chapters throughout the country provide services to patients and families such as counseling, referral, and equipment loaning. Publications include booklets for professional education (e.g., "The Nurse And Multiple Sclerosis"), patients and lay people, and six educational films on multiple sclerosis.

National Safety Council
444 North Michigan Avenue
Chicago, Ill. 60611

The Safety Council's functions include public education on the prevention of accidents and the promotion of safe working conditions for all workers. The Council also offers a Safety Training Institute for professionals working in occupational safety, which includes a hospital safety training course. The Council has available many publications, films and posters on all aspects of safety and safety education. Write for catalog.

National Sickle Cell Disease Program
Division of Blood Diseases And Resources
National Heart and Lung Institute
National Institutes of Health
Room 5A-03, Building 31
Bethesda, Md. 20019

This is a program for screening for sickle cell disease, research into it, and public and professional education on this hereditary blood disease. Listings of Sickle Cell Disease Centers throughout the U.S. are available, along with several other publications including "So, I Have The Sickle Cell Trait," "Sickle Cell Fundamentals," "Adolescents With Sickle Cell Anemia And Sickle Cell Trait," bibliographies and films on sickle cell anemia.

Parkinson's Disease Foundation
William Black Medical Research Building
Columbia University Medical Center
640 W. 168th Street
New York, N.Y. 10032

The Foundation promotes research into the causes and treatment of Parkinson's disease and serves as an information source for patients and health care workers. Publications include "Exercises For The Parkinson Patient," "The Parkinson Patient At Home," and a film entitled "Management Of Parkinson's Disease And Syndrome With Levodopa."

Pharmaceutical Manufacturers Association
1155 Fifteenth Street, N.W.
Washington, D.C. 20005

This group of drug manufacturers and makers of medical and diagnostic products, publishes *Health Care And The Consumer, A Guide To Informational Materials,* which lists films and publications available from its member companies.

United Ostomy Association, Inc.
1111 Wilshire Blvd.
Los Angeles, Calif. 90017

This is a national organization with many local chapters, whose members have had colostomies, ileostomies, or urostomies. It functions as a support group on the local and national levels and a source of education on ostomies. A list of local chapters is available on request. Publications include *Ostomy Quarterly, The Ostomy Handbook* by Edith Lenneberg, ET, and Miriam Weiner, MA (a book for health professionals), booklets on sex and the ostomate, and guides to ostomy care.

Publications on Medical-Surgical Nursing and Related Topics

This is HEW, a booklet on the functions and structure of the U.S. Department of HEW is available from the U.S. Department of Health, Education and Welfare, Washington, D.C. 20201. The names and addresses of some of the H.E.W. agencies of interest to nurses (as listed in this publication) are given below:

Health Care Financing Administration
Office of Information
Room 5218, Switzer Building
330 C Street, S.W.
Washington, D.C. 20201

Bureau Of Education For The Handicapped
U.S. Office of Education
400 Maryland Avenue, S.W.
Washington, D.C. 20202

Public Health Service
Office Of Public Affairs
Room 731, Humphrey Building
200 Independence Avenue, S.W.
Washington, D.C. 20201

National Institutes Of Health
Office Of Public Affairs
Room 309, Building 1
9000 Rockville Pike
Bethesda, Md. 20014

Food And Drug Administration
Consumer Inquiries
HFG-20
5600 Fishers Lane
Rockville, Md. 20857

Health Resources Administration
Office Of Communications
Room 10-44, Center Building
3700 East-West Highway
Hyattsville, Md. 20782

(The Division Of Nursing comes under the auspices of the Health Resources Administration. Write here for information on its functions and for a copy of the catalog, *Division Of Nursing Selected Publications,* DHEW Pub. No. (HRA) 78-58, revised 1978.)

Health Services Administration
Office Of Communications And Public Affairs
Room 14A-55, Parklawn Building
5600 Fishers Lane
Rockville, MD. 20857

Alcohol, Drug Abuse And Mental Health
Administration
5600 Fishers Lane
Rockville, Md. 20857

Center For Disease Control
Office Of Information
Atlanta, Ga. 30333

Office Of Human Development Services
Public Information Office
Room 329D, Humphrey Building
200 Independence Avenue, S.W.
Washington, D.C. 20201

Administration On Aging
Office Of Public Information
Room 4553, North Building
330 Independence Avenue, S.W.
Washington, D.C. 20201

Administration For Children, Youth And Families
Office Of Public Information
Room 3853, Donohoe Building
400 Sixth Street, N.W.
Washington, D.C. 20201

HEW/Office For Civil Rights
Room 5400 North Building
330 Independence Avenue, S.W.
Washington, D.C. 20201

"Nurse's Pocket Reference," a 30-page pocket guide with useful information for nurses, can be obtained free of charge from Becton Dickinson Pharmaceuticals, Rutherford, N.J. 07070.

Medifacts, copyright 1978 by Eli Lilly and Company, Indianapolis, Indiana, 46206, is a pocket-size, 88-page booklet on lab values, measurements, diseases and other useful information for nurses.

Blueprint: A Patient Education Program For The Hospital, a booklet, and other materials on patient education, are available from Professional Research, Inc., 660 South Bonnie Brae Street, Los Angeles, Calif. 90057.

Patient Education, a booklet on patient education concepts and resources, is available from Metropolitan Life Insurance Co., Health and Welfare Division, One Madison Avenue, New York, N.Y. 10010.

A "Patient Education Series" consisting of flipcharts, 35mm slides and pamphlets on various topics (such as diabetes, heart disease, stroke, mastectomy, hypertension, lung disease, renal disease and others) is available from the Robert J. Brady Co., A Prentice-Hall Co., Bowie, Md. 20715.

Help Yourself, ed. by Eddie Miller (92 pages), on health prevention, and *Stress,* also ed. by Eddie Miller (96 pages), are materials for health education available for free, from Blue Cross, 840 North Lake Shore Drive, Chicago, Ill. 60611. (This material is adapted from *Medical Self-Care,* Number 5, 1978.)

"The Enigmas Of Essential Hypertension," a 30-page brochure, is available from Roche Laboratories, Professional Services Department, Nutley, N.J. 07110.

"High Blood Pressure: A Positive Approach" (pamphlets in English or Spanish), and "Hypertensive Management Chart" for record keeping, are available from Boehringer Ingelheim, Ltd., 90 East Ridge, P. O. Box 368, Ridgefield, Conn. 06877.

"How To Extend Your Life Span," a booklet by Dr. Paul Dudley White on heart disease, part of the Prudential Health Series, is available from Prudential Insurance Co. of America, 5 Prudential Plaza, Newark, N.J. 07101.

"Sphygmomanometers: Principles And Precepts" and "The Clinical Measurement Of Blood Pressure" are booklets for health professionals available from W. A. Baum Co., Inc., Copiague, New York 11726.

"Heart Sounds: Pocket Reminder For Nurses," a six-page guide to auscultation of the heart, is available from Merck Sharp and Dohme, Division of Merck and Co., Inc., West Point, Pa. 19486. The material is adapted from *Methods Of Clinical Exami-*

nation: A Physiologic Approach, 3rd edition, by Judge and Zuidema, Little Brown and Co., 1974.

"Arrhythmias Complicating Cardiac Infarction," by James E. Muller, M.D., copyright 1978, American Optical Corporation, is a large plastic wall chart showing ECG patterns for all types of arrhythmias. It is a useful guide for posting in intensive and cardiac care units. Copies may be obtained from American Optical Medical Division, Crosby Drive, Bedford, Mass. 01730.

"Troublesome Traces," a booklet on the prevention and cure of ECG monitoring problems, and "How To Take The Strain Out Of Stress Testing," an introduction to ECG monitoring techniques, are available from NDM Corporation (New Dimensions in Medicine), 3040 East River Road, P. O. Box 1408, Dayton, Ohio 45401.

Several pamphlets for patient education on Chronic Obstructive Pulmonary Disease are available free of charge from Breon Laboratories, Inc., 90 Park Avenue, New York, N.Y. 10016.

"The 'Ins and Outs' Of Better Breathing," a patient education booklet, and "Postural Drainage Positions," an instructional chart for patients or health care personnel, are available from Boehringer Ingelheim, Ltd. (see address under "High Blood Pressure. . ." above).

"Regional Guide To Seasonal Airborne Pollens," a wall chart, and "How To Create A Clean Room," a booklet for allergic persons, are available from Dome Division of Miles Laboratories, 400 Morgan Lane, West Haven, Conn. 06516.

Programmed Instruction In Asepsis, a book for professional education which includes a final exam with answers, and "Asepsis Newsletter, Continued Education In Asepsis," are available from Arbrook, Inc., Arlington, Texas 76010.

"Effective Infectional Control Tips," a booklet; posters on infection prevention and proper hygiene; patient instruction pamphlets on isolation; booklets for patients with I.V.'s and foley catheters on infection prevention; are all available from M. J. White Company, 2211 Pleasant Drive, Missoula, Mont. 59801.

"Range Of Joint Motion Exercises, A Study Guide For Nurses," and "The Decubitus Ulcer, Its Causes, Treatment and Prevention," a booklet, are available free of charge from Westwood Pharmaceuticals, Inc., 468 Dewitt Street, Buffalo, N.Y. 14213.

A booklet on the causes, prevention and treatment of decubitus ulcers, a number of forms for the assessment of decubitus ulcer potential, a flow sheet, position chart and bath and skin report, are all available from Knoll Pharmaceutical Co., 30 North Jefferson Road, Whippany, N.J. 07981.

"Bowel Evacuation, An Illustrated Teaching Manual" for nurses, and "Bowel Retraining Record," are available from Boehringer Ingelheim, Ltd., "on a gratis basis depending on availability of supply." (See address above under "High Blood Pressure...")

"Nurse's Aid to Understanding Constipation," "Nurse's Guide to Bowel Retraining," pamphlets, and "The Enema: Indications And Technique," a booklet, are available from C. B. Fleet Co., Inc., P. O. Box 11349, Lynchburg, Va. 24506.

Several publications on physical therapy, including the *Journal Of The American Physical Therapy Association,* and audio visual materials on patient transfers and other related topics, are available from American Physical Therapy Association, 1156 15th Street, N.W., Washington, D.C. 20005.

Spanish-Language Health Communication Teaching, a list of printed materials and their sources, is available free of charge from the U.S. Department of HEW, Health Services and Mental Health Administration, Office Of Communication And Public Affairs, 5600 Fishers Lane, Rockville, Md. 20857.

Travenol Guide To Fluid Therapy (price: $4) and *The Fundamentals Of Body Water And Electrolytes,* a visual review (price: $2), are available from Travenol Laboratories, Inc., Deerfield, Ill. 60015.

The *Nursing 80 Photobook Series* (The Skillbook Company, 6 Commercial St., Hicksville, N.Y. 11801) consists of excellent photobooks illustrating nursing procedures. Titles in the series include *Dealing With Emergencies, Using Monitors, Caring for Cardiac Patients, Providing Respiratory Care, Managing I.V. Therapy,* and others. The books cost $9.95 each plus shipping and handling, and are available on a 10-day free trial basis.

General Nursing Periodicals

Advances In Nursing Science is a quarterly journal dealing with up-to-date research and practices in nursing. Each issue covers one topic in depth. From Aspen Systems Corporation. (Cost: $29.75 per year.)

The American Journal Of Intravenous Therapy is a journal published bimonthly by McMahon Publishing Co. (Cost: $14 per year.)

Archives Of Surgery is a monthly specialty journal published by the American Medical Association (see address in index of publishers). (Cost: $18 in the U.S., $28 for foreign.)

Clinical Symposia (By CIBA Pharmaceutical Co., Summit, N.J. 07901) is published five times yearly and distribution by CIBA is limited to physicians and medical students. It consists of practical information on medical topics with full-color illustrations accompanying the text. Nurses interested in obtaining reprints of specific volumes may do so for $1.50 each. Write to CIBA for a list of reprints available.

Critical Care Quarterly is a journal with each issue covering in depth, one topic of interest to health professionals in critical care. A sampling of previous titles includes "Acute Respiratory Failure," "Neurological Injuries," "Cardiopulmonary Resuscitation," and "Burn Management." Available from Aspen Systems Corporation. (Cost: $29.75 per year.)

Dialysis And Transplantation (By Creative Age Publications, 12849 Magnolia Boulevard, North Hollywood, Calif. 91607) is a monthly journal for all health professionals involved with dialysis and renal transplantation. (Cost: $25 per year in the U.S. and $35 for foreign.)

Emergency Nurse Legal Bulletin is a quarterly publication with a newsletter format containing information on the legal implications of emergency department nursing. From Med/Law Publishers. (Cost: $18 per year.)

Health Services Manager (By AMACOM, a division of American Management Associations, 135 West 50th Street, N.Y. 10020) is a monthly newsletter on health care management for directors of nursing, hospital administrators and directors of inservice training. (Cost: $18 per year.)

Hospital Topics (By Hospital Topics, Inc., 3807 Bond Place, Sarasota, Fla. 33582) is the "official journal of the National Hospital Nursing Supervisor Management Conference and the National Central Service Conference." It is published bimonthly and contains articles of interest to supervisors in operating rooms, central service, infection control and inservice education. (Cost: $20 per year.)

Image: Sigma Theta Tau (Image: Sigma Theta Tau, 1232 West Michigan, Indianapolis, Ind. 46223) is the official journal of Sigma Theta Tau, the National Honor Society of Nursing. It is published three times a year and features articles on nursing leadership and promotes scholarship and excellence in nursing. (Cost: $5 per year.)

Infusion (Infusion, 12 High Street, Andover, Mass. 01810) is a bimonthly interdisciplinary journal on I.V. therapy. (Cost: $12 per year.)

International Nursing Index is a quarterly publication of the American Journal Of Nursing Co., which indexes "over 240 nursing magazines published in the United States and abroad." (Cost: $50 per year.)

Journal Of Allied Health is a quarterly journal for allied health professionals from Charles B. Slack, Inc.

The Journal Of Nursing Administration is a monthly journal for nursing supervisors and administrators. It deals with current and relevant issues in this field. Available from Concept Development, Inc. at a cost of $19.95 per year in the U.S. and $25 per year for foreign subscriptions.

Journal Of Surgical Practice is a bimonthly publication of McMahon Publishing Co., aimed at surgeons but also of interest to surgical nurses at a cost of $14 per year.

The Lancet (The Lancet, 7 Adam Street, Adelphi, London WC2N 6AD or for American Subscriptions, 34 Beacon Street, Boston, Mass.) is a medical journal aimed at physicians in a wide field, especially those affiliated with universities and medical schools, at a cost of $38.50 in the United States and $29.50 for interns and residents.

Life Support Nursing, "The Digest Of Equipment, Apparatus And Technique" (at 5535 Balboa Boulevard, Suite 101, Encino, Calif. 91316) is published bimonthly. This journal is aimed at E.R., I.C.U., C.C.U., O.R., and recovery room nurses. It contains information on equipment and instruments used in these fields as well as articles on critical care practice at a cost of $12 a year.

Medical Anthropology, Cross Cultural Studies In Health and Illness is a quarterly journal of interest to nurses and other health professionals concerned with cultural influences on health and illness. Available from Redgrave Publishing Company at a cost of $17 per year.

The New England Journal Of Medicine (at 10 Shattuck, Boston, Mass. 02115) is a prestigious medical journal with articles of interest to nurses as well as physicians. (Cost: $25 per year, worldwide.)

Nursing Clinics Of North America is a hard-cover quarterly publication of W. B. Saunders Company. Each issue contains articles covering two symposia on topics of interest to nurses.

Nursing Digest is a quarterly journal which deals in depth with a single topic of nursing care in each issue. From Concept Development, Inc. at a cost of $12 a year in the U.S. and $15 for a foreign subscription.

Nursing Forum is a quarterly journal available from Nursing Publications, Inc. at a cost of $18 per year.

Nursing '80 (From Intermed Communications, Inc., P. O. Box 3744, One Health Road, Marion, Ohio 43302) is a monthly nursing journal which focuses on patient care and practical information for nurses. It contains many helpful illustrations and is both informative and interesting at a cost of $16 per year.

Nursing Leadership is a quarterly journal for nursing administrators and leaders in all fields of nursing, from Charles B. Slack, Inc. at a cost of $10 per year.

Nursing Mirror (From Surrey House, 1 Throwley Way, Sutton, Surrey SMI 4QQ, England) is a publication aimed at nurses at all levels and with all interests.

Orthopedics is a bimonthly specialty journal from Charles B. Slack, Inc. at a cost of $28 a year.

RN is a monthly magazine published by Medical Economics Co. It includes articles pertinent to all fields of nursing at a cost of $13.50 a year in the U.S., $18.50 per year in Canada and $23.50 a year in all other countries.

Supervisor Nurse (From Circulation Department, Box F, Concord, Mass. 01742) is a monthly journal devoted to topics of interest to nursing administrators at a cost of $18 per year in the U.S. and $25 in foreign countries.

Surgical Clinics of North America is a publication of W. B. Saunders Co., published every other month ($39.00/year).

Today's OR Nurse is a monthly specialty journal available from Charles B. Slack, Inc. at a cost of $12 per year.

Topics In Clinical Nursing is a quarterly journal which considers one topic in clinical care in each issue. It takes a holistic approach and emphasizes the client's part in his/her health care. From Aspen Systems Corporation at a cost of $26 a year.

Topics In Emergency Medicine is a new quarterly journal for emergency care nurses, physicians and allied health professionals, from Aspen Systems Corporation at a cost of $36 a year.

Audiovisual Materials

General Medical-Surgical Nursing and Health

"Nonverbal Communication in Nursing" and "Nurse-Patient Interaction" are series of filmstrips and sound cassettes for students and practicing nurses from Concept Media.

"Communication Skills In The Health Care Institution," a filmstrip for nurses, is from Eye Gate Media.

Audiotape and filmstrip lessons on the fundamentals of nursing care are available from Multi Media Office. They are useful in nursing schools, particularly for independent study.

"Fundamental Nursing Skills" is a multiprogram for independent study on the basics in nursing care. From Lippincott's Audiovisual Media.

"Fundamental Concepts In Nursing," a series of filmstrips and sound cassettes or records, is available from Concept Media.

The American Journal Of Nursing Company has an extensive listing of films on all aspects of nursing care. Write for complete catalog.

"This Is Nursing," a film on the nurse as a member of the health team is available from University of California Extension Media Center.

"Shock: Recognition And Management" is a film from Association-Sterling Films.

"Run Dick, Run Jane" is a film on the value of regular exercise to prevent heart disease. Available in English and Spanish, from Brigham Young University.

"Human Heart Transplants" is a film on the ethics of organ transplants and includes interviews with transplant patients and surgeons. From the Graphic Curriculum.

"Silent Countdown" is a film on high blood pressure and its control, from West Glen Films.

"High Blood Pressure—If Only It Hurt A Little" is a film on the dangers of high blood pressure, from West Glen Films.

"Live Or Die" is a gripping film for health education for all age groups. It portrays the life and death of a man and a woman who both died at age 47. The film shows how their poor eating habits, stress and lack of exercise contributed to their deaths. It is an excellent film for motivating people to live health-promoting life styles. From Perennial Education, Inc.

"Heart Care," "Shock And Hemorrhage," "Intravenous Therapy," "Wound Care And Dressing Techniques" and "How to Give An Injection" are examples of the educational filmstrips for nursing students available from Eye Gate Media.

"Home Care—An Approach To The Treatment Of Chronic Disease" is a film for professionals from the American Heart Association.

"Coronary Counterattack" is a film on prevention of coronary disease, with emphasis on keeping physically fit, from Brigham Young University.

"An Introduction To Nursing In A Coronary Care Unit" is a film from the American Heart Association.

"Critical Care Nursing—Eight Videocassettes" is a series dealing with various aspects of critical care. From American Journal of Nursing Co.

"Nursing Care: Myocardial Infarction" is a film available from C. B. Fleet Co., Inc.

Medical Illustration slides (for 35mm projectors) of illustrations from *The CIBA Collection Of Medical Illustrations* and *Clinical Symposia* are available from CIBA-GEIGY. There are over 2300 color slides on anatomy and pathology.

"Hospital," a moving film on life in a metropolitan hospital and the indignities and dehumanization people face there, is available from Zipporah Films.

"Pain And Its Alleviation," a film on the nurse's role in alleviating pain, is available from the University of California Extension Media Center.

"The Decubitus Ulcer," a film on the prevention and care of decubitus ulcers, is available from Westwood Pharmaceuticals.

Films on intravenous infusion techniques and venous blood collection are available from Becton-Dickinson, Co.

"Rendezvous With Life," an educational film on the use of an artificial kidney in the home, is available from Baxter Laboratories.

"Functional Anatomy Of The Human Kidney" is a film from Association-Sterling Films.

"Asepsis In Respiratory Therapy" is a film available from Arbrook, Inc.

First Aid Audiovisual Materials

"Choking: Saving A Life," a film on saving a choking victim, is available from American Educational Films.

"CPR Quiz: Basic Life Support," "CPR Trainer," "CPR Filmstrip," "First Aid Quiz Number 1/Saving A Life," "First Aid Quiz Number 2/Treating An Injury," and "Deep Water Rescue: Artificial Respiration," are all available from American Educational Films.

"Cardiopulmonary Resuscitation Emergency Technics And Training," a film, is available from Ayerst Laboratories.

"External Cardiac Massage," a film, available from Association-Sterling Films.

"Choking: A First Aid Film," and "CPR Trainer" are films from Professional Research, Inc.

"CPR (Cardiopulmonary Resuscitation): A Life At Stake" is a film from Aims Instructional Media, Inc.

"Medical Emergency Procedures (CPR And The Heimlich

Maneuver)" is a series of two filmstrips and cassettes from Eye Gate Media.

"Mouth-To-Mouth Resuscitation" is a film demonstrating this procedure on victims of various ages, from the University of California Extension Media Center.

"New Breath Of Life" is a film on the most recent recommendations for managing choking, including the Heimlich maneuver and mouth-to-mouth resuscitation, from Pyramid Films.

"How To Save A Choking Victim: The Heimlich Maneuver" is a film from Paramount Communications.

Several films and slide series on first aid, safety and disaster management are available from the American National Red Cross. Write for Audio Visual Catalog.

"Disaster Nursing—Meeting The Challenge" is a film designed for courses in disaster nursing, also from the American National Red Cross.

"They Called It Fireproof," a film on the need for concern for hospital safety, is available from the National Film Board of Canada.

Resources on Burns and Burn Care

The International Society For Burn Injuries
c/o Dr. John Doswick, Jr., M.D., F.A.C.S.
4200 East Ninth Avenue, Box C-309
Denver, Colo. 80262

The Society sponsors the International Congress on Burns. It will be held in San Francisco in 1982. Materials available from the Society include a directory of burn care facilities in the United States and Europe.

National Fire Protection Association
470 Atlantic Avenue
Boston, Mass. 02210

This organization publishes many educational materials on fire protection and fire safety. Especially of interest to nurses are *Firesafety In Hospitals,* a "slide-tape training program," *Handling Radiation Emergencies,* a 184-page book, *Fire Safety For Nursing Home Employees,* and *Health Care Safety.*

Audiovisual Materials

"Eleven West" is a film documenting treatment on the burn unit of Cleveland Metropolitan Hospital, from Films Incorporated.

Resources on Cancer

American Cancer Society, Inc.
National Headquarters
777 Third Avenue
New York, N.Y. 10017

The American Cancer Society local units provide research, counseling, sick room supplies, transportation, rehabilitation, and support groups, along with educational programs and conferences. Partial payment for limited services for indigent patients is also available.

The American Cancer Society has numerous pamphlets and posters on cancer available for the lay public and health professionals. One excellent pamphlet is "Listen With Your Heart" by Marion Stonberg, A.C.S.W., on talking with cancer patients, for family and friends. Contact local chapters for this and the many other educational materials available. (See list below for addresses.)

Alabama Division, Inc.
2926 Central Avenue
Birmingham, Alabama 35209
(205) 879-2242

Alaska Division, Inc.
1343 G Street
Anchorage, Alaska 99501
(907) 277-8696

Arizona Division, Inc.
634 West Indian School Road
P.O. Box 33187
Phoenix, Arizona 85067
(602) 264-5861

Arkansas Division, Inc.
5520 West Markham Street
P.O. Box 3822
Little Rock, Arkansas 72203
(501) 664-3480-1-2

California Division, Inc.
731 Market Street
San Francisco, California 94103
(415) 777-1800

Colorado Division, Inc.
1809 East 18th Avenue
P.O. Box 18268
Denver, Colorado 80218
(303) 321-2464

Connecticut Division, Inc.
Barnes Park South
14 Village Lane
P.O. Box 410
Wallingford, Connecticut 06492
(203) 265-7161

Delaware Division, Inc.
Academy of Medicine Bldg.
1925 Lovering Avenue
Wilmington, Delaware 19806
(302) 654-6267

District of Columbia Division, Inc.
Universal Building, South
1825 Connecticut Avenue, N.W.
Washington, D.C. 20009
(202) 483-2600

Florida Division, Inc.
1001 South MacDill Avenue
Tampa, Florida 33609
(813) 253-0541

Georgia Division, Inc.
1422 W. Peachtree Street, N.W.
Atlanta, Georgia 30309
(404) 892-0026

Hawaii Division, Inc.
Community Services Center Bldg.
200 North Vineyard Boulevard
Honolulu, Hawaii 96817
(808) 531-1662-3-4-5

Idaho Division, Inc.
1609 Abbs Street
P.O. Box 5386
Boise, Idaho 83705
(208) 343-4609

Illinois Division, Inc.
37 South Wabash Avenue
Chicago, Illinois 60603
(312) 372-0472

Indiana Division, Inc.
4755 Kingsway Drive, Suite 100
Indianapolis, Indiana 46205

(317) 257-5326

Iowa Division, Inc.
Highway #18 West
P.O. Box 980
Mason City, Iowa 50401
(515) 423-0712

Kansas Division, Inc.
3003 Van Buren Street
Topeka, Kansas 66611
(913) 267-0131

Kentucky Division, Inc.
Medical Arts Bldg.
1169 Eastern Parkway
Louisville, Kentucky 40217
(502) 459-1867

Louisiana Division, Inc.
Masonic Temple Bldg., Room 810
333 St. Charles Avenue
New Orleans, Louisiana 70130
(504) 523-2029

Maine Division, Inc.
Federal and Green Streets
Brunswick, Maine 04011

(207) 729-3339
Maryland Division, Inc.
200 East Joppa Road
Towson, Maryland 21204
(301) 828-8890
Massachusetts Division, Inc.
247 Commonwealth Avenue
Boston, Massachusetts 02116
(617) 267-2650
Michigan Division, Inc.
1205 East Saginaw Street
Lansing, Michigan 48906
(517) 371-2920
Minnesota Division, Inc.
2750 Park Avenue
Minneapolis, Minnesota 55407
(612) 871-2111
Mississippi Division, Inc.
345 North Mart Plaza
Jackson, Mississippi 39206
(601) 362-8874
Missouri Division, Inc.
715 Jefferson Street
P.O. Box 1066
Jefferson City, Missouri 65101
(314) 636-3195
Montana Division, Inc.
2820 First Avenue South
Billings, Montana 59101
(406) 252-7111
Nebraska Division, Inc.
Overland Wolfe Centre
6910 Pacific Street, Suite 210
Omaha, Nebraska 68106
(402) 551-2422
Nevada Division, Inc.
953-35B East Sahara
Suite 101 ST&P Bldg.
Las Vegas, Nevada 89104
(702) 733-7272
New Hampshire Division, Inc.
22 Bridge Street
Manchester, New Hampshire
(603) 669-3270
New Jersey Division, Inc.
2700 Route 22, P.O. Box 1220
Union, New Jersey 07083
(201) 687-2100

New Mexico Division, Inc.
525 San Pedro, N.E.
Albuquerque, New Mexico 87108
(505) 262-1727
New York State Division, Inc.
6725 Lyons Street
P.O. Box 7
East Syracuse, New York 13057
(315) 437-7025
☐ **Long Island Division, Inc.**
535 Broad Hollow Road
(Route 110)
Melville, New York 11747
(516) 420-1111
☐ **New York City Division, Inc.**
19 West 56th Street
New York, New York 10019
(212) 586-8700
☐ **Queens Division, Inc.**
111-15 Queens Boulevard
Forest Hills, New York 11375
(212) 263-2224
☐ **Westchester Division, Inc.**
246 North Central Avenue
Hartsdale, New York 10530
(914) 949-4800
North Carolina Division, Inc.
222 North Person Street
P.O. Box 27624
Raleigh, North Carolina 27611
(919) 834-8463
North Dakota Division, Inc.
Hotel Graver Annex Bldg.
115 Roberts Street
P.O. Box 426
Fargo, North Dakota 58102
(701) 232-1385
Ohio Division, Inc.
453 Lincoln Bldg.
1367 East Sixth Street
Cleveland, Ohio 44114
(216) 771-6700
Oklahoma Division, Inc.
1312 N.W. 24th Street
Oklahoma City, Oklahoma 73106
(405) 525-3515

Oregon Division, Inc.
910 N.E. Union Avenue
Portland, Oregon 97232
(503) 231-5100
Pennsylvania Division, Inc.
Route 422 & Sipe Avenue
P.O. Box 416
Hershey, Pennsylvania 17033
(717) 533-6144
☐ **Philadelphia Division, Inc.**
21 South 12th Street
Philadelphia, Pennsylvania 19107
(215) 665-2900
Puerto Rico Division, Inc.
(Avenue Domenech 273
Hato Rey, P. R.)
GPO Box 6004
San Juan, Puerto Rico 00936
(809) 764-2295
Rhode Island Division, Inc.
345 Blackstone Blvd.
Providence, Rhode Island 02906
(401) 831-6970
South Carolina Division, Inc.
2442 Devine Street
Columbia, South Carolina 29205
(803) 787-5623
South Dakota Division, Inc.
1025 North Minnesota Avenue
Hillcrest Plaza
Sioux Falls, South Dakota 57104
(605) 336-0897
Tennessee Division, Inc.
2519 White Avenue
Nashville, Tennessee 37204
(615) 383-1710
Texas Division, Inc.
3834 Spicewood Springs Road
P.O. Box 9863
Austin, Texas 78766
(512) 345-4560
Utah Division, Inc.
610 East South Temple
Salt Lake City, Utah 84102
(801) 322-0431

Vermont Division, Inc.
13 Loomis Street, Drawer C
Montpelier, Vermont 05602
(802) 223-2348
Virginia Division, Inc.
3218 West Cary Street
P.O. Box 7288
Richmond, Virginia 23221
(804) 359-0208
Washington Division, Inc.
2120 First Avenue North
Seattle, Washington 98109
(206) 283-1152
West Virginia Division, Inc.
Suite 100
240 Capital Street
Charleston, West Virginia 25301
(304) 344-3611
Wisconsin Division, Inc.
611 North Sherman Avenue
P.O. Box 1626
Madison, Wisconsin 53701
(608) 249-0487
☐ **Milwaukee Division, Inc.**
6401 West Capitol Drive
Milwaukee, Wisconsin 53216
(414) 461-1100
Wyoming Division, Inc.
Indian Hills Center
506 Shoshoni
Cheyenne, Wyoming 82001
(307) 638-3331
Affiliate of the
American Cancer Society
Canal Zone Cancer Committee
Drawer A
Balboa Heights, Canal Zone

University Hospitals Cancer Center
At-Home Rehabilitation Project
University Hospitals of Cleveland
2074 Abington Road
Cleveland, Ohio 44106

This project, funded by the National Cancer Institute, was established to show "the value of team home care services to cancer patients and their families." Materials available from the project include *At-Home Cancer Rehabilitation: A Team Manual,* Dobos, J. (ed), 1979 ($10.00); *At-Home Rehabilitation for Cancer Patients: Team Training Curriculum,* Dobos, J., 1979 ($10.00); a slide-tape program, "A Better Life," Dobos, J., ed., 1978, on rehabilitation for cancer patients and families; and bibliographies on pediatric cancer and on cancer and employment.

Cancer Counseling And Research Center
1300 Summit Avenue—Suite 710
Fort Worth, Tex. 76102

This center, founded by O. Carl Simonton, M.D., and Stephanie Matthews-Simonton, psychotherapist, has developed innovative methods to study and treat the emotional/psychological needs of cancer patients and their families. The center combines counseling and "relaxation/visual imagery" with medical treatment.

The Center has become a model for the rest of the country and both Dr. Simonton and Ms. Matthews-Simonton have published several articles on their research and treatment programs. Printed materials available from the Center include *Getting Well Again* (Subtitle: "A Step-By-Step Self-Help Guide To Overcoming Cancer For Patients And Their Families") by O. Carl Simonton, Stephanie Matthews-Simonton and James Creighton ($8.95); "Belief Systems And Management Of The Emotional Aspects Of Malignancy" ($2); and several reprints of lectures.

Cancer Information Clearinghouse
Office Of Cancer Communications
National Cancer Institute
7910 Woodmont Avenue, Suite 1320
Bethesda, Md. 20014

This clearinghouse disseminates information on cancer education materials to organizations involved in public, patient, and professional education. Bibliographies are provided as well as referrals to sources for cancer information materials. Bibliographies available include "Breast Cancer: Annotated Bibliography Of Public, Patient, And Professional Information On Educational Materials" (NIH Publication No. 79-2002); "Nutrition For The Cancer Patient," 2nd edition; "Patient Education Materials For Ostomates"; "Public And Patient Cancer Education Materials in Spanish"; and "Cancer Information In The Workplace."

DES Action, Inc.
Long Island Jewish-Hillside Medical Center
New Hyde Park, N.Y. 11040

DES Action is an organization concerned with providing education to professionals and the general public on the problems caused by DES use in pregnant women. A main goal of the group is to reach people who are not aware of their exposure to DES and to educate them as to the health care needed to diagnose and treat any problems resulting from this exposure. The organization also supports legislation concerning the DES problem. It publishes educational pamphlets (including one entitled "From One DES Teenager To Another"), a list of Doctors in various parts of the country skilled in diagnostic procedures needed, and a regular Newsletter available for $15 for individuals, and $25 for groups.

International Association Of Laryngectomees (IAL)
777 Third Avenue
New York, N.Y. 10017

IAL is an organization sponsored by the American Cancer Society, and it is an excellent resource for people having a laryngectomy and the nurses working with them. Extensive literature is available, including: "Helping Words For The Laryngectomee," a booklet; "First Aid For (Neck Breathers) Laryngectomees"; "Laryngectomees At Work"; "Your New Voice"; "IAL News," a bimonthly newsletter; and "IAL Directory Of Instructors of Alaryngeal Voice," listing names and addresses of instructors throughout the United States, Canada and Jamaica. Also available are emergency cards for the neck breather to carry to inform anyone of his/her condition in case of emergency, instructions for making bibs to wear over the stoma, and a directory of sources for materials of use to laryngectomees.

Leukemia Society Of America, Inc.
211 East 43rd Street
New York, N.Y. 10017

This is a national organization (with several local chapters) for research into, and education and patient-aid in leukemia, the lymphomas and Hodgkin's disease. Publications include an "Annual Report" on the activities of the Society, "Patient Aid Program," a pamphlet on the aid available to patients unable to meet the cost of treatment, "What Is Leukemia?" "Leukemia: A Guide To The Management Of The Disease" and "Hodgkin's Disease."

Living With Cancer
P.O. Box 3060
Long Island City, N.Y. 11103

Living With Cancer is a self-help support group for cancer victims through which they share information and experiences. The organization conducts meetings for members, offers information and referrals.

This material is adapted from "Self-help for cancer patients" by Ricki Fulman in *The New York Daily News*, October 30, 1979, p. 41.

Sources on Mastectomy Information

"After Mastectomy: Finding the Right Prosthesis." Reprints available from Consumers Union, Orangeburg, New York 10962.
Companies that produce special clothes and prostheses. You can write for the name or names of stores near you that carry their products:
Accentuette, 8520 Warner Drive, Culver City, California 90230.
Airway, Inc., Erie Avenue at Pennsylvania Railroad, Cincinnati, Ohio 45209.
Camp International, Inc., 109 W. Washington Street, Jackson, Michigan 49201.
Confidante, Berger Bros. Company, 135 Derby Avenue, New Haven, Connecticut 06507.
Jobst Institute, Inc., 653 Miami Street, Toledo, Ohio 43694.
Jodee, Inc., 200 Madison Avenue, New York, New York 10016.
Profile, Medical Research Associates, Inc., 744 Walnut Avenue, Andalusia, Pennsylvania 19020.
Reach to Recovery, American Cancer Society.
Silveco Products, Inc., 2502-14 Milwaukee Avenue, Chicago, Illinois 60647.
Simone, Inc., 3748 East 91st Street, Cleveland, Ohio 44115.
Stryker, 420 Alcott Street, Kalamazoo, Michigan 49001.

From *The Hospital Experience* by Judith Nierenberg, R.N., and Florence Janovic, copyright © 1978 by the Bobbs-Merrill Co. Reprinted by permission of the publisher.

Periodicals on Cancer

Cancer Nursing—An International Journal For Cancer Care is a new journal devoted to all aspects of cancer nursing. It covers information on current practices in the field, and on new research. Available from Masson Publishing, Inc. at a cost of $18.50 per year in the United States and $25 in foreign countries.

Audiovisual Materials on Cancer

"Nursing The Person With Cancer: An Overview" and "Relief Of Pain: The Nurse's Role" are two audiocassette courses available for registered nurses from the University of Wisconsin. Continuing education units can be earned by taking these courses. Contact UW-Extension for information.

"Pain And Its Alleviation" is a videocassette tape series on pain available from the University of Wisconsin Extension.

"Research To Prevent Cancer," a film presented by the Department of H.E.W., Cancer Institute, is available from Association-Sterling Films, Inc.

"Progress Against Cancer" is a film dealing with the cause, prevention, and treatment of cancer, presented by the Cancer Institute of the Department of H.E.W., and available from Association-Sterling Films.

"Make Today Count" is the film story of the organization of the same name, an organization for people with terminal illnesses, founded by a cancer victim. From Brigham Young University.

"Learning To Live Without Cancer" by Robert Gilley, M.A., and "Role Of The Mind In Cancer Therapy" by O. Carl Simonton, M.D., and Stephanie Matthews-Simonton, are two tape cassettes on "psychological intervention" in cancer treatment. Both are available from Communication Enterprises, Inc.

"Relaxation And Mental Imagery As Applied To Cancer Therapy" and "The Role of Emotions In The Development And Treatment of Cancer" are a few of the tapes and records available from the Cancer Counseling and Research Center. Write for brochure of complete listings.

"Cancer I—The Nature Of Cancer And Its Diagnosis," "Cancer II—Focusing On Feelings," and "Cancer III—Treatment Modalities With Implications For Nursing Care," are filmstrips plus sound cassettes or records, from Concept Media.

"Cancer Studies: A Basic Review," and "Breast Cancer Studies" are sound-filmstrips available from Eye Gate Media.

"Soon There Will Be No More Me" is a film of a young woman with cancer, dealing with her thoughts and feelings, from Churchill Films.

"Breast Self-Examination: A Plan For Survival—A Lifetime Habit," a film for women on the need for breast self-exam and a demonstration on how to do it, and "Man And Woman's Guide To Breast Examination," are two films from University Of California Extension Media Center.

"Nature Of Leukemia," a slide/script presentation consisting of eight slides showing both normal and leukemic blood cells, is available from the Leukemia Society Of America, Inc.

"Cancer Detection: Routine Proctosigmoidoscopy" is available from C. B. Fleet Co., Inc.

The American Cancer Society has several films and filmstrips available on all aspects of cancer for all age groups. The Society also provides a projector and projectionist without charge for large groups. Contact the local chapter of the Cancer Society.

Resources on Communicable Diseases

Educational materials on communicable diseases are available from the Department of H.E.W., Center For Disease Control, Atlanta, Ga. 30333.

An extensive guide to "Communicable Diseases," including information on 30 common communicable diseases, is available in the American Red Cross' textbook, *Family Health and Home Nursing,* © 1979 by the American National Red Cross, pages 568–585. It is a useful guide for nurses and clients alike.

Audiovisual Materials

"VD Quiz," "VD: A New(er) Focus," and "VD Prevention" are three films from American Educational Films.

"VD 'A Plague On Our House' " is a film available from Association-Sterling Films.

"More Common Than Measles Or Mumps," an animated film for teenagers on VD, is available from Films Incorporated.

"VD. And Women" is a patient education program from Professional Research, Inc.

"VD: Twentieth Century Plague" is a filmstrip for early adolescents on the medical aspects of venereal disease from Marshfilm.

Resources on Diabetes

American Diabetes Association, Inc.
600 Fifth Avenue
New York, N.Y. 10020

This is a non-profit voluntary health organization for patient, professional and public education and research. Publications for patients include "What You Need To Know About Diabetes," "What Everyone Should Know About Diabetes," "Exchange Lists for Meal Planning," and several other pamphlets on diabetes. Publications for professionals include *Diabetes: The Journal Of the American Diabetes Association,* a monthly scientific journal; *Diabetes Mellitus,* 4th edition, a 300 page volume; *Diabetes Care,* The Association's Clinical Journal; and *Diabetes Forecast,* a bimonthly publication for patients and professionals.

Joslin Diabetes Foundation, Inc.
One Joslin Place
Boston, Mass. 02215

This is a foundation for services and education on diabetes which is affiliated with the Joslin Clinic (a group of physicians treating diabetics) and the Diabetes Treatment Unit of New England Deaconess Hospital. Publications include educational booklets on diabetes, covering treatment and emotional aspects, a *Diabetes Teaching Guide* in English or Spanish, and the *Joslin Diabetes Manual*.

Publications

Body Map For Diabetics, a booklet on giving insulin injections which includes a body map for alternating sites, is available from Baptist Hospitals Foundation of Birmingham, Inc., 3201 Fourth Avenue, South Birmingham, Ala. 35222. (Cost: $2 each, bulk rates available.)

A "Getting Started" kit for diabetics which includes a booklet, "Getting Started At Home," a site selector for insulin injections, "Proper Injection Technique" and "The Importance Of Proper Dosage Accuracy For The Diabetic," is available from Becton-Dickinson, Advertising Department, Rutherford, N.J. 07070.

Diabetes as a Way of Life, 4th edition, by T. S. Danowski, M.D., Coward, McCann and Geoghegan, Inc., New York, 1979. This book for diabetics describes the condition and how to live with it. It covers emotional adjustments as well as physical treatment and control of diabetes.

Managing Your Diabetes (a patient handbook) by Jean Ranch, R.N., B.S.N. and Mae McWeeny, R.N., B.S.N., Abbott-Northwestern Hospital, Inc., 1978, is available from Sister Kenny Institute (see address under "Resources on the Handicapped").

Audiovisual Materials on Diabetes

"Diabetes—Discussion Of An Etiology" is a film on current research, from Hoechst.

"Diabetes (The History Of)," a film on the history of diabetes to the present, from Hoechst.

"Diabetes—What You Don't Know Can Hurt You," and "The Modern Diabetic" are films from Ames Company.

"Giving An Insulin Injection" is a teaching film for diabetics, from Upjohn.

"Understanding Diabetes," a filmstrip for patients, is available from Eye Gate Media.

"Live With It" is a film for newly diagnosed diabetics showing ten diabetics and how they adjusted, from Teach 'em, Inc.

"The New Diabetic Counseling Series," a series of ten filmstrips on all aspects of diabetes for patient education, is available from Trainex Corporation.

"Diabetes—The Doctor Talks To You About Diabetes" is a cassette for patients by Max Ellenberg, M.D., from Soundwords, Inc.

Resources in Environmental and Occupational Health

American Occupational Medical Association
150 N. Warker Drive
Chicago, Ill. 60606

The Association publishes the *Journal Of Occupational Medicine* ($20 a year in U.S., $25 foreign) and reprints from the Journal are available on request.

Coalition For The Reproductive Rights Of Workers
1636 Champa Street
P. O. Box 2812
Denver, Colo. 80201

This is a group of individuals and organizations working towards eliminating hazards to the reproductive capacity of workers exposed to toxic materials.

Environmental Action
Suite 731
1346 Connecticut Avenue
Washington, D.C. 20036

This organization works toward improvement of environmental problems through legislation, lobbying and education. It publishes a monthly magazine, *Environmental Action.*

Industrial Health Foundation, Inc.
5231 Centre Avenue
Pittsburgh, Pa. 15232

IHF is an organization which promotes healthful working conditions by providing information, literature searches and bibliographies, and holding meetings and training courses for occupational health nurses. Publications include *Industrial Hygiene Digest,* which contains literature abstracts and occupational health news.

National Clean Air Coalition
530 7th St. S.E.
Washington, D.C. 20003

This Coalition is a group of organizations and individuals concerned about clean air which works for clean air legislation and implementation of clean air laws.

National Institute For Occupational Safety And Health (NIOSH)
Parklawn Building
5600 Fisher Lane
Rockville, Md. 20852

This is a Federal agency which focuses on research into "on-the-job hazards to the health and safety" of workers, recommending safety standards, and training occupational health workers. The Institute has numerous publications on occupational and environmental health. Write for *NIOSH Publications Catalog:* 2nd edition, Charlene B. Maloney, 1978 (DHEW (NIOSH) Pub. No. 78-123). For information on courses in occupational health, request "NIOSH Schedule Of Courses" in this field.

Professional Health Services, Inc. (PHS)
83 S. Eagle Road
Havertown, Pa. 19083

PHS is a mobile health service which offers industrial health testing for companies. The tests include x-rays and pulmonary function, audiometry, cardiology, visual screening and laboratory testing. The testing services are suited to the individual needs of the company. Equipment plus trained personnel are provided for the tests.

Science For The People
897 Main Street
Cambridge, Mass. 02139

This is a group of people concerned about the effects of technology which works toward making science and technology responsive to the needs of people. There are over 20 local chapters in the United States and Canada. The group organizes workshops and debates to educate people on the effects of technology and how they can have a say in the steps taken in science and technology. Publications include *Science For The People,* a bimonthly magazine, books and articles on genetics, nutrition, nuclear power, and related topics.

Society For Occupational And Environmental Health
Suite 308
1341 G. Street, N.W.
Washington, D.C. 20005

The Society provides a forum for exchanging information on occupational and environmental health hazards and finding ways to alleviate them. Membership is open to professionals and lay people who share a strong interest in this area. (Annual dues for active membership: $30, students: $6.) Publications include the Society's Newsletter and books on the Society's conference proceedings ("Women And The Workplace," "Dust And Disease," "Pesticides And Human Health," and "Health Hazards In The Arts And Crafts").

Union Of Concerned Scientists
1208 Massachusetts Avenue
Cambridge, Mass. 02138

This is a group of scientists, concerned about the effects of nuclear power, which works toward control of its use and better safety practices in nuclear power plants. Publications include *Nucleus,* a newsletter, and books on the use and dangers of nuclear power.

Women's Occupational Health Resource Center
School of Public Health
Columbia University
60 Haven Avenue, B-1
New York, N.Y. 10032

This is an organization focusing on women's occupational health issue which provides information and literature on women's occupational health. Publications include the bimonthly *Newsletter,* the quarterly *Technical Bulletin* and several *Factsheets.*

Publications

Accident Prevention Manual For Industrial Operations, 7th

edition, is available from the National Safety Council, 444 North Michigan Ave., Chicago, Ill. 60611.

The New Nurse In Industry, A Guide For The Newly Employed Occupational Health Nurse, by Jane A. Lee, R.N., B.S., published by the U.S. Department of H.E.W., is available from the Superintendent of Documents, U.S. Government Printing Office, Washington, D.C. 20402. (DHEW (NIOSH) Pub. No. 78-143). It is an excellent resource in this field with extensive bibliographies and listings of further resources.

Common Knowledge
Box 316-M
Bolinas, CA 94924

This is a quarterly publication on environmental hazards and recent studies in the promotion of health ($10.00/year). (This listing is adapted from MEDICAL SELF-CARE, Number 7, 1979, © 1979, MEDICAL SELF-CARE.)

East West Journal, 233 Harvard St., Brookline, Mass. 02146, is a magazine concernd with protecting the environment, healthful living, nutrition and similar themes. Cost of subscription is $12.00 per year.

Audiovisual Materials on Environmental and Occupational Health

"Song Of The Canary," a documentary "film about the dangers of the American Workplace" by John Hunig and David Davis is available from Manteca Films, P. O. Box 315, Franklin Lakes, N.J. 07417.

"Getting The Lead Out" is a film discussing lead in the environment as a threat to good health, from Syntex Laboratories.

Resources on the Handicapped

American Coalition of Citizens With Disabilities, Inc.
1346 Connecticut Ave, N.W.
Washington, D.C. 20036

A national, non-profit organization which promotes the rights of disabled citizens through advocacy, education, and referral services. Publications include *The Coalition*, a newsletter.

Amputee Shoe and Glove Exchange
c/o Dr. and Mrs. Richard E. Wainerdi
1635 Warwickshire Drive
Houston, Tex. 77077

This Exchange matches amputees with similar sizes and tastes for utilizing spare gloves and shoes (both economical and a way to put amputees in touch with someone else with similar concerns).

"International Disabled Expo"
32 West Randolph Street
Chicago, Ill. 60601

This is an annual exposition of products and services for people with physical handicaps. It is sponsored by the Paralyzed Veterans of America and is open to professionals and the disabled. The Expo includes exhibits of the latest equipment, talks by experts in the field, and audiovisual materials.

Reprinted from *National Resource Directory*, 1979, by the National Spinal Cord Injury Foundation.

National Spinal Cord Injury Foundation
369 Elliot Street
Newton Upper Falls, Mass. 02164
(617) 964-0521

Formerly the National Paraplegia Foundation, the National Spinal Cord Injury Foundation was incorporated in July 1948 to improve services for persons with spinal cord injury disease and to promote research in the field of spinal cord injury. Based on this initial focus, the Foundation has three major program areas known most widely as CARE, CURE, and COPING.

CARE refers to a commitment to assist in the development of integrated and comprehensive systems of quality care, including the areas of prevention, acute care, physical and emotional rehabilitation, return to independent living, and lifetime follow-up services. In addition, CARE refers to promoting research in the areas of improved clinical care and the development of necessary equipment and special devices.

CURE refers to the effort to discover a way to cure the effects of spinal cord injury or, more specifically, to identify a way to regenerate the human spinal cord. The FOUNDATION's Research Division manages this activity which includes the annual awarding of research fellowships to deserving young neuroscientists.

COPING refers to the FOUNDATION's efforts to break down barriers to independent life styles for persons who have spinal cord injuries and others who use wheelchairs for mobility. Examples of these barriers are seen in attitudes, architecture, employment, housing, and transportation. Through the advocacy efforts of the national organization and local chapters, the National Spinal Cord Injury Foundation fights for the civil rights of all these individuals.

Within these general program parameters, the FOUNDATION offers more specific services to individuals and to groups. These include programs to:
1. prevent spinal cord injuries.
2. promote ideal standards and criteria of care.
3. identify resources available for the use of individuals who have experienced spinal cord injuries.
4. provide case consultation services to persons who have recently been spinal cord injured.
5. develop and implement independent living rehabilitation programs that assist high-level quadriplegics to make the transition from dependent life styles in institutional settings to more independent settings at the community level.
6. conduct educational programs for professionals that result in improved care and to promote ideal standards of care.

Reprinted from *National Resource Directory*, published by the National Spinal Cord Injury Foundation, 1979.

Rehabilitation International, U.S.A.
20 West 40th Street
New York, N.Y. 10018

Rehabilitation International is a national voluntary organization which provides needed services to disabled people throughout the world. Its publications include *Rehabilitation/World,* a quarterly journal; the *International Rehabilitation Film Review Catalogue,* a catalog of films on rehabilitation from all over the world, including reviews and ordering information and *International Directory Of Access Guides,* 1978–79, an aid for handicapped travelers.

Sister Kenny Institute
Chicago Avenue at 27th Street
Minneapolis, Minn. 55407

Sister Kenny Institute is a center for rehabilitation for disabled individuals. The Institute publishes educational materials on rehabilitation and offers continuing education workshops for professionals several times a year. It has an Outreach Education Department which sends rehabilitation educators to other institutions to conduct workshops for the staff. Write for *Educational Materials Catalog* for information on excellent books and audiovisual aids for nurses in this field.

Publications on the Handicapped

Pamphlets and Books

Affirmative Action For Disabled People, a guide available from the President's Committee on Employment of the Handicapped, Washington, D.C. 20210.

"Amputee's Guide-Below-the-Knee," "Amputee's Guide Above-The-Knee," "Crutches On The Go" (in English or Spanish), "Amputee's Manual-March," and "Back Care" are excellent booklets for patient education, available from Medic Publishing Company, P. O. Box O, Issaquah, Wash. 98027.

Fire Safety For You—A Guide For Handicapped People is available from the National Fire Protection Association, 470 Atlantic Avenue, Boston, Mass. 02210.

Functional Aids For The Multiple Handicapped, a paperback book, and "Human Sexuality," an annotated bibliography on disability and sexuality, are available from United Cerebral Palsy Associations, 66 East 34th Street, New York, N.Y. 10016.

In A Nutshell, A Guide For Stroke Rehabilitation In The Community Hospital is a guide for hospitals working with people with strokes and other disabilities. It is available for 25¢ plus 25¢ postage and handling from the National Easter Seal Society, 2023 West Ogden Avenue, Chicago, Ill. 60612.

National Resource Directory, A Guide To Services And Opportunities For Persons With Spinal Cord Injury Or Disease And Others With Severe Physical Disabilities, published in 1979 (166 pages, paperback) by the National Spinal Cord Injury Foundation, 369 Elliot Street, Newton Upper Falls, Mass. 02164.

This book is an invaluable resource for people with spinal cord injuries and other handicaps. It provides information on the practical aspects of living with spinal cord injury, in a positive and realistic manner. It covers everything from physical care measures and sources for equipment to education and seeking employment. The emotional and psychological adjustments are emphasized throughout the book, in a similarly supportive manner. Perhaps one of the best things a nurse could do for her spinal cord injured patients is to give them access to this book. Nurses can learn much from it themselves.

The National Spinal Cord Injury Foundation also has available the following publications: *Handbook Of Care: Paraplegic And Quadraplegic Individuals* (for nurses), *Nursing Management Of Spinal Cord Injuries,* and *Paraplegia Life Magazine,* a bimonthly publication.

Several booklets on programs for handicapped persons are available from the Office of Human Development Services, Room 3380, Hubert H. Humphrey Building, Washington, D.C. 20201.

Directory of Organizations Interested in the Handicapped, 6th edition, 1980, is an excellent guide to resource groups working with handicapped people. Cost is $2.00 for the handicapped and their families and $3.00 to all others, with bulk rates available. To obtain this Directory write: People-to-People Committee for the Handicapped, 1522 K St., N.W., Suite 1130, Washington, D.C. 20005.

Financial Assistance for the Disabled, published by the INA MEND Institute to assist the newly disabled person to be aware of what financial benefits are available. Includes workers' compensation, insurance policies, social services, medicare, medicaid, health, vocational rehabilitation, veterans, and community agencies. Available from the INA MEND Institute, Human Resources Center, Albertson, L.I., New York 11507; $1.00 per copy plus $.25 for postage and handling.

Reprinted from *National Resource Directory, 1979,* published by the National Spinal Cord Injury Foundation.

A Guide to Sexuality for Spinal Cord Injured People

One of the better illustrated guides explaining the techniques of sexual expression for the spinal cord injured adult is a book entitled "Sexual Options For Paraplegics and Quadriplegics" by Thomas O. Mooney, Theodore M. Cole, M.D., and Richard A. Chilgren, M.D. This explicit guide focuses on the sheer joy and exuberance of sexuality and shows that a spinal injury need not preclude satisfactory sexual expression. For the health professionals involved in severe physical disability and the spinal cord injured person, this book is a fine source of useful information and brings an important message about the courage, determination and basic humanity which we all share. It is available by writing to:

> Little, Brown and Company
> Medical Division
> 34 Beacon Street
> Boston, Massachusetts 02106

The listed price of this book is $7.95.

Reprinted from *National Resource Directory, 1979,* published by the National Spinal Cord Injury Foundation.

Excellent Sources Providing In-Depth Examinations of Special Aids are:

Aids to Independent Living: Self-Help for the Handicapped, Edward Lowman, Judith Klinger, McGraw-Hill Book Co., Order Services, Princeton-Hightstown Road, Hightstown, New Jersey 08520. The cost is $42.50, plus postage. This book can be obtained through:

> Massachusetts Institute of Technology (MIT)
> Humanities Library, 145-224
> Interlibrary Loan
> Cambridge, Massachusetts 02139
> (617) 253-5682

GREEN PAGES: A news magazine with large directory of products and services for the disabled, including exercise equipment, communicating aids, eating aids, clothing, automotive equipment, books, clubs, transportation, etc. Broken down into service categories and by state.

Green Pages
641 W. Fairbanks
Winter Park, Florida 32789

Reprinted from *National Resource Directory, 1979,* published by the National Spinal Cord Injury Foundation.

Bibliography on Higher Education and the Handicapped

The College Guide for Students with Disabilities, A directory of 500 educational facilities and services throughout the United States for the college bound disabled student. The guide includes:

- specific handicapped programs and services of each campus
- building by building accessibility information, as well as information on the accessibility of a particular field of study.
- information on current handicapped student populations and organizations.
- information on a wide range of non-campus based resources: sources of financial aid, state and federal activities, etc.

   Cost: $12.00 single copy for disabled individual
   $20.00 single copy for agencies

For further information, contact:
Abt Associates, Inc.
55 Wheeler St.
Cambridge, Mass.
(617) 492-7100

"Accessibility of Junior Colleges for Handicapped," President's Committee on Employment of the Handicapped, Washington, D.C., 20210.

"Accommodating Students Who Have Physical Disabilities: A Resource Guide for Massachusetts Community Colleges," Technical Education Research Centers, Inc., 44 Brattle St., Cambridge, Mass. 02138.

"**A Preliminary Report on the Facilities for Physically Limited Students at the University of California General Campuses,**" printed in February 1976—can be obtained by writing: Mark Rapaport, University of San Diego, CA.

Directory of National Associations Relating to the Education of the Crippled and/or Health Impaired," request the most recent directory from the Department of Health, Education and Welfare, Washington, D.C.

"**Education of the Handicapped Student,**" Reprint—$.50 Rehabilitation Literature, 2023 West Ogden Ave., Chicago, Illinois

"**First Ponder, Then Dare,**" Booklet of college and universities barrier free. Presidents Committee on Employment of the Handicapped, Washington, D.C. 20201.

"**Guiding the Physically Handicapped College Student,**" Herbert Rusalem, 1962, $3.00 from Teacher's College Press, Columbia Univ., 1234 Amsterdam Ave., N.Y. 10027.

"**Higher Education and Handicapped Students,**" Free from Harry Waters, Ed.D., Kansas State Teachers College, Emporia, Kansas 66801.

"**Mobility for Handicapped Students,**" Free from Rehabilitation Services Administration, Department of Health, Education and Welfare, Washington, D.C. 20210.

"**Wheelchairs on Campus,**" Reprint of May, 1966 **Performance,** Free, The President's Committee on Employment of the Handicapped, Washington, D.C. 20210.

Reprinted from *National Resource Directory*, 1979, published by the National Spinal Cord Injury Foundation.

Periodicals

Sexuality And Disability is a quarterly journal for health professionals which deals with topics related to sex in individuals with physical and mental illness. Published by Human Sciences Press at a cost of $18 a year.

Audiovisual Materials on the Handicapped

"Angela's Island" is a film which deals with the rehabilitation of an 11-year-old paraplegic girl and the problems of the handicapped. From Films Incorporated.

"Exceptional Films About Exceptional Children" is a brochure on 17 films dealing with handicapped children. The brochure may be obtained from Films Incorporated.

"Adjusting To Amputation" shows three teen-agers sharing their experiences in adjusting to amputation. From Health Sciences Communication Center.

"The Human Race" is a film story of a man born with deformed hands and no feet who runs in 26-mile marathons ("on the stubs of his feet") and is a successful teacher, father, and author. It is a positive film for showing what can be done in spite of handicaps. From Brigham Young University.

"They Can Be Helped" is a film for professionals working with handicapped children. It shows how special care and stimulation can make a difference in their progress. From Brigham Young University.

Four films on "sexuality and the spinal cord injured person" are available from Multi Media Resource Center.

"Like Other People" is a film "dealing with the sexual, emotional and social needs of the mentally or physically handicapped." From Perennial Education, Inc.

"Access" is a film on helping the handicapped participate fully in society. From Polymorph Films.

"Gravity Is My Enemy" and "Walter" are two positive films on coping with physical handicaps, from Churchill Films.

"Teaching The Handicapped To Dress" is a film from the American Journal of Nursing Co.

"To Live As Equals" is a film intended to change negative attitudes toward the handicapped, from American Journal Of Nursing Co.

"Walk Awhile ... In My Shoes" is a film on the need for improved facilities for the handicapped. From the National Film Board Of Canada.

"Get It Together" is a positive film about a paraplegic and his struggle for rehabilitation, from Pyramid Films.

Several slides and films on mental retardation are available from the National Association for Retarded Citizens.

"Language Of The Deaf" is a film showing how the deaf enjoy all aspects of life, from Carousel Films.

"Deaf Child Speaks" is a film on the work of the Oral Education Center in Southern California in teaching the deaf to function in the hearing world. From the University Of California Extension Media Center.

"Deafness And Communication" is a film on the ways in which the deaf can learn to communicate. From the University Of California Extension Media Center.

Several videotape cassettes and tape/slide shows on deafness and related topics are available from the Alexander Graham Bell Association For The Deaf.

Resources on Self-Help and Consumer-Oriented Health Care

Center For Medical Consumers And Health Care Information, Inc.
237 Thompson Street
New York, N.Y. 10012

This is a non-profit organization which functions as an educational resource for people on health care issues and encourages them to play an active role in their own health care by being informed. Publications include *Health Facts,* a bimonthly newsletter for consumers ($6 a year). Services include workshops and a "Telephone Health Library" offering tapes on health issues.

Consumer Coalition For Health
1511 K Street, N.J. Suite 220
Washington, D.C. 20005

This is a national consumer health activist organization with agency and individual members. The group, in conjunction with Public Citizen Health Research Group, publishes *Consumer Health Action Network,* a newsletter for members. (Membership is $15 a year for individuals.)

Health Activation Network™
P. O. Box 923
Vienna, Va. 22180

This is a non-profit organization for health professionals and consumers which promotes health education and "self-care skills," and is "committed to the concept that each of us has the responsibility for promoting good health." The Network offers counseling and training in health activation, aids individuals in establishing local health activation groups, advises on sources for funding, and provides educational materials and equipment on self-help. The Network offers a "Black Bag Learning Series"™ which includes a "Black Bag" containing equipment for monitoring vital signs and conducting a preliminary physical exam, as well as educational materials on the use of the equipment. Publications include "Health Activation News," a quarterly newsletter, and several self-help guides.

Health/PAC
Health Policy Advisory Center
17 Murray Street
New York, N.Y. 10007

This is a non-profit center for change in the established health care system. It acts as a resource center for health activists and works to prevent discrimination against health care workers and consumers, and to make good, low-cost health care available to all. Publications include the Health/PAC Bulletin, published six times a year, which covers such issues as women's health, primary care, health care workers, environmental health and other topics (cost: $10 a year, $8 for students), and several pamphlets on health care issues.

National Health Federation
212 West Foothill Blvd.
P. O. Box 688
Monrovia, Calif. 91016

The National Health Federation is a "non-profit consumer-oriented" group which promotes the rights of individuals to choose their system of health care. It does not espouse any one means of treatment but rather advocates that all legal and safe health care practices be available. The NHF has educational and legislative programs at work to aid in its role of advocate for health care consumers. Publications from NHF include the *NHF Bulletin,* published monthly, a monthly "NHF Newsletter," and several reprints of articles on health care.

National Self-Help Clearinghouse
Graduate School And University Center
City University Of New York
33 West 42nd Street, Room 1227
New York, N.Y. 10036

This Clearinghouse functions to support self-help groups and to provide information on them to professionals. Publications include: *Self-Help Reporter,* a newsletter published five times yearly; *Self-Health And Health: A Report, Self-Help Groups: Perspectives And Directions* by Elinor Bowles, a manual for establishing self-help groups, and a directory of existing self-help groups.

Books on Self-Care

In recent years there has been a proliferation of consumer-oriented books on health care. The following list is a sample of the types of books available in this area.

Drakeford, John W., *People to People Therapy,* Harper and Row, 1978. This is a book on self-help groups, their history, how they function, and information on forming groups.

Hendin, David, *The World Almanac Whole Health Guide,* New American Library, New York, 1977.

Nierenberg, Judith, and Florence Janovic, *The Hospital Experience,* Bobbs-Merrill Co., 1978. This is an excellent book for patients explaining what goes on in a hospital, including tests and procedures and the reasons for them, patients' rights, and how to ask questions. The book goes a long way in dispelling the mystique of the hospital and allaying patients' fears through education.

Rosenfeld, Isadore, *The Complete Medical Exam,* Simon and Schuster, New York, 1978. This book explains the medical exam for lay people, including procedures, information on prevention of illness, and methods of self-exam, such as breast self-exam.

Samuels, Mike, and Hal Bennett, *The Well Body Book,* Random House, New York, 1973. This book describes a plan for medical care consumers on how to take charge of their own state of health.

Sehnert, Keith W., with Howard Eisenberg, *How to Be Your Own Doctor Sometimes,* Grosset and Dunlap, New York, 1975. This is a resource for people who want to be "activated patients" and learn how to check their own symptoms (blood pressure, pulse, heart beat, etc.) and play an active role in their own health care.

Taylor, Robert B., *Dr. Taylor's Self-Help Medical Guide,* Arlington House Publishers, New Rochelle, N.Y., 1977. This book deals with self-care measures in treating minor health problems and offers information on how to determine when it is necessary to see a doctor.

Vickery, Donald, and James F. Fries, *Take Care of Yourself, a Consumer's Guide to Medical Care,* Addison-Wesley Publishing Co., Menlo Park, Ca., 1976.

Periodicals

Medical Self-Care, Access To Medical Tools, P. O. Box 718, Inverness, Calif. 94937. *Medical Self-Care* is a quarterly Whole Earth Catalog-type magazine on resources in health care. It contains reviews of medical books and other tools and is intended for lay people to help them take responsibility for their own health. Nurses can utilize this excellent periodical both as a resource to recommend to clients and for their own information. It is not only innovative and informative, but also a joy to read. (Cost: $10/year.)

The Harvard Medical School Health Letter, 79 Garden St., Cambridge, Mass. 02138. This is a monthly newsletter for consumers, offering health information, published by the Harvard Medical School. ($12.00/year).

Resources on Smoking

Action On Smoking And Health (ASH)
P. O. Box 19556
Washington, D.C. 20006

This is a non-profit political action group against smoking. To raise funds to support its activities and to enlighten people on the effects of smoking, ASH sells t-shirts, buttons, stickers and signs with anti-smoking slogans on them. (Of use to nurses is their "Thank You For Not Smoking" sign which can be placed in hospitals or offices.)

The National Interagency Council On Smoking And Health
419 Park Avenue South, Suite 1301
New York, N.Y. 10016

This is a coalition of agencies concerned about the dangers of smoking. Member organizations include the American Nurses

Association, National League For Nursing and the National Student Nurses Association, along with 31 other organizations. The Council promotes education on the hazards of smoking, aimed especially at young people.

Smokenders
International Headquarters
Prospect Street at Rt. 22
Phillipsburg, N.J. 08865

This is an organization with affiliates in several areas which helps people to stop smoking by educating them on why people smoke and how to quit. Founded by Dr. Jon Rogers and Jacqueline Rogers in 1968, it has helped several thousands of people stop smoking. Write for listing of geographical locations of Smokenders groups.

Publications

Smoking And Health, An Annotated Bibliography Of Public And Professional Education Materials, 1978, is prepared by the Cancer Information Clearinghouse (see address under section on Cancer Resources), DHEW Pub. No. (NIH) 78-1841.

Audiovisual Materials on Smoking

"Smoking: A New Focus" is a film aimed at preventing or stopping smoking, available in Spanish or English, from American Educational Films.

"The Feminine Mistake" and "Smoking: How To Stop" are films on smoking for patient education from Pyramid Films.

Several films on smoking are available from the American Cancer Society.

"Smoking: A Report On The Nation's Habit," and "Smoking and Health—A Report To Youth," are among the many films on smoking and its effects available from Narcotics Education, Inc.

NCI Makes Available Smokers "Quit Kit"

Although 9 out of 10 smokers say they would like to kick the habit, two-thirds of them claim they have never received any advice from their physicians on how to quit smoking, according to the Department of Health, Education, and Welfare and the National Cancer Institute.

To answer this need, NCI has a "Helping Smokers Quit" kit for health care professionals.

The kit includes take-home tests designed to help the smoker identify his reasons for smoking, a collection of the latest tips on quitting, a description of the benefits of nonsmoking, special information for nurses to aid patients involved in quitting, and several wall posters.

For further information about the kits, or to obtain one, write: Helping Smokers Quit Kit, Dept. K-13, National Cancer Institute, Bethesda, Md. 20014.

Reprinted from *The American Journal of Nursing,* September, 1979, Vol. 79, No. 9, p. 1502,

Resources on Speech and Hearing Disorders

Alexander Graham Bell Association For The Deaf, Inc.
3417 Volta Place, N.W.
Washington, D.C. 20007

This is a private, non-profit organization which serves as an information center and advocate for the deaf, and sponsors conferences and educational programs. The Bell Association has three divisions, the American Organization for the Education of the Hearing Impaired, International Parents' Organization, and the Oral Deaf Adults Section. Publications include *The Volta Review,* a journal published six times a year, *Annual Monograph, Newsounds,* a newsletter, and several books and booklets on deafness and related topics.

American Speech-Language-Hearing Association
10801 Rockville Pike
Rockville, Md. 20852

This is the national scientific organization for professionals concerned with speech and hearing behavior and disorders. Publications include two quarterly journals, *Journal Of Speech And Hearing Disorders and Journal Of Speech And Hearing Research,* a monthly newsletter, ASHA, and a directory of speech pathologists and audiologists.

Gallaudet College
Kendall Green
Washington, D.C.

The only accredited liberal arts college for the deaf, Gallaudet College has excellent educational programs for the deaf and materials for people working with the hearing impaired. An extensive list of publications on deafness is available from the College Bookstore. The College publishes a journal, *Gallaudet Today,* which has articles on deafness.

Innovations In Nursing Care of the Deaf

The University of Rochester Medical Center conducted a survey of the needs of deaf patients and the value of having a nurse specialist in the care of the deaf. The position of nurse specialist was established and this nurse functions in two main roles; as "nurse interpreter" for deaf patients and their families and in "nursing intervention," which includes direct treatment, emotional support, patient teaching, and inservice training for staff on the needs of the deaf.

For further information on this program contact: Ellen Wolf, M.N.P., Administrative Director, Student Health Service, Rochester Institute Of Technology, One Tomb Memorial Drive, Rochester, N.Y. 14623.

The above material is adapted from *Survey Of Needs Of Deaf Patients At University Of Rochester Medical Center* by Ellen Wolf, R.N., M.N.P., 1975.

Resources on Vision and Blindness

American Association Of Ophthalmology
1100 17th Street, N.W.
Washington, D.C. 20036

Several pamphlets on eye care and disorders can be obtained from the Association.

American Foundation For The Blind
15 West 16th Street
New York, N.Y. 10011

The Foundation is a non-profit agency for research and education which promotes improved services to the blind. Publications include booklets, manuals and flyers on blindness and related topics; a catalog of *Aids And Appliances For The Blind And Visually Impaired;* a professional journal, *New Outlook For The Blind;* and a legislative newsletter, the *Washington Report.*

American Printing House For The Blind, Inc.
1839 Frankfort Avenue
Louisville, Ky. 40206

This is a publishing house for the blind and visually handicapped which publishes in Braille, and produces talking books, educational aids, and large type books. Catalogs of publications are available on request.

Better Vision Institute, Inc.
230 Park Avenue
New York, N.Y. 10017

This is an educational organization which publishes several pamphlets for public education on eye care and the need for eye exams.

National Library Service For The Blind And Physically Handicapped
The Library Of Congress
1291 Taylor Street, N.W.
Washington, D.C. 20542

The library provides a free library service for the blind and physically disabled who can't read standard books. It includes talking books and books and magazines in Braille.

National Society For The Prevention Of Blindness, Inc.
79 Madison Avenue
New York, N.Y. 10016

The Society has available many pamphlets on eye care, screening and safety, as well as posters, charts, and *The Sight-Sharing Review: Quarterly Professional Journal.*

Recording For The Blind, Inc.
215 East 58th Street
New York, N.Y. 10022

This is a free loan service of recordings of books to individual handicapped persons. The blind or handicapped person must be registered with the service, then he/she may borrow recordings.

The Seeing Eye, Inc.
Morristown, N.J. 07960

This is the national organization which provides guide dogs for the blind. Applications for a dog should be sent to this address. The Seeing Eye also has available "If Blindness Occurs," a booklet for those working with the newly blinded, films on blindness, and other publications.

Audiovisual Materials

Educational films on the prevention of blindness, for both professional and general audiences (including screening tests for eye problems, eye safety for children and industry), are available from the National Society For The Prevention Of Blindness, Inc. Write for catalog.

5 Nutrition

Nutrition is currently receiving much-deserved and widespread attention by health professionals and lay people alike. Scientists are learning more and more about the role played by the foods we eat in the prevention and treatment of illness and the maintenance of health.

Because nurses are so often the health professionals who spend the most time in patient education, it is necessary to have an understanding of the essential nutrients and their sources as well as special diets that clients may be placed on. The following material includes information on these topics.

Also of growing concern is the effect of additives in our food. The chart on the "Safety of Common Food Additives" answers many questions of nurses and patients in this area.

An increasing number of people are turning away from meat as the source of dietary protein and following various forms of vegetarian diets. In order for nurses to offer adequate teaching to these clients, we must first have a basic understanding ourselves of what constitutes an adequate vegetarian diet. Thus information on these diets is included here.

Obesity is a major health problem in the United States. There are many fad diets and weight loss programs available, and it is important for nurses to have a working knowledge of treatments for obesity, in order to better advise clients. The Protein Sparing Modified Fast has been receiving much attention in nursing literature, and so a detailed description of it is included here.

Nutrition is an area in which cultural patterns and attitudes play an important role. Any nutrition education provided by nurses must take into account the client's financial means and culturally determined preferences. Information on the eating habits of two ethnic groups is included here as examples of the importance a person's culture plays in what he/she eats. Many other groups have different dietary laws and habits. These two are included to stimulate thought in this area and as a reminder to consider cultural preferences when working with people from any ethnic group.

The resource section of this chapter contains information on sources for educational aids in this field. Another excellent resource to keep in mind for nutrition information is the nutritionist or dietician in health care settings. If your clinical facility has a nutritionist this person can be invaluable to you and your clients.

I. **Nutrients For Health**

II. **Other Important Nutrients**

III. **Recommended Daily Dietary Allowances**

IV. **Safety of Common Food Additives**

V. **Special Diets**

    Liquid Diets
        Clear Liquid
        Full Liquid
        Bland Liquid

    Soft Diets
        Soft Solid
        Mechanically Soft

    Restricted Sodium Diet
    Low- or Minimal-Fiber Diet
    Bland Diet
    Restricted Fat Diets
    Diets For Diabetics
    Diet During Pregnancy and Lactation
    Vegetarian Diets

VI. **The Calorie**

VII. **Obesity**

    Treatments for Obesity
    Compulsive Eating Cycle
    The Protein Sparing Modified Fast

VIII. **Dietary Habits of Two Ethnic Groups**

    Oriental Dietary Habits
    Jewish Dietary Laws

IX. **Nutrition Resources**

    Organizations
    Publications and Educational Materials
    Audiovisual Aids

Nutrients for Health

Nutrient	Important Sources of Nutrient	Some major physiological functions		
		Provide energy	Build and maintain body cells	Regulate body processes
Protein	Meat, Poultry, Fish Dried Beans and Peas Egg Cheese Milk	Supplies 4 Calories per gram	Constitutes part of the structure of every cell, such as muscle, blood, and bone; supports growth and maintains healthy body cells.	Constitutes part of enzymes, some hormones and body fluids, and antibodies that increase resistance to infection.
Carbohydrate	Cereal Potatoes Dried Beans Corn Bread Sugar	Supplies 4 Calories per gram. Major source of energy for central nervous system.	Supplies energy so protein can be used for growth and maintenance of body cells.	Unrefined products supply fiber—complex carbohydrates in fruits, vegetable, and whole grains—for regular elimination. Assists in fat utilization.
Fat	Shortening Oil Butter, Margarine Salad Dressing Sausages	Supplies 9 Calories per gram.	Constitutes part of the structure of every cell. Supplies essential fatty acids.	Provides and carries fat-soluble vitamins (A, D, E, and K).
Vitamin A (Retinol)	Liver Carrots Sweet Potatoes Greens		Assists formation and maintenance of skin and mucous membranes that line body cavities and	Functions in visual processes and forms visual purple, thus promoting healthy eye tissues and

Continued on next page

| Nutrient | Important Sources of Nutrient | Some major physiological functions |||
		Provide energy	Build and maintain body cells	Regulate body processes
	Butter, Margarine		tracts, such as nasal passages and intestinal tract, thus increasing resistance to infection.	eye adaptation in dim light.
Vitamin C (Ascorbic Acid)	Broccoli Orange Grapefruit Papaya Mango Strawberries		Forms cementing substances, such as collagen, that hold body cells together, thus strengthening blood vessels, hastening healing of wounds and bones, and increasing resistance to infection.	Aids utilization of iron.
Thiamin (B$_1$)	Lean Pork Nuts Fortified Cereal Products	Aids in utilization of energy.		Functions as part of a coenzyme to promote the utilization of carbohydrate. Promotes normal appetite. Contributes to normal functioning of nervous system.
Riboflavin (B$_2$)	Liver Milk Yogurt Cottage Cheese	Aids in utilization of energy.		Functions as part of a coenzyme in the production of energy within body cells. Promotes healthy skin, eyes, and clear vision.
Niacin	Liver Meat, Poultry,	Aids in utilization of energy.		Functions as part of a coenzyme in fat synthesis, tis-

	Fish Peanuts Fortified Cereal Produts	sue respiration, and utilization of carbohydrate. Promotes healthy skin, nerves, and digestive tract. Aids digestion and fosters normal appetite.	
Calcium	Milk, Yogurt Cheese Sardines and Salmon with Bones Collard, Kale, Mustard, and Turnip Greens	Combines with other minerals within a protein framework to give structure and strength to bones and teeth.	Assists in blood clotting. Functions in normal muscle contraction and relaxation, and normal nerve transmission.
Iron	Enriched Farina Prune Juice Liver Dried Beans and Peas Red Meat	Combines with protein to form hemoglobin, the red substance in blood that carries oxygen to and carbon dioxide from the cells. Prevents nutritional anemia and its accompanying fatigue. Increases resistance to infection.	Aids in utilization of energy. Functions as part of enzymes involved in tissue respiration.

Reproduced by permission of the National Dairy Council from *Nutrition Source Book*, © 1978. National Dairy Council.

Other Important Nutrients

Nutrient	Important Sources of Nutrient	Some major physiological functions
Vitamin D, The Sunlight Vitamin	Vitamin D Milk Fish liver oils Sunshine on skin (not a food)	Helps absorb calcium from the digestive tract and build calcium and phosphorus into bone.
Vitamin E	Vegetable oils Green leafy vegetables Whole grain cereals Wheat germ Egg yolk, butter milkfat	Protects vitamin A and unsaturated fatty acids from destruction by oxygen. Exact biochemical mechanism by which it functions still unknown.
Vitamin B$_6$	Beef liver, pork, ham Soybeans, lima beans Bananas Whole grain cereals	Assists in red blood cell regeneration. Helps regulate the use of protein, fat and carbohydrate.
Folic Acid (Folacin)	Green, leafy vegetables Liver, dry legumes, nuts Whole grain cereals Some fruits as oranges	Assists in normal blood formation. Helps enzyme and other biochemical systems function.
Vitamin B$_{12}$	Only in animal foods— Liver, meat, fish, shellfish Milk, milk products Eggs, poultry Vegetarian diets should include milk or a B$_{12}$ supplement.	Assists in the maintenance of nerve tissues and normal blood formation.

Biotin **(No RDA-NRC)**	Kidney and liver Milk and eggs Most fresh vegetables	Helps regulate the use of carbohydrate. Assists body in forming and using fatty acids.
Pantothenic Acid **(No RDA-NRC)**	Liver, kidney, egg yolk Meat, milk Whole grain cereals, legumes	Helps regulate the use of carbohydrate, fat, and protein for the production of energy.
Phosphorus	Milk and milk products Meat, poultry, fish, eggs Whole grain cereals Legumes	Combines with calcium to give bones and teeth strength. Helps regulate many internal activities of the body.
Iodine	Seafoods Iodized salt	Helps regulate the rate at which the body uses energy.
Magnesium	Legumes, whole grain cereals Milk, meat, seafood Nuts, eggs Green vegetables	Helps regulate the use of carbohydrate and production of energy within the cells. Helps nerves and muscles work.
Zinc	Meat, liver, eggs, oysters Other seafoods, milk Whole grain cereals	Becomes part of several enzymes and insulin.
Copper **(No RDA-NRC)**	Seafood, meat, eggs, legumes Whole grain cereals Nuts, raisins	Assists with iron storage and its release to form red blood cells.

Reproduced by permission of the National Dairy Council from *Nutrition Source Book*, © 1978. National Dairy Council.

Recommended Daily Dietary Allowances

FOOD AND NUTRITION BOARD, NATIONAL ACADEMY OF SCIENCES–NATIONAL RESEARCH COUNCIL
RECOMMENDED DAILY DIETARY ALLOWANCES,[a] Revised 1980

Designed for the maintenance of good nutrition of practically all healthy people in the U.S.A.

	Age (years)	Weight (kg)	Weight (lb)	Height (cm)	Height (in)	Protein (g)	Vit-A (µg RE)[b]	Vit-D (µg)[c]	Vit-E (mg α-TE)[d]	Vit-C (mg)	Thiamin (mg)	Riboflavin (mg)	Niacin (mg NE)[e]	Vit B-6 (mg)	Folacin[f] (µg)	Vit B-12 (µg)	Calcium (mg)	Phosphorus (mg)	Magnesium (mg)	Iron (mg)	Zinc (mg)	Iodine (µg)
Infants	0.0–0.5	6	13	60	24	kg × 2.2	420	10	3	35	0.3	0.4	6	0.3	30	0.5[g]	360	240	50	10	3	40
	0.5–1.0	9	20	71	28	kg × 2.0	400	10	4	35	0.5	0.6	8	0.6	45	1.5	540	360	70	15	5	50
Children	1–3	13	29	90	35	23	400	10	5	45	0.7	0.8	9	0.9	100	2.0	800	800	150	15	10	70
	4–6	20	44	112	44	30	500	10	6	45	0.9	1.0	11	1.3	200	2.5	800	800	200	10	10	90
	7–10	28	62	132	52	34	700	10	7	45	1.2	1.4	16	1.6	300	3.0	800	800	250	10	10	120
Males	11–14	45	99	157	62	45	1000	10	8	50	1.4	1.6	18	1.8	400	3.0	1200	1200	350	18	15	150
	15–18	66	145	176	69	56	1000	10	10	60	1.4	1.7	18	2.0	400	3.0	1200	1200	400	18	15	150
	19–22	70	154	177	70	56	1000	7.5	10	60	1.5	1.7	19	2.2	400	3.0	800	800	350	10	15	150
	23–50	70	154	178	70	56	1000	5	10	60	1.4	1.6	18	2.2	400	3.0	800	800	350	10	15	150
	51+	70	154	178	70	56	1000	5	10	60	1.2	1.4	16	2.2	400	3.0	800	800	350	10	15	150
Females	11–14	46	101	157	62	46	800	10	8	50	1.1	1.3	15	1.8	400	3.0	1200	1200	300	18	15	150
	15–18	55	120	163	64	46	800	10	8	60	1.1	1.3	14	2.0	400	3.0	1200	1200	300	18	15	150
	19–22	55	120	163	64	44	800	7.5	8	60	1.1	1.3	14	2.0	400	3.0	800	800	300	18	15	150
	23–50	55	120	163	64	44	800	5	8	60	1.0	1.2	13	2.0	400	3.0	800	800	300	18	15	150
	51+	55	120	163	64	44	800	5	8	60	1.0	1.2	13	2.0	400	3.0	800	800	300	10	15	150
Pregnant						+30	+200	+5	+2	+20	+0.4	+0.3	+2	+0.6	+400	+1.0	+400	+400	+150	[h]	+5	+25
Lactating						+20	+400	+5	+3	+40	+0.5	+0.5	+5	+0.5	+100	+1.0	+400	+400	+150	[h]	+10	+50

[a] The allowances are intended to provide for individual variations among most normal persons as they live in the United States under usual environmental stresses. Diets should be based on a variety of common foods in order to provide other nutrients for which human requirements have been less well defined. See text for detailed discussion of allowances and of nutrients not tabulated. See Table 1 (p. 20) for weights and heights by individual year of age. See Table 3 (p. 23) for suggested average energy intakes.

[b] Retinol equivalents. 1 retinol equivalent = 1 µg retinol or 6 µg β carotene. See text for calculation of vitamin A activity of diets as retinol equivalents.

[c] As cholecalciferol. 10 µg cholecalciferol = 400 IU of vitamin D.

[d] α-tocopherol equivalents. 1 mg d-α tocopherol = 1 α-TE. See text for variation in allowances and calculation of vitamin E activity of the diet as α-tocopherol equivalents.

[e] 1 NE (niacin equivalent) is equal to 1 mg of niacin or 60 mg of dietary tryptophan.

[f] The folacin allowances refer to dietary sources as determined by *Lactobacillus casei* assay after treatment with enzymes (conjugases) to make polyglutamyl forms of the vitamin available to the test organism.

[g] The recommended dietary allowance for vitamin B-12 in infants is based on average concentration of the vitamin in human milk. The allowances after weaning are based on energy intake (as recommended by the American Academy of Pediatrics) and consideration of other factors, such as intestinal absorption; see text.

[h] The increased requirement during pregnancy cannot be met by the iron content of habitual American diets nor by the existing iron stores of many women; therefore the use of 30–60 mg of supplemental iron is recommended. Iron needs during lactation are not substantially different from those of nonpregnant women, but continued supplementation of the mother for 2–3 months after parturition is advisable in order to replenish stores depleted by pregnancy.

Reproduced from *Recommended Dietary Allowances* (1980), with the permission of the National Academy of Sciences, Washington, D.C.

Safety of Common Food Additives

The following is based on "Chemical Cuisine," a poster prepared by Nutrition Action, a project of Center for Science in the Public Interest. A full-color poster may be obtained for $1.75 from C.S.P.I., 1755 S Street N.W., Washington, D.C. 20009.

AVOID

Artificial Colorings: Most are synthetic chemicals not found in nature. Some are safer than others, but names of colorings are not listed on label. Used mostly in foods of low nutritional value, usually indicating that fruit or natural ingredient omitted.

Additive	Use	Comment
Blue No. 1	In beverages, candy, baked goods.	Very poorly tested.
Blue No. 2	Pet food, beverages, candy.	Very poorly tested.
Citrus Red No. 2	Skin of some Florida oranges.	May cause cancer. Does not seep through into pulp.
Green No. 3	Candy, beverages.	Needs better testing.
Orange B	Hot dogs.	Causes cancer in animals.
Red No. 3	Cherries in fruit cocktail, candy, baked goods.	May cause cancer.
Red No. 40	Soda, candy, gelatin desserts, pastry, pet food, sausage.	Causes cancer in mice. Widely used.
Yellow No. 5	Gelatin dessert, candy, pet food, baked goods.	Poorly tested; might cause cancer. Some people allergic to it. Widely used.
Brominated Vegetable Oil (BVO)	Emulsifier, clouding agent. Citrus-flavored soft drinks.	Residue found in body fat; safer substitutes available.
Butylated Hydroxytoluene (BHT)	Antioxidant. Cereals, chewing gum, potato chips, oils, etc.	May cause cancer; stored in body fat; can cause allergic reaction. Safer alternatives.
Caffeine	Stimulant. Naturally in coffee, tea, cocoa; added to soft drinks.	Causes sleeplessness; may cause miscarriages or birth defects.
Quinine	Flavoring. Tonic water, quinine water, bitter lemon.	Poorly tested; some possibility that may cause birth defects.
Saccharin	Noncaloric sweetener. "Diet" products.	Causes cancer in animals.
Sodium Nitrite, Sodium Nitrate	Preservative, coloring, flavoring. Bacon, ham, frankfurters, luncheon meats, smoked fish, corned beef.	Prevents growth of botulism bacteria, but can lead to formation of small amounts of cancer-causing nitrosamines, particularly in fried bacon.

Continued on next page

CAUTION

Artificial Coloring: Yellow No. 6	Beverages, sausage, baked goods, candy, gelatin.	Appears safe, but can cause allergic reactions.	**Monosodium Glutamate (MSG)**		drome" (headache and burning or tightness in head, neck, arms) in some sensitive adults.
Artificial Flavoring	Soda, candy, breakfast cereals, gelatin deserts, etc.	Hundreds of chemicals used to mimic natural flavors, almost exclusively in "junk" foods; indicates "real thing" is left out. May cause hyperactivity in some children.	**Phosphoric Acid; Phosphates**	Acidifier, chelating agent, buffer, emulsifier, nutrient, discoloration inhibitor. Baked goods, cheese, powdered foods, cured meat, soda, breakfast cereals, dried potatoes.	Useful chemicals that are not toxic, but their widespread use creates dietary imbalance that may be causing osteoporosis.
Butylated Hydroxyanisole (BHA)	Antioxidant. Cereals, chewing gum, potato chips, oils.	Appears safer than BHT but needs better testing. Safer substitutes available.	**Propyl Gallate**	Antioxidant. Oil, meat products, potato sticks, chicken soup base, chewing gum.	Not adequately tested; use is frequently unnecessary.
Heptyl Paraben	Preservative. Beer.	Probably safe, has not been tested in presence of alcohol.	**Sulfur Dioxide, Sodium Bisulfite**	Preservative, bleach. Sliced fruit, wine, grape juice, dried potatoes, dried fruit.	Can destroy vitamin B-1, but otherwise safe.
Monosodium Glutamate (MSG)	Flavor enhancer. Soup, seafood, poultry, cheese, sauces, stews, etc.	Damages brain cells in infant mice; causes "Chinese restaurant syn-			

SAFE

Alginate, Propylene & Glycol Alginate	Thickening agent, foam stabilizer. Ice cream, cheese, candy, yogurt.	Derived from seaweed.	**Gums: Locust Bean, Guar, Furcelleran, Arabic, Karaya, Tragacanth, Ghatti**	pudding, salad dressing, dough, cottage cheese, candy, drink mixes.	
Alpha Tocopherol	Antioxidant, nutrient. Vegetable oil.	Vitamin E.	**Hydrolyzed Vegetable Protein (HVP)**	Flavor enhancer. Instant soups, frankfurters, sauce mixers, beef stew.	Vegetable (usually soybean) protein chemically broken down into constituent amino acids.
Ascorbic Acid, Erythorbic Acid	Antioxidant, nutrient, color stabilizer. Oily foods, cereals, soft drinks, cured meats.	Ascorbic acid and its salt, sodium ascorbate, provide nutrient vitamin C; erythorbic acid has no value as vitamin. All help	**Lactic Acid**	Acidity regulator. Spanish olives, cheese, frozen desserts	Naturally occurring in almost all living organisms.

Additive	Use	Description
Beta Carotene	Coloring, nutrient. Margarine, shortening, nondairy creamers, butter.	Body converts it to Vitamin A.
Calcium (or Sodium) Propionate	Preservative Bread, rolls, pies, cakes.	Prevents mold growth; calcium a nutrient.
Calcium (or Sodium) Stearoyl Lactylate	Dough conditioner, whipping agent. Bread dough, cake fillings, artificial whipped cream, processed egg white.	Sodium stearoyl fumerate, also safe, serves same function.
Carrageenan	Thickening and whitening agent. Ice cream, jelly, chocolate milk, infant formula.	From "Irish moss" seaweed.
Casein, Sodium Caseinate	Thickening and whitening agent. Ice cream, ice milk, sherbet, coffee creamers.	Nutritious, the principal protein in milk.
Citric Acid, Sodium Citrate	Acid, flavoring, chelating agent. Ice cream, sherbet, fruit drink, candy, carbonated beverages, instant potatoes.	Citric acid is abundant in citrus fruits and berries; an important metabolite.
EDTA	Chelating agent. Salad dressing, margarine, sandwich spreads, mayonnaise, processed fruits and carbonated beverages.	Traps metallic impurities that would otherwise cause rancidity and discoloration.
Lactose	Sweetener. Whipped topping mix, breakfast pastry.	Slightly sweet carbohydrate from milk.
Lecithin	Emulsifier, antioxidant. Baked goods, margarine, chocolate, ice cream.	Common in animals and plants; a source of the nutrient choline.
Mannitol	Sweetener. Chewing gum, low-calorie foods.	Less sweet than sugar but because it is poorly absorbed by body, has only half the calories of sugar.
Mono- and Diglycerides	Emulsifiers. Baked goods, margarine, candy, peanut butter.	Safe, but used mostly in foods that are high in sugar or fat.
Polysorbate 60, 65 and 80	Emulsifiers Baked goods, frozen desserts, imitation dairy products.	Synthetic but appear to be safe.
Sodium Benzoate	Preservative. Fruit juice, carbonated drinks, pickles, preserves.	Used more than 70 years to prevent growth of micro-organisms.
Sodium Carboxy-methylcellulose (CMC)	Thickening, stabilizing agent, prevents sugar from crystallizing. Ice cream, beer, pie fillings, icings, diet foods, candy.	Made by reacting cellulose with acetic acid (vinegar) studies indicate safety.
Sorbic Acid, Potassium Sorbate	Prevents mold, bacterial growth. Cheese, syrup, jelly, cake, wine, dried fruits.	From berries of mountain ash. Sorbate may be safe substitute for

Continued on next page

245

Ferrous Gluconate	Coloring, nutrient. Black olives.	A source of nutrient iron.
Fumaric Acid	Tartness agent. Powdered drinks, pudding, pie fillings, gelatin desserts.	Safe, but to enhance solution in cold water, DSS added, a poorly tested, detergent-like additive.
Gelatin	Thickening, gelling agent. Powdered dessert mix, yogurt, ice cream, cheese spread, beverages.	From animal bones, hooves and other parts. Little nutritional value as protein.
Glycerin (Glycerol)	Maintains water content. Marshmallow, candy, fudge, baked goods.	Natural backbone of fat molecules. Used as energy or to build complex molecules.
Gums: Locust Bean, Guar, Furcelleran, Arabic, Karaya, Tragacanth, Ghatti	Thickening, stabilizing agents. Beverages, ice cream, frozen	Derived from bushes, trees or seaweed; poorly tested but probably safe.
		vegetables, canned shellfish, soft drinks.
		sodium nitrite in bacon.
Sorbitan Monostearate	Emulsifier. Cakes, candy, frozen pudding, icing.	Keeps oil and water mixed.
Sorbitol	Sweetener, thickening agent, moisturizer. Dietetic drinks and foods; candy, shredded coconut, chewing gum.	From fruits and berries, half as sweet as sugar; slowly absorbed, thus safe for diabetics.
Starch, Modified Starch	Thickening agent. Soup, gravy, baby foods.	From flour, potatoes, corn; Modified chemically to improve solution in cold water. Used to make foods look thicker and richer.
Vanillan, Ethyl Vanillan	Substitute for vanilla flavoring. Ice cream, baked goods, beverages, chocolate, candy, gelatin desserts.	Vanillan, synthetic version of main flavor in vanilla bean, is safe; ethyl vanillan has more authentic taste but needs more testing.

SPECIAL CONSIDERATIONS

Salt (Sodium chloride)	Flavoring. Most processed foods: soup, potato chips, crackers, cured meat, etc.	Large amounts of sodium may cause high blood pressure in susceptible people and increase risk of heart attack and stroke.
Sugars: Corn Syrup, Dextrose, Glucose, Invert Sugar, Sugar	Sweeteners. Candy, soft drinks, cookies, syrups, toppings, sweetened cereals and many other foods.	Mostly in foods with low, if any, nutritional value. Excess sugars may promote tooth decay and precipitate diabetes in susceptible persons, condensed source of calories.

Reprinted from *The New York Times*, July 12, 1978, © 1979 by The New York Times Company. Reprinted by permission.

Liquid Diets

Clear Liquids	**Full Liquids**	**Bland Liquids**
Water	All liquids allowed on the clear liquid diet and the following additions:	The full liquid diet with the following exceptions:
Ice		
Tea	Milk, cream	No tea
Regular or decaffeinated coffee		No coffee
Carbonated beverages		No colas
Clear bouillon, consomme, broth	Strained, canned, or homemade soups as tolerated	No meat soups and broths or highly seasoned soups
Plain gelatin desserts	Simple puddings (liquid at body temperature) such as custard, vanilla pudding, ice cream without nuts or fruits	
Water ice	Refined cooked cereal	
Juices (apple, grape, lemonade)	Strained fruit and vegetable juices as tolerated	
Sugar, salt		

SOFT DIETS

Two types of soft diets (soft solid and mechanically soft) are available. Either may be used as a transition from liquid to house diet.

Soft Solid Diet

This transitional diet between the liquid and the house diet is not necessarily mechanically soft. To the full liquid diet are added a limited variety of relatively low-fiber foods that are considered easy to digest. If these solid foods are tolerated by the patient, it is hoped that a house diet will be ordered. The diet is considered to be adequate, but may soon become monotonous.

Continued on next page

Allowed	Avoided
Milk Whole, skim, buttermilk, yogurt. Milk drinks flavored with moderate amounts of syrups (chocolate, coffee, strained fruit), malt	Milk drinks or yogurt containing whole fruits or berries with seeds or skins
Beverages Tea, coffee, cocoa, decaffeinated or cereal beverages, powdered fruit drinks, carbonated beverages	
Eggs Hard-cooked, pasteurized, or other salmonella-free egg preparations such as approved eggnog mixes (see page 151)	Raw eggs, soft-cooked eggs unless pasteurized, fried eggs
Meats Broiled, baked, roasted chicken, turkey, beef, lamb, veal, liver, white fish, crisp bacon	Fried, highly seasoned items such as cold cuts, sardines
Cheese Mild cheese such as cottage, cream, American, cheddar, Swiss	Strongly flavored, pungent cheeses
Breads Refined, enriched white bread, plain or toasted; plain muffins, rolls; white flour crackers such as common, oyster, soda, saltines; melba toast, rusk, zwieback	Freshly baked hot breads; whole grain breads or crackers; those containing raisins or other fruits, nuts, bran, seeds; fried breads such as crullers and doughnuts
Cereals Refined (ready-to-eat or cooked) made from refined wheat, rice, corn; cereals prepared for babies; noodles, macaroni, spaghetti; strained oatmeal	Whole grain cereals other than strained oatmeal. Prepared cereals with bran, berries, raisins
Vegetables Cooked asparagus tips, beans (green and wax beans only), beets, broccoli buds, carrots, tomato juice, winter squash. If desired, strained peas, spinach, or summer squash may be added.	Other vegetables, strongly flavored sauces
Fruits Cooked or canned without seeds and skins, such as applesauce, baked apple, peeled apricots, peaches, pears; ripe	Berries, raw fruits other than those listed
Fruits (continued) bananas, orange sections, grapefruit sections	
Juices Fresh, frozen, or canned as tolerated	

Allowed	Avoided
Desserts Simple puddings without nuts or fruits such as custard, tapioca, plain ice cream, sherbet, water ice; plain, simple cakes and cookies	Pastries, cakes, cookies, and puddings made with nuts or fruits containing seeds and skins
Fats Butter, cream, margarine, crisp bacon, mayonnaise, mayonnaise-type salad dressing	

Mechanically Soft Diet

This diet differs from the house diet in that modifications of texture or consistency, or both, are made to enable the individual to ingest foods with relative comfort and in sufficient amounts. No restrictions in seasonings are imposed unless specified.

If modification other than in texture is indicated, it should be included in the diet order.

This diet may be appropriate for patients who are edentulous or have wired jaws or other conditions that impede chewing or swallowing.

Patients with esophageal injury or obstructive disease will likely need particular attention and encouragement. Frequent feedings of thoroughly blenderized foods and liquids, seasoned to the individual's taste, help the patient to secure sufficient nourishment.

The diet is adequate when foods are eaten in amounts usually planned.

Reprinted with permission of Little, Brown and Co. from *Diet Manual, Massachusetts General Hospital Dietary Department*, © 1977, Little, Brown and Company.

RESTRICTED SODIUM DIET

Characteristics and Principles. Foods high in sodium are restricted or limited and salt is not added as foods are cooked and served. This diet reduces water retention (edema). The diet prescription specifies 250, 500, 700, and 2000–4500 mg of sodium. (A person in health may eat 6–12 gm or even 20 gm of salt daily.) Tables showing the sodium content of foods must be used in planning diets according to prescription. The diet should be complete and may be made more palatable for some persons by the use of a salt substitute.

Type of Food	Foods Allowed	Foods Restricted
Beverages	Coffee, tea, Postum, and most carbonated drinks	Whole milk may be restricted and sodium-free milk prescribed
Breads	Salt-free breads	All breads made with salt
Cereals and cereal products	Most cereals can be used freely if not prepared with salt	No cooked cereals if prepared with salt. A few dry cereals are restricted that have an appreciable sodium content
Dairy products	500 ml milk daily. Unsalted butter or margarine	Low-sodium milk may be prescribed and foods made with milk limited or restricted
Desserts	Most desserts if prepared without salt. Fruits recommended	Commercial desserts made with salt
Eggs	One daily	
Fats	Unsalted butter or fortified margarine. Mayonnaise (unsalted)	Commercial salad dressing prepared with salt
Fruits	All—amounts served are determined by sodium content	None
Meats, fish, and poultry	None, if prepared with salt	Canned meats put up with salt and all dried and salted meats and fish
Seasonings	Salt substitutes may be prescribed. Herbs may be used to flavor foods so that salt-free dishes are more palatable	Salt (sodium chloride)
Soups and broths	All if made at home or commercially without salt	Most canned broths and soups restricted unless low sodium is specified
Sweets, candy, honey, jelly, and syrup	All in discreet amounts, if made at home or commercially without salt	Commercial candies containing salt
Vegetables	All that have low-sodium content and that are cooked without salt. Amount served depends on sodium content	Frozen or canned if processed with salt—vegetables high in sodium (see lists giving sodium content)

Note. Light salting of foods may be allowed for diets prescribing more than 2000 mg of sodium.

LOW- OR MINIMAL-FIBER DIET

Characteristics and Principles. A diet designed to reduce residue or fecal bulk in the intestines and to reduce mechanical irritation of the intestinal wall. It may be prescribed before and after surgery on the gastrointestinal tract and during inflammation of the intestines where distention causes pain or in ulcerative conditions where perforation is feared. (In constipation, chronic diverticulitis, and some other bowel disorders a high-fiber diet is believed by many to be indicated (see Note). A minimal-fiber diet may be deficient in thiamine and vitamin B6. Both of them may be prescribed.

Type of Food	Foods Allowed	Foods Restricted
Beverages	Any	None
Breads	Any breads, pancakes, or waffles made	Bran breads made with coarsely ground

Continued on next page

Type of Food	Foods Allowed	Foods Restricted
Cereals and cereal products	with refined flour or meal Cooked and raw cereals made with finely ground grains	flour or meal Cereals made with bran or any coarsely ground grain
Dairy products	Any	None
Desserts	Any without skin and seed of fruit, nuts, or coarsely ground grain	Any with skin or seeds of fruit, nuts, or coarsely ground grain
Eggs	Any	None
Fats	Any	None
Fruits	Strained fruit juices	All whole fruits
Meat, fish, and poultry	Any	None
Seasonings	Any	Pickles, relishes, olives
Soups and broths	Any clear or strained soup	Soups made with vegetables or any restricted food
Sweets, candy, honey, jelly, and syrup	Any without nuts, seeds, or skins of fruit	Any with nuts, seeds, or skins of fruits
Vegetables	None	All vegetables

Note. A *high-fiber diet* is one in which the restricted foods on the *low-fiber* diet (fruits, vegetables, and whole-grain breads and cereals) are not only allowed but stressed.

BLAND DIET

Characteristics and Principles. This diet is a regular diet from which foods are omitted that mechanically or chemically irritate the gastrointestinal tract. Some institutions have dropped the designation "bland," but all provide a non-irritating dietary regimen which may start with frequent small feedings of milk, dishes made with milk, cereals, starches, and jello. Other foods are added, as tolerated, until the diet meets the Recommended Dietary Allowances of the Food and Nutrition Board of the National Research Council. Some institutions list bland diets I through IV.

Type of Food	Foods Allowed	Foods Restricted
Beverages	Milk, whole or skim, and drinks made with milk	Coffee, tea, carbonated beverages, and seasoned broths, chocolate drinks
Breads	Toasted bread and crackers made of refined flour, rusk, and zweiback	Whole-grain breads and crackers. Freshly baked bread
Cereals and cereal products	Cereal gruel, strained	Whole-grain cereals unless strained
Dairy products	Whole or skim milk, yogurt, butter, junket, cheese—cottage, cream, Cheddar	Rich cheeses
Desserts	Custards, jello, ice cream, sherbet	Any desserts made with nuts or fruit with skins or seeds. Rich pastries
Eggs	One or two daily, soft boiled, poached, or in eggnog	Fried egg
Fats	Butter, fortified margarine	All fried foods and fatty meats
Fruits	Strained fruit juices. Fresh or cooked peeled fruits without seeds as tolerated	Unpeeled fruits and fruits with seeds and fibers like pineapple; some raw fruits may not be tolerated
Meat, fish, and poultry	All omitted at first but tender nonfatty meats, fish, and poultry are added as tolerated	Tough, fried, spiced, or fatty meats, fish, or poultry
Seasonings	Salt to taste	Spices and condiments generally
Soups and broths	None allowed at first but gradually added if made without irritating foods	Commercial soups containing spices, or any restricted seasonings

Continued on next page

Type of Food	Foods Allowed	Foods Restricted
Sweets, candy, honey, jelly, and syrup	Clear candies, honey, jelly, and syrup in small amounts	Chocolate candies, coconut candies, and excessive use of concentrated sweets
Vegetables	Rice, potato (without skin) added first with gradual addition of carrots, peas, spinach, asparagus, and other non-irritating vegetables	Gas-forming vegetables such as the cabbage family, beans, corn, cucumber, peppers, onions
Miscellaneous		Nuts, pickles

RESTRICTED FAT DIETS (HYPERLIPOPROTEINEMIA DIETS)

Characteristics and Principles. Restricted fat diets are of five types with slightly different characteristics and used for different purposes as follows: *Type I*—To decrease the dietary fat available and so lower the triglyceride concentration of the blood plasma. *Type IIa*—To decrease the dietary fat so that the level of triglyceride is lowered in the blood plasma. *Type IIb*—To decrease the dietary cholesterol and carbohydrate, to control the cholesterol and triglyceride concentration in the blood plasma. *Type III*—To decrease the amount of dietary cholesterol and carbohydrate, to control the concentration of cholesterol and triglyceride in the blood plasma. *Type IV*—To control weight, to restrict the amount of carbohydrate and cholesterol in the diet and so reduce the level of prebetalipoproteins of the blood plasma. *Type V*—To restrict calories, fat, and cholesterol to reduce chylomicron and prebetalipoprotein in the blood plasma.

For detailed directions the reader should refer to booklet prepared by the National Heart and Lung Institute. See page 2051 for references listed at the beginning of this section on diets.

	Type I	Type IIa	Type IIb and Type III	Type IV	Type V
Diet Prescription	Low fat—25–30 gm (¾ to 1 oz)	Low cholesterol—polyunsaturated fat increased	Low cholesterol—about 20% protein, 40% fat, 40% carbohydrate	Controlled carbohydrate—45% of calories—moderately restricted cholesterol	Low fat—30% of calories, carbohydrate 50%—moderately restricted cholesterol
Calories	Unrestricted	Unrestricted	Sufficient to maintain or reach "ideal" weight		
Protein	Unrestricted	Unrestricted	Increased protein	Limited to amount that maintains or achieves "ideal" weight	Increased protein
Fat	Kind unrestricted; Amount restricted to 25–30 gm (¾ to 1 oz)	Limited amount of saturated fat allowed; polyunsaturated fat increased	Controlled so that 40% of calories come from polyunsaturated fats	Limited to amount that maintains or achieves "ideal" weight (polyunsaturated fats recommended)	Limited so that 30% of calories come from (polyunsaturated) fats
Cholesterol	Unrestricted	Limited; only that in meat allowed	Limited to less than 300 mg from meat in diet	Limited to 300–500 mg (5–8 gr)	
Carbohydrate	Unrestricted	Unrestricted	Restricted—concentrated sweets not allowed		
Alcohol	Restricted	Discreet amount allowed	2 drinks allowed if substituted for carbohydrates		Restricted

Reprinted with permission of Macmillan Publishing Co., Inc., from *Principles and Practice of Nursing*, 6th edition, by Virginia Henderson and Gladys Nite, Copyright © 1978, Macmillan Publishing Co., Inc.

Dietary Strategies for the Two Main Types of Diabetes

Dietary Strategy	Obese Patients Who Do Not Require Insulin	Insulin-Dependent Nonobese Patients
1. Decrease calories	Yes	No
2. "Protect" or improve beta-cell function	Very urgent priority	Seldom important, because beta cells are usually extinct
3. Increase frequency and number of feedings	Usually not	Yes
4. Day-to-day consistency of intake of calories, CHO, protein, and fat	Not crucial if average caloric intake remains in low range	Very important
5. Day-to-day consistency of the ratios of CHO, protein, and fat for each of the feedings	Not crucial	Desirable
6. Consistency of timing of meals	Not crucial	Very important
7. Extra food for unusual exercise	Not usually appropriate	Usually appropriate
8. Use of food to treat, abort, prevent hypoglycemia	Not necessary	Important

Reprinted with permission of Little, Brown and Co., from *Manual of Medical Therapeutics*, 22nd edition, edited by Nicholas Costrini and William Thomson, © 1977 Little, Brown and Company.

Quantities of Food Needed During Pregnancy and Lactation

Food Group	Active Nonpregnant Woman	Pregnant Woman	Lactating Woman
Meat	2 servings of meat, fowl, or fish daily; 3–5 eggs per week	2–3 servings of meat, fowl or fish daily; 1 egg per day	3–4 servings of meat, fowl, or fish daily; 1 egg per day
Vegetables:			
Dark green or deep yellow	1 serving (at least 3 times per week)	1 serving per day	1 serving per day
Other vegetables	2 or more servings per day	2–3 servings per day	2–3 servings per day
Fruits:			
Citrus, melon, strawberry, tomato	1 serving per day	1 or more servings per day	2 or more servings per day
Other fruits	1 serving per day	1 serving per day	2 servings per day
Bread and cereals	4 or more servings per day	4 servings per day	4 servings per day
Milk	1 pint (two 8-oz glasses) per day	1 quart (four 8-oz glasses) per day	Four 8-oz glasses per day
Additional fluid	Ad lib.	At least two additional glasses per day	At least two additional glasses per day

Reprinted by permission of Little, Brown and Co. from *Nursing Care of the Growing Family* by Adele Pillitteri, © 1977, Little, Brown and Co.

Vegetarian Diets

Vegetarians may be divided into four groups:

1. *Strict vegetarians,* the "Vegans." They eat no food of animal sources: meat, fish, poultry, milk, eggs, or cheese.

2. *Lacto-ovo vegetarians.* These include eggs, milk, and milk products in their diets.

3. *Lacto-vegetarians.* They allow themselves milk and milk products in their diets.

4. *Ovo-vegetarians.* Eggs are included in this diet.

The "Vegans" are the only ones of the above four groups in danger of malnutrition. The effects of strict avoidance of food of animal origin may not be apparent for many years, perhaps twelve to fifteen. Long-term "Vegans" are relatively rare, but they are likely sooner or later to suffer the destruction of certain nerve fibers. This condition is irreversible, caused by a lack of vitamin B_{12}. There is no adequate source of B_{12} in the vegetable kingdom. However, this important vitamin could be taken as medication.

Another hazard of the strict vegetarian diet is calcium deficiency, which doesn't show up until late in life in the form of bone fractures. All *strict* vegetable diets are likely to be low in calcium, and the calcium from medication is not as efficiently utilized as from food. Such calcium deficient diets are especially hazardous for the infant, the growing child and adolescent, and the pregnant or lactating mother. Other possible nutritional deficiencies of the "Vegans" are iron and iodine. There are relatively few food sources of vitamin D. Food sources of vitamin D are cod liver and other fish liver oils. Increasingly, milk is being fortified with vitamin D, but not everywhere. Where there is very little opportunity for exposure to the sun, vitamin D, which is necessary for calcium utilization, may be lacking. Vitamin D may be supplied by medication.

Despite the above seemingly ominous warnings, it is possible to obtain an adequate diet from the vegetable world by supplementing it with vitamin B_{12}. However, this requires a broad knowledge of the dietary properties of foods.

Amino acids, and there are 22 of them, are the building blocks of protein. The word "protein" is of Greek origin, meaning "primary" or "of first importance." Protein is essential for every living organism. If vegetarianism is to be your route, the lacto-ovo vegetarian diet is the wisest, the diet that includes, along with vegetables, eggs, milk, and milk products.

The healthy individual can synthesize within his or her own body 14 amino acids. The other 8 (leucine, lysine, valine, isoleucine, threonine, phenylalanine, methionine, and tryptophan) must be obtained from food. These 8 have been labeled "essential amino acids." All 8 are present in foods of animal origin except gelatin. In foods of vegetable origin, such as cereal grains, nuts, legumes, vegetables, and fruit, one or more of these essential amino acids may be missing. However, by eating certain *combinations* of foods, our amino acid needs may be met. That is, the presence of an amino acid in one food may supply that amino acid in which another food is lacking. One of the more classic examples of this complementing action is found in beans and rice.

Reprinted by permission of G. P. Putnam's Sons from *The House and Garden Book of Total Health*, Mary Jane Pool, Caroline Seebohm, editors, Copyright 1978, G. P. Putnam's Sons.

SOME SOUND GUIDELINES FOR VEGETARIANS:

Be sure your calorie needs are met: 2,000 calories for a healthy woman aged twenty-three to fifty whose weight is within normal limits, and 2,700 for a man aged twenty-three to fifty. Choose your diet from a wide variety of whole cereal grains, nuts, soybeans, and other "oil seeds," thin dark green leaves, other vegetables, millets, legumes, and fruits.

Be sure your protein needs are met: 46 grams of protein each day for a healthy woman aged twenty-three to fifty and 56 grams for a man aged twenty-three to fifty. These are the recommended daily dietary allowances from the Food and Nutrition Board of the National Research Council. For example, a typical day's meals might include:

	Grams of Protein
3 glasses of milk	24
4 slices of whole grain bread	8
⅔ cup cooked dried beans, peas or lentils *	10
2 ounces cheese	14

(The inclusion of milk, milk products, and eggs enhances the quality of the vegetarian diet in all probably deficient areas except iodine. Using iodized salt provides this important trace element.)

* or 1 egg

Reprinted by permission of G. P. Putnam's Sons, from *The House and Garden Book of Total Health*, Mary Jane Pool, and Caroline Seebohm, Editors, Copyright 1978, G. P. Putnam's Sons.

FOOD GUIDE FOR PREGNANT VEGETARIANS.

Food Group	No. Serv./Day	Nutrients
I. PROTEIN FOODS		

A. Animal Foods
  1. Milk & Milk Products .... 4†
  Serv. Size: 1 c. milk (whole, skim, buttermilk, yogurt)
  ¼ c. dried milk solids
  1½ oz. cheddar cheese
  1⅓ c. creamed cottage cheese
  2. Eggs, 1 per serv.
B. Plant Foods 3*
  1. Beans (soybeans, kidney, pinto, black, garbanzo, lima, navy, blackeyed peas, lentils, etc.)
  2. Nuts (walnuts, pecans, Brazil, peanuts, cashews, filberts, almonds, and nut butters)
  3. Seeds (sunflower, sesame, pumpkin, squash, etc.)
  4. Grains (wheat, oats, rice, corn, barley, millet, etc.)

Milk & Cheeses: calcium, Vit. D, riboflavin, Vit. A, protein, phosphorus, Vit. E, B-6, B-12, Mg, Zn.

Complementary Protein Combinations: protein, Fe, thiamine, riboflavin, niacin, Vit. B-6, P, Mg, Zn & fiber (roughage).

II. GRAIN PRODUCTS .... 3†
A. Cereals, Hot: rolled oats, cracked wheat, malted barley, ½ c.
B. Cereals, Ready-to-eat: shredded wheat, corn & wheat flakes, ¾ c.
C. Breads, rolls, bagels, cornbread, 1 sl. or one piece.
D. Pasta: macaroni, spaghetti, noodles, ½ c.
E. Cooked rice, millet, bulgur, whole wheat berries, etc., ½ c.

Grain Products: *Whole grain* items have Vit. E, B-6, folacin, Mg, Zn, & fiber; refined cereals & bread lost these in milling.
"Enriched" *and* whole grain products have thiamin, riboflavin, niacin, Fe & protein.

III. DARK GREEN VEGETABLES 2
Serv.: 1 c. raw, ¾ c. cooked.
Asparagus, broccoli, cabbage, greens (beet, collards, kale, mustard, swiss chard, spinach, turnip), dark green lettuce as chicory, endive, escarole, romaine (not head or iceberg lettuce)

Dark Green Vegetables: folacin, Vit. A, E, B-6, riboflavin, Fe, & Mg. Also Vit. C (below).

Continued on next page

Food Group	No. Serv./Day	Nutrients
IV. FRUITS & VEG. RICH IN VIT. C .... 1 1 orange, ½ grapefruit, 4 oz. orange or grapefruit juice, 12 oz. tomato or pineapple juice, ½ cantaloupe, ¼ guava, ¾ c. strawberries, ¾ c. raw cabbage, ½ gr. pepper, 2 tomatoes, 1 stalk broccoli, ¾ c. greens, 3-4 Brussels sprouts.		*Group IV:* specifically for Vit. C.
V. OTHER FRUITS & VEGETABLES 1		

* Refers to 3 servings of complementary protein combinations to obtain "complete" protein.

† Part of the servings noted for these groups can be included in complementary protein dishes.

Reprinted by permission of *Birth and the Family Journal* from "Vegetarian Diets in Pregnancy" by Eleanor R. Williams, Ph.D., R.D., in *Birth and the Family Journal*, Vol. 3, No. 2, Summer, 1976, © 1976.

The Calorie – A Brief Summary of Basic Facts

I. The calorie (Latin, *calor*, heat) is a measure of heat.
   A. In nutritional terms, the calorie measures the energy value that a definite proportion of food will yield upon oxidation within the body or upon being burned within a laboratory.
   B. The large calorie or kilocalorie is the unit of measurement used in dietetic laboratories and studies. The kilocalorie is equal to the amount of heat needed to raise 1 kg. of H_2O 1° C.

II. Calories are drawn from the following three major groups of nutrients.
   A. Proteins:
      1. One gram of protein is equivalent to 4 calories. This is termed the "fuel factor" or average caloric value of protein.
      2. Proteins supply approximately 15 per cent of the average daily caloric intake.
   B. Fats:
      1. One gram of fat is equivalent to 9 calories.
      2. Fats supply 40 per cent of the average daily caloric intake.
   C. Carbohydrates:
      1. One gram of carbohydrate is equivalent to 4 calories.
      2. Carbohydrates supply approximately 45 per cent of the average dietary intake.

III. The caloric needs of the healthy individual vary with the following factors:
   A. Basal metabolic rate (BMR):
      1. Defined as the amount of energy that a physically, mentally, and emotionally relaxed person must expend in order to maintain the basic physical processes of life.
      2. Metabolic rates are determined by measuring the number of calories produced during a certain time period, e.g., over 24 hours.
      3. The BMR is higher in men than in women; it is increased during periods of growth, during pregnancy and lactation, and during emotional upsets.
      4. The BMR is lower in elderly persons, and in conditions of starvation and malnutrition.
   B. Surface area of the body:
      1. Surface area is a measurement that takes both height and weight into account. It can be computed from specially designed tables.
      2. A large person has a greater surface area, greater metabolic rate, and greater need for calories than a smaller individual.
   C. Activity:
      1. Sedentary activity requires fewer calories than physical activity.
      2. Mental activity, however difficult and demanding, requires very few calories.
   D. Age:
      1. A younger person has a greater metabolic rate and higher caloric needs than does an older person.

Reprinted by permission of W. B. Saunders Co. from *Medical-Surgical Nursing: A Psychophysiological Approach*, by Joan Luckmann and Karen Sorenson, © 1974, W. B. Saunders Co.

Summary of Treatments for Obesity

Therapy	Components	Comments on Effectiveness
Human Chorionic Gonadotropin (Simeon's Diet)	Low kcal diet (500 kcal) in conjunction with daily injections of HCG, a hormone extracted from the urine of pregnant women. Action of hormone is well understood.	Double-blind studies have shown that effectiveness is due to placebo effect, daily reinforcement, and 500 kcal diet. Patients frequently say they do not feel hunger.
Acupuncture	Staple placed in ear supposedly to stimulate a point affecting urge to eat.	Not proved to be effective.
Amphetamines	Daily or every-other-day administration of pill to reduce appetite. Used alone or in conjunction with diet.	Pills reduce appetite, but for many a tolerance develops at the end of several weeks. Side effects are stimulation, mouth dryness, insomnia, possible dependence, and abuse. Fenfluramine has least number of stimulant side effects but can cause depression.
Thyroid Hormone	Given in pharmacologic doses to induce hypermetabolism, particularly after long-term dieting; T_3 is low in long-term dieters.	Does cause increased weight loss but only temporarily. Some increased protein catabolism.
Diuretics	Daily administration, often hidden in diet control "plans" or "packages."	Causes diuresis and loss of water and thus temporary weight loss. Chronic use may lead to K^+ depletion.
Gastric Bypass Surgery	The stomach is reduced in size, with the result that the patient can no longer consume the same amount of food as before. Food intake is reduced because of discomfort, which eventually leads to vomiting.	Reserved for the morbidly obese (100 lbs. above ideal weight). Effective in promoting weight loss, but "dumping" syndrome may be a side effect. Patient must learn to accommodate to small stomach by eating small amounts of food more frequently.
Jejunoileal Bypass Surgery	A large portion of the small intestine is bypassed so that the absorptive capacity of the intestines is decreased. Result: fewer calories absorbed and tremendous weight loss.	Reserved for the morbidly obese. Effective for weight loss, although some clients regain weight as intestine adapts. Complications include: hypokalemia and electrolyte imbalance, liver disease, hyperoxaluria and kidney stones, protein malnutrition, and multiple vitamin deficiencies.

Continued on next page

Therapy	Components	Comments on Effectiveness
Jaw Wiring	Jaws are wired closed or held closed with rubber bands. Person can only take liquids through a straw.	Depending on liquids taken, intake may be nutritionally inadequate. Patient loses weight because he cannot take same number of calories as usual. Dental attention necessary. Could be dangerous in event of nausea—need wire cutters handy. No long-lasting behavior change.
Fasting	Patient usually hospitalized, removed from environment, and placed on complete fast with electrolyte and vitamin supplements.	Effective for rapid weight loss, 3 to 5 lbs. per week. BMR drops as loss progresses so that rate of weight loss also slows down. Effectiveness pales when patient begins eating again and has not learned new eating behaviors to maintain low weight.
Protein Sparing Modified Fast (PSMF)	Fasting with protein supplementation of 1.5 Gm. protein/kg. ideal body weight (IBW). Protein in form of lean meat, fish, or poultry, or as "liquid protein"—protein isolate or amino acids. Nitrogen loss is reduced; lean body mass is maintained. Mineral and vitamin supplementation is mandatory. The resulting ketosis seems to reduce feelings of hunger.	Effective for weight loss, 3 to 4 lbs. per week, and reducing loss of lean body mass. However, there may be reversal to old eating habits and overweight after the fast is terminated.
Behavioral Modification — Self-monitoring — Environmental changes	Patient learns to observe eating behaviors through record-keeping, and to make changes in his environment and behavior that result in a smaller energy intake. Focus is on the behaviors related to food, not the food itself.	Fairly effective, especially in terms of long-term weight loss. Weakness is that some patients may uncover psychologic problems that must be dealt with. Requires much motivation and attention, especially in the beginning.
Behavioral Modification — Aversive conditioning — Hypnosis — Positive imagery	Through techniques of covert conditioning or internal control, mental suggestions for eating behavior change are made.	These techniques are successful in reducing food intake only for as long as they are maintained. Have a tendency to become less strong with time.
Exercise	Aerobic, energy-expending exercise is most effective for cardiovascular training, improvement of muscle tone, and improvement of psychologic well-being.	Effective as an addition to calorie-reduction program to cause greater weight loss. Alone can produce weight loss of ½ lb. per week if done daily. Positive aspect of a weight control program. Helps to control appetite in overweight persons.

Low carbohydrate, high protein diets, high or moderate in fat (ketogenic)
- Pennington Diet, 1953
- "Calories Don't Count Diet," 1961
- The Drinking Man's Diet, 1964
- Dr. Stillman's Diet, 1967
- Dr. Atkin's Diet, 1972

Balanced, low calorie diets
- Many names and variations

Diet usually 1000 kcal or less, with less than 50 Gm. CHO. Protein is usually 120 Gm. or more. Based on fact that if CHO restricted, body metabolizes ketones, which decreases hunger and causes diuresis and water loss. Usually low in calories because one cannot eat enough protein to make up for calories previously obtained from carbohydrate.

Protein meets the RDA, carbohydrate is moderate, and fat is low. Calories restricted, but usually not less than 1000 kcal. Carbohydrate at least 80 Gm. Protein 1.0 Gm/kg. IBW.

Effective for short-term weight loss. Unappetizing, so patients can not stay with it. Do not know effects of long-term ketosis. Does result in less hunger and menstrual dysfunction, but may include aggravation of gout and osteoporosis. Short-term losses of 2 to 3 lbs. per week are seen; much is due to water loss. Long-term weight loss is from calorie deficit. Can cause increase in blood fat and cholesterol levels.

Diet continues to meet the RDA. Carbohydrates prevent ketosis. Patient usually experiences hunger. Diet can be made to fit in with existing eating patterns; can be lifetime change. Weight loss due to calorie deficit is 1 to 2 lbs. per week.

Reprinted by permission of W. B. Saunders Co. from "A Sensible Approach to the Obese Patient" by Kathleen Mahan in *Nursing Clinics of North America*, June, 1979, Vol. 14, No. 2, © 1979, W. B. Saunders Co.

Compulsive Eating Cycle

Reasons for compulsive eating vary, but the vicious circle illustrated is common to many women.

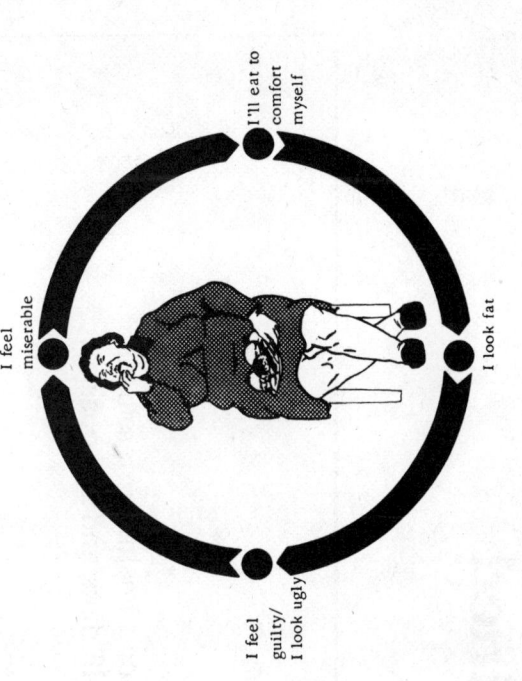

I'll eat to comfort myself

I look fat

I feel guilty/ I look ugly

I feel miserable

Reprinted from *Woman's Body, An Owner's Manual*, The Diagram Group, © 1977 Paddington Press, Ltd., New York, N.Y. Reprinted with permission.

The Protein Sparing Modified Fast–What Is It?

A number of questions have arisen among health professionals concerning the general efficacy of PSMF diets and the possible hazards associated with their uses.

by C. Jean Poulos

Considerable concern has recently been voiced in the matter of fat diets, particularly those involving liquid protein. While the public eagerly jumps at any new diet that is introduced, many family physicians pay little heed to these "lose-weight-with-no-effort" advertisements until they are confronted in their offices with the medical problems resulting from such diets.

Weight control, a problem which no individual patient should attempt to solve, belongs in the armamentarium of every family physician. His office nurse must have a thorough knowledge of nutrition and be trained in diet counseling either through school, seminars, workshops, or by her/his physician-employer. It is the nurse who holds the key to an effective weight control program by providing emotional support as well as making the patient aware of dietary changes.

A number of questions have arisen among health professionals concerning the general efficacy of these kinds of diets and the possible hazards associated with their uses. As early as February, 1976, the American Society of Bariatric Physicians was concerned about possible ill consequences from inadequately monitored PSMF programs being offered by commercial weight loss clinics where physician supervision was minimal. In response to this concern, the ASBP adopted the following position:

"It is the official opinion of the American Society

Protein Quality

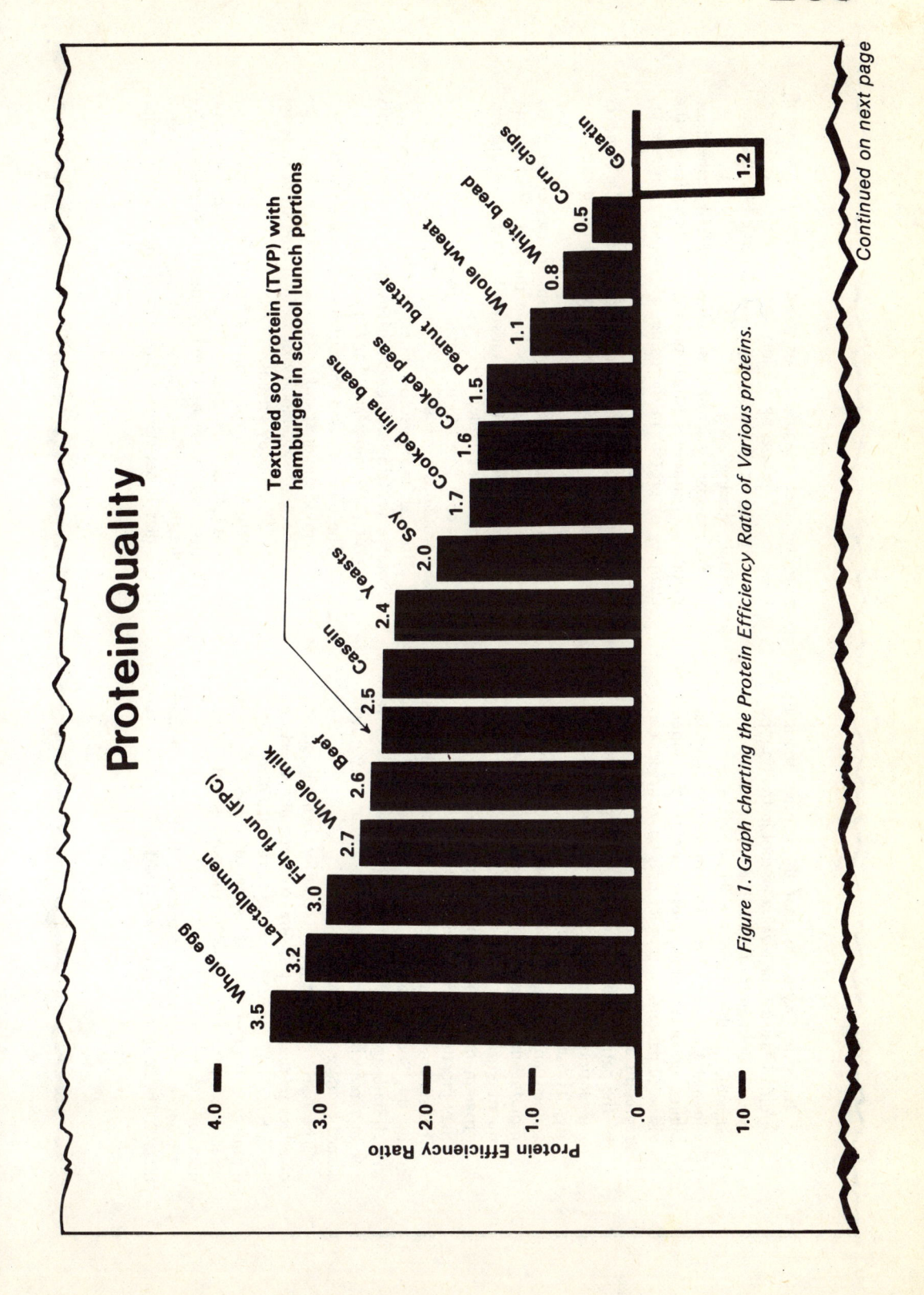

Food	PER
Whole egg	3.5
Lactalbumen	3.2
Fish flour (FPC)	3.0
Whole milk	2.7
Beef	2.6
Casein	2.5
Yeasts	2.4
Soy	2.0
Cooked lima beans	1.7
Cooked peas	1.6
Peanut butter	1.5
Textured soy protein (TVP) with hamburger in school lunch portions	1.2
Whole wheat	1.1
White bread	0.8
Corn chips	0.5
Gelatin	0

Figure 1. Graph charting the Protein Efficiency Ratio of Various proteins.

Continued on next page

263

of Bariatric Physicians that the protein sparing modified fast can be a valuable tool in treating the obese in the hands of a qualified physician knowledgeable in this technique. However, the casual administration of this program by commercial clinics or other organizations where the supervision of patients by physicians is only cursory can represent a serious threat to the health and welfare of the patient. Because of the severity of this unconventional approach to the treatment of obesity, its use should be reserved solely, to specially trained and qualified physicians who personally monitor the progress of patients on a very frequent and regular basis. The administration of this program by anyone other than such a physician may threaten the well-being of the patient."

This statement was incorporated into news releases sent out by the Society as well as into correspondence with several state agencies requesting these agencies to investigate any breach of proper medical care and any potential hazard to the general public.

The ASBP must be given credit for their high standards of ethics by repeatedly refusing to accept any advertising in its publication, *Obesity and Bariatric Medicine*, for any liquid protein product which is marketed by the manufacturer directly to the public for the purposes of weight reduction.

What is the meaning of the so-called "protein-sparing diets"? The protein-sparing modified fast is a severe intake-restricted diet intended to promote the maximum loss of body fat, while sparing the loss of lean body mass. Hence, this type of weight-loss program is identified by the term "Protein-Sparing".

Protein-sparing action is the term used to describe those metabolic conditions which favor the preservation of the quantity of protein in the tissues of the body. In essence, these are conditions in which:

1) Normal loss of tissue protein from metabolic turnover is completely replaced by uptake from dietary protein, and
2) All of the body's energy needs are met either a) By the supply of nutrients from the diet, or b) By the breakdown of tissue substance other than protein (fats, for example).

A diet is considered to be protein-sparing if no net loss of tissue protein is experienced when the diet is employed.

Although many factors enter into the establishment of favorable protein-sparing conditions, two of these factors are particularly important. They are:

1) The quantity and the nutritional quality of the proteins in the diet; and
2) The ready availability of cellular fuel to provide for all of the body's needs.

Proteins in nature are formed from large, complex combinations of approximately 20 different kinds of amino acid sub-units. Of these, 8 are considered to be essential for the adult human; that is, they must be provided in the diet. If the diet is deficient in any one of the essential amino acids, little protein-sparing action would be promoted.

On the other hand, dietary proteins which contain a good balance of the essential amino acids are of high nutritional quality and subsequently their use favors protein-sparing conditions. Needless to say, if the protein in the diet is of high nutritional quality, but ingested in insufficient quantity to provide the body's minimum requirements for the essential amino acids, the diet will not be protein-sparing.

The human body has a very high requirement for energy. By far the greatest energy requirement in the normal individual is for the support of basal functions, such as respiration, circulation, and neurological functions. Because the basal metabolic functions are all essential to life, the supply of energy for basal metabolism has the highest priority. Thus, if insufficient cellular fuel is provided in the diet, the body will satisfy its energy needs by breaking down tissue substance. As some of these energy needs cannot be satisfied by using fat as a fuel, and the body's capability to store carbohydrates is very limited, an insufficient diet can result in the breakdown of tissue protein to supply the energy needed for basal metabolic functions. Metabolic conditions which eliminate the necessity for such degradation of tissue protein would be considered protein-sparing conditions.

The regulation of fat deposition and mobilization in the body has a close relationship to the regulation of blood glucose levels. In general, the synthesis of fatty acids and the storage of fat occurs when blood glucose levels are elevated and insulin is present in higher concentrations. On the other hand, when blood glucose is depressed, insulin concentrations decrease, and fat, which is the body's alternative fuel supply, is mobilized from storage to provide a continuing source of cellular fuel. Thus, we can say in general that the presence of high levels of insulin in the system favors fatty acid synthesis and fat deposition, while the absence of elevated insulin concentrations tends to favor fat mobilization and the catabolism of the resultant fatty acids.

Just as the name implies, the Protein-Sparing Modified Fast was designed as a modification of a complete fasting diet, with the intent of eliminating, or substantially reducing, the loss of lean body mass normally associated with the total fast. This was accomplished by providing a diet restricted in content to protein alone, supplemented with necessary amounts of vitamin and minerals. The absence of carbohydrate in the diet eliminated the insulin response normally associated with glucose ingestion and, thus, removed the potential interference with fat mobilization caused by the hormone. In addition, by providing amino acids needed to replace tissue proteins lost in normal metabolic turnover, and to supply the energy needs which cannot be supplied by fat, the diet could be made truly protein-sparing. This point was confirmed in the initial work by comparing nitrogen intake with loss of nitrogen through excretion. [1, 2, 3, 4]

However, it is not clear whether or not all of the currently-popular applications of PSMF can be considered to be really protein-sparing diets. Unfortunately, in the time since Blackburn and his coworkers first introduced the concept of PSMF, little work has been done to determine if all applications (particularly those which employ proteins or protein hydrolysates that are deficient in certain of the essential amino acids) promote the same non-negative nitrogen balance as was initially reported. Certainly, this question deserves some scientific investigation before all applications of PSMF are endorsed as safe and effective.

Even in the absence of clear scientific evidence, however, certain preliminary conclusions can be drawn on theoretical grounds alone. This can be done by calculating the maximum possible rate of weight loss on this kind of diet, assuming complete protein-sparing action, and comparing this rate with that actually observed when the diet is followed. If the steady-state rate of weight loss is significantly greater than the theoretical value, loss of lean body mass has to be involved, and the diet cannot be considered to be protein-sparing.

For example, consider a female subject of 150 pounds body weight with an ideal body weight of 110 pounds. Assume further that her average daily energy requirement is 2000 calories. If she is on a PSMF providing 65 grams per day of protein as the sole source of major nutrient, she will have an average daily calorie deficit of about 1740 calories. At 9 calories per gram, this translates into 193 grams or about 0.42 pounds of fat per day; that is, if the energy requirement is to be satisfied solely from mobilized body fat, only slightly less than one-half pound of fat loss would occur for this purpose.

It could be argued, of course, that because such subjects are normally in a state of ketosis, fat loss from ketonuria could account for additional weight reduction without consideration for energy requirements. However, Cahill and his coworkers [5] have shown that ketonuria in fasting subjects account for very little loss of mass. In fact, the subjects' urine would have to be constantly greater than 5% in ketone bodies before any significant fat loss could be attributed to ketonuria.

Thus, loss of weight in this subject at a rate greater than 0.42 pounds per day has to be the result of factors other than fat mobilization. One such potential factor is, of course, loss of lean body mass through mobilization of tissue protein.

The 1740 calorie energy deficit of this subject translates, at 4 calories per gram, into 435 grams of protein or about 0.96 pounds. The subject can lose almost one pound per day as protein, but she cannot lose as much as one-half pound per day and have it accountable as fat loss. For this reason, loss of tissue protein appears to be almost a requirement of rapid-weight-loss diet regimens, and loss of weight at rates in excess of theoretical limits can be taken as presumptive evidence that the diet employed is not really protein-sparing.

Some applications of PSMF would certainly appear to favor such protein-depleting conditions. Many of those based on the use of collagen or collagen hydrolysates have not corrected for the severe deficiency in methionine (an essential amino acid) and, of course, little protein-sparing action can be expected in a diet which is deficient in any essential amino acid.

We have heard many reports from practitioners employing the PSMF that patients frequently respond to the diet with one or more symptoms of hypoglycemic stress. This should not be particularly surprising when you consider the metabolic burden involved in generating glucose in required

P.E.R. (Protein Efficiency Ratio) proteins, such as egg albumin, latalbumin, or casein would be preferred (See Chart 1).

Although predigestion of the protein might be desirable in isolated cases of specific protein allergies or proteolytic insufficiency of the digestive system, it does not seem the predigestion protein is generally necessary for the success of the diet program.

Some crude fiber is needed in the diet to assure normal intestinal function, yet the majority of these diets are fiber-deficient.

A search of the market was made in anticipation of finding the same quantity of prescription diet products available to the physician as the profusion of fad diets which are currently available to the lay public. Such was not to be — only two prescription products were unearthed which are nutritionally-balanced diet programs designed to give the body the precise physiological tuning needed to attain maximum loss of body fat.

One — AMINOSYN, developed by Abbott Laboratories, is a crystalline amino acid solution for intravenous protein-sparing total parenteral nutrition. Requiring hospitalization and constant monitoring, this product does not purport to maintain good health and normal energy.

The second product, MILCO-TRIM, developed by Miller Pharmacal, Inc. of Chicago, has many applications in addition to weight control that are of great interest to the nurse. It is widely used in hospitals and convalescent hospitals because it provides a completely balanced diet in a form easily utilized in tubal feedings. Numerous geriatric facilities are utilizing MILCO-TRIM as a supplemental feed-

quantities from a diet consisting of only a small amount of protein, most of which is needed for tissue replacement. And, of course, such a regimen can place a severe burden on those who, under normal circumstances, have difficulty maintaining adequate blood sugar supplies, or those who manifest diminished glucogenic capability.

Often such individuals are required to terminate use of the diet. As an alternative, some practitioners have recommended supplementing the diet with a non-insulin-stimulating carbohydrate, such as levulose (also called fructose). [7] This makes it possible to establish more normal blood sugar levels while maintaining the desired state of fat mobilization fostered by a continuing depression in insulin level.

In addition, because levulose has the highest protein-sparing action of any carbohydrate, [8] protein-sparing conditions can be improved through the proper use of this sugar in the diet program.

No diet should be considered to be "protein-sparing" merely because it specifies the use of a small daily intake of protein or protein hydrolysates as the sole source of major nutrient. In fact, unless correct amounts of protein of good nutritional quality are used, a substantial portion of any weight loss can be at the expense of lean body mass. The addition to the diet of a non-insulin-stimulating carbohydrate such as levulose may be useful in avoiding some side effects resulting from hypoglycemic stress, without upsetting the fat-reduction pattern of the program.

With so many high-quality nutritional proteins available, it is difficult to understand why collagen (gelatin) has become the protein of choice in most of the modified fasting diets in use today. The use of one or more of the high

Continued on next page

HYPERKALEMIA

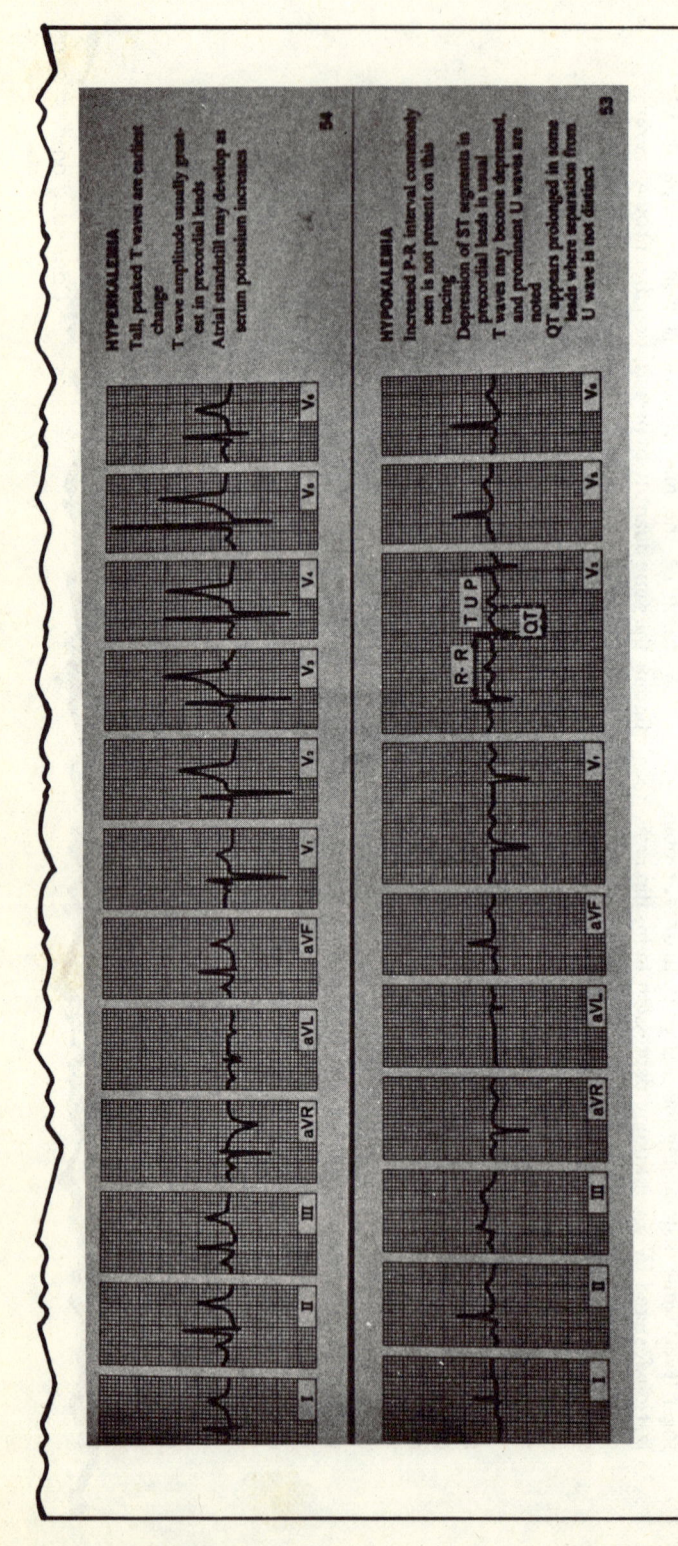

Tall, peaked T waves are earliest change

T wave amplitude usually greatest in precordial leads

Atrial standstill may develop as serum potassium increases

HYPOKALEMIA

Increased P-R interval commonly seen is not present on this tracing

Depression of ST segments in precordial leads is usual

T waves may become depressed, and prominent U waves are noted

QT appears prolonged in some leads where separation from U wave is not distinct

ing for their elderly patients. Many internists are using this product with great success in the treatment of their ulcer patients by providing diet feedings broken down into many small portions to be dispensed during the day. Surgeons have used MILCO-TRIM in reducing patients' weight while keeping nutrition at a maximum level prior to surgery. The dentist, too, has found this product beneficial to his patients undergoing full extractions for dentures in that they are provided proper nutrition. MILCO-TRIM is not a PSMF diet but rather a reduced caloric diet, although it retains the behavioral modifications of the PSMF. Requiring a minimal amount of monitoring, this is the safest product available.

For additional information on this prescription product, contact Miller Pharmacal, Inc., P.O. Box 299, 245 W. Roosevelt Road, West Chicago, Illinois 60185. Also available is a physicians' handbook directed toward the use of MILCO-TRIM.

Of great importance to the nurse working with any patient on a diet is the awareness of the possibility of potassium deficiency, and also *hyperkalemia*, wherein some patients tend to overcompensate for potassium loss. Hypokalemia is a serious complication of fasting modified by protein-sparing therapy. It can lead to cardiac disturbances to include atrial and ventricular arrhythmias, and a potentiation of digitalis effects. If it develops gradually, potassium depletion, even when severe in degree, may be virtually asymptomatic. Most often, however, patients will note at least some vague malaise, weakness, and fatigue. Very severe depletion may cause marked generalized motor weakness of muscles, especially in the lower extremities, often associated with considerable aching and stiffness. Abrupt development of sudden exacerbation of potassium depletion may result in virtual paralysis of all peripheral skeletal musculature, even including the muscles of respiration. Polyuria and polydipsia are very common symptoms along with postural hypotension.

On physical examination, potassium-deficient patients sometimes have slight peripheral edema. They may also demonstrate decreased motor power, diminished or absent deep tendon reflexes, and occasionally signs of tetany. The cardiovascular manifestations of potassium depletion include hypotension and cardiac arrhythmias, the latter especially in patients taking digitalis.

Most offices and hospitals take a laboratory test for plasma potassium and an electrocardiogram. (See Chart 2 for characteristic changes, particularly in T and U waves. The T wave is flattened, diphasic, or inverted, whereas the U wave remains upright and becomes more prominent. These alterations are only roughly correlated with the severity of the disturbance in potassium metabolism and do not appear to be clearly related either to serum concentration or to total body deficit. [11]) For the office or clinic nurse it would behoove her to memorize these patterns as many offices routinely run EKG lead as part of the monitoring of all weight reduction patients, and the nurse is responsible for the taking of the EKG test.

On the other hand, hyperkalemia's major clinical manifestations are cardiac arrhythmias and occasionally peripheral muscle weakness or paralysis. On the EKG peaking of the T wave is the earliest change; later the QRS segment widens, the P-R interval lengthens, and the P waves disappear. The laboratory test, of course, will show an elevated serum potassium level.

With a complete understanding of nutrition, counseling techniques, and complications that may arise from reduction diets, the nurse is an important ally to the physician in his care of the weight reduction patient.

References

1. Blackburn, G.L., et al. "Protein-Sparing Therapy during Periods of Starvation with Sepsis or Trauma," Ann. Surg. 177:588 (1973).

2. Blackburn, G.L., et al. "Peripheral Intravenous Feeding with Isotonic Amino Acid Solutions," Amer. J. Surg. 125:477 (1973).

3. Blackburn, G.L. and J.P. Flatt, "Preservation of Lean Body Mass during Weight Reduction," Fed. Pro. 32:916 (1973).

4. Flatt, J.P. and G.L. Blackburn. "The Metabolic Fuel Regulatory System Implications for Protein-Sparing Therapy during Calorie Deprivation and Disease," Amer. M. Clinic. Nutr. 27:175 (1974).

5. Owen, O.E., H.P. Morgan, H.G. Kemp, J.M. Sullivan, M.G. Herrera, and G.F. Cahill. "Brain Metabolism during Fasting," J. Clin. Invest. 46:1589–1595 (1967).

6. Lindner, P.G. and G.L. Blackburn. "Multidisciplinary Approach to Obesity Utilizing Fasting Modified by Protein-Sparing Therapy," Obesity/Bariatric Med., Vol. 5, No. 6 (1976).

7. Palm, J.D. Diet Away Your Stress, Tension and Anxiety. Doubleday and Company, Inc., Garden City, New York (1976).

8. Albanese, A.A., W.C. Felch, R.A. Higgons, B.L. Vestal, and L. Stephanson. "Utilization and Protein-Sparing Action of Fructose in Man," Metabolism 1:20–25 (1952).

9. Stegink, L.D., J.B. Freeman, J. Wispe, and W.E. Connor. "Absence of the Biochemical Symptoms of Essential Fatty Acid Deficiency in Surgical Patients Undergoing Protein-Sparing Therapy," Amer. J. Clin. Nutr. 30:388–393 (1977).

10. Williams, R.J. Physicians' Handbook of Nutritional Science, Charles C. Thomas Co., Springfield, Illinois (1975).

11. Keefer, C.S. and R.W. Wilkins. Medicine Essentials of Clinical Practice, Little, Brown Co. pp. 842–848 (1970).

C. Jean Poulos, Sc.D., is Director of Research at Monterey Bay Research Institute, Santa Cruz, California.

Dietary Habits of Two Ethnic Groups

Oriental Dietary Habits

Dietary difficulties and restrictions are problems for Oriental patients that the hospital nurse may encounter, especially on the maternity floor.

The dietary habits of an ethnic group are the product of the group's present environment as well as a long tradition. Although the group may be subjected to outside influences, the dietary habits that have become meaningful to the group for many generations are persistently cherished and not easily changed. Consequently the nurses may often experience an ungrateful response from the Oriental patient when they encourage her to take "nutritious" and "delicious" American food. For example, many Oriental people are not accustomed to milk and milk products. Frequently mentioned reasons for objecting to milk and milk products are stomach ache, gas, and diarrhea.

In Oriental society there are traditional health foods that are very important for the patient's psychologic as well as physical well-being. A pregnant mother in such a cultural group is encouraged to eat special herbs and foods to insure the baby's health as well as her own. In the home country, various kinds of health foods with long traditional usage are carefully prepared and provided for the mother. Ginseng herb, one of the most commonly used, highly valued, and expensive herbs, is usually sought as a general strength tonic for the expectant mother and postpartum mother of Oriental tradition.

The classic postpartum diet for Korean mothers is seaweed soup with rice. The soup is highly valued among them since they believe it cleans the blood and increases the mother's milk production. Traditionally, this soup is served hot to new mothers in Korea soon after delivery.

The classic Chinese postpartum diet is high in hot foods. Most fruits and vegetables, considered cold, are avoided. Basic mainstays of a postpartum and lactating diet generally consist of rice and eggs and a chicken soup containing pig knuckles, vinegar ginger, and sometimes peanuts. Because the vinegar in the soup helps to transfer tricalcium phosphate from the bone of pig knuckles into solution, the traditional soup may supply some of the calcium essential in the diets of postpartum and lactating women. Some Chinese women may refuse to take prescribed iron supplements because they believe that this hardens the bones and makes delivery difficult.

Because of the difficulty of finding these traditional foods on the American maternity floor, the patient may not feel comfortable.

It is also noteworthy that because of religious beliefs some Oriental patients are vegetarians. By failing to recognize this belief, a staff can create enormous discomfort for the patient. For example, a postpartum patient from India was served bacon, egg, cereal, milk, and juice for her diet. The patient drank only a glass of juice, because she was a vegetarian.

Food habits should be given serious consideration during hospitalization of Oriental patients for their welfare as well as the advancement of hospital care. A considerate nurse will ask her Oriental patient about her food preference before making a menu. A considerate staff will give the patient explanations about American dishes and their ingredients in detail, hoping the patient may find suitable substitutes from the hospital menu. A considerate nurse will allow the patient's relatives or friends to bring their ethnic foods for her patient, if they are not medically contraindicated. A considerate nurse will be supportive to her patient by allowing her to eat her native foods while giving her encouragement to try American foods that are culturally acceptable as well as nutritious.

Reprinted by permission of W. B. Saunders Co. from "Understanding the Oriental Maternity Patient" by Hyo Jin Chung in *Nursing Clinics of North America*, March, 1977, 12:1, © 1977, W. B. Saunders Company.

Jewish Dietary Laws

by Bonnie Gordon

Jewish dietary laws are based on certain restrictions set down in the Bible and although there are many fine points and disagreements about detail the basic tenets of "keeping kosher" (kosher means "fit" or "proper") refer to the following: (1) It is forbidden to eat the meat of certain animals such as the pig or the horse, certain deep sea foods, and particular kinds of birds. Pork, bacon, ham, shrimp, lobster, and oysters, therefore, are some popular foods that are *not* kosher. (2) Meat that *is* permissible, such as beef from a cow or chicken, must be slaughtered according to Jewish ritual and must meet specific health standards. This means that meat that comes packaged in the local supermarket—unless specifically noted otherwise—is *not* kosher. Kosher meat may be obtained from special "kosher" butchers who are supervised by rabbis who oversee the slaughtering of the animal. The written laws on the method of slaughter are quite detailed and explicit. (3) The separation of milk and meat is another major factor in determining "kashruth" (the laws relating to kosher food). Observant Jews keep separate dishes and utensils for meat and dairy meals. The distinction includes not just meat and dairy products per se but any food which contains meat or milk, respectively, or the by-products of milk or meat. Cheese and yogurt, for example, would be considered dairy; a vegetable soup that uses a beef stock would be considered meat. Also, one would not eat a kosher hot dog or corned beef sandwich on a roll that contained milk as one of its ingredients, however minor. A third category is food that is "pareve" or neutral. Pareve food can be eaten with either meat or dairy meals, and include such foods as all fruits and vegetables, eggs, fish, and grains.

The reasons given by those Jews who observe kashruth vary. The most important, some say, is that kashruth is something God set forth as one of the commandments and, as such, needs no logical explanation but must be taken on faith. It is regarded as an important symbol of the distinctive Jewish heritage. Another attitude is that the self-control and limitations set in the preparing and eating of foods represents a way that one determines boundaries for oneself, in order to regulate one's own life; it is a way of taking responsibility for one's actions, a reminder that one is the master of one's own life, one's own body. Finally, the laws of kashruth are very much tied to a reverence for life. The slaughter of an animal for food is considered a serious act and must be done in a specific manner, with no pain for the animal; it must be done by a God-fearing person who takes care to follow the letter of the law. The laws of kashruth also specify that Jews are forbidden to eat the blood of the animal which represents life itself; part of the kashering process is a draining of the blood from the animal so that it can be eaten. Also, the basis of the separation of milk and meat laws is the injunction "You shall not boil a kid in its mother's milk," underlining the basic cruelty of combining the elements of life (the milk) with the element of death (the flesh). The meat of all carnivorous animals is forbidden, as is meat derived from the sport of hunting.

Sources: *The Jewish Catalog*, compiled and edited by Richard Siegel, Michael Strassfeld, and Sharon Strassfeld, The Jewish Publication Society of America, Philadelphia, Pa.

What is a Jew? by Rabbi Morris N. Kertzer, The MacMillan Co., N.Y., N.Y.

AMERICAN DIETETIC ASSOCIATION
430 N. Michigan Avenue
Chicago, Illinois 60611

A professional association of registered dieticians and others with shared concerns, dedicated to improving nutrition and providing education in this field.

Publications include: "Exchange Lists For Meal Planning"; "Interactions Of Selected Drugs With Nutritional Status In Man," by Donna March; *The ADA Journal,* published monthly at $24.00/year; *Handbook Of Diet Therapy,* by D. Turner; Nutrition booklets for patient education and pamphlets on nutrition knowledge for nurses.

CSPI
Center For Science In The Public Interest
1755 South Street, N.W.
Washington, D.C. 20009

A non-profit organization for the improvement of the American diet through public education, research and lobbying.

Educational materials available from CSPI include: *Nutrition Action Magazine,* a monthly journal; posters on chemical additives in foods; books and pamphlets on food for health (including the book *Food For People Not For Profit,* by Lerza and Jacobson; T-shirts with "Food For People Not For Profit" or "Give Peas A Chance" written on them).

NATIONAL DAIRY COUNCIL
6300 North River Road
Rosemont, Illinois 60018

An organization of the dairy industry for nutrition research and education.

Materials available from the Dairy Council include: "Comprehensive List Of Foods," a booklet with nutrient information on several common foods; *Nutrition Sourcebook,* a handy 40-page guide to nutrients; *Dairy Council Digest,* a bimonthly periodical; *Nutrition News,* a quarterly periodical; several nutrition education booklets and posters.

There is a small fee for each of these materials and they may be ordered through your local division of the Dairy Council or if there is no local one in the area, through the national office.

NUTRITION TODAY SOCIETY
101 Ridgely Avenue
P. O. Box 1829
Annapolis, Maryland 21404

An organization for distributing nutrition information made up of professionals and lay people.

Publications and Educational Materials

"Nutrition Facts To Guide Your Food Choices," a poster, and "See The Facts About The Foods You Eat," a pamphlet, are available free from Cereal Institute, Inc., 135 South La Salle Street, Chicago, Illinois 60603.

"A Daily Food Guide," "Nutrition, Food At Work For You," and "There's More To Food Than Eating," are available from Prudential Insurance Co., 5 Prudential Plaza, Newark, N.J. 07101.

"Nutrition Slide Guide," a useful slide-rule, pocket guide to over 300 foods, their calorie count and nutrients ($2.98 each, less for bulk orders), available from Dunn and Reidman, P.O. Box 241, Pacific Palisades, California 90272.

The DIETician consists of a booklet on nutrition and the components of hundreds of foods and a calculator for keeping track of the calories and grams of protein, fat and carbohydrate consumed in a day. It is useful for people on diets for weight loss or those who must control fat and carbohydrate intake. The cost is $13.95 plus $1.00 for postage and handling. It is available from Franklin J. Scott Co., 6070 S. Belvedere, Tucson, Arizona 85706.

Prenatal and postnatal educational materials on infant feeding, diet plans for pregnancy, reducing and specific diseases, can be obtained in quantity free of charge for patient education from Carnation Company, Medical Marketing Division, 5045 Wilshire Boulevard, Los Angeles, California 90036.

Booklets on sodium restricted diets are available from the American Heart Association, 44 East 23rd Street, New York, New York.

"Meal Planning Guide," a 12-page colorful booklet on nutrition and several recipe booklets are available at no cost for up to 100 copies of each, for the use in nutrition education from Pet, Inc., Grocery Products Division, Office of Consumer Affairs, P.O. Box 392, St. Louis, Missouri 63166.

Several books and reports on nutrition are published by the World Health Organization. Send request for "Nutrition" catalog to the World Health Organization, Distribution and Sales, 1211 Geneva 27, Switzerland.

A *Catalog of Nutrition Education Material* compiled by *Family Circle Magazine* with the Food Council of America, copyright 1973, The Family Circle, Inc., is available from *Family Circle Magazine*, 488 Madison Avenue, New York, New York 10022.

Infant Nutrition, Feeding the Infant . . . Building the Man is a 64-page guide to infant nutrition for professionals prepared for Wyeth Laboratories by Medcom, Inc., copyright 1972, Medcom, Inc., available from Medcom, Inc., 2 Hammarskjöld Plaza, New York, New York 10017.

The Kitchen Book: Notes From A Child Care Center, copyright Karen Hewitt and Andrew Simon, 1978. Available from Ethan Allen Child Care Center, Inc., 600 Dalton Drive, Fort Ethan Allen,

Winooski, Vermont 05404 ($5.00/copy). This paperback book on the use of nutritious, healthful foods for feeding children in a day care setting, is an informative (and fun) resource for anyone involved with nutrition programs and nutrition education for young children. The ideas set forth in the book can be applied to children's nutrition in health care institutions and other settings as well as day care centers. The book is divided into sections on children and food, "the politics of food," sample menus and recipes and a bibliography which includes resources in children's nutrition.

"Nutritive Value of Foods," revised 1977, a 40-page guide to the nutrients in several common foods, is published by the U.S. Department of Agriculture and prepared by Agricultural Research Service. Available from Superintendent of Documents, U.S. Government printing Office, Washington, D.C. 20402.

Nutrition Today Magazine, a quarterly publication on all aspects of nutrition. For subscription information write to *Nutrition Today,* 1140 Connecticut Avenue, N.W., Washington, D.C. 20036.

The Journal of Applied Nutrition is the official journal of the International College of Applied Nutrition (a non-profit organization for those working in nutrition or nutrition research), located at Box 386, La Habra, California 90631. This journal focuses on the application of nutrition for health professionals. ($10.00/year for two/three issues per year.)

Nutrition—Applied Personally, also from the International College of Nutrition (see address above), is a guide for patients which includes menus and information on good nutrition. ($3.00 each, less for bulk orders.)

"Talking Food Pamphlets," from Talking Food Company, 12 Gifford Court, Salem, Ma. 01970, are 4-page pamphlets, each covering one topic on nutrition and "natural" foods. Titles include, "Sugar And How It Gets That Way," "Our Daily Flour," "Natural Foods Are the Best Buy," and 17 others (Cost: $3.00 for the set of 20 pamphlets, bulk packs of 50 of any one pamphlet, $4.00). Talking Food also makes available books on natural foods and is currently preparing a newsletter, *Fanatics' Monthly.*

Diet For A Small Planet, Frances Lappé. *"Diet For A Small Planet* is in part a nutrition book but even more an exposition of our responsibilities to the rest of the planet, as well as to ourselves. The concern for energy conservation, for wise allocation of our natural resources, and for living better lower on the food chain mark *Diet For A Small Planet* as superb reading in the area of environmental sensitivity."

Reprinted from *High Level Wellness* © 1977 by Donald B. Ardell. Permission granted by Rodale Press, Inc., Emmaus, Pa. 18049.

This book is an excellent resource for vegetarians since it explains combining non-meat proteins to get the complete protein necessary for health.

Nutrition Films and Audiovisual Aids

"Nutrition: The Inner Environment," especially for teenagers, available in Spanish and English, from Educational Films.

"What Is This Thing Called Food," deals with chemical additives in foods and their effects on the human body. From Films Incorporated.

A series of audiotape and film strip lessons on nutrition for independent study are available from Multi Media Office.

"Diet For A Small Planet," based on the book by Frances Moore Lappé, discusses protein, particularly non-meat sources for it. From Bullfrog Films.

"Maintaining Nutrition in the Critically Ill Patient" and "Nutrition in the Injured Patient" are agailable from Norwich-Eaton Pharmaceuticals.

"The Junk Food Man," an animated educational film for children on the evils of "junk food." From Aims Instructional Media, Inc.

"Food For Health," an educational film on proper nutrition from World Health Organization Films.

"Nutrition," a film on the disastrous effects of the widespread problem of malnutrition. From Tricontinental Film Center.

"Bottle Babies," a moving film on the devastating effect of feeding powdered milk formulas to infants in underdeveloped countries. From Tricontinental Films.

A series of filmstrips and records or cassettes on nutrition for school children is available from Marshfilm. The series is useful to school nurses and nurses involved in health education.

Several films and filmstrips on nutrition education are available from the National Dairy Council.

Nutrition Today makes available several useful nutrition education teaching aids on various topics. They consist of slides plus a syllabus.

6 Maternity Nursing

Maternal-Child health care is an area of rapid growth and change from the traditional practices of the past. Many technological advances have made it possible to greatly reduce the risks of childbearing to mother and child. They have enabled women to sustain pregnancies who several years ago would not have been able to, and infants who could not have survived 20 years ago can now thrive. Psychological research on bonding and the importance of early parent-child interation (particularly the work of John Kennell and Marshall Klaus at Case Western Reserve University) has influenced attitudes and practices in maternity settings.

At the same time a growing awareness on the part of consumers of their needs and the range of possibilities in the childbearing experience has necessitated a reevaluation of traditional hospital-oriented childbirth. Consumer demands have influenced the development of family-centered care and the whole home-birth movement.

The material in this section includes reference guides for nurses and information on some of the technological advances mentioned above, such as amniocentesis. The resource section is a sampling of the many organizations promoting informed parent participation in the childbirth process. This combination of material from both of these areas of advancement in maternity care is included here in the belief that both advances have value, that they can enhance each other, and that nurses in this field must be aware of both the innovations in technical skills and the needs and desires of families.

In line with the awareness of the need for optimal birthing experiences, the role of the nurse-midwife has been rapidly gaining in prominence. A growing number of physicians are seeing the value of nurse-midwife-physician teams in which the nurse-midwife manages the uncomplicated pregnancy and birth and the physician manages high-risk patients. A listing of schools training nurse-midwives is included here for nurses interested in pursuing this field.

I. The Pregnant Patient's Bill of Rights
II. Family-Centered Care—A Sample Pattern
III. Diagnosis of Pregnancy
IV. Weight Gain in Pregnancy
V. Fundal Height
VI. Leopold's Maneuvers
VII. Childbirth Education
- Childbirth Educator's Role
- Innovations in Prenatal Education
VIII. Adolescent Pregnancy
IX. Alcohol and Pregnancy—Fetal Alcohol Syndrome
X. High Risk Pregnancy—Identification
XI. Medications Having Adverse Effects on Fetus and Infant
XII. Amniocentesis
- Conditions Diagnosed by Amniocentesis
- Nurse's Role During Amniocentesis
XIII. Intrauterine Growth Retardation—Causal Factors
XIV. Preeclampsia-Eclampsia
- Signs and Symptoms
- Treatment
XV. Diabetes and Pregnancy
XVI. Labor
- Cervical Dilatation
- Normal Labor Graph
- Labor Abnormalities
- Mechanism of Labor—LOA
- Fetal Monitoring
  - FHR Deceleration Patterns
  - Diagnosis of Acute Fetal Distress
  - Treatment of Fetal Distress
- Apgar Scoring
- Emergency Childbirth

XVII. **Postpartum**
      Hypovolemic Shock—Treatment and Observations
      Disorders of Mothering
      Estimation of Gestational Age
         Examination First Hour
         Examination After 24 Hours
      Common Variations in the Neonate
      Danger Signs in the Newborn

XVIII. **Innovations in Maternity Care**

XIX. **SISTER STELLA'S BABIES—A Review**

XX. **MINDS, MOTHERS AND MIDWIVES—A Review**

XXI. **Resources in Maternity Nursing**

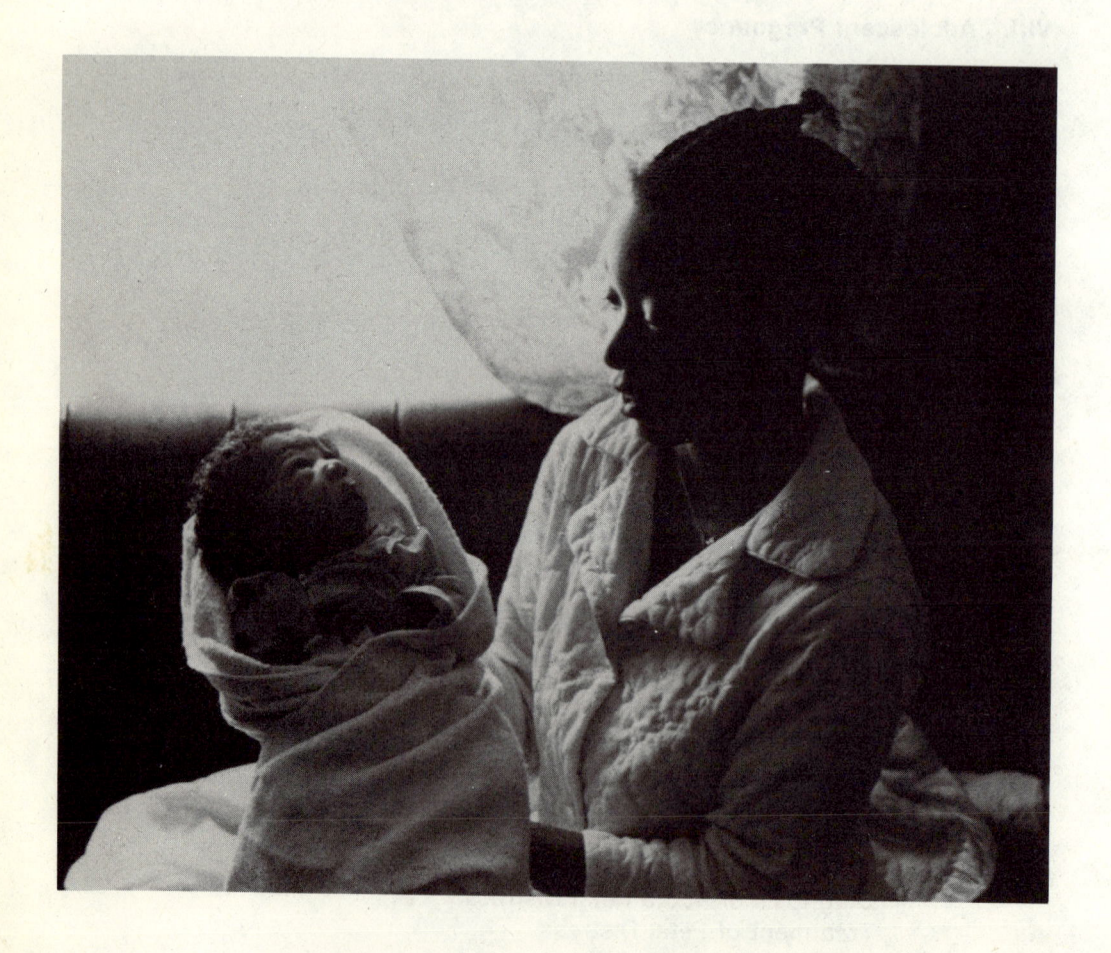

© 1978, American Journal of Nursing Co., from *Sister Stella's Babies,* pp. 94, 95, by Sister Mary Stella Simpson, D.C., R.N., C.N.M. Reprinted by permission of the American Journal of Nursing Co.

"We have organized a society in which responsibility for healing, education and birthing has been handed over to the professions. As a result the motherhood role has become impoverished. All too often the only personal satisfaction and social recognition that a woman can find is in a job outside the home. We have lost something precious. For being a mother is one of the most important jobs anyone can do. The future lies in the hands of the mothers of today."

Reprinted by permission of Random House Inc. from Women As Mothers by Sheila Kitzinger. Copyright 1978 by Random House Inc., New York.

THE PREGNANT PATIENT'S BILL OF RIGHTS

American parents are becoming increasingly aware that well-intentioned health professionals do not always have scientific data to support common American obstetrical practices and that many of these practices are carried out primarily because they are part of medical and hospital tradition. In the last forty years many artificial practices have been introduced which have changed childbirth from a physiological event to a very complicated medical procedure in which all kinds of drugs are used and procedures carried out, sometimes unnecessarily, and many of them potentially damaging for the baby and even for the mother. A growing body of research makes it alarmingly clear that every aspect of traditional American hospital care during labor and delivery must now be questioned as to its possible effect on the future well-being of both the obstetric patient and her unborn child.

One in every 35 children born in the United States today will eventually be diagnosed as retarded; in 75% of these cases there is no familial or genetic predisposing factor. One in every 10 to 17 children has been found to have some form of brain dysfunction or learning disability requiring special treatment. Such statistics are not confined to the lower socioeconomic group but cut across all segments of American society.

New concerns are being raised by childbearing women because no one knows what degree of oxygen depletion, head compression, or traction by forceps the unborn or newborn infant can tolerate before that child sustains permanent brain damage or dysfunction. The recent findings regarding the cancer-related drug diethylstilbestrol have alerted the public to the fact that neither the approval of a drug by the U. S. Food and Drug Administration nor the fact that a drug is prescribed by a physician serves as a guarantee that a drug or medication is safe for the mother or her unborn child. In fact, the American Academy of Pediatrics' Committee on Drugs has recently stated that there is no drug, whether prescription or over-the-counter remedy, which has been proven safe for the unborn child.

The Pregnant Patient has the right to participate in decisions involving her well-being and that of her unborn child, unless there is a clearcut medical emergency that prevents her participation. In addition to the rights set forth in the American Hospital Association's "Patient's Bill of Rights," (which has also been adopted by the New York City Department of Health) the Pregnant Patient, because she represents TWO patients rather than one, should be recognized as having the additional rights listed below.

1. *The Pregnant Patient has the right*, prior to the administration of any drug or procedure, to be informed by the health professional caring for her of any potential direct or indirect effects, risks or hazards to herself or her unborn or newborn infant which may result from the use of a drug or procedure prescribed for or administered to her during pregnancy, labor, birth or lactation.

Continued on next page

2. *The Pregnant Patient has the right*, prior to the proposed therapy, to be informed, not only of the benefits, risks and hazards of the proposed therapy but also of known alternative therapy, such as available childbirth education classes which could help to prepare the Pregnant Patient physically and mentally to cope with the discomfort or stress of pregnancy and the experience of childbirth, thereby reducing or eliminating her need for drugs and obstetric intervention. She should be offered such information early in her pregnancy in order that she may make a reasoned decision.

3. *The Pregnant Patient has the right*, prior to the administration of any drug, to be informed by the health professional who is prescribing or administering the drug to her that any drug which she receives during pregnancy, labor and birth, no matter how or when the drug is taken or administered, may adversely affect her unborn baby, directly or indirectly, and that there is no drug or chemical which has been proven safe for the unborn child.

4. *The Pregnant Patient has the right* if Cesarean section is anticipated, to be informed prior to the administration of any drug, and preferably prior to her hospitalization, that minimizing her and, in turn, her baby's intake of nonessential pre-operative medicine will benefit her baby.

5. *The Pregnant Patient has the right*, prior to the administration of a drug or procedure, to be informed of the areas of uncertainty if there is NO properly controlled follow-up research which has established the safety of the drug or procedure with regard to its direct and/or indirect effects on the physiological, mental and neurological development of the child exposed, via the mother, to the drug or procedure during pregnancy, labor, birth or lactation — (this would apply to virtually all drugs and the vast majority of obstetric procedures).

6. *The Pregnant Patient has the right*, prior to the administration of any drug, to be informed of the brand name and generic name of the drug in order that she may advise the health professional of any past adverse reaction to the drug.

7. *The Pregnant Patient has the right* to determine for herself, without pressure from her attendant, whether she will accept the risks inherent in the proposed therapy or refuse a drug or procedure.

8. *The Pregnant Patient has the right* to know the name and qualifications of the individual administering a medication or procedure to her during labor or birth.

9. *The Pregnant Patient has the right* to be informed, prior to the administration of any procedure, whether that procedure is being administered to her for her or her baby's benefit (medically indicated) or as an elective procedure (for convenience, teaching purposes or research).

10. *The Pregnant Patient has the right* to be accompanied during the stress of labor and birth by someone she cares for, and to whom she looks for emotional comfort and encouragement.

11. *The Pregnant Patient has the right* after appropriate medical consultation to choose a position for labor and for birth which is least stressful to her baby and to herself.

12. *The Obstetric Patient has the right* to have her baby cared for at her bedside if her baby is normal, and to feed her baby according to her baby's needs rather than according to the hospital regimen.

13. *The Obstetric Patient has the right* to be informed in writing of the name of the person who actually delivered her baby and the professional qualifications of that person. This information should also be on the birth certificate.

14. *The Obstetric Patient has the right* to be informed if there is any known or indicated aspect of her or her baby's care or condition which may cause her or her baby later difficulty or problems.

15. *The Obstetric Patient has the right* to have her and her baby's hospital medical records complete, accurate and legible and to have their records, including Nurses' Notes, retained by the hospital

until the child reaches at least the age of majority, or, alternatively, to have the records offered to her before they are destroyed.

16. *The Obstetric Patient*, both during and after her hospital stay, has the right to have access to her complete hospital medical records, including Nurses' Notes, and to receive a copy upon payment of a reasonable fee and without incurring the expense of retaining an attorney.

It is the obstetric patient and her baby, not the health professional, who must sustain any trauma or injury resulting from the use of a drug or obstetric procedure. The observation of the rights listed above will not only permit the obstetric patient to participate in the decisions involving her and her baby's health care, but will help to protect the health professional and the hospital against litigation arising from resentment or misunderstanding on the part of the mother.

Endorsed by the International Childbirth Education Association

Bulk orders: $.03 each plus $.40 postage and handling.
For a complimentary copy send a stamped, self-addressed envelope to the
Committee on Patient's Rights • Box 1900 • New York, New York 10001

Reprinted with permission of Doris Haire, for the International Childbirth Education Association.

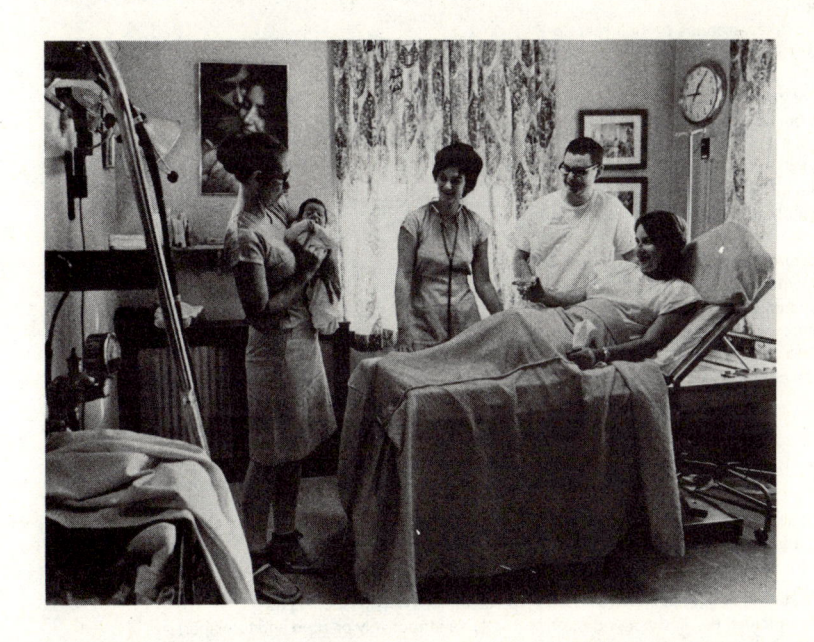

An example of a home-like birthing room, with the new parents toasting the baby with champagne while the nurse-practitioner and monitrice—Bella Mae Carlson—wraps the baby. Reprinted with permission from "Six Years' Experience of Prepared Childbirth in a Home-Like Labor-Delivery Room," by E. Sumner, M.D., in *Birth and the Family Journal*, Vol. 3, No. 2, Summer, 1976.

Family-Centered Maternity Care

Recommended Family-Centered Approach;

I. Preparation of Patients: Have available to consumers: two or more types of preparation for Childbirth Classes taught by Certified Nurse-Midwives and other personnel.

    A. A psychophrophylactic method, i.e. Lamaze

    B. A psychophysical method, i.e. Grantly Dick-Read method of abdominal breathing as a technique

    C. A comprehensive course incorporating education about pregnancy and childbirth, breathing and relaxation techniques with aspects of parenting and child care

All class approaches should include a bibliography of reading materials. These classes:

    1) increase the consumers' awareness of their responsibility toward insuring a healthy outcome for mother and child

    2) serve as opportunities for consumers and providers to match expectations and achieve mutual goals from the childbirth experience

    3) serve as criteria to assist the consumers to be eligible for participation in the full family-centered program

        (a) a tour of the obstetrical suite and post-partum units should be:

            (1) offered as an integral part of the preparation for childbirth programs

            (2) available to consumers by appointment

        (b) a "hot line" telephone should be available in the obstetrical suite where patients could call in to request information or have their inquiries answered

II. Preparation of Hospital Staff:

    A. In-depth continuing education programs for all levels of staff including medical and administrative, are to be conducted on an ongoing basis to:

        1) Educate *all levels* of staff including janitorial and office clerks, medical, nurse-midwifery and nursing staff, supervisory and administrative personnel on the objectives of the Family-Centered Maternity Program which may include but are not limited to:

            (a) current trends in childbirth practices

            (b) alternative childbirth practices: safe and unsafe, as they are being practiced

            (c) "The Pregnant Patient's Bill of Rights"

            (d) needs of childbearing families to share the total experience

            (e) explanation of the term "family" so that it includes any "significant" or "supporting others" individual to the expectant mother

            (f) the advantages to families and to the larger society of establishing the parenting bond immediately after birth

            (g) the responsibilities of the consumer patients toward insuring a healthy outcome of the childbirth experience

            (h) the economic advantage to the hospital for initiating the program and how this could benefit each employee

            (i) the satisfaction to be gained by each employee toward assisting families to adjust to the new family member

            (j) how the Family-Centered Maternity Program is to function and the role each level employee is to perform to insure its success

III. Family-Centered Program

    A. *Family Waiting Room* and *Early Labor Lounge* should be available in or near the obstetrical suite where:

        1) patients in early labor could walk and visit with children and husbands

        2) the "significant other" person could go for a "rest break," if necessary

        3) a small kitchen could be available for preparation of nourishments and for placement of snack machines

This Family Waiting Room is to:

    1) be attractively painted and furnished
    2) include reading materials
    3) include a nursery play area
    4) include a telephone/intercom connection with the labor area

B. *A Diagnostic-Admitting Room* is to be adjacent to or near the family waiting room where:

    1) patients could be examined to ascertain their status in labor without being formally admitted and put to bed if they're in early labor
    2) any pregnant patient past 20 weeks gestation could be evaluated for any health problem during pregnancy

Concept: The "supporting other or others" remain with the client/patient throughout the childbirth process as long as her progress is normal

C. *"Birthing Room"* which is designed to be:
    1) a combination labor and delivery room for patient and supporting others
    2) brightly and attractively painted and furnished to include:
        (a) wall pictures
        (b) colorful drapes and throw rug
        (c) casual and comfortable lounge chairs or large floor cushions
        (d) colorful commercial sheets, pillow-cases and spreads to match the room decor
    3) stocked for medical emergencies but concealed behind wall cabinets or drapes or readily available to be wheeled in when needed
    4) wired for soft music to be "piped" in, if desired
    5) contain —
        (a) modern hospital bed which can be totally lowered to floor to height of home bedding or which can be raised to "hospital height" for the delivery
        (b) combination labor/delivery bed equipment if it is both safe and appealing
        (c) whichever equipment that allows the patient to be in semi-Fowler's (head raised) position for the actual delivery
    6) have space for an infant cribbette, and
    7) equipment for a normal spontaneous vaginal delivery

Concept: Breastfeeding and handling of the baby by the mother and "supporting other" is encouraged to foster parenting bond

D. *Other Labor Rooms*:
    1) "supporting other" or "others" can be with laboring patient whether progress in labor is normal or abnormal
    2) may contain regulation hospital equipment including fetal monitors, but concealed as much as possible
    3) should be attractively painted and furnished with colorful drapes and paintings
    4) to include a lounge chair comfortable enough for sleeping
    5) are equipped for the performance of deliveries

E. *Delivery Rooms*: (Lighting can be dimmed, according to need)

    1) are for patients who do not desire to use the "Birthing Room" for normal spontaneous vaginal deliveries
    2) who need forceps deliveries or
    3) who require Cesarean sections
    4) delivery tables are to include adjustable back-rests and an overhead mirror is to be available
    5) breastfeeding and handling of the baby is encouraged immediately after delivery

Concept: The "supporting other" can accompany the patient into the delivery room as long as progress is expected to include a normal spontaneous vaginal delivery

F. *Recovery Room*: (For those not using the "Birthing Room"); Patients may be returned to their original labor rooms, depending upon the demand, or to a Recovery Room where in addition to medical monitoring —
    1) the infants are allowed to be with the mothers and fathers for a minimum of 30 minutes after delivery
    2) the "supporting other" or "others" are allowed to visit with the new mother in privacy
    3) a "pass" is given to the father of the baby to allow him extended visiting privileges on the "new family" unit

G. *The "New Family Unit"* is to:
    1) contain flexible rooming-in with a central nursery to allow for:
        (a) optional "rooming-in"
        (b) babies to be returned to the central nursery for professional nursing care when desired by the mother
        (c) newborns being separated from their mothers no more than a maximum of 10 hours in the first 24 hours

Continued on next page

2) have extended visiting hours for fathers of the new babies to allow them to assist with the care and feeding of their babies
3) have prescribed visiting hours for friends since the emphasis of the family-centered approach is on the family
4) contain a family room where —
   (a) children can visit with their mothers and fathers, and
   (b) where professional staff are available to answer questions about parenting and adjustment issues of the enlarged family
   (c) where cafeteria-like meals can be served and eaten restaurant-style by the mothers
5) have classes taught by nurse-midwives and professional nurses and other personnel on infant feeding, infant care and parenting
6) allow visiting and feeding by the mothers in the special nurseries such as:
   (a) newborn, intensive care nursery
   (b) and isolation nursery
7) allow for breastfeeding on demand with professional personnel available for assistance

Reprinted by permission of the American College of Nurse-Midwives from "A Sample Pattern For Family Centered Maternity Care" by Betty Carrington, C.N.M., M.S., in *Journal of Nurse-Midwifery*, Vol. XXII, No. 1, Spring, 1977, © 1977, American College of Nurse-Midwives.

Diagnosis of Pregnancy

Presumptive Manifestations		Probable Manifestations		Positive Manifestations
Symptoms	Signs	Symptoms	Signs	Signs
Amenorrhea	Bluish coloration of vagina, cervix	Same as presumptive	Abdominal enlargement	Fetal heart tones
Nausea, vomiting	Softened uterocervical junction		Uterine contractions	Palpation of fetal outline
Mastodynia				
Quickening	Irregular softened fundus		Ballottement of object in abdomen	Sonography of gestational sac or fetal shape
Urinary symptoms				
Fatigue	Uterine enlargement		Uterine souffle	Fetal electrocardiogram
Constipation	Breast changes		Agglutination pregnancy tests	Radioimmunoassay for HCG
Weight gain	Skin changes			
	Basal body temperature elevation			X-ray examination of fetal skeleton
	Gingival hypertrophy			

Reprinted with permission from *Health Care of Women*, Leonide Martin, Copyright 1978, J. B. Lippincott, Co.

Weight Gain in Pregnancy

In general, it is suggested that pregnant women should gain about 24 pounds (11 kilograms). A woman who is underweight at the time that pregnancy begins might be advised to gain 30 or more pounds (17 kilograms), while a woman who is definitely obese might be advised to gain only 22 pounds (10 kilograms).

Pregnancy is not the time to lose weight; however, chemical changes in the mother's body during weight loss can damage the baby's developing brain. The weight gain should be gradual: only 1.5–3 pounds (.07–1.4 kilograms) should be gained in the first 3 months, and about .5 to 1 pound (.02–.05 kilograms) per week after 3 months. The following information gives an idea of the general distribution of the weight just before delivery.

	Pounds	Kilograms
Baby	7.5	3.4
Placenta	1.4	.7
Amniotic fluid	2.2	1.0
Uterus	2.2	1.0
Breast growth	1.1	.5
Blood volume	3.3	1.5
Extracellular fluid	3.3	1.5
Maternal stores (fat and protein to support lactation)	3.0	1.5

Reprinted by permission of the American Red Cross from *Family Health and Home Nursing,* © 1979, by the American National Red Cross, Washington, D.C.

Fundal Height at Various Times During Pregnancy

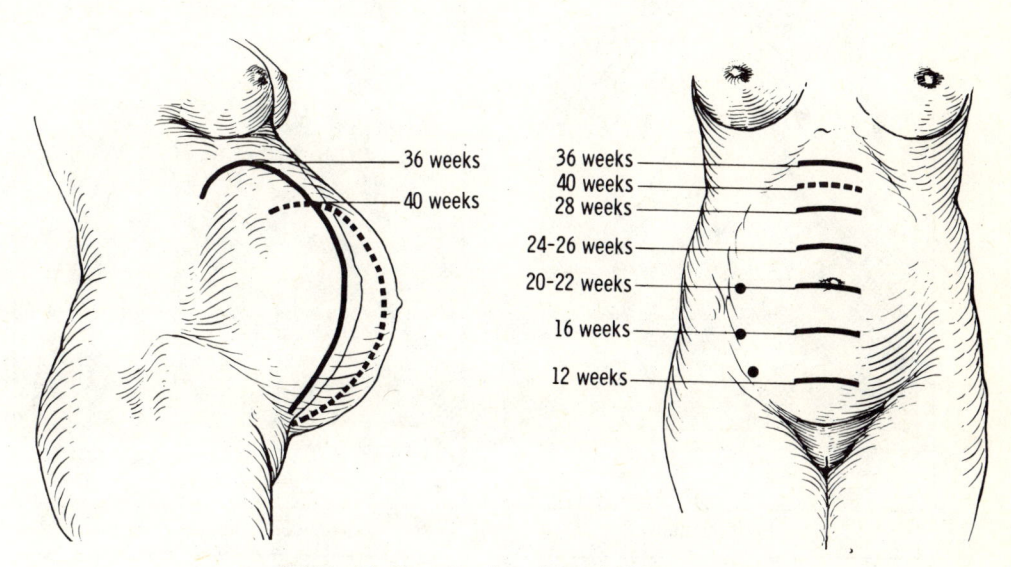

Height of fundus at various times during pregnancy.

Reproduced, with permission, from Benson, R. C. (editor): *Current Obstetric & Gynecologic Diagnosis & Treatment,* 2nd ed. Copyright 1978 by Lange Medical Publications, Los Altos, California.

Leopold's Maneuvers

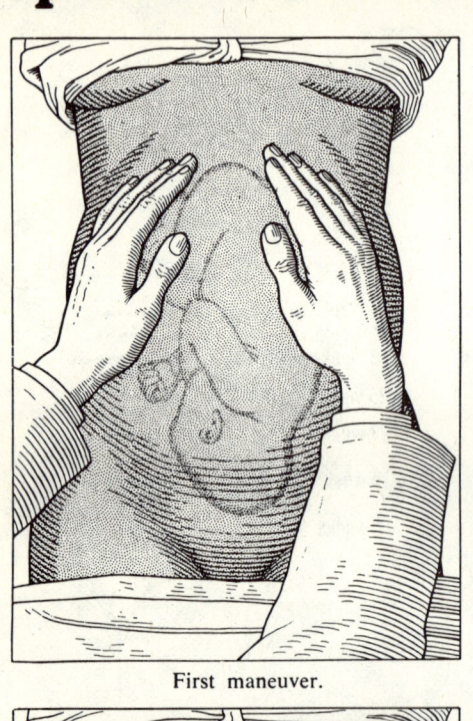

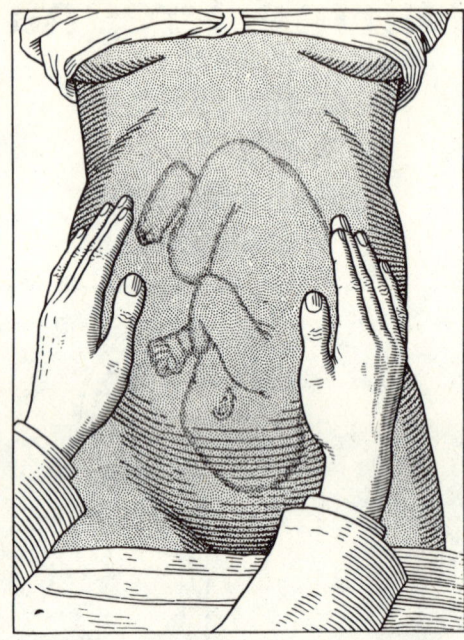

First maneuver.

Second maneuver.

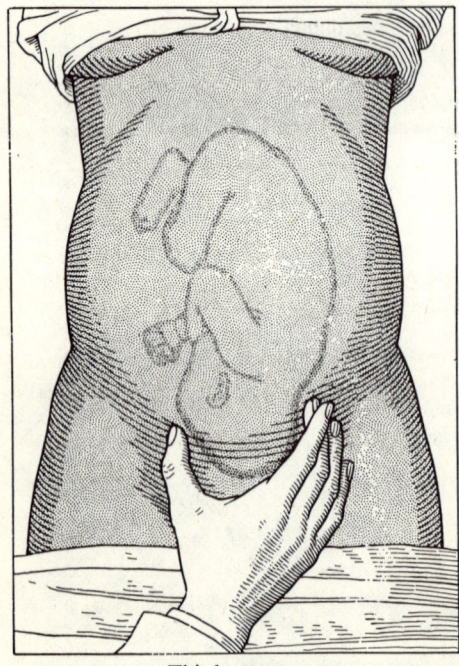

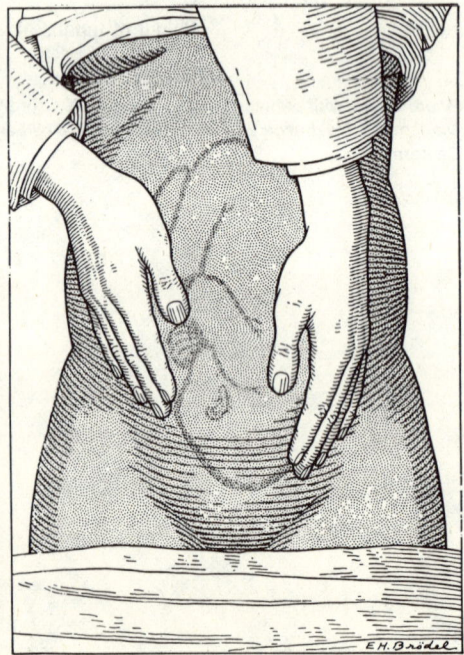

Third maneuver.

Fourth maneuver.

Reprinted by permission of Appleton-Century-Crofts from *William's Obstetrics*, 14th edition, by Louis Hellman and Jack Pritchard, Copyright 1971, Appleton-Century-Crofts.

CHILDBIRTH EDUCATOR'S ROLE IN RELATION TO CHILDBIRTH TEAM MEMBERS

The following chart illustrates how the childbirth educator relates to the different team members during the ante, intra and postpartum phases of childbirth.

CHILDBIRTH EDUCATOR'S ROLE

Team Members	Antepartum	Intrapartum	Postpartum
Mother	Resource person. Teaches relaxation, breathing, comfort measures. Assesses physiologic and psychologic state.	During labor, the childbirth educator works with the mother, father, physician and labor nurse. Properly trained parents are able to function with sufficient independence so that they require only intermittent support from the labor staff. Occasionally, the husband-coach is not present at the labor, and the childbirth educator acts as monitrice.*	Follow-up visit to assess early parenting adjustment.
Father	Establishes role of coach. Helps develop team concept and effort. Assesses ability to work with wife and cope with stress.		Follow-up report to obtain feedback on delivery experience.
Physician	Communicates any unusual findings relative to mother's status or father's ability to cope.		Solicit feedback on individual couple performance.
Labor Nurse	Communicates class performance. Predicts area where support of nurse is needed for mother or father.		Solicit feedback on individual couple performance.
Postpartum Nurse	Communicates any concerns parents may have that might influence early parenting.		Solicit feedback about postpartum adjustment.
Nursery Nurse	Communicates any concerns parents may have that might influence early parenting.		Solicit information about newborn status.

*Monitrice is the French word used to designate the trainer who becomes the labor coach in traditional Lamaze settings. Whether paid or voluntary, the monitrice is not a hospital employee and does not relieve the hospital staff of its responsibilities for monitoring the safety of mother and baby. Also, the monitrice has no authority to dictate medical or nursing intervention necessary for safety of mother and/or baby. If monitricing is a regular practice, specific policies must be developed governing responsibilities and behavior as well as stipulating qualifications of those persons eligible to monitrice. This should be a joint medical-nursing committee decision based on awareness of needs of the local situation.

From NAACOG Technical Bulletin No. 3, Nov., 1978, "Preparation for Parenthood." Reprinted with permission, The Nurses' Association of The American College of Obstetricians and Gynecologists.

"It is terribly easy to tell people how they ought to have their babies and run their lives and bring up their children. To give advice seems such a simple, obvious thing to do when people are confused and muddled, especially when they are eager to be given a formula for success. In my work as a childbirth educator, preparing couples not only for labour but also to some extent, I hope, for parenthood and the birth of the family, I have learned that telling people how they ought to behave creates more problems than it solves and all too often means that they are unable to adapt to challenges confronting them, because instead of flexibility they are armed with a series of magic formulae which they hope will work when the going gets difficult.

It is much more valuable to give people information and *self-confidence* so that they can make their own informed choices in terms of the reality they face. To do that it is also important to get to know yourself, be honest about your own feelings and start from inside awareness rather than external mechanical acts. This is as true for bathing a baby comfortably and being able to enjoy doing it as it is for breathing through contractions at the end of the first stage of labour, or facing the sense of uselessness and the longing which a mother may feel when her child goes off to the first long day at school, leaving the house empty. It applies equally to all the varied and chaotic, frustrating, tantalizing, and satisfying experiences of bringing up a family and coping with the vivid kaleidoscope of changing relationships within it."

From: *Women As Mothers* by Sheila Kitzinger, © 1978 by Sheila Kitzinger, published in the United States by Random House, Inc., New York. Reprinted by permission.

Innovations in Prenatal Education

It has become standard practice in most hospitals and clinics to offer prenatal classes for expectant parents. But in the last few years some health care institutions have been recognizing the needs of family members other than the pregnant couple to be educated in the childbirth experience. Innovations in this area include prenatal classes for children offered at the University of Minnesota (see "Prenatal Classes Especially for Children" by Philothea T. Sweet, *MCN, The American Journal of Maternal Child Nursing,* March/April, 1979, pp. 82–3) and at the Denver Birth Center (see "Answering A Child's Questions About Sex and a New Baby" by Janet Malinowski, *American Journal of Nursing,* November, 1979, pp. 1966–7). Classes for grandparents-to-be are offered at St. Francis Hospital in Port Jervis, N.Y. (see "Prenatal Classes for Expectant Grandparents" by Sister Marie James McCallen and Rosemary Lamb, *MCN, The American Journal of Maternal Child Nursing,* Nov./Dec., 1978, pp. 336–8).

Adolescent Pregnancy

Teens Having Babies

Reprinted by permission of Anthony J. Janetti, Inc., from PEDIATRIC NURSING, May/June 1978, vol. 4, no. 3 © 1978, Anthony J. Janetti, Inc.

by Mildred Abbott, C.N.M.

Prologue

Although the number of pregnancies among teen-agers in the United States has been increasing steadily for some years now, the problem has only recently gained the attention it deserves. In 1976, government agencies and concerned groups such as Planned Parenthood Foundation declared the adolescent pregnancy rate to be in epidemic proportions; this conclusion was based on 1974 statistics.

In my opinion, this new interest is stimulated in part by the increased premarital birth rate among white teenagers. A New York Times reporter verified this suspicion in an interview in which she was seeking information about the Adolescent Prenatal Program to be described in this article. During the interview, I provided her with details about the program, its goals and accomplishments. She expressed interest in meeting and interviewing a young couple but, when she learned that couples who might consent to an interview were black or hispanic, she explained that she preferred a white couple. According to her, people who read The New York Times are not interested in minority teens who become pregnant; this would not be considered news, but white girls now having and keeping babies would interest the readers.

This seemed to parallel the history of the drug problem that existed in poor communities for years but gained widespread attention only when white teen-agers began "experimenting" with **drugs.**

Although the reporters remarks angered me, I knew her comments were all too true, and, since our discussion, two articles both dealing with the increasing pregnancy rate among white

Continued on next page

teen-agers have appeared in The New York Times Magazine. This publicity is undoubtedly focusing attention on a situation that is more prevalent in the United States than in most other industrialized countries.

The Scope of the Problem

What does the term "epidemic proportions" connote? In 1974, one million women, ages 15 to 19, and an additional 30,000 under 15 became pregnant; 41 percent of these pregnancies were terminated voluntarily or ended in miscarriage, while the remaining 608,000 pregnancies were continued until delivery.

Teen-age childbearing is a serious social, economic and health problem because all women in this age group are considered at risk when pregnant. Compared with women in their twenties, the teen-agers have twice the chance of developing complications leading to infant and maternal mortality or morbidity. Among the reasons for this high risk status are:
1. The teen-ager's biologic immaturity, supposedly making them more susceptible to cephalopelvic disproportion, low-birth-weight or premature infants pre-eclampsia, anemia, and post-datism.
2. The psychologic impact of trying to cope with motherhood while still coping with her own maturing process.
3. Society's attitude.
4. Financial instability.
5. Inability to obtain good obstetric care.

Until I began the practice of nurse-midwifery at Columbia-Presbyterian Medical Center in 1969, I was unaware of the adolescent pregnancy rate and, as I became more familiar with this problem, I decided to work primarily with sexually active and pregnant adolescents.

With no support except that of nursing and the hospital's Department of Social Service, plans were formulated to implement an Adolescent Prenatal Program to provide the specialized obstetric care teen patients need but, for a variety of reasons, were not then receiving. Many teen-agers would come in seeking care but were quickly "turned off" by hospital bureaucracy and by medical personnel who were so judgmental that the patient, who wanted an excuse not to seek care, left the clinic and frequently was not seen again until she was admitted in active labor.

So, in 1969 Mrs. Elizabeth Graham, a highly competent social worker, and I initiated the Adolescent Prenatal Program without special funding and without support from the hospital's administration. For the first six years we ran the program but, since the initial six-year period, new members have been added to the team.

The Program

The Adolescent Prenatal Program has now evolved into a five-part program consisting of:
1. The Teen-age Prenatal Clinic, where these young patients receive prenatal care from nurse-midwives, with medical supervision when needed;
2. a Young Parents Group;
3. a Young Parents Parenting Group;
4. a Well Baby Clinic staffed by pediatric nurse practitioners; and
5. a Young Adults Family Planning Clinic.

The *Young Parents Group,* originally started by the OB/GYN Department of Social Service meets in a two-hour counseling session held in conjunction with the Teen Prenatal Clinic. The educationally and therapeutically oriented sessions are designed to expose the young people to information about anatomy, nutrition, the physiology of pregnancy, labor and delivery, child care, abortion, contraception, family life and human sexuality. We endeavor

FIGURE I
AGE OF PATIENTS SAMPLED FROM ADOLESCENT PRENATAL PROGRAM AT COLUMBIA PRESBYTERIAN HOSPITAL

N = 220 *

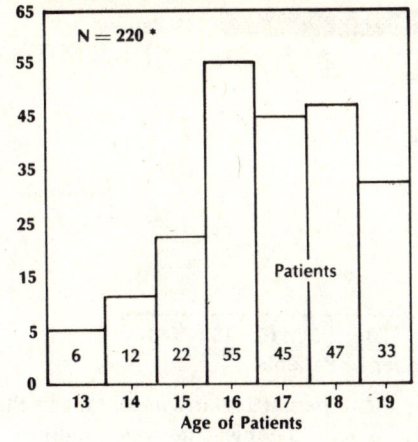

Age of Patients	Number of Patients
13	6
14	12
15	22
16	55
17	45
18	47
19	33

* There were 226 charts reviewed, 5 patients were omitted for a variety of reasons, 2 were omitted because they reached 20th birthday before they delivered.

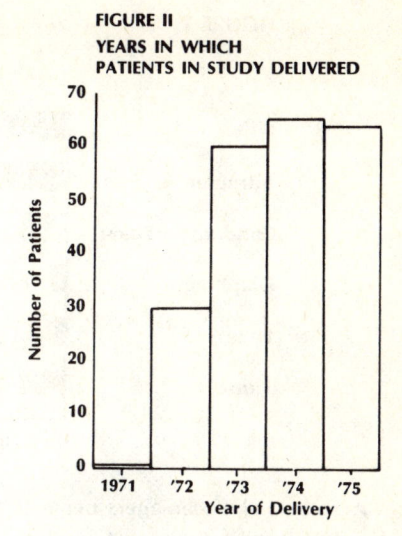

FIGURE II
YEARS IN WHICH PATIENTS IN STUDY DELIVERED

Year of Delivery	Number of Patients
1971	0
'72	30
'73	59
'74	64
'75	63

FIGURE III
METHOD OF DELIVERY

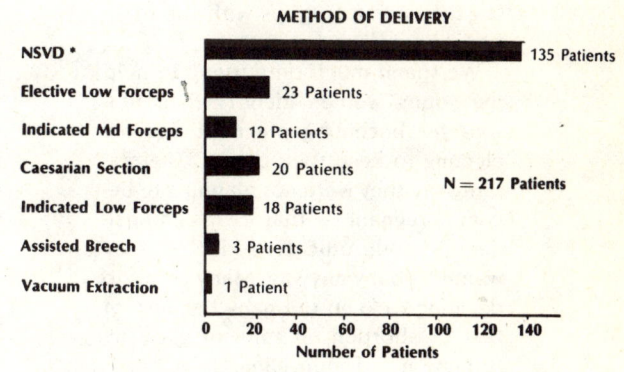

	Patients
NSVD *	135
Elective Low Forceps	23
Indicated Md Forceps	12
Caesarian Section	20
Indicated Low Forceps	18
Assisted Breech	3
Vacuum Extraction	1

N = 217 Patients

* Normal Spontaneous Vaginal Delivery. Forty-two patients were delivered by nurse midwives.

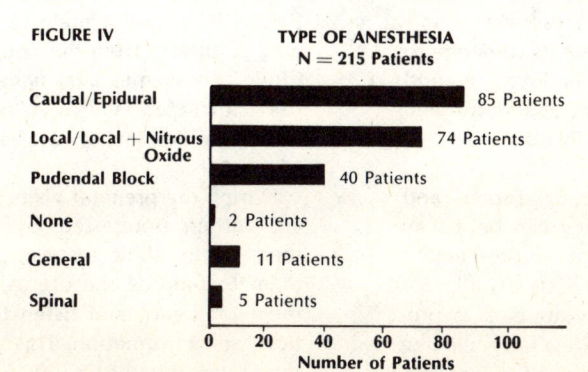

FIGURE IV
TYPE OF ANESTHESIA
N = 215 Patients

	Patients
Caudal/Epidural	85
Local/Local + Nitrous Oxide	74
Pudendal Block	40
None	2
General	11
Spinal	5

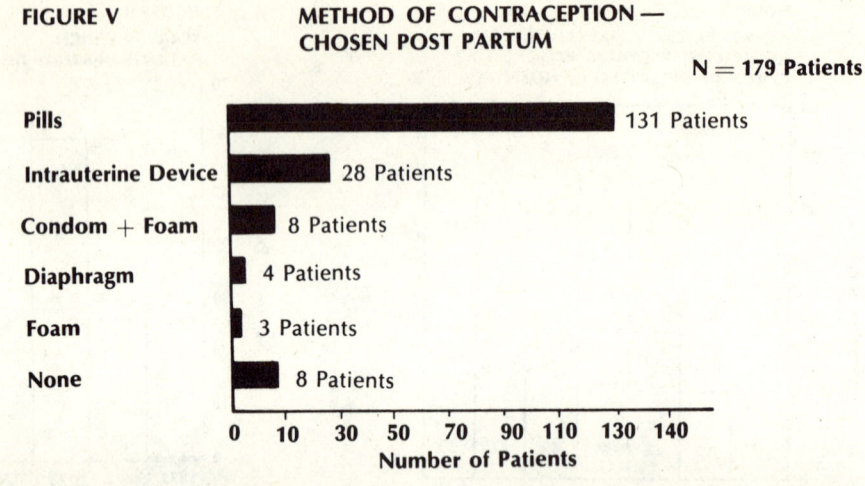

FIGURE V   METHOD OF CONTRACEPTION —
                  CHOSEN POST PARTUM

                                          N = 179 Patients

Method	Patients
Pills	131 Patients
Intrauterine Device	28 Patients
Condom + Foam	8 Patients
Diaphragm	4 Patients
Foam	3 Patients
None	8 Patients

0 10 30 50 70 90 110 130 140
         Number of Patients

to help the teen-agers begin to get in touch with their own feelings about these issues.

At the Clinic and at these Group sessions we try to reach these young people who have elected to carry their pregnancies to term — to help them begin to come to grips with the realities of parenthood.

We spend much time trying to help the young women identify their reasons for becoming pregnant and for electing to keep their babies. The majority say they were not planning to become pregnant — that it was an accident — but quickly add that they wanted a baby anyway. Many admit to deciding to keep the baby because of fear of abortion, in spite of good information and counseling.

For many, the baby represents a cure (probably a temporary one) for some problems in their lives, especially loneliness; the baby represents someone to have, to love and to be loved by, and someone who will not abandon them. A baby can temporarily bolster self-esteem.

For both the young father and mother, the pregnancy can be a way (again probably temporary) to cement their relationship. Most of all, for many, having a baby appears to provide a chance to create a fairy-tale-like family unit consisting of a mother, father and a baby. Such make-believe can be particularly important to these young people, the vast majority of whom have come from one-parent homes.

We spend much time discussing the seriousness of being pregnant, the risks of adolescent pregnancy and the importance of teen-agers using contraception. Frequently friends and siblings of groups members attend these sessions and such discussions may prevent some pregnancies, but, equally important, they provide these young people with information "to put on the streets" since this is where many teens receive a great deal of their initial information on sex.

The *Young Parents Parenting Group* meets for a two-hour session, with leaders from four disciplines — a social worker, a nurse-midwife, a pediatric nurse practitioner from the Well Baby Clinic, and a male family planning counselor from the Young Adults Clinic. These meetings have successfully attracted and involved young fathers, some of whom are as young as 15.

During the prenatal visits, we try to get fathers interested by involving them in the clinic session, permitting them to palpate the uterus, listen to the fetal heart, and listen to instructions and information. This stimulates their interest in the Groups. Fathers are permitted in both the labor and delivery rooms, and we feel that our program has been very successful in helping many of these young men realize that a baby needs two parents when possible and that, although they may not be able to support the child financially, they can support the young mother and baby with love and attention.

The Parenting Group has been a way to let the young mothers and fathers know that we do not stop caring about them when the pregnancy is completed, and we take cognizance of the fact that they now have different needs. This group attempts to help the young parents deal with the realities of being teens with babies. We discuss baby care, including what can be defined as child abuse, how it feels to be a mother or a father, what their expectations of this role had been and what differences they have found. We also try to help them define and pursue careers or educational goals they may have established for themselves.

The *Young Adults Clinic,* a free program for all young people under 21, is for family planning and family life services, and is funded by a grant from USDHEW.

Accomplishments

Although there have been repeat pregnancies among our younger teens more so than in the 17-to-19-year-old group, the program's overall results can be considered highly satisfactory. We have never tried to reduce recidivism but rather, through education and emotional support, to build the teen's self-esteem by helping her discover herself. We believe that a person, really in tune with her body and herself, would prefer to plan her life and her future in a more constructive way.

Over the years, there has been some change in terms of increased sophistication with participants more willing to accept some responsibility for their behavior, such as: acknowledging that they have been sexually active and must, therefore, accept some responsibility for planning either for an abortion or for care of the infant, and at the same time planning for their own education and economic future. There have been nearly 1000 pregnant teens in our program since its inception. With our primary focus on patient care and with very limited staff, we have not been able to do extensive research, but in 1975 I did review data on 220 patients, facts from this review, which lend themselves to graphic representation, are presented in Figures I through V, with other information summarized as follows:

average education: 10th grade
married: 23   *single:* 173
living with or had both parents at home: 39
on public assistance: nearly 90 percent
received Medicaid: nearly 90 percent
average weeks pregnant at registration: 16 weeks
average weeks of pregnancy at delivery: 39.4 weeks
average weight gain: 24.8 pounds (based on 90 whose prepregnancy weight was known)
previously pregnant: 30

(These patients were 13 to 18 years old. One, age 17, had delivered a full-term infant at 15; another, age 20 at time of this delivery, had had three other children; six had had spontaneous abortions.)

hematocrits: average initial, 33.5 mg/percent; average at last visit, 35.8 mg/percent.
pre-eclampsia: severe, two; both had good obstetric outcomes.
average time in labor: for entire group, 11 hours, 30 minutes. (92 primagravida averaged six hours, 35 minutes)
average weight of infants: 3200 grams (14 weighed less than 2500 grams; seven of these, weighed 2200 grams or more.)

average Apgars:
one minute — 8
five minutes — 9

All babies were kept by the teen-age mothers, the majority of whom returned to school with help from the baby's grandmother or other relatives.

To break a potential cycle of repeated pregnancies, these young people need many things — better schools and more assistance during the pregnancy, good day care centers, and, most of all, jobs. Most want to work but either cannot find suitable jobs for their limited education or are unable to find trustworthy baby sitters. Memories of their own childhood make many fearful of child abuse.

Epilogue

Among our observations, there are two factors that are very disturbing to our group — the increasing numbers of 13-to-15-year-old girls who are becoming pregnant, and teen-agers who seek no care until they come to the hospital in active labor.

In 1976, 46 teen-age patients who had received little or no prenatal care were admitted to our hospital. Several had been seen once or twice to have the pregnancy confirmed, but had never followed up with prenatal care. Three or four never acknowledged being pregnant and, only when labor began, did some parents discover the condition. Two teen-agers delivered at home and were brought in by amazed and shocked families.

When the obstetric nurse-specialist, responsible for keeping statistics on unregistered patients, interviewed these 46 patients, she received a variety of reasons from them for not having sought prenatal care; among them were:

"I did not have any money or Medicaid so the hospital would not accept me for prenatal care." (this was the most frequent comment)

"I did not want my family to know I was pregnant."

"I was too scared."

"I did not like hospitals."

"I just moved to town."

The obstetric outcomes for these women were as follows:

Eight, most of whom delivered prematurely, had infants under 2500 grams.

One severely anemic mother required two units of blood postpartum.

Five mothers were hospitalized six to eleven days for cesarean section, toxemia and/or infection.

Six babies had to be placed in Babies Hospital Intensive Care Unit.

Three babies were too sick or too small to survive.

These unregistered teen-agers were prime examples of patients at risk, and may, in my opinion, be responsible for the statistics that label all teen-agers "high risk." It is urgent that this group be reached. They must be identified when they come to the Pediatric Clinic for nausea and vomiting and not misdiagnosed because pregnancy in a 12- or 13-year-old is the last thing in the medical person's mind. They must be identified by teachers who notice symptoms and be encouraged to tell their parents and seek prenatal care. Parents, even though busy just surviving, must take more interest in the physical appearance and changes in emotional state of their daughters. Parents must provide more information on sex and contraception or encourage the school system to take over this task and do it in a manner that will have meaning for a very young person.

Finally, health care providers must be given the funds necessary to eradicate the excuse of "I did not have any money or Medicaid so the Hospital would not accept me for prenatal care." □

Reprinted by permission of Anthony J. Janetti, Inc., from *Pediatric Nursing*, May/June, 1978, Vol. 4, No. 3. © 1978, Anthony J. Janetti, Inc.

Recommended References on Adolescent Pregnancy

Abbott, Mildred, "Teen Group—Medical Student Seminars," *Journal of Nurse-Midwifery,* Vol. XX, No. 1, Spring, 1975, p. 20.

Aiman, J., "X-ray pelvimetry of the pregnant adolescent. Pelvic size and frequency of contractions," *Obstetrics and Gynecology,* September, 1976, 48(3): 281–6.

Badger, E. et al., "Education for adolescent mothers in a hospital setting," *American Journal of Public Health,* May, 1976, 66(5): 469–72.

Blos, Peter, *On Adolescence,* Macmillan Publishing Co., New York, 1962.

Bryan-Logan, B.N. et al., "Unwed Pregnant Adolescents: Their Mothers' Dilemma," *Nursing Clinics of North America,* March, 1974, 9(1).

Corbett, Margaret-Ann and Burst, Helen V., "Nurse-Midwives and Adolescents: The South Carolina Experience," *Journal of Nurse-Midwifery,* Vol. XXI, No. 4, Winter, 1976, pp. 13–17.

Curtis, Frances, "Observations of Unwed Pregnant Adolescents," *American Journal of Nursing,* Vol. 74, No. 1, January, 1974.

Dott, A.B. et al., "Medical and Social Factors Affecting Early Teenage Pregnancy," *American Journal of Obstetrics and Gynecology,* January 15, 1976, 125(4).

Evans, Jerome, et al., "Teenagers: Fertility Control Behavior and Attitudes Before and After Abortion, Childbearing or Negative Pregnancy Test," *Family Planning Perspectives,* July/August, 1976, 8(4).

Fischman, S.H., "The Pregnancy-Resolution Decisions of Unwed Adolescents," *Nursing Clinics of North America,* June, 1975, 10(2).

Frye, B.A. et al., "Reaching Out To Pregnant Adolescents," *American Journal of Nursing,* September, 1975, 75(9).

Furstenberg, Frank F., "The Social Consequences of Teenage Parenthood," *Family Planning Perspectives,* July/August, 1976, 8(4).

Graham, Elizabeth H., "Young Parents' Group," *Journal of Nurse-Midwifery,* Spring, 1975.

Howard, Marion, *Only Human: Teenage Pregnancy and Parenthood,* The Seabury Press, New York, 1975.

Huyck, N.I., "Nutrition services for pregnant teenagers," *Journal of the American Dietetic Association,* July, 1976, 69(1): 60–2.

McAnarney, E.R., "Adolescent Pregnancy—A Pediatric Concern?" *Clinical Pediatrics,* January, 1975, 14(1): 19–22.

McRae, Maureen, "An Approach to the Single Parent Dilemma," *MCN, American Journal of Maternal Child Nursing,* May/June, 1977, 2(3).

Mercer, Ramona, "Becoming a Mother at Sixteen," *MCN, American Journal of Maternal Child Nursing,* Jan./Feb., 1976, 1(1).

Millar, Hilary, E.C., *Approaches to Adolescent Health Care in the 1970's,* U.S. Dept. of H.E.W., Public Health Service, Health Services Administration, 1975.

Trussell, T. James, "Economic Consequences of Teenage Childbearing," *Family Planning Perspectives,* July/August, 1976, 8(4).

ALCOHOL AND PREGNANCY
Fetal alcohol syndrome

Since 1971, there has been renewed attention given to the effects of chronic alcohol use during pregnancy. At that time, a researcher reported his observations of infants born to alcoholic mothers. The constellation of features observed have since been termed the *fetal alcohol syndrome.* Alcohol can pass through the placenta to the developing fetus and interfere with prenatal development. At birth, infants with fetal alcohol syndrome are smaller, both in weight and length. There is a decrease in head size, probably related to a decrease in brain growth. These infants also have a "dysmorphic appearance," that is, they are strange looking, just appear "different," although the difference is not easily described. At birth the infants are jittery and tremulous. Whether this jitteriness is the result of nervous system impairment from the long-term exposure to alcohol and/or miniwithdrawal is unclear. There have been reports of newborn infants having the scent of alcohol on their breath. Cardiac problems and retardation are also associated with the fetal alcohol syndrome. This syndrome is now being seen as the third leading cause of mental retardation.

Other dangers to the fetus

Perhaps even more worrisome than the fetal alcohol syndrome are recent reports on the effects of as little as two drinks (1 ounce of pure alcohol) on the unborn baby. As little as two drinks a day may lead to increased risk of abnormalities. This two-drink figure is *not* a numerical average. It refers to the amount of alcohol consumed on any one day. As the amount of alcohol consumed on any given day rises, the risk also increases:

Less than two drinks	Very little risk
Two to four drinks	10% risk of abnormalities
Ten drinks	50% risk of abnormalities
Over ten drinks	75% risk of abnormalities

Based on this information, in the summer of 1977 the National Institute on Alcohol Abuse and Alcoholism issued a health warning, advising expectant mothers not to have more than two drinks a day.

How alcohol interferes with normal prenatal growth is not fully understood. Nor is it known if there are critical periods during pregnancy when alcohol is especially hazardous. Research with animals suggests the alcohol level of some of the fetus' tissues may be ten times higher than that of the mother. If this is the case, the mechanisms have not been identified. One would guess that the alcohol, since it can pass through the placenta to the fetus, could exit as easily. Therefore both would have equivalent blood alcohol levels.

However, *if* there is this difference in alcohol levels, if the fetus' is ten times greater than the mother's, consider the following possibility. A 140-pound expectant mother has two highballs, consuming 1 ounce of pure alcohol. Her blood alcohol level would be 0.045 and that of certain organs in the baby would be 0.45. The fetal alcohol concentration is reaching the level that produces coma in an adult. Although the fetus doesn't have to breathe on its own, that's still a whopping amount of alcohol.

What is clear from case reports of women who drank alcohol during delivery, and in whom blood alcohol level studies were done, is that the newborn baby's blood alcohol level did not drop as fast as the mother's. The reason presumably is that the infant has an immature liver. Newborns don't have the fully developed enzyme systems (alcohol dehydrogenase) necessary to metabolize alcohol.

Reprinted with permission of the C. V. Mosby Company from Price, Trevor: Medical complications. In Kinney, Jean, and Leaton, Gwen: *Loosening the Grip,* St. Louis, 1978, The C. V. Mosby Co.

Identification of High Risk Pregnancy: Factors Associated with Increased Risk

Maternal Characteristics

Age less than 15 and over 35
Lower socioeconomic status
Unmarried
Family or marital conflicts
Emotional illness or family history of mental illness
Persistent ambivalence or conflicts about the pregnancy

Stature under 5 feet
20 percent underweight or overweight
Inadequate diet

Reproductive History

Parity greater than 8
Two or more previous abortions
Previous stillborn or neonatal death
Previous premature labor or low birth weight infant (<2500 Gm.)
Previous excessively large infant (>4000 Gm.)
Infant with isoimmunization or ABO incompatibility
Infant with congenital anomaly, genetic disorder, or birth damage
Preeclampsia or eclampsia
Uterine fibroids >5 cm. or submucous
Abnormal Pap smear
Infertility
Prior cesarean section
Prior fetal malpresentations
Contracted pelvis
Ovarian masses
Genital tract abnormalities (incompetent cervix, subseptate or bicornate uterus)

Substances Abuse

Drugs
Alcohol
Heavy smoking >2 packs/day

Medical Problems

Chronic hypertension
Renal disease (pyelonephritis, glomerulonephritis, polycystic kidney)
Diabetes mellitus
Heart disease (aortic insufficiency, pulmonary hypertension, diastolic murmur, cardiac enlargement, heart failure, arrhythmia)

Sickle cell trait or disease
Anemias with hemoglobin <9 Gm. and hematocrit <32 percent
Pulmonary disease (tuberculosis, COPD)
Endocrine disorders (hypo- or hyperthyroidism, family history of cretinism, adrenal or pituitary problems)
Gastrointestinal or liver disease
Epilepsy
Malignancy (including leukemia and Hodgkin's disease)

Complications of Present Pregnancy

Low or excessive weight gain
Hypertension (mean arterial pressure >90, BP 140/90, increase >30 mm. Hg systolic or >20 mm. Hg diastolic)
Recurrent glycosuria and abnormal FBS or glucose tolerance test
Uterine size inappropriate for gestational age (either too large or too small)
Recurrent urinary tract infections
Severe varicosities or thrombophlebitis
Recurrent vaginal bleeding
Premature rupture of membranes
Multiple pregnancy
Hydramnios with a single fetus
Rh negative with a rising titer
Late or no prenatal care
Exposure to teratogens (medications, x-ray, radioactive isotopes)
Viral infections (rubella, cytomegalovirus, herpes, mumps, rubeola, chickenpox, shingles, smallpox, vaccinia, influenza, poliomyelitis, hepatitis, Western equine encephalitis, Coxsackie B virus)
Syphilis, especially late pregnancy
Bacterial infections (gonorrhea, tuberculous listeriosis, severe acute infection)
Protozoan infections (toxoplasmosis, malaria)
Postmaturity

Reprinted with permission from *Health Care of Women*, Leonide Martin, copyright 1978, J.B. Lippincott Co.

THE FETUS AND THE NEWBORN INFANT

MATERNAL MEDICATIONS WHICH MAY ADVERSELY AFFECT THE FETUS AND NEWBORN INFANT

DRUG	EFFECT ON FETUS	DEPENDABILITY OF EVIDENCE
Adrenal corticosteroids	Cleft palate	Suggestive
Amphetamines	Congenital heart disease, transposition of the great vessels	Conclusive
Aminopterin	Abortion, malformations	Conclusive
Azathioprine	Abortion	Suggestive
Busulfan (Myleran)	Stunted growth, corneal opacities, cleft palate, hypoplasia of ovaries, thyroid and parathyroids	Doubtful
Chlorambucil	Renal agenesis	Suggestive
Chloroquine	Deafness	Doubtful
Chlorothiazide	Thrombocytopenia	Conclusive
Cigarette smoking	Low birth weight for gestational age	Suggestive
Cyclophosphamide	Multiple malformations	Suggestive
Dicumarol	Fetal bleeding and death, hypoplastic nasal structures	Conclusive
Insulin shock	Death	Conclusive
Lysergic acid diethylamide (LSD) or impurities in commercial preparations	Skeletal defects	Doubtful
	Chromosome damage	Suggestive
Meclizine (Bonine)	Congenital malformations	Doubtful
Mepivacaine	Bradycardia, death	Conclusive
6-Mercaptopurine	Abortion	Suggestive
Methimazole	Goiter	Conclusive
Methyltestosterone	Masculinization of female fetus	Conclusive
17-Alpha-ethinyl-19-nortestosterone (Norlutin)	Masculinization of female fetus	Conclusive
Phenmetrazine (Preludin)	Defect of diaphragm	Doubtful
Potassium iodide	Goiter	Conclusive
Progesterone	Masculinization of female fetus	Suggestive
17-Alpha-ethinyl testosterone (Progestoral)	Masculinization of female fetus	Conclusive
Propylthiouracil	Goiter	Conclusive
Quinine	Abortion, thrombocytopenia	Conclusive
	Deafness	Doubtful
Radioactive iodine (^{131}I)	Destruction of fetal thyroid	Conclusive
Stilbestrol	Masculinization of female fetus	Suggestive
	Vaginal adenocarcinoma in adolescence	Conclusive
Streptomycin	Deafness	Suggestive
Tetracycline	Retarded skeletal growth	Suggestive
	Pigmentation of teeth, hypoplasia of enamel	Conclusive
	Cataract, limb malformations	Doubtful
Thalidomide	Phocomelia, other malformations	Conclusive
Trimethadione and Paramethadione	Abortion, multiple malformations, mental retardation	Conclusive
Tolbutamide	Congenital malformations	Doubtful
Vitamin D	Supravalvular aortic stenosis, hypercalcemia	Doubtful

Reprinted by permission of W.B. Saunders from *Nelson Textbook of Pediatrics,* 10th edition, Vaughan and McKay, Copyright 1975, W.B. Saunders Co.

> **TABLE 6–8. CONDITIONS IN WHICH ANTENATAL DIAGNOSIS BY AMNIOCENTESIS HAS BEEN MADE**
>
> Adrenal cortical hyperplasia
> Chromosomal translocations
> Down dyndrome
> Fabry's disease
> Galactosemia
> Gaucher's disease
> Glycogen-storage disease (type II)
> G_{M1} gangliosidosis, Type I
> G_{M1} gangliosidosis, Type II
> Hunter syndrome
> Hurler syndrome
> Krabbe's disease
> Lesch-Nyhan syndrome
> Lysosomal acid phosphatase deficiency
> Maple syrup urine disease
> Methylmalonic acidemia
> Metachromatic leukodystrophy
> Niemann-Pick disease
> Sex determination
> Tay-Sachs disease (G_{M2} gangliosidosis)

Reprinted by permission of W.B. Saunders from *Nelson Textbook of Pediatrics*, 10th edition, Vaughan and McKay, Copyright 1975, W.B. Saunders Co.

The Role of the Nurse During Amniocentesis

KATHLEEN HOGAN, RN, MS, and DONNA TCHENG, RN, BSN

Amniocentesis is a relatively simple, safe, and accurate diagnostic tool which is being performed with increased frequency in local hospitals. The maternity nurse has a responsibility to know the clinical applications, the role of the nurse during the procedure, and the potential risks associated with amniocentesis.

Amniocentesis is the procedure by which a sample of amniotic fluid is aspirated from the amniotic sac, usually transabdominally, occasionally transvaginally. This same procedure is also used to inject substances such as radiocontrast materials for amniography and hypertonic solutions to induce abortion.

Amniocentesis was suggested as

early as 1882, but the first report of performing the procedure was in 1919 by Henbel in a case of polyhydramnios. Due to complications associated with the procedure, amniocentesis was abandoned for several years. Renewed interest in its use was initiated by the work of Bevis in 1952 and Liley in 1961, who reported analyses of amniotic fluid in cases of Rh isoimmunization.[1]

INDICATIONS AND APPLICATIONS

Indications for amniocentesis include:
1. Early prenatal detection of genetic disorders;
   a. Cell culture for karyotype to determine chromosomal aberrations,
   b. Sex chromatin for detection of sex-linked disorders,
   c. Cell culture for biochemical studies of inborn errors of metabolism,
   d. Alpha-feto protein levels for diagnosis of neural tube defects;
2. Assessment of fetal maturity;
3. Follow-up of isoimmune disease;
4. Amniography: the injection of radiopaque substance for early detection of myelocele has been abandoned; however, it is still useful for immediate detection of fetal death;
5. Intrauterine fetal transfusion; and
6. Second trimester abortion induced with the injection of hypertonic saline.

Currently there are several clinical applications of amniocentesis. This procedure may be performed anywhere from 14 weeks' gestation to beyond term depending on the diagnostic information required.

1. *Genetic Counseling.* Advanced maternal age has become the most common indication for amniocentesis due to the risk of chromosomal abnormality found to be 1–2% at 35–38 years of age, 2% at 39–40 years, and 10% at 45 years of age.[2] The second most common indication is a previous child with Down's Syndrome. Amniotic fluid analysis is one of the best indices of fetal status. The chief source of information is cast off fetal cells which can be cultured in 3–4 weeks for chromosome studies or biochemical analysis. As a result of karyotyping, all presently recognized chromosomal anomalies can be identified in utero.[3] More than 60 inborn errors of metabolism, which generally result in severe physical and mental retardation, can be detected antenatally through biochemical studies of enzymes of such cultured fetal cells. Determination of fetal sex can provide some guidance relative to the risk factor in sex-linked hereditary diseases since only males are afflicted with such disorders. Open neural tube defects such as encephalocele, anencephaly, and spina bifida can be detected by an appreciable increase in alpha-1-fetoprotein (AFP) in the amniotic fluid. Normally alpha-1-fetoprotein is high at 15 weeks' gestation, 18.5 μg per ml, decreasing markedly during the second and third trimesters to 0.26 μg per ml at term. There is a 5% recurrence rate of open neural tube defects.[4] It should be noted that determination of AFP is associated with a diagnostic accuracy rate of 90% in mothers at high risk.

2. *Isoimmunization.* The quantity of bilirubin found in the amniotic fluid is used to determine the severity of hemolytic anemia in the fetus. Amniocentesis is indicated when maternal isoimmune titers are above 1:8 to 1:16. The initial analysis is usually performed at 24–25 weeks' gestation because intrauterine transfusion is impractical before this time.[5]

3. *Assessment of Fetal Maturity.* The use of amniocentesis late in pregnancy for the purpose of estimating fetal maturity has enabled the physician to determine when to terminate a pregnancy in the presence of such maternal conditions as diabetes, toxemia, uncertain due date, Rh incompatibility, and postdatism. Four parameters are commonly used to determine gestational age:

   a. Cytology: Nile blue sulfate causes fetal fat cells found in amniotic fluid to turn orange. If 10–20% of the cells found in the sample are orange-stained, the fetus is usually 35–36 weeks' gestation and 2500 gm in weight.[6]
   b. Creatinine: The amount of creatinine increases with age after 32 weeks' gestation. A level over 1.7 mg/100 ml indicates gestational age to be 35 weeks or more.
   c. Bilirubin: Bilirubin disappears from the amniotic fluid of normal infants by 38 weeks' gestation. Therefore absence of bilirubin is supportive evidence of a mature fetus.
   d. Phospholipids: Fetal lung maturity is determined by an increased production of surfactant. Since respiratory distress syndrome (RDS) is the most common cause of death in the premature neonates, this test of pulmonary maturity is of critical importance. The main components of surfactant are the phospholipids, lecithin and sphingomyelin. The absolute concentration of surfactant is variable, but the ratio of lecithin to sphingomyelin (L/S ratio) is proportional to the ability of the lungs to expand normally and to resist atelectasis on expiration. An L/S ratio of 2:1 indicates pulmonary maturity. The relatively simple and inexpensive Shake or Foam Test introduced in 1971 is another way to measure the presence of surfactant. Exact amounts of amniotic fluid, 95% ethyl alcohol, and isotonic saline are shaken for 15 seconds. A foamy layer which persists after 10 minutes at the top of the test tube indicates an L/S ratio of 2 or greater.[5,7] An advantage of the Shake Test is that the results are immediately available. However, the accuracy rate is not very high.

COMPLICATIONS

Amniocentesis causes both maternal and fetal risks. The incidence of combined maternal and fetal complications is reported at 1% or less, indicating the rarity of occurrence. Fetal risks occur more often than maternal risks. Current research reports that amniocentesis should be considered a highly accurate (99.4%) and safe procedure.[3] Possible maternal risks include the following:
1. Amniotic fluid embolism,
2. Hemorrhage secondary to perforation of uterine or other abdominal vessels,
3. Infection,
4. Induced labor,
5. Abruptio placentae,
6. Puncture of the intestine or bladder, and
7. Rh isoimmunization.

Possible fetal risks include the following:
1. Fetal death,
2. Amnionitis,
3. Injuries directly induced by the needle,
4. Leakage of amniotic fluid,
5. Bleeding, and
6. Abortion or premature delivery.

It must be emphasized to the

client that complications are rare and if they do occur they tend to be relatively mild. The high level of safety now evident with this procedure may be due to the degree of skill exhibited by the practitioner, maintenance of asepsis, and placental localization prior to amniocentesis.

PROCEDURE
Nursing Objectives
1. To insure client understanding of the purpose and procedure of amniocentesis.
2. To provide the necessary equipment for the procedure.
3. To assist the physician with the procedure.
4. To monitor the client carefully after the procedure.
5. To insure obtaining an uncontaminated specimen of amniotic fluid.

Client Education
It is the responsibility of the attending physician to discreetly review with the expectant couple the risk of the disorder under investigation, the nature of the information to be obtained, and the risks of the procedure, including possible pitfalls such as failure to obtain amniotic fluid, the possibility of erroneous diagnosis, and the 5–10% incidence of culture failure, perhaps necessitating repeating the procedure. When amniocentesis is performed for the purpose of genetic counseling, it is usually recommended that the physicians discuss pregnancy termination in the event an affected fetus should be found. It should be pointed out that studies indicate the most predominant outcome of genetic tests done on amniotic fluid was a prediction of normality.

A key therapeutic nursing intervention is to keep the client informed throughout the procedure. By reducing client anxiety, physical discomfort and stress perception are minimized. The chief complaint of discomfort during the procedure is due to the local infiltration. Some clients describe a sensation of pressure deep in the pelvis. Clients may fear injury to the fetus from the needle puncture or loss of amniotic fluid. The nurse should emphasize the rarity of such an occurrence. Reassurance can be provided by explaining that the fetus floats freely and usually moves away if the needle should come close. Explain that amniotic fluid is constantly being manufactured and the removal of small amounts will not harm the baby. Occasionally a client will complain of lower abdominal cramping for a few hours after the procedure. This has not been proven to have an adverse effect on the pregnancy. The nurse should inform the client that any vaginal spotting or leakage of amniotic fluid that occurs at home should be reported to her physician. Generally no difficulties are incurred as a result of the procedure; consequently the client may resume normal activities without any restrictions.

Facilities
Virtually all amniocenteses are carried out on an outpatient basis unless the client lives a long distance away or unless any complication arises, either during or directly after amniocentesis. This procedure is often done in the ultrasonography room after placental localization, but has been successfully completed in various other places, such as the delivery room or recovery room areas of the obstetric department or in the doctor's office. Most important is that the procedure should be carried out under full antiseptic conditions in order to avoid the complication of amnionitis.

EQUIPMENT NEEDED FOR AMNIOCENTESIS[10]

The following equipment should be ready for use during an amniocentesis:

1. Amniocentesis tray containing the following items:
   a. 1 scrub gown for physician,
   b. 1 pair sponge-holding forceps,
   c. Several gauze sponges (4 inches by 4 inches),
   d. 1 cup for skin antiseptic,
   e. 4 sterile towels,
   f. 1 #20 or #21 gauge 4-inch spinal needle with stylus,
   g. 1 glass 20 ml syringe (plastic disposable syringes have been reported to cause chromosomal aberrations *in vitro*).
2. Added to tray after opening:
   a. 1 pair surgeon's gloves,
   b. 1 #22 or #25 gauge needle (for local anesthesia),
   c. 1 10 ml disposable syringe (large enough to hold enough local anesthesia for a second or third infiltration should the first amniocentesis attempt fail).
3. To hand to physician:
   a. Skin antiseptic (Betadine° solution),
   b. Local anesthetic (Xylocaine† 1% plain),
   c. 3 sterile capped glass specimen tubes labeled with patient's name, doctor, and "amniotic fluid," (Light-excluding containers are often used if bilirubin is to be measured).
4. Miscellaneous extras:
   a. Fetal monitor to apply after procedure,
   b. Flashlight to use during procedure,
   c. Razor for shaving abdomen if necessary,
   d. Aluminum foil to wrap specimen in for transport to laboratory,
   e. Bandaid to cover insertion area,
   f. pHisoHex° and sterile warm water to cleanse area after procedure,
   g. Caps and masks for attendants during procedure.

PROCEDURAL STEPS

Placental Localization

Amniocentesis preceded by placental localization carries a significantly reduced morbidity rate due to avoidance of the placental site. Ultrasonography to localize the placenta and confirm fetal age is often standard practice prior to genetic amniocentesis and has been shown to reduce the incidence of bloody taps, thereby increasing safety.

Explanation

A certain amount of anxiety is caused by contemplating amniocentesis; therefore the procedure should be explained to the patient in some detail.[5]

Surgical Permit

Amniocentesis is usually considered a surgical procedure and requires that an operation permit be signed before the procedure is carried out.

Bladder

The patient should be instructed to void prior to amniocentesis if the procedure is carried out past the 20th

---

°Povidone-iodine, Purdue-Frederick Co., Norwalk, Connecticut.

†Lidocaine, Astra Pharmaceutical Products, Inc., Worcester, Massachusetts.

° Sudsing antibacterial skin cleanser, Winthrop Laboratories, New York, New York.

week of gestation. (Prior to 20 weeks, a full bladder will hold the uterus steady and out of the pelvis).

Premedication

No premedication is used if local infiltration at the site of insertion is to be used. If not, a sedative may be ordered.

Maternal Blood Pressure

If the procedure is being carried out on an out-patient basis, it is wise to record the maternal blood pressure to have this information available should any complications arise during the procedure such as supine hypotensive syndrome.

Detecting Fetomaternal Hemorrhage

In checking for fetomaternal hemorrhage, the physician will often order a specimen of maternal blood taken before amniocentesis to compare with a specimen taken after the procedure, since fetal cells do occur in varying amounts in maternal blood[1] during pregnancy.

Fetal Heart Rate

Fetal heart rate is checked before and after amniocentesis to insure that the fetus is viable before the amniocentesis is carried out and that no fetal distress has been caused by the procedure.

Positioning

The patient should be made as comfortable as possible on a firm surface. She should be given one pillow so that she is not tempted to sit up to see the procedure, thereby tightening her abdominal muscles.

Abdominal Preparation

The lower abdomen is then bared and shaved if necessary. If placental localization has been done previously, the nurse should have the results available at this time.

Gowning

In order to avoid the hazards of infection or chromosomal aberration due to contamination, the procedure should be carried out under full antiseptic conditions. Currently there is disagreement concerning the usage of gowns and masks for physician and attendant.

Equipment

The amniocentesis tray is opened and the necessary items added. (For contents of tray, see section "Equipment Needed for Amniocentesis.")

Site Selection

Using the results of the placental localization, the physician selects the site for insertion. The patient is asked to place her hands behind her head in order to avoid using them and thus contaminating the area. Betadine solution is poured into the cup and the physician preps the abdomen using the sponges and sponge-holding forceps. He then drapes the area with the four sterile towels.

Local Anesthesia

The Xylocaine is opened and held for the physician while he obtains the necessary amount for skin infiltration using the 10 ml syringe and the small gauge needle.

Fluid Withdrawal

After local skin infiltration, the 20- or 21-gauge needle with stylus is inserted at the same point, the stylus withdrawn, the 20 ml glass syringe attached to the needle, and the specimen of amniotic fluid withdrawn and placed into the three sterile, labeled tubes which are handed to the physician at this time.

Light Protection

If fluid is being obtained for bilirubin determination, the actual withdrawal is often done under indirect lighting from a flashlight only. The specimen tubes are then immediately wrapped in aluminum foil to eliminate any excess light which could cause inaccurate bilirubin determination.

Termination

The physician then quickly withdraws the needle, and the Betadine solution is cleansed from the abdomen with pHisohex and sterile warm water, dried with a sterile gauze square, and covered with a bandaid. (A skin burn may occur unless the Betadine is thoroughly washed off before covering with the bandaid).

Specimen

The properly labeled specimen is sent to the laboratory with the proper requisition form.

Fetal Monitor

At some institutions, the external fetal monitor is then applied to the patient for 30 minutes, and if no contractions are noted, the patient may be discharged.

Recording

The procedure is promptly recorded and pertinent charges made.

ACKNOWLEDGMENTS

The authors wish to thank David Chow, MD, Section Head of Obstetrics at St. Joseph Hospital Medical Center, Bloomington, Illinois, for his assistance in the preparation of this article.

References

1. Emery, A. E. H.: *Antenatal Diagnosis of Genetic Disease*. Baltimore, The Williams and Wilkins Company, 1973, pp 12, 15, 16
2. Bond E.: "Genetic Counseling Protocol." 1976
3. The NICHD National Registry for Amniocentesis Study Group: "Midtrimester Amniocentesis for Prenatal Diagnosis." *JAMA* 236 (13): 1471, 1475, 1976
4. Pritchard, A. and P. C. MacDonald: *Williams Obstetrics*. New York, Appleton-Century-Crofts, 1976, p 273
5. Reeder S. R., et al.: *Maternity Nursing*. Philadelphia, J. B. Lippincott, 1976, pp 538, 546, 558
6. Dickason, E. J. and M. O. Schult: *Maternal and Infant Care*. St. Louis, McGraw-Hill Book Company, 1975, p 494
7. Werch, A., et al.: "The Role of Amniotic Fluid Analysis." *JOGN* 3 (3):43–46, 1974

Kathleen Hogan has a BSN from St. John College at Cleveland, Ohio, and her MS is from Illinois State University, Normal, Illinois. She is course chairperson of maternal–child nursing at Mennonite Hospital School of Nursing, Bloomington, Illinois. She is a member of INA.

Donna Tcheng is a graduate of the University of Iowa School of Nursing at Iowa City. She is an instructor of maternal–child nursing at Mennonite Hospital School of Nursing and a member of Sigma Theta Tau.

Reprinted by permission of J.B. Lippincott/Harper from *JOGN Nursing*, Sept./Oct., 1978, © 1978, Harper and Row Publishers.

FACTORS IMPLICATED IN THE ETIOLOGY OF INTRAUTERINE FETAL GROWTH RETARDATION

Fetal Factors
    Chromosomal disorders (e.g., autosomal trisomies)
    Chronic fetal infections (e.g., cytomegalic inclusion disease, congenital rubella, syphilis)
    Radiation injury
    Multiple gestation
    Pituitary failure (?)
Placental Factors
    Decreased placental weight or cellularity or both
    Decrease in surface area
    Villous placentitis (bacterial, viral, parasitic)
    Infarction
    Tumor (chorioangioma, hydatidiform mole)
    Placental separation
    Twin transfusion syndrome (parabiotic syndrome)
    Localized transfer lesions (?)
Maternal Factors
    Toxemia
    Hypertensive or renal disease or both
    Hypoxemia (high altitude, cyanotic, cardiac, or pulmonary disease)
    Malnutrition or chronic illness
    Sickle cell anemia
Experimental Factors
    Maternal uterine ischemia — rat
    Fetal placental ischemia — sheep and monkey
    Maternal protein deprivation — rat, guinea pig, and pig

Reprinted by permission of W.B. Saunders from *Nelson Textbook of Pediatrics*, 10th edition, Vaughan and McKay, Copyright 1975, W.B. Saunders Co.

Signs and Symptoms of Preeclampsia-Eclampsia

mild	moderate	severe preeclampsia-eclampsia
Weight gain—edema More than 1–2 lb/wk No visible edema	More than 1–2 lb/wk Some edema above waist in abdomen, fingers, face, and extremities	Excessive weight gain; usually face puffy, rings hard to get off, etc.
Hypertension 30/15 rise over baseline reading	Diastolic, 90 or above; 140/90 or above	Systolic, 160 or above; diastolic, 110 or above; with preexisting hypertension—may be very high
Feels some lethargy, fatigue	Complains of headaches, lethargy, fatigue	Complains of frontal headache, lasting, unrelieved by analgesics. Cerebral and visual disturbances, ringing in ears, fainting episodes Grand mal convulsion may occur in sleep
Check status by roll-over test		May experience amnesia up to 48 h before convulsion. Patient appears alert and functions normally unless heavily sedated Epigastric girding pain, result of edema/hemorrhage in liver capsule
Urine—quality/quantity No proteinuria or just a trace	+1, +2 proteinuria	Proteinuria +3, +4, 5 g or more in 24-h specimen
Not much change	Scanty concentrated urine, DHEA-S reduced clearance	Oliguria—1000 mL or less in 24 h, progressing to severe oliguria; sometimes anuria—400 mL or less in 24 h
Blood changes Some increase in plasma volume	Blood estriols may be reduced, reflecting impaired placental-fetal function	Hematocrit elevated because of hemoconcentration; plasma volume lowered; platelets lowered Uric acid above 5 mg/100 mL
Fundal changes Some retinal arteriolar spasm	More extensive spasm can be seen	Edema—papilledema, ischemia of retina
Infant If delivered at this time, usually no problem	Usually no major problems if delivered at this phase	Infants may be malnourished or "small-for-dates" babies because of placental changes Precipitate delivery may occur; infant anoxic, stillborn. Premature separation may occur

Reprinted by permission of McGraw-Hill from *Maternal and Infant Care*, Elizabeth Dickason and Martha Schult, Copyright © 1975, McGraw-Hill.

Treatment for Preeclampsia-Eclampsia

mild	moderate	severe preeclampsia-eclampsia
Home care Rest in bed as much as possible. Stay home—no shopping, tiring activities, etc.	*Hospitalize* Bed rest in side-lying position, with bathroom privileges	*Hospitalize* Strict bed rest, padded side rails, tongue blade at bedside, close observation. Check levels of consciousness
Diet Moderate salt intake; high protein; limit carbohydrates if overweight; fluids	Fluids, high protein, moderate salt intake	Clear fluids or IV fluids only
Intake and output Record not necessary	Careful output record	Measured intake and output; balance intake against output q4h. Hourly output from Foley catheter
Vital signs Roll-over test	q4h while awake; FHT bid	May be more often than q4h, depending on medication and condition Oxygen by mask prn, tracheostomy set at bedside. Suction at bedside
Medical supervision See doctor 1–2 times a week	Daily Ophthalmoscope exam	Prn Ophthalmoscope exam
Tests Urine for protein DHEA-S clearance Estriols	Urine for protein (24 h)/estriols Blood uric acid Vanillylmandelic acid (VMA) Serum electrolytes Creatinine Blood uric acid	Same as for moderate preeclampsia Hematocrit, platelets
Medication None, or low dose phenobarbital, 30 mg, tid	Phenobarbital, 30–60 mg, q6h Diuretic: short trial to see effect(?)	Phenobarbital, 30–60 mg, q6h Depending on condition: Magnesium sulfate IV, IM, Diazepam IV

Reprinted by permission of McGraw-Hill from *Maternal and Infant Care*, Elizabeth Dickason and Martha Schult, Copyright © 1975, McGraw-Hill.

Interaction of Diabetes and Pregnancy

diabetes changes pregnancy	pregnancy changes diabetes
Oversized babies (metabolic acceleration: true skeletal growth, fat, water retention)	Subclinical (latent) diabetes may become clinical (overt, gestational) diabetes
Fetal death after 36 weeks likely (because of acidosis or placental dysfunction)	Renal glucose threshold is increased: a. Glucose tolerance test is changed b. 2-h postprandial level is elevated
Fetal anomalies more common (3% are lethal)	
Infertility and spontaneous abortion rate higher	Glucose tolerance is changed: a. Elevated needs for insulin, but sometimes b. Lowered needs for insulin if fetal pancreas functions to provide mother's need
Higher incidence of hypertension	
Higher incidence of preeclampsia (one-third to one-half of patients are affected)	Status of diabetes changes because of differing metabolic needs throughout pregnancy
Placenta ages more rapidly	Metabolic complications (hyperemesis, nausea) difficult to treat
Abruptio placentae more common; hemorrhage more common	Work of labor depletes glycogen stores; ketosis may result
Premature labor more common	
Hydramnios 10 times more common in the diabetic	Anabolic activity changes to catabolic activity after delivery, upsetting diet and insulin needs
Higher incidence of infection	High estrogen levels may affect glucose tolerance of liver

Reprinted by permission of McGraw-Hill from *Maternal and Infant Care*, Elizabeth Dickason and Martha Schult, Copyright © 1975, McGraw-Hill.

Cervical Dilatation

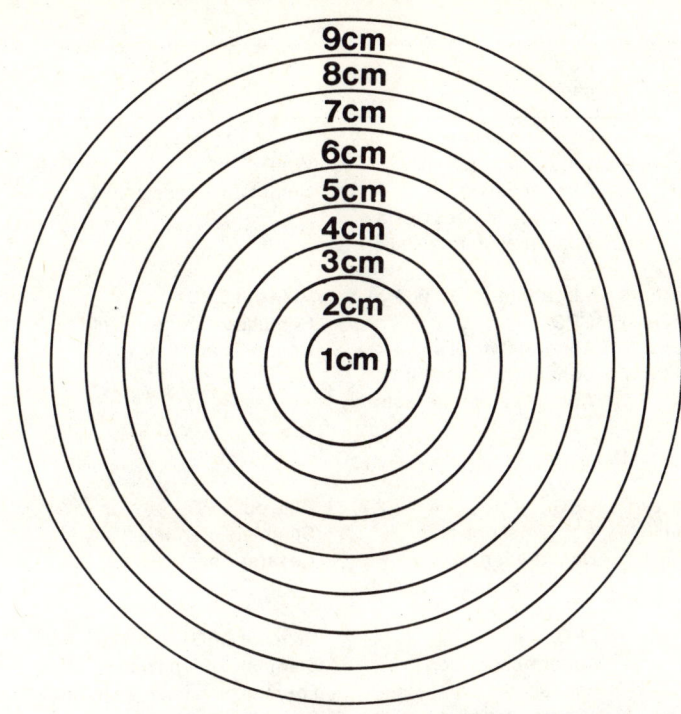

Diagrammatic representation of dilatation of the cervix in centimeters to scale.

Normal Labor Graph

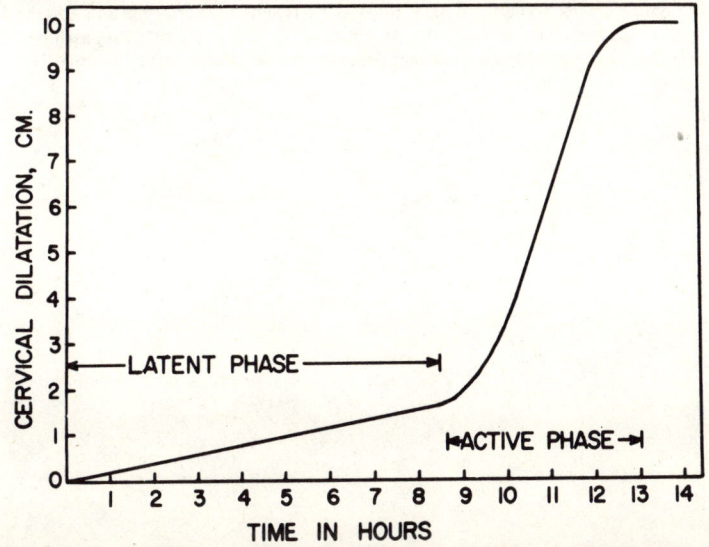

Reprinted from "Patterns of Uterine Activity and Cervical Dilatation in Normal and Abnormal Labor," by R. Laros and M. Margules, in JOGN, Vol. 5, No. 5, Sept./Oct., 1976 (Supplement), pp. 61s and 62s, Copyright 1976, Harper and Row Publishers. Reprinted by permission.

Labor Abnormalities

Abnormality	Definition	Possible causes	Possible treatments
Prolonged latent phase	17 hr (primipara) 11.5 hr (multipara)	Question of onset Unfavorable cervix Over-sedation Conduction anesthesia Abnormal uterine activity	Recognize false labor Wait Stimulate uterine activity
Slow slope active phase	0.7 cm/hr (primipara) 1.1 cm/hr (multipara)	Large infant (≥4,000 g) CPD Abnormal position Conduction anesthesia Abnormal uterine activity	Rule out CPD Stimulate uterine activity Cesarean section
Active phase arrest	No change in dilatation for 2 hr	CPD Abnormal position Dehydration Abnormal uterine activity	Rule out CPD Stimulate uterine activity Cesarean section
Prolonged second stage	>2 hr	CPD Abnormal position Poor secondary forces Abnormal uterine activity	Rule out CPD Stimulate uterine activity Forceps or vacuum extraction Cesarean section

CPD = cephalopelvic disproportion

Reprinted from "Patterns of Uterine Activity and Cervical Dilatation in Normal and Abnormal Labor," by R. Laros and M. Margules, in JOGN, Vol. 5, No. 5, Sept./Oct., 1976 (Supplement), pp. 61s and 62s, Copyright 1976, Harper and Row Publishers. Reprinted by permission.

Mechanism of Labor-LOA

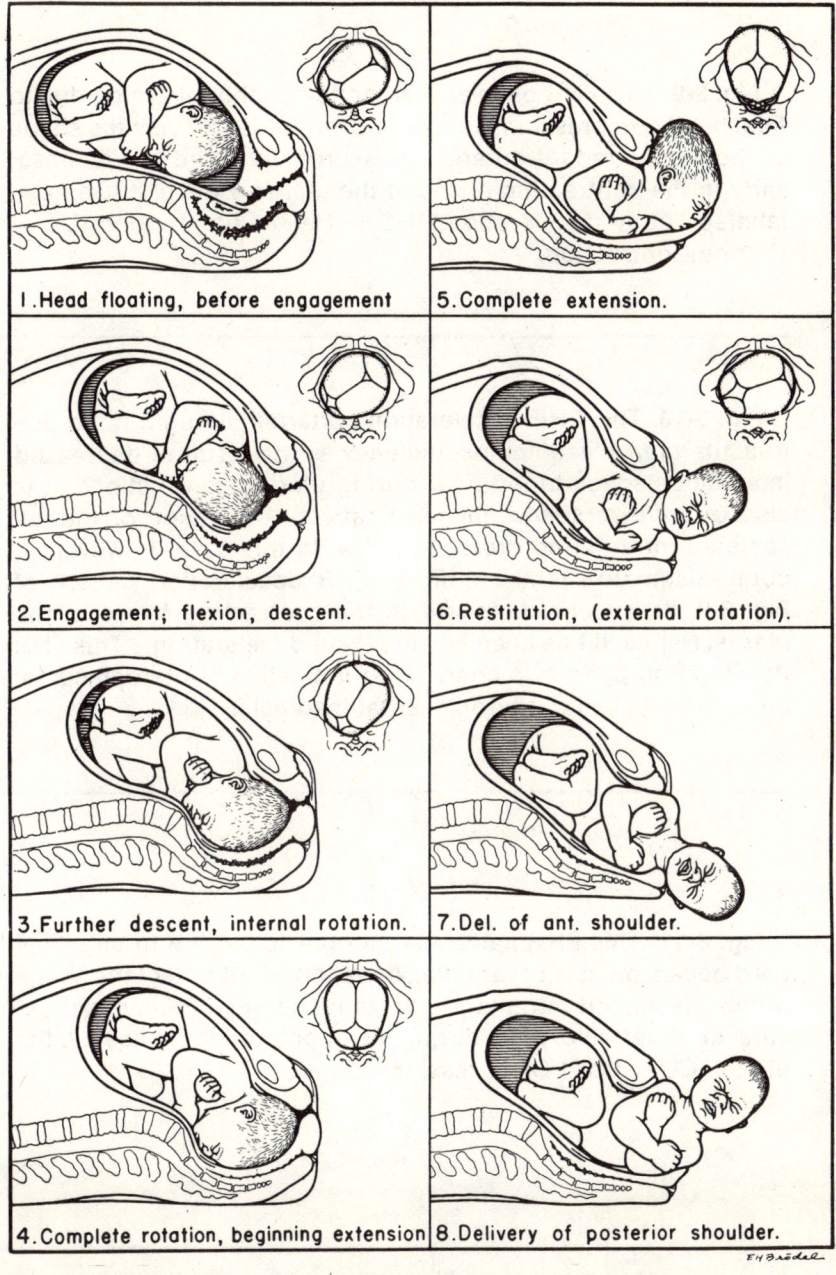

1. Head floating, before engagement
2. Engagement; flexion, descent.
3. Further descent, internal rotation.
4. Complete rotation, beginning extension
5. Complete extension.
6. Restitution, (external rotation).
7. Del. of ant. shoulder.
8. Delivery of posterior shoulder.

Principal movements in the mechanism of labor and delivery; LOA position.

Reprinted by permission of Appleton-Century-Crofts from *William's Obstetrics*, 14th edition, by Louis Hellman and Jack Pritchard, Copyright 1971, Appleton-Century-Crofts.

Fetal Monitoring

THE MECHANISMS OF FHR DECELERATION PATTERNS

Fig. 3-9. This FHR deceleration pattern is thought to be due to fetal head compression. It is of *uniform shape,* reflects the shape of the associated intrauterine pressure curve, and has its onset *early* in the contracting phase of the uterus. Hence, it has been labeled "early deceleration." HC = Head Compression, UC = Uterine Contraction.

Fig. 3-10. This FHR deceleration pattern is thought to be due to acute uteroplacental insufficiency as the result of decreased intervillous space blood flow during uterine contractions. It is also of *uniform shape* and also reflects the shape of the associated intrauterine pressure curve. In this case, however, in contradistinction to the uniform FHR deceleration pattern of Fig. 3-9, its onset occurs *late* in the contracting phase of the uterus. Hence, it has been labeled "late deceleration." This FHR deceleration pattern is considered indicative of uteroplacental insufficiency. UPI = Uteroplacental Insufficiency.

Fig. 3-11. This FHR pattern is thought to be due to umbilical cord occlusion. It is of *variable shape,* does not reflect the shape of the associated intrauterine pressure curve, and its onset occurs at a variable time during the contracting phase of the uterus. CC = Cord Compression.

HEAD COMPRESSION

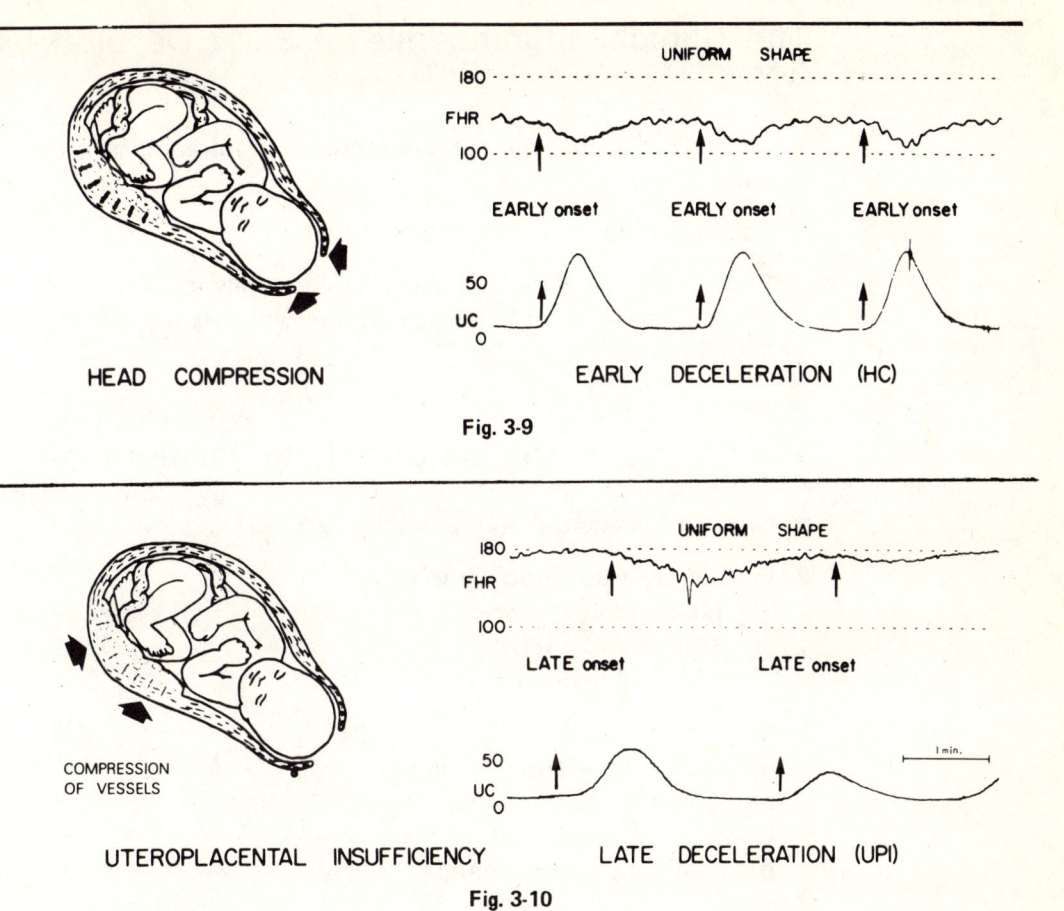

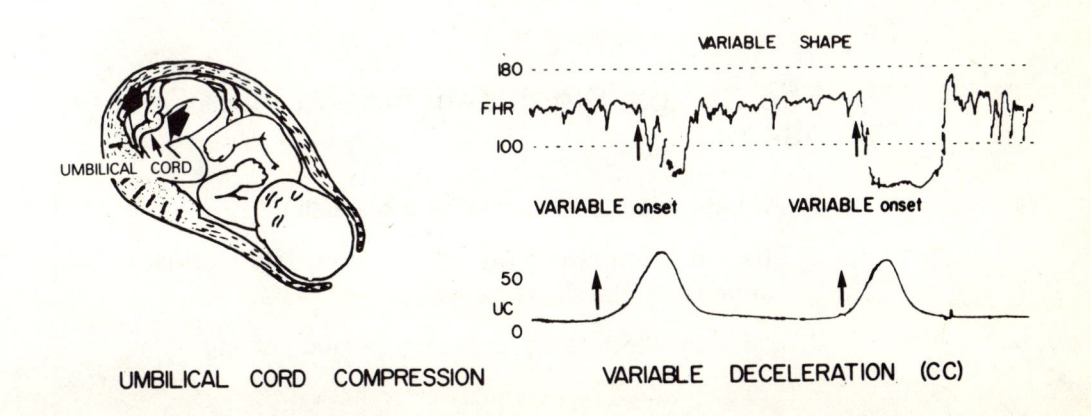

EARLY DECELERATION (HC)

Fig. 3-9

COMPRESSION OF VESSELS

UTEROPLACENTAL INSUFFICIENCY

LATE DECELERATION (UPI)

Fig. 3-10

UMBILICAL CORD COMPRESSION

VARIABLE DECELERATION (CC)

From Hon, Edward H.: *An Introduction to Fetal Heart Rate Monitoring*, 2nd edition, Copyright 1975 by Edward H. Hon.

The Clinical Significance of Early Deceleration

1. Probably due to a momentary increase in intracranial pressure.

2. Appears to be an innocuous FHR pattern.

3. Present clinical significance is related largely to the need to differentiate it from late deceleration which is an ominous FHR pattern.

The Clinical Significance of Late Deceleration

1. Due to decreased maternal-fetal exchange.

2. Frequently associated with:
    a) high-risk pregnancies
    b) uterine hyperactivity
    c) maternal hypotension.

3. May be alleviated by:
    a) decreasing uterine activity
    b) correcting maternal hypotension
    c) maternal hyperoxia
    d) maternal position change.

4. *This ominous FHR pattern is usually found in the normal FHR range.*

The Clinical Significance of Variable Deceleration

1. Probably due to umbilical cord occlusion.

2. The most common FHR pattern associated with clinically diagnosed fetal distress.

3. Markedly alleviated by maternal position change.

From Hon, Edward H.: *An Introduction to Fetal Heart Rate Monitoring*, 2nd edition, Copyright 1975 by Edward H. Hon.

The Diagnosis of Acute Fetal Distress*

1. *Warning signals are:*
   a) mild variable deceleration
   b) progressive increase in baseline FHR level
   c) tachycardia of 160 beats per minute or greater
   d) progressive decrease in baseline FHR variability *

2. *Ominous signs are:*
   a) variable deceleration which lasts more than one minute and falls to less than 60 beats per minute or less and getting progressively worse.
   b) late deceleration of *any* magnitude, with or without tachycardia. If it is associated with a very smooth baseline FHR, the situation is more serious.
   c) smooth baseline FHR.

3. Intermittent auscultation of the FHR between contractions is of little value for the early detection of fetal distress.

4. *An FHR which is clinically considered normal, i.e., one which is within the range of 120–160 beats per minute is not necessarily a normal FHR pattern, since late deceleration which is ominous is found frequently within these clinically normal limits. Additionally, average FHR variability must also be present for an FHR pattern to be considered normal.*

* Whenever there is a decrease in FHR variability, the most important clinical factors to be considered are the effects of:
   a) Drug administration, e.g., narcotics, hypnotics, tranquilizers.
   b) Fetal sleep usually lasts 20–30 minutes and alternates with periods of average or moderate variability.
   c) Acidosis or asphyxia which are associated with ominous FHR patterns.

From Hon, Edward H.: *An Introduction to Fetal Heart Rate Monitoring*, 2nd edition, Copyright 1975 by Edward H. Hon.

The Treatment of Fetal Distress

1. Change the position of the patient.
2. Correct maternal hypotension.
3. Decrease uterine activity.
4. Administer oxygen at the rate of 6–7 liters per minute with a tight face mask.
5. Prepare for operative delivery.

6. If ominous FHR patterns persist for thirty minutes after the institution of the above measures, labor should be terminated operatively.

From Hon, Edward H.: *An Introduction to Fetal Heart Rate Monitoring,* 2nd edition, Copyright 1975, Edward H. Hon.

A "Fetal File" for storing fetal monitor records is available from Ludlow Recording Products, Ludlow Corporation, P.O. Box 300, Ware, MA 01082. It is a handy and convenient file system. Write for further information.

Shock Hazards from Monitoring Equipment

The following list is presented to provide a quick source of reference as to what symptoms may be indicative of shock hazards and what practices should be avoided:

A. Suspect shock hazards if:
 1. A staff member or patient complains of receiving an electrical shock.
 2. Two-wire cords or plugs are used on equipment.
 3. Three-wire adapters are used.
 4. Power cords are frayed or plugs are broken.
 5. Noise on an EKG wave form cannot be eliminated by changing the electrodes.
 6. The equipment malfunctions or blows a fuse.
 7. An unconscious patient jumps or twitches when monitoring equipment is attached.

B. Precautions to guard against shock hazards:
 1. Never use three-wire adapters.
 2. Never use equipment unless it is equipped with a three-wire plug and cord. (The hospital maintenance service can install the proper cords.)
 3. Before an electrical device is plugged in, inspect the plug for broken pins or shell, power cord for fraying or cuts, and the receptacles for breaks or cracks.
 4. Never remove a plug from a receptacle by pulling on the power cord. Always grip the plug shell to remove the plug.
 5. If an electrical device is dropped, have it checked before placing it in operation.
 6. If multiple monitoring devices are to be connected to a patient, it is advisable to plug all equipment into the same group of wall outlets. If this is not

possible, use of a multiple outlet extension cord approved by local fire inspectors is recommended.

7. If any liquid is spilled on an electrical device, it should immediately be unplugged and checked for damage.

8. When in doubt about electrical safety, contact someone who can check the equipment and power wiring.

Reprinted from "Are Babies Dying of Electrocution?" by Neil Edwards and Doris Edwards in *Nursing Clinics of North America*, March, 1971, pg. 91, © 1971, W. B. Saunders Co.

Apgar Scoring

This is a means of standardizing the method of evaluating and recording the condition of newborns in numerical terms at one minute and five minutes after birth, based on the work of Dr. Virginia Apgar.

Signs	Score		
	0	1	2
Color	Blue-pale	Body pink, limbs blue	completely pink
Respiratory effort	absent	slow, irregular, weak cry	strong cry
Heart rate	absent	slow, less than 100	over 100
Muscle tone	limp	some flexion of limbs	active movement
Response to stimuli	absent	facial grimace	crying

The five signs are each given a score of 0, 1 or 2 points, the total of the five is the apgar score.

One Minute Score

Severe 0–2   Moderate 3–4   Mild 5–7   No asphyxia 8–10

Five Minute Score

The score at five minutes gives a more accurate prediction regarding survival: a low score at five minutes being more serious than a low score at one minute.

EMERGENCY CHILDBIRTH

Signs and symptoms of impending childbirth
1. Nausea and vomiting
2. Mother displays intense anxiety
3. Heavy show of blood
4. Intense desire by mother to defecate
5. Rapidly occurring contractions with increasing intensity and desire to bear down by mother
6. Bulging of membranes from vulva and/or spontaneous rupture
7. Dilatation of anus with expulsion of feces
8. Crowning of the fetal head (figure 1)

Necessary equipment
1 large basin (for placenta)
1 pair of scissors
2 medium Kelly clamps
1 bulb syringe
1 double grip cord clamp
3 small sterile towels
1 pack 4x4's
1 baby blanket

All of the above instruments and equipment should be placed in the basin, double wrapped and sterilized. One or two pairs of prepackaged sterile gloves should be taped to the top of the sterile set.

The following should also be available:
Infant resuscitation equipment (Ambu-bag, airway, suction, O_2, infant intubation tray)
Heated Isolette, if possible
Warm blankets
Name bands for both mother and infant.

Delivery of infant
Maintain sterile technique whenever possible, but do not endanger mother or infant with undue delay.

1. Place mother in dorsal position, with legs bent and hands grasping knees. Assign assistant to stand at head of bed to monitor vital signs and offer verbal support and encouragement to the mother.
2. Remain calm. Attempt to gain mother's confidence and cooperation by explaining what you are doing and what you expect of her.
3. If time permits, apply sterile gloves and drape perineal area with sterile towels from delivery pack.
4. Apply gentle pressure with palm of hand to crowning head and perineal area to prevent rapid expulsion of the head. **Never try to stop delivery by pushing forcefully against the head.**
5. Encourage mother to pant during contractions to allow for slow, gentle delivery.
6. As head is delivered, provide support with both hands and allow the head to rotate naturally to the side.
7. Immediately slip finger around infant's neck and feel for cord that may be wrapped around the neck and choking the infant. If present, attempt to gently slip it off over the head. If it is not possible to remove cord, clamp and cut cord at once (see step 13).

(Figure 1) Crowning

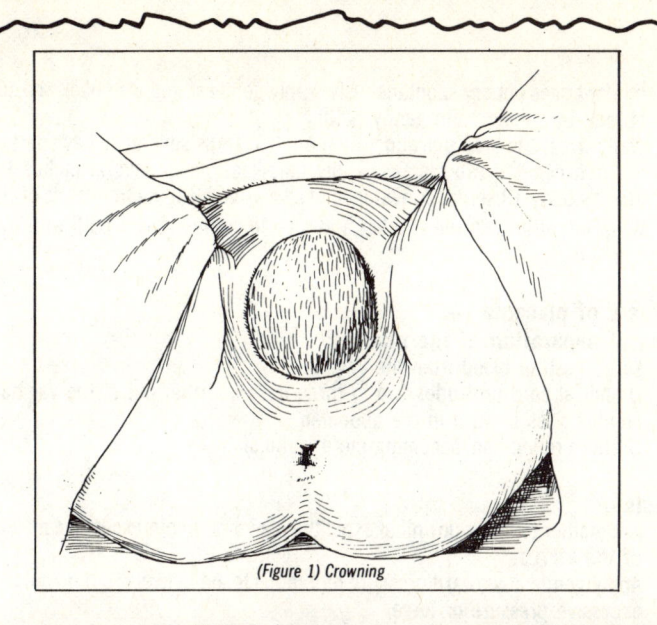

8. If membranes are still intact over infant's face, remove by snipping them at the nape of the neck and pulling away from face and airway at once.
9. Suction nose then mouth gently with bulb syringe to insure adequate airway. (Newborns are obligate nose breathers).
10. After insuring patent airway, proceed to deliver the shoulders. Place hands on either side of head and exert gentle downward pressure (toward the floor) to deliver the anterior shoulder. Then pull upward to permit delivery of the posterior shoulder. Support the rest of the body as it is born.
11. With firm grip on body, hold infant along length of arm, (figure 2) with head lower then feet and again suction the nose and mouth. Keep the infant below or equal to the level of the mother until the cord stops pulsating. **Do not hang infant by feet.**

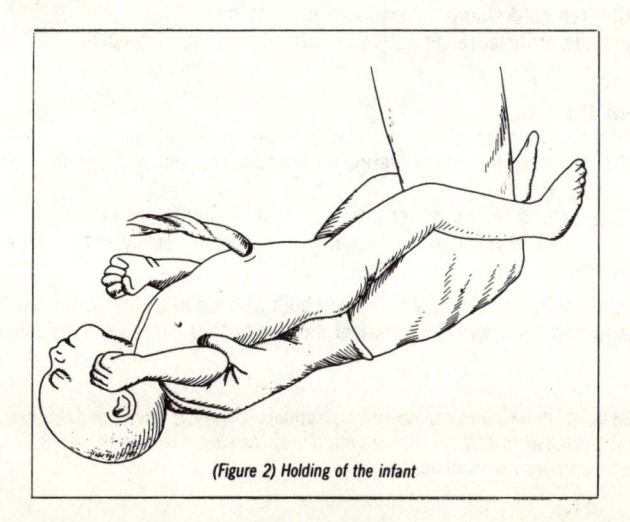

(Figure 2) Holding of the infant

Continued on next page

12. If infant does not cry spontaneously, apply gentle stimulus to back and soles of feet, by rubbing and gently patting.
13. Wait for cord to stop pulsating, then apply clamps several inches apart and cut *between* the two clamps. Apply umbilical clamp several inches from infant's body. Observe for evidence of excessive bleeding from ends of cord.
14. Wrap infant in a sterile blanket and give to mother. Cover both with warm blankets.

Delivery of placenta —
signs of separation of the placenta
1. Large gush of blood from the vagina
2. Umbilical cord protrudes two to three inches farther out of the vagina
3. Fundus rises upward in the abdomen
4. Uterus firming and becoming more globular

Expulsion
1. Ask mother to "bear down" to expel the placenta. **Avoid excessive massage of the uterus.**
2. Apply gentle downward pressure on fundus to aid delivery, but do not apply excessive pressure or force.
3. Save the placenta for future inspection by physician. Observe for evidence of missing portions of the placenta.

Care of the newborn
1. Maintain patent airway. Place infant on side, either with mother or in Isolette, in plain view.
2. Administer eye care (silver nitrate or penicillin prophylaxis) according to hospital policy.
3. Administer hypoprothrombinemia prophylaxis—phytonadione (AquaMephyton)—according to hospital policy.
4. Assess Apgar score at one minute after birth and again at five minutes. (See any text on maternity nursing.)
5. Observe cord stump for evidence of bleeding.
6. Provide artificial respiratory and cardiac support as needed.

Care of the mother
1. Observe for signs of excessive vaginal bleeding and shock.
2. Prevent relaxation of the uterine muscles by frequent massage and close observation.
3. Be prepared to administer intravenous fluid therapy as indicated.
4. Administer oxytocic agents according to hospital policy and doctor's preference.

Keep both mother and child warm, band both with identification bands (apply two to infant) and transport to obstetrical unit for further care and observation.

Reprinted from "Emergency Childbirth" by Kathleen Schrader and Susan Budassi, artwork by Charles S. Wellek, in *JEN Journal of Emergency Nursing*, March/April, 1979, Vol. 5, No. 2. Reprinted with permission of *JEN*.

Postpartum

Hypovolemic Shock

physiologic changes	patient symptoms	interventions
cardiac/circulatory status *Deceased* venous pressure, cardiac output, pulse pressure, arterial pressure	Feels weak, dizzy; may feel rapid heartbeat	Record vital signs; if necessary, take apical pulse. Monitor CVP; if severe hypotension persists, line should be inserted by doctor. Support blood volume with plasma expanders, whole blood, Ringer's lactate.
Peripheral vasoconstriction To protect vital organs; adrenal medulla stimulated to produce catecholamines, adding to vasoconstriction	Feels cold, peripheral tissues are pale, nails blanch slowly; feels restless, anxious, fearful	Keep patient warm, check skin color, turgor, mucous membrane moisture, temperature. Reassure patient, stay with her. Record expressed statements, observations.
respiratory status Tachypnea Respiratory center stimulated by hypoxia	Complains of "air hunger," shortness of breath	Note rate, rhythm, depth of respirations. Administer oxygen by mask (do not use Trendelenburg position during pregnancy; instead, place patient in side-lying position).
gastrointestinal status Fluid shift from interstitial tissues and intestinal tract to vascular compartment (takes several hours to shift).	Sensation of thirst increases	Drop in hematocrit observed after shift. Draw blood for serial hemoglobin/hematocrit determinations. Keep NPO if returning to OR or delivery room for correction of bleeding.
Decreased parasympathetic activity + reduced GI motility, secretions	Nausea may occur	
renal status Conservation of fluids and salts stimulated by vasoconstriction of renal arterioles (needs 70 mmHg pressure to effectively filtrate blood)	May have no sensation of need to void	Observe closely for oliguria (lower limit of normal 30 mL/h). Record hourly output and specific gravity, from Foley catheter.

Reprinted by permission of McGraw-Hill from *Maternal and Infant Care*, Elizabeth Dickason, Martha Schult, Copyright © 1975, McGraw-Hill.

FIXED
1. Mothers care by her own mother
2. Endowment or genetics of mother
3. Practices of culture
4. Relations with family and husband
5. Experiences with previous pregnancies
6. Planning course and events during pregnancy

ALTERABLE
1. Behavior of doctors, nurses and hospital personnel
2. First days of life, separation of mother and infant
3. Practices of hospital

PARENT ↔ INFANT

EFFECTIVE CARETAKING AND ATTACHMENT

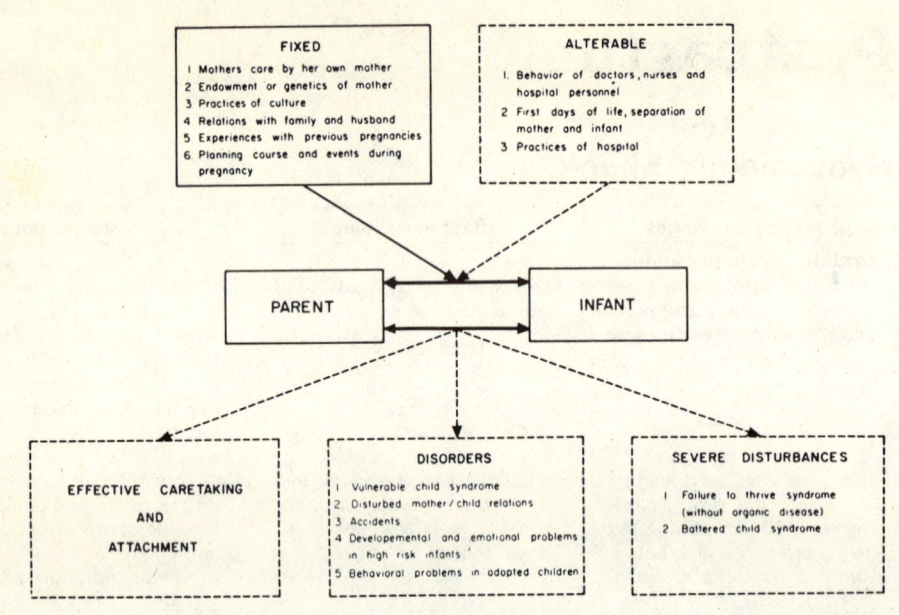

DISORDERS
1. Vulnerable child syndrome
2. Disturbed mother/child relations
3. Accidents
4. Developmental and emotional problems in high risk infants
5. Behavioral problems in adopted children

SEVERE DISTURBANCES
1. Failure to thrive syndrome (without organic disease)
2. Battered child syndrome

Disorders of mothering: a hypothesis of their aetiology. Solid lines indicate determinants that are ingrained; dashed lines indicate factors that may be altered or changed

Reprinted from Klaus, Marshall H., and Kennell, John H., "Parent-to-Infant Attachment" in *Recent Advances in Paediatrics,* Number 5, David Hull, editor, Copyright 1976, Churchill Livingstone. Reprinted with permission.

Estimation of Gestational Age

Clinical estimation of gestational age. An approximation based on published data.
Adapted from Lubchenco LO: P Clin North America 17:125, 1970.

Examination First Hours

PHYSICAL FINDINGS		20	21	22	23	24	25	26	27	28	29	30	31	32	33	34	35	36	37	38	39	40	41	42	43	44	45	46	47	48
Vernix		Appears				Covers body, thick layer														On back, scalp, in creases		Scant, in creases		No vernix						
Breast tissue and areola		Areola and nipple barely visible no palpable breast tissue															Areola raised			3–5 mm	5–6 mm	7–10 mm				?12 mm				
Ear	Form	Flat, shapeless														Beginning incurving superior		Incurving upper 2/3 pinnae		Well-defined incurving to lobe										
	Cartilage	Pinna soft, stays folded												Cartilage scant returns slowly from folding				Thin cartilage, springs back from folding				Pinna firm, remains erect from head								
Sole creases		Smooth soles without creases													1–2 anterior creases		2–3 anterior creases	Creases anterior 2/3 sole			Creases involving heel				Deeper creases over entire sole					
Skin	Thickness & appearance	Thin, translucent skin, plethoric, venules over abdomen, edema														Smooth, thicker, no edema			Pink			Some desquamation pale pink			Thick, pale, desquamation over entire body					
	Nail plates	Appear												Nails to finger tips												Nails extend well beyond finger tips					
Hair		Appears on head			Eye brows and lashes						Fine, woolly, bunches out from head							Silky, single strands, lays flat						?Receding hairline or loss of baby hair, short, fine underneath						
Lanugo		Appears	Covers entire body													Vanishes from face				Present on shoulders					No lanugo					
Genitalia	Testes													Testes palpable in inguinal canal						In upper scrotum			In lower scrotum							
	Scrotum													Few rugae				Rugae, anterior portion					Rugae cover	Pendulous						
	Labia & clitoris													Prominent clitoris, labia majora small, widely separated				Labia majora larger, nearly cover clitoris						Labia minora and clitoris covered						
Skull firmness		Bones are soft									Soft to 1" from anterior fontanelle						Spongy at edges of fontanelle, center firm			Bones hard, sutures easily displaced					Bones hard, cannot be displaced					
Posture	Resting	Hypotonic, lateral decubitus					Hypotonic				Beginning flexion, thigh			Stronger hip flexion			Frog-like					Hypertonic			Very hypertonic					

Continued on next page

334

Confirmatory Neurologic Examination To Be Done After 24 Hours

Weeks Gestation

		20	21	22	23	24	25	26	27	28	29	30	31	32	33	34	35	36	37	38	39	40	41	42	43	44	45	46	47	48
Recoil - leg		No recoil																	Partial recoil				Prompt recoil							
	Arm	No recoil														Begin flexion, no recoil			Prompt recoil, may be inhibited			Prompt recoil after 30" inhibition								
Tone																														
Physical Findings	Heel to ear							No resistance				Some resistance									Impossible									
	Scarf sign	No resistance											Elbow passes midline					Elbow at midline				Elbow does not reach midline							
	Neck flexors (head lag)	Absent																			Head in plane of body		Holds head							
	Neck extensors														Head begins to right itself from flexed position				Good righting cannot hold it		Holds head few seconds		Keeps head in line with trunk > 40"		Turns head from side to side					
	Body extensors															Straightening of legs			Straightening of trunk			Straightening of head and trunk together								
	Vertical positions									When held under arms, body slips through hands					Arms hold baby, legs extended?			Legs flexed, good support with arms											
	Horizontal positions									Hypotonic, arms and legs straight							Arms and legs flexed				Head and back even, flexed extremities			Head above back					
Flexion angles	Popliteal	No resistance								150°				110°		100°					90°		80°							
	Ankle												45°				20°					0		A pre-term who has reached 40 weeks still has a 40° angle						
	Wrist (square window)									90°			60°			45°			30°			0								
Reflexes	Sucking							Weak, not synchronized with swallowing				Stronger, synchronized		Perfect				Perfect, hand to mouth											
	Rooting							Long latency period slow, imperfect			Hand to mouth			Brisk, complete, durable																
	Grasp							Finger grasp is good, strength is poor				Stronger						Can lift baby off bed, involves arms											
	Moro	Barely apparent						Weak, not elicited every time						Complete with arm extension, open fingers, cry				Arm adduction added				Hands open			?Begins to lose Moro				
	Crossed extension							Flexion and extension in a random, purposeless pattern				Extension, no adduction				Still incomplete			Extension, adduction, fanning of toes			Complete						

Automatic walk			Minimal	Begins tiptoeing, good support on sole	Fast tiptoeing	Heel-toe progression, whole sole of foot	A pre-term who has reached 40 weeks walks on toes	?Begins to lose automatic walk
Pupillary reflex	Absent	Appears	Present					
Glabellar tap	Absent		Appears	Present				
Tonic neck reflex	Absent		Appears	Present				
Neck-righting	Absent				Appears	Present after 37 weeks		
	20 21	22 23 24 25 26 27 28 29	30 31	32 33	34 35	36 37	38 39 40 41	42 43 44 45	46 47 48

Reproduced, with permission, from Kempe, C. H., Silver, H. K., O'Brien, D. (editors): *Current Pediatric Diagnosis & Treatment*, 5th ed. Copyright 1978 by Lange Medical Publications, Los Altos, California.

COMMON VARIATIONS IN THE NEONATE

Milia

Cephalhematoma / Caput Succedaneum

Nevus Flammeus

Continued on next page

336

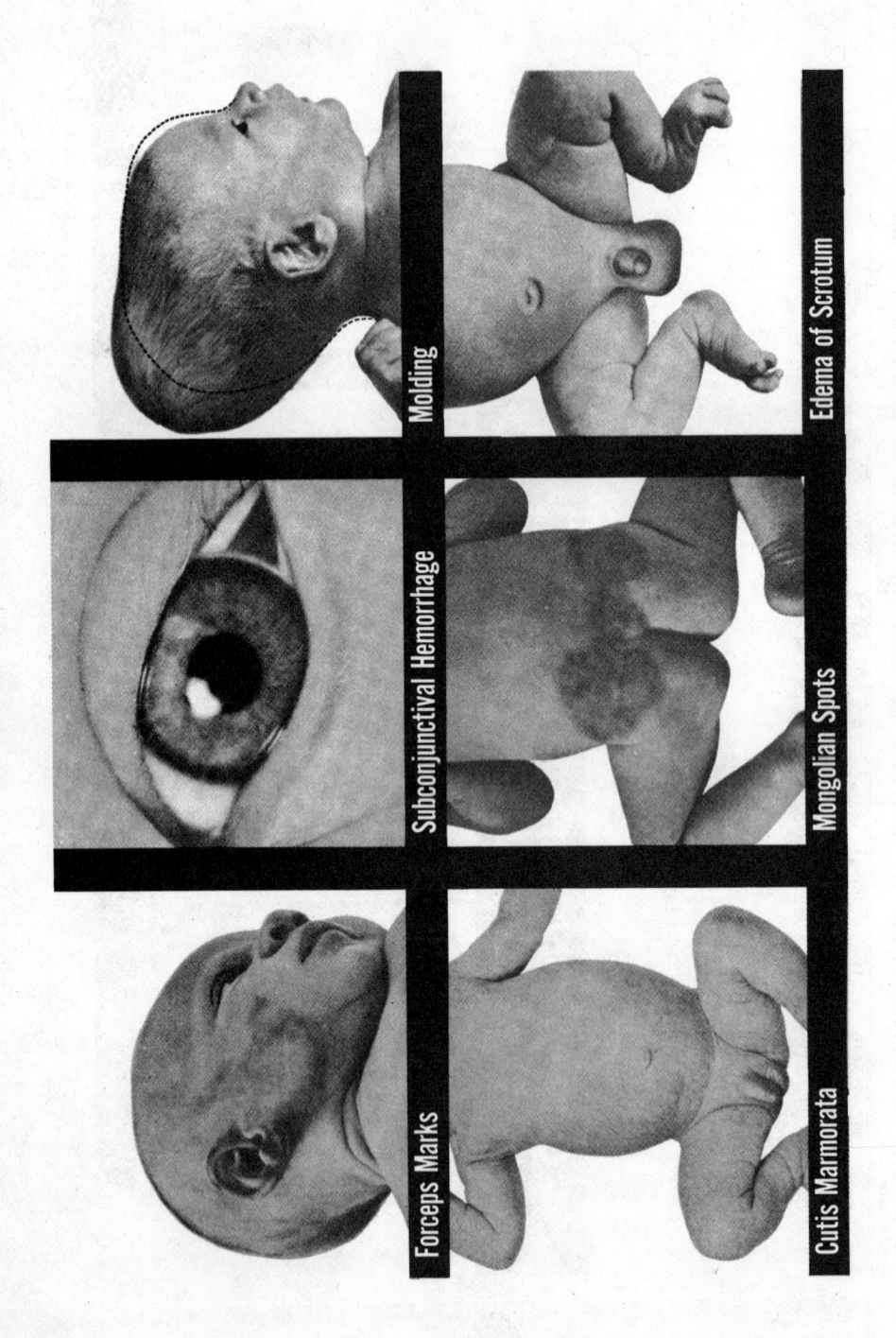

Molding

Edema of Scrotum

Subconjunctival Hemorrhage

Mongolian Spots

Forceps Marks

Cutis Marmorata

337

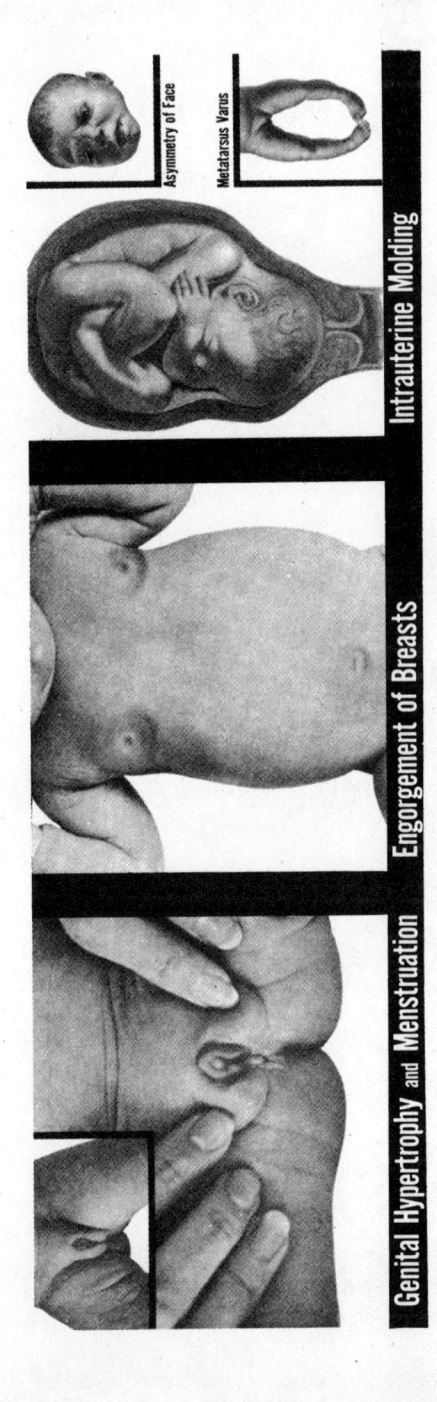

Asymmetry of Face

Metatarsus Varus

Intrauterine Molding

Engorgement of Breasts

Genital Hypertrophy and Menstruation

Clinical Education Aid No. 8, © 1961 & 1975, Ross Laboratories, Columbus, Ohio, reprinted with permission.

DANGER SIGNS in the newborn

Positive family history of hereditary disease
Complications of gestation and delivery
Congenital malformations
Low Apgar score
Rapid or difficult respiration
Apnea
Rapid, slow or irregular pulse
Cyanosis
Prematurity
Low birth weight
Small head for size

Single umbilical artery
Sweating
Edema
Fever or hypothermia
Jaundice
Pallor
Petechiae
Excessive salivation
Vomiting of bile
Diarrhea
Abdominal distention
Bleeding from circumcision or cord
Cord odor or exudate
Sudden changes in behavior and condition ("not looking right")

Abnormal cry
Cough
Excessive irritability
Twitching
Convulsions
Lethargy
Paralysis
Full fontanelle
Delayed or inadequate voiding (beyond 24 hours)
No meconium (beyond 48 hours)

Adapted from a chart of The Newborn Center — Denver Children's Hospital

Nursing Inservice Aid No. 4, © 1973, Ross Laboratories, Columbus, Ohio, reprinted with permission.

For further data on assessment and care of the neonate, see the following chapter, "Nursing Care of Children."

References on Breastfeeding

Books
(These books are recommended for new and expectant parents as well as for nurses)

Eiger, Marvin S. and Sally W. Olds, *Complete Book of Breast-Feeding*, Bantam Books, New York, 1973.

Ewy, Donna and Rodger Ewy, *Preparation for Breastfeeding*, Doubleday and Co., Inc., New York, 1975.

Gerard, A., *Please Breast Feed Your Baby*. Hawthorn Books, 1970.

ANNOUNCING

TRU-BREAST
A REVOLUTIONARY NEW METHOD OF INFANT FEEDING!
IT'S READY IN AN INSTANT!
LESS WORK FOR MOTHER!

WITH THESE PATENTED FEATURES:

LUL-A-BYE Sound Unit. Baby hears same soothing heartbeat he or she has grown accustomed to. While nursing, baby is lulled to sleep.

TRU-BREAST Unit is unbreakable, since baby can't drop it on the floor.

KWICK-FIL Holding Tank stores baby's milk at just the right temperature. Never too hot. Never too cold. Features automatic refill. Never bother with formulas again.

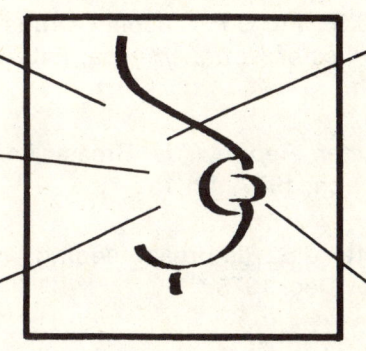

Baby less hungry than usual? No need to refrigerate left-overs. Milk stays warm and sterile in Unit. Ready when baby is.

TRU-BREAST Nursing Units never need sterilizing.

KWICK-KLEEN Nipple. No need to boil this nipple. Made of guaranteed lifetime materials *and* it can't be accidentally pulled off!

BUT THAT'S NOT ALL!
TRU-BREAST Units solve the problem of storage of baby items until the next baby comes along. They are decorative as well as functional! They come in all sizes, shapes and colors and outward appearance has nothing to do with ability of Units to function. Units come in pairs and improve with use. **TRU-BREAST** makes traveling with baby easier--the no-mess, no worry way!

With TRU-BREAST Around, Why Bother With Other Methods?

NOTICE: The above announcement may be given to friends, handed out in classes, laid out in waiting rooms, distributed at meetings, or included in conference packets. Available from NAPSAC, P.O. Box 267, Marble Hill, MO 63764. (314) 238-2010. Printed 8½x5½ in size on colored paper. Prices (including postage): $1 per 20 copies. $2 per 50 copies. $4 per 125. $10 per 500. $18 per 1000. NAPSAC also publishes a Directory of Alternative Birth Services, as well as other books & a newsletter for members. Write for free literature about NAPSAC.

Reprinted by permission of NAPSAC from NAPSAC NEWS, Vol. 4, Number 4, Winter, 1979.
The author of "Tru-Breast" is Margaret Nelson, a former La Leche League Leader.

Jelliffe, Derrick, and E.F. Patrice Jelliffe, *Human Milk in the Newborn World: Psychosocial, Nutritional and Economic Significance,* Oxford University Press, 1978.

La Leche League, *The Womanly Art of Breastfeeding,* Franklin Park, Ill., Interstate Printers and Publishers, 1963.

Pryor, Karen, *Nursing Your Baby,* Pocket Books, New York, 1973.

Articles

Applebaum, R.M., "Modern Management of Successful Breast Feeding," *Pediatric Clinics of North America,* February, 1970, Vol. 17, No. 1, p. 203.

Baum, J. David, "Nutritional Value of Human Milk," *Obstetrics and Gynecology,* January, 1971, Vol. 37, No. 1.

BRIEFS, December, 1978, 42: 152–4, "Testing Breast Milk for Contaminants."

Brown, R.E., "Breast Feeding in Modern Times," *American Journal of Clinical Nutrition,* May, 1973, Vol. 26, p. 556.

Catz, C.S., and G.P. Ciacoia, "Drugs and Breast Milk," *Pediatric Clinics of North America,* February, 1972, Vol. 19, No. 1, p. 151.

Consumer Report, "Is Breast Feeding Best For Babies?," March, 1977, 42: 152–7.

Doucette, J.S., "Is Breast-feeding Still Safe For Babies?," *MCN,* Nov/Dec, 1978.

Dutton, M.A., "A Breastfeeding Protocol," *JOGN Nursing,* May/June, 1979, pp. 151–155. (This is an excellent in-depth article on a protocol established at Women's Hospital at the University of Michigan for teaching and assisting new mothers in establishing breastfeeding.)

Goodman, N., "In-Depth Breastfeeding Class," *Keeping Abreast Journal of Human Nurturing,* July/Sept., 1978, 3: 214–9.

Hall, J.M., "Influencing Breastfeeding Success," *JOGN Nursing,* Nov./Dec., 1978.

Henderson, K.J., L.D. Newton, "Helping Nursing Mothers Maintain Lactation while Separated from Their Infants," *MCN,* Nov./Dec., 1978.

Ilfrig, Sr. M.C., "Nursing Care and Success in Breast Feeding," *Nursing Clinics of North America,* June, 1968, Vol. 3, No. 2, p. 345.

Jelliffe, D.B. and E.F.P. Jelliffe, "Lactation, Conception, and the Nutrition of the Nursing Mother and Child," *Journal of Pediatrics,* Vol. 81, No. 4, p. 829.

Leighton, N.S., "Initiating and Supporting the Early Breastfeeding Relationship," *Keeping Abreast Journal of Human Nurturing,* July/Sept., 1978, 3: 214–9.

Murdaugh, Sr. A. and L.E. Miller, "Helping the Breast Feeding Mother," *American Journal of Nursing,* 121:465, 1975.

Newton, M., and N. Newton, "Normal Course and Management of Lactation," *Clinical Obstetrics and Gynecology,* March, 1962, Vol. 5, No. 1, p. 44.

Newton, M. and N. Newton, "Psychological Aspects of Lactation," *New England Journal of Medicine,* Nov. 30, 1967, Vol. 277, No. 22, p. 1179.

* Parsons, Lee Jarvis, "Weaning From the Breast," *JOGN Nursing,* May/June, 1978, Vol. 7, No. 3.

Perez, A., et al., "First Ovulation After Childbirth: The Effect of Breastfeeding," *American Journal of Obstetrics and Gynecology,* 1972, 114:1041.

Taif, B., "Breast-feeding: Is It Better?," *Journal of Practical Nursing,* January, 1977, 27:32–4.

Thompson, M., "Establishment of Lactation," *Nursing Forum,* 1971, 10:292.

Whitley, N., "Barriers to Effective Breastfeeding Counseling," *Hospital Topics,* May/June, 1977, 55:40.

Keeping Abreast Journal is an excellent resource on breast feeding information for nurses and parents alike. It is available from Resources in Human Nurturing, International, 3885 Forest St., P.O. Box 6861, Denver, Co. 80206.

* *Lee Parsons' article on weaning is excellent and one of the few resources for professionals and lay people on this important topic. As nurses and midwives we encourage mothers to breastfeed and offer support in initiating the process but unfortunately mothers are usually left to fend for themselves in the weaning process. Far too little emphasis has been given to the importance of weaning both to mother and child. It is a very real separation process and as such can cause problems for both members of the nursing couple. For the mother, weaning her child may call to mind old feelings about previous separations and losses, and the way the weaning is handled can have a great impact on how the child handles separation and loss in the future. It is hoped that more research will be done on the weaning process and that more literature will be available for nurses and the families they work with.*

Innovations in Maternity Care

MATERNITY CARE ASSOCIATION CHILDBEARING CENTER
New York, New York

Background: Growing numbers of women in all socioeconomic groups have become disenchanted with traditional hospital maternity care. The increased cost and dehumanizing personal care that are characteristic of hospitals make home deliveries an attractive alternative. However, home deliveries may not be the safest care for the mother and the infant. Therefore, an alternative having the advantages of the institution and the personal touch of home delivery was established in New York City.

The objective of the Maternity Care Association Childbearing Center is to show the public how the need for satisfying, yet safe and low-cost, maternity care can be provided for a low-risk childbearing population. Care is provided by an obstetrician-nurse midwife team in a home-like setting surrounded by family. The option to go home with the baby within 12 hours of delivery is available.

Families anticipating a normal childbearing experience will be accepted, and patients will be carefully screened to allow only those low in risk to participate. A nearby acute-care hospital provides back-up in an emergency. In addition, emergency equipment is available at the center.

Nursing Role: There are five full-time nurse midwives at the center. The families have a full range of services, including prenatal care, classes in preparation for childbirth and infant care, and labor, delivery, and postpartum checkups. Most mothers will return home with their infants within 12 hours of delivery. The follow-up care is provided by public-health nurses in the home during the postpartum period. Regular telephone contact is kept with the new mothers. (The public-health nurses are under a contract between the Maternity Center Association and the Visiting Nurse Service of New York.)

Contact for Further Information:
Ruth Watson Lubic, RN, MA, CNM
General Director, Maternity Center Association
48 East Ninety-second Street
New York, New York 10028
(212) 369-7300

MATERNITY SHORT STAY—HOME VISITING SERVICES
Yakima, Washington

Purpose: About two and one-half years ago, a program was started to allow maternity patients and their infants to be discharged on the first postpartum day and followed up at home by registered nurses. It was believed that this program of early discharge would allow nurses time to teach patients on an individual basis, save patients $100 to $200 on the hospital bill, and provide better and longer follow-up care in the setting in which the mother would be taking care of her own child. It also would provide the family unit with as much time together as possible and discourage home deliveries by reuniting families sooner.

The target consumer population varies. Welfare clients do not qualify because of legal restrictions. To be eligible, a client must have prearranged the service with her physician's office; she must have adequate help at home to allow time for rest; she must have an uncomplicated course of labor and delivery; and she must live within a reasonable proximity of Yakima.

Nursing Role: The nurse visits the home of the patient three times, usually the day after discharge, again two days later, and finally about a week after the delivery. In addition, there is a follow-up phone call after two weeks. The nurse assesses both mother and child for physical and psychological status. She is available to answer questions and give support, teaching, and counseling. She works with the physician by referral when necessary. This service is private, and the director is a certified nurse mid-wife.

Contact for Further Information:
Tamara J. Baker, RN, CNM
Maternity Short Stay—Home Visiting Services
205 C North Sixty-Third Avenue
Yakima, Washington 98902
(509) 966-9818

Reprinted from *Analysis and Planning for Improved Distribution of Nursing Personnel and Services*, Sheila Kodadek, Editor, 1976, Division of Nursing, Health Resources Administration, U.S. Department of H.E.W.

Sister Stella's Babies
by Sister Mary Stella Simpson, D.C., R.N., C.N.M.

Published by American Journal of Nursing Company,
Copyright © 1978, American Journal of Nursing Co.,
10 Columbus Circle, New York, N.Y. 10019 (cost: $9.95)

Written informally and excerpted from her letters home to the Sisters of her order, this book details the work of Sister Stella as a nurse-midwife among impoverished people in Bolivar County, Mississippi. It is a pictorial essay with many exquisite photographs of the people she worked with. Sister Stella's accounts of the difficulties providing adequate health care with poor facilities to a population lacking in health education are an inspiration to all nurses. Her adaptability and ingenuity will be especially appreciated by maternity nurses, public health nurses, and nurses working with people from different cultures than their own. The dedication and warmth that is conveyed in her descriptions of her work will make enjoyable reading for nurses in other fields as well.

Minds, Mothers And Midwives

Prince, Joyce and Margaret Adams
New York: Churchill Livingstone, 1978
Reviewed by Bethea Brost, R.N., B.S.N.

Concerned consumers and providers of maternal and infant care will gain valuable insight into some of the psycho-social factors affecting pregnancy, the delivery, and integration of the infant into the family unit. This continuous period has been coined "maternalizatum" by the authors. The importance of a working knowledge of this period is emphasized, if one is to effectively support the family. Pertinent and meaningful research studies are cited throughout. The entire book is informative, but the chapters on neonatal abilities, handicaps, and post-natal events are especially thought-provoking. This book is highly recommended for health professionals and parents.

Maternity Nursing Resources

General Resources In Maternity Care

The International Childbirth
Education Association (I.C.E.A.)
P. O. Box 20852
Milwaukee, Wisc. 53220

This is an organization of health care providers and consumers. I.E.C.A. promotes family centered maternity care and education for childbirth and parenthood. The group disseminates information to the lay public and professionals on childbirth and related topics and conducts conferences and seminars. There are many local childbirth education associations throughout the country.

The I.C.E.A. manufactures cloth fetal models for use with a pelvis model in childbirth education. These are available from Sue Lange, 423 Sagamore Drive, Rochester, N.Y. 14617.

A branch of the I.C.E.A., The International Childbirth Education Association Bookcenter, has available a wide variety of literature on pregnancy and birth, childbirth preparation, Cesarean birth, alternatives to hospital birth, family planning, women's health, food and nutrition, breastfeeding, parenthood, child care and development, child health, and books for children on childbirth. For a complete listing of these excellent resources write: The I.C.E.A. Bookcenter, P. O. Box 70258, Seattle,

Maternity Center Association
48 East 92nd Street
New York, N.Y. 10028

This is a nonprofit agency which promotes improved maternity care by conducting research; providing education to both expectant couples and professionals, training childbirth educators; and by developing and running demonstration projects in family centered care (currently the Center is running the Childbearing Center, an alternative to both hospital and home delivery, as a demonstration project. See page 66 for further information on the Childbearing Center). The Maternity Center publishes several classic materials for use in childbirth education, including the *Birth Atlas* ($20), the book *A Baby Is Born*, *Briefs,* a monthly magazine, and instructions for making a knitted uterus for use in classes. Write for full information on publications and on two-week training programs for nurses in childbirth education.

"The Maternity Center Association is now offering a demonstration program in primary health care to couples enrolled in its childbirth education classes.

The new program, Self-Help Education Initiated in Childbirth, or SHEIC, is supported by a grant from the New York Community Trust. It covers three major areas: preventive health care (nutrition, hygiene, physical fitness, environmental control), health assessment during and after pregnancy, and premedical treatment (emergency first-aid, home remedies, comfort measures during pregnancy).

Routine prenatal care is carried out by the couples themselves. They take and analyze urine specimens, check the woman's blood pressure and weight, measure the height of the uterine fundus, and listen to fetal heart tones. Each procedure is checked by one of the center's nurse-midwives until the couple is proficient.

Learning units developed from the classes will be made available to interested childbirth education groups."

Reprinted from *American Journal of Nursing*, July, 1978, "Creative Care Unit," p. 1206.

National Association of Parents and Professionals
For Safe Alternatives In Childbirth (NAPSAC)
P. O. Box 267
Marble Hill, Missouri 63764

NAPSAC is a nonprofit organization of parents and professionals (about 10% of the members are physicians, 20% nurses, 20% midwives, 20% childbirth educators, and 30% interested parents) interested in family-centered maternity care, childbirth education, and safe alternatives to traditional hospital birthing. Publications include a quarterly newsletter for members, and the following books: *Safe Alternatives In Childbirth,* ed. by David Stewart and Lee Stewart (paperback, $5); *21st Century Obstetrics Now!,* by Lee Stewart and David Stewart (2 volumes, paperback, $11 for set); *NAPSAC Directory of Alternative Birth Services* by Penny Simkin ($3.50); *Birth Goes Home* by Lester Hazell (paperback, $3.50); and a three volume set, *Compulsory Hospitalization Or Freedom Of Choice In Childbirth?* ($18 for the three books). Discounts are available for bulk orders.

Resources In Human Nurturing, International
Advocates For Infants, Children And Families
3885 Forest Street
P.O. Box 6861
Denver, Colo. 80206

This is an organization of "professionals, paraprofessionals, students and parents dedicated to promoting and protecting human nurturing." The group focuses its concerns particularly on "the perinatal period and early childhood." Members include groups and individuals who work with children and families. The organization conducts seminars and workshops on breastfeeding, family-centered maternity care, and related topics. Publications include *Keeping Abreast, Journal of Human Nurturing,* the quarterly journal of RHNI, a unique journal aimed at health care workers concerned with infant nutrition, the family, public health, and maternal and child health; *RHNI Bulletin,* a quarterly newsletter; and *Resources In Human Nurturing 1977–78,* a directory of members. RHNI also has available for purchase "Lact-Aid Nursing Supplementer" kits for use in stimulating lactation in a non-lactating mother. It is useful for mothers of premature and sick infants.

Resources on Breast and Bottle Feeding

The Evenflo Company
771 North Freedom Street
Ravenna, Ohio 44266

The Evenflo Company makes available breast pump kits, breast feeding sets, nursing pads, nipple shields, breast cream, and a brochure, *"The Joy Of Nursing,"* and a booklet, *"Bright Beginnings"* (on bottle feeding).

The Human Lactation Center, Ltd.
666 Sturges Highway
Westport, Conn. 06880

This is a non-profit organization which functions as "a scientific research institute" and provides education on lactation. (Membership fee is $10 for individuals, $25 for institutions). Publications include *The Lactation Review,* the Center's periodical, reports of the proceedings of the International Conferences on Human Lactation, and reports of research conducted worldwide by the Center.

La Leche League International, Inc.
9616 Minneapolis Avenue
Franklin Park, Ill. 60131

La Leche League is an organization which promotes breast feeding through personal support groups and instruction from nursing mothers. For people wishing to contact a local group, La Leche League has a directory of its League Leaders in various locations. It also has available many publications for both the health professional and nursing mothers. These include: *The Womanly Art Of Breastfeeding*, the League manual; *Mothers In The Kitchen*, a cookbook for mothers; a bi-monthly journal, *La Leche League News; Nursing Your Baby* by Karen Pryor; *The Tender Gift: Breastfeeding* by Dana Raphael; and several pamphlets and leaflets including "Father To Father—On Breastfeeding," and "How The Maternity Nurse Can Help The Breastfeeding Mother," by B. A. Countryman, R.N., M.N. Bulk order discounts are available.

Childbirth Education Association Of
Greater Philadelphia, Inc.
814 Fayette Street
Conshohocken, Pa. 19428

The Association has available "Confi-Dry Milk Cups," aids for women with inverted nipples who want to nurse or for collecting leaking milk. Information on "Collection Of Breastmilk" and a manual for counselors of breastfeeding mothers, can also be obtained from here.

Ortho Pharmaceutical Corporation
Raritan, N.J. 08869

Ortho has available a pamphlet, "The Bond Of Love, A Guide For The Nursing Mother."

Resources on Cesarean Birth

C/Sec, Inc. (Cesareans/Support Education and Concern)
66 Christopher Road
Waltham, Mass. 02154

This organization provides education on cesarean birth, supports families experiencing it, and conducts workshops for hospital staffs in an attempt to change attitudes and hospital policies regarding cesarean births. Anyone interested in promoting the goals of the organization may become a member ($8). Publications include "Frankly Speaking, A Pamphlet For Cesarean Couples" (56 pages), "Manual For Setting Up Prepared Childbirth Classes For Cesarean Parents," "Guide For Establishing A Cesarean Support Group," a C/Sec Newsletter, and others, all for small fees, which are reduced for members. This is a very useful group serving a long neglected population of maternity patients.

Resources on Genetics

National Genetics Foundation, Inc.
9 West 57th Street
New York, N.Y. 10019

This is a foundation providing information, support and services to people with possible genetic disorders. The foundation coordinates a network of genetic counseling and treatment centers throughout this country and Canada. It makes referrals for individuals to the closest appropriate center for their problem. Pamphlets available include: "Genetic Counseling And Treatment Network," "Can Genetic Counseling Help You?," and "How Genetic Disease Can Affect Your Family."

"Genetic Counseling," a 22-page booklet is available from The National Foundation For The March Of Dimes, 1275 Mamaroneck Avenue, White Plains, N.Y. 10605.

Informed Homebirth
P.O. Box 788
Boulder, Colorado 80306

Informed Homebirth is a national organization with chapters in several states. It offers classes for expectant parents who wish to give birth at home or in alternative birthing centers; a cassette tape course for couples who live where classes are not available; a program for training people interested in teaching the Informed Homebirth series of classes; and publications which include a bi-monthly newsletter, "Special Delivery," and the book *Special Delivery: The Complete Guide to Informed Birth* by Rahima Baldwin (Cost: $9.95 plus 75¢ postage and handling). Membership is available to those wishing to support the homebirth movement and costs $10.00/year.

Resources on Home Birth

Whatever a nurse's feelings about home deliveries, many maternity nurses, at some point in their work, come into contact with couples who want information on home deliveries and others who are determined to deliver at home, in spite of any arguments favoring hospital delivery which a nurse may present. Because the home birth and alternative birth movements are growing, nurses should be able to advise expectant parents on resources available to them, wherever they choose to deliver. The following organizations provide educational materials and other services to persons interested in alternative birthing settings and methods.

American College Of Home Obstetrics
664 North Michigan Avenue
Suite 610
Chicago, Ill. 60611

This is an organization of physicians who attend home births. The organization was established to share knowledge in this field, to publish information, and to promote the highest possible standards in home obstetrics. The college also provides support and aid to physicians active in home obstetrics who are subject to the disapproval of their local medical communities. Publications include a quarterly "Newsletter."

Association For Childbirth At Home International
National Headquarters
Box 1219
Cerritos, Calif. 90701

This is a group of parents and professionals which support parents' rights to choose their birthing place and attendant. A.C.H.I. offers numerous services to parents and professionals working in home birth. Publications include "Birth Notes," the journal of A.C.H.I. Many books and other publications on home birth and all aspects of childbearing are available from the A.C.H.I. Bookstore. Request the catalog from the A.C.H.I. Bookstore, P. O. Box 2232, 6840 Orangethorpe, Suite E, Buena Park, Calif. 90621.

Birth Day
Box 388
Cambridge, Mass. 02138

Birth Day is a group of parents and others concerned about a couple's right to choose their place of giving birth, their birth attendant, and the manner of giving birth. The group "exists to promote and protect the normal in all births wherever those births occur: at home, in a hospital or in a maternity home." (Quoted from Birth Day brochure.) It provides mutual support and encouragement and seeks to change attitudes towards birth and to improve maternity care. Birth Day is working for the development of emergency back-up for home births. Publications include a quarterly Newsletter and bibliographies for parents desiring a home birth. Birth Day also provides classes for couples planning home births, referrals to professionals, and speakers on home birth and alternatives to hospital delivery.

H.O.M.E. (Home Oriented Maternity Experience)
511 New York Avenue
Takoma Park
Washington, D.C. 20012

H.O.M.E. is a national organization which supports parents who want to give birth at home. It offers courses to parents through local groups and resource literature is available, including *Home Oriented Maternity Experience: A Comprehensive Guide To Home Birth* ($3 plus 75¢ for postage), and a quarterly newsletter.

Homebirth
Boston University Station
P. O. Box 355
Boston, Mass. 02215

Homebirth, an organization of parents who want control over their birthing experience, provides parents with resources and educational materials. Classes are given to help parents prepare for alternative birthing experiences and the *Homebirth Newsletter* is published quarterly. Also available are several educational materials including "Contraindications For Childbirth At Home," "Suggested Supplies For A Homebirth," and "Choosing A Birth Attendant."

Informed Homebirth
P.O. Box 788
Boulder, Colorado 80306

Informed Homebirth is a national organization with chapters in several states. If offers classes for expectant parents who wish to give birth at home or in alternative birthing centers; a cassette tape course for couples who live where classes are not available; a program for training people interested in teaching the Informed Homebirth series of classes; and publications which include a bi-monthly newsletter, "Special Delivery," and the book *Special Delivery: The Complete Guide to Informed Birth* by Rahima Baldwin (Cost: $9.95 plus 75¢ postage and handling). Membership is available to those wishing to support the homebirth movement and costs $10.00/year.

Resources for Infant Care

Baby Care Lambskins, lambskin rugs for infants to cuddle and sleep on, are used in some hospitals and birthing centers as well as in homes. For information on purchasing them, write Health Care Products, Inc., P. O. Box 26221, Dept. ABP, Denver, Colo. 80226.

The *Infant Development Guide,* a loose leaf manual (over 400 pages) of infant development in the first year of life, is available from Johnson and Johnson Baby Products Company, Professional Products Division, Piscataway, N.J. 08854. It is useful in teaching expectant and new parents. Johnson and Johnson also has several booklets on infant care and development for parents. Write for Educational Services Guide.

"A New Parent's Guide To Bathing Baby," is a booklet available from Winthrop Laboratories, 90 Park Avenue, New York, N.Y. 10016.

Andrea's Baby Pack is a carrier for infants which is useful to parents. Some of these packs have been used in hospital nurseries and pediatric units to provide extra cuddling of infants while enabling nurses to do charting or other work at the same time. Write Andrea's Baby Pack, 2441 Hilyard Street, Eugene, Ore. 97405.

Resources on Nutrition in Pregnancy

SPUN (Society for the Protection of the
Unborn Through Nutrition)
Suite 603
17 N. Wabash
Chicago, Ill. 60602

SPUN is an organization which provides literature for expectant parents and professionals on the importance of good nutrition in pregnancy. Publications include a newsletter, *The Pregnant Issue: Medicate Or Educate?,* and *Preventing Nutritional Complications Of Pregnancy: A Manual For SPUN Counselors.*

Books

What Every Pregnant Woman Should Know: The Truth About Diet And Drugs In Pregnancy, by Dr. Tom Brewer and Gail Sforza Brewer, copyright 1977, Random House.

Resources on Pregnancy and Prenatal Care

Coping With The Overall Pregnancy/Parenting Experience
(C.O.P.E.)
37 Clarendon Street
Boston, Mass. 02116

"Intrinsic to pregnancy and infant parenting adjustment are major physical, hormonal, emotional and life-style changes that span more than a two-year period. Ambivalence about having children is a common reaction even among those who have planned their pregnancies. At the same time, a range of emotional turbulence can be triggered internally by physical and hormonal changes and externally by the cultural image that at least some 'craziness' is inherent in the pregnancy experience.

"Coping with the Overall Pregnancy/Parenting Experience (COPE) support groups exist to bridge these conflicts and enable a woman to focus on her needs, motivations, and questions surrounding her experience. They draw pregnant women and new mothers together in small groups to share their mutual experiences and knowledge under the guidance of a group leader, herself a parent trained by COPE in perinatal psychology. Other groups include pregnant teenagers, single parents, fathers, couples, mothers of toddlers, all of whom share and learn under the direction of a new specialist *who has been there.* The COPE model also encompasses groups for postabortion women.

"Founded in 1972 by psychiatric nurse group therapist Maureen F. Turner, COPE's birth coincided with that of her second child and her realization that, despite months spent in the intimacy of a consciousness-raising group, she and others ignored her pregnancy, impending birth, and postpartum issues. Sisterhood at that time did not necessarily include motherhood. An important psychological preparation had been eclipsed in favor of more militant concerns. And for her, new motherhood rested on its traditional foundations. 'One was alone, tired, and isolated.'

"COPE groups evolved with enthusiastic media attention and support that, in turn generated the first of (to date) over 12,000 phone calls. More than 600 women have participated in peer-led support groups."

Nurses and others interested in forming local COPE groups should write the above address for information on the COPE Model and on becoming a licensed COPE group. COPE now functions as a "perinatal mental health center" and has made important contributions "to the new field of perinatal psychology."

Reprinted by permission of Plenum Publishing Corporation from "The COPE Story: A Service To Pregnant And Postpartum Women" by Maureen F. Turner, R.N. and Martha H. Izzi, B.S., in The Woman Patient, Vol. 1, edited by Malkah T. Notman and Carol C. Nadelson, copyright 1978, Plenum Publishing Corporation.

Publications

"Your Pregnancy," a booklet for expectant parents, is available from Ortho Pharmaceutical Corporation, Raritan, N.J. 08869.

"Expectant Mother's Guide" is a booklet from Gerber Products Co., Fremont, Mich. 49412.

"Having Children ... A Guide For The Diabetic Woman," by Richard Hansknecht, M.D., is available from the Juvenile Diabetes Foundation, 23 East 26th Street, New York, N.Y. 10010.

"Information About Rh Hemolytic Disease Of The Newborn," a brochure for expectant mothers, is available from Parke-Davis and Co., Detroit, Mich. 48232.

The First Gifts, a 68-page prenatal guide for teenaged parents, is especially designed for this age group. It is useful in schools and clinics as well as prenatal classes for teenagers. Contact Caring Mothers Cooperative, Box 211, Tuckerton, N.J. 08087. Also available from here are pamphlets on vaginal hygiene, simple instructions for sewing a "Cozy Carrier" infant carrier, and "Steppin Stones To Mom-Hood," a board game for young expectant parents.

The Birth Primer by Rebecca Rowe Parfitt, copyright 1977, Running Press, Philadelphia, Pa. (Paperback, 259 pages at $5.95). This is a very useful book for expectant parents which, as its subtitle indicates, is "A Source Book Of Traditional And Alternative Methods In Labor And Delivery." Ms. Parfitt presents the alternatives available to parents and offers detailed information on associations, books, films and other childbirth education resources. It serves as a guide for further study and decision making on the type of birthing experience desired.

Resources on Preparation for Childbirth

American Academy Of Husband-Coached Childbirth
P. O. Box 5224
Sherman Oaks, Calif. 91413

An organization which provides childbirth education information and services, this group trains childbirth educators in the Bradley Method of childbirth, which focuses on relaxation and abdominal breathing with the husband as coach. Workshops for educators are given at locations in various parts of the country. *Husband-Coached Childbirth,* the book by Dr. Robert Bradley, and other publications may be obtained through the Academy, as well as a list of Bradley-trained childbirth educators.

American Society For Psychoprophylaxis In Obstetrics (A.S.P.O.)
1411 K Street, N.W.
Washington, D.C. 20005

A.S.P.O. is a national, non-profit organization which promotes psychoprophylactic preparation for childbirth. It has a training and certification program for childbirth educators. (Write for information on becoming A.S.P.O. certified.) The group is made up of health professionals and parents. A.S.P.O. publications include childbirth education materials, the *A.S.P.O. National Directory* (which lists names and addresses of certified teachers and physicians), "Conceptions," a quarterly newsletter, and "Professional Bulletin," a quarterly publication for professional members.

Childbirth Without Pain Education League, Inc.
3940 Eleventh Street
Riverside, Calif. 92501

The League offers Lamaze classes in preparation for childbirth locally in California and also offers educational materials and a correspondence course for those in other areas where classes are not offered.

National Childbirth Trust (NCT)
Education For Parenthood
2 Queensborough Terrace
Bayswater, London W2 3TB
Great Britain

The NCT is a "registered charity" which prepares couples for childbirth and parenthood through prenatal classes. It also has postnatal support groups for new parents in many areas and a Breastfeeding Promotion Group which offers support to mothers who are breast feeding. NCT has available many leaflets and books on all aspects of childbearing for parents and professionals and it markets a special bra for pregnancy and nursing and nipple shields. It is an excellent resource for nurses and midwives in Great Britain.

Publications on Preparation for Childbirth

Preparation For Childbearing is a book for expectant parents from the Maternity Center Association, 48 East 92nd Street, New York, N.Y. 10028.

Fathering: Participation In Labor And Birth, by Celeste R. Phillips, R.N., M.S. and Joseph T. Anzalone, M.D., 1978, is available from The C. V. Mosby Co. (160 pages, $7.95).

The Natural Childbirth Workbook, by Panchita MacNeil, C.B.E., is an 80-page manual for students in childbirth classes. (Cost: $4.95, with a quantity discount for instructors of $3 each for ten or more copies.) Contact MacNeil, 7526 Penfield Avenue, Canoga Park, Calif. 91306.

Childbirth Instructor manuals and training guides are available from the Childbirth Education Association of Greater Philadelphia, Inc., 814 Fayette Street, Conshohocken, Pa. 19428.

An educational program for prenatal and infant care classes consisting of educational aids from various suppliers, sent free of charge to childbirth education instructors, is available from *American Baby Magazine,* Inc., 575 Lexington Avenue, New York, N.Y. 10022.

The Pennypress
1100 23rd Ave., East
Seattle, Washington 98112

The Pennypress publishes and distributes "materials on childbearing and parenting." These include a series of pamphlets, "The Better Babies Series" (4-page pamphlets for handouts in childbirth or parenting classes and clinics and hospitals with such titles as "Planning Your Baby's Birth," "Sex During Pregnancy," Childbirth—A Teenager's Guide," "Cesarean Birth—A Special Delivery," and others, all written by experts in these areas, and available at low cost), and several books, including *Mom and Dad and I Are Having A Baby!* by Maryann Malecki, R.N., for children who will be present at a birth; *Without Spanking or Spoiling,* by Elizabeth Crary, for parents of young children, *The New Parent Class* by Margot Edwards R.N., a book for professionals working with pregnant teenagers, and other books on related topics. All of the materials from The Pennypress are inexpensive and very worthwhile.

Orange Cat Goes to Market
442 Church St.
Garberville, CA 95440

Orange Cat Goes to Market is a marvelous bookstore with an especially good selection of books on pregnancy, birthing, and parenting. Kathy Epling publishes a delightful catalog of books on these topics which the store carries. The catalog includes brief descriptions of the books and their usefulness, and information on placing mail orders. It would be well placed in every office or clinic frequented by expecting or new parents. For a copy write Kathy Epling at the above address.

Publications on Exercise and Childbearing

Essential Exercises For The Childbearing Year, by Elizabeth Noble, R.P.T., from Houghton Mifflin Co., Dept. BFJ, 2 Park Street, Boston, Mass. 02107.

Moving Through Pregnancy, The Complete Exercise Guide For Today's Woman, by Elisabeth Bing, from Bobbs-Merrill, 4 West 58th Street, New York, N.Y. 10019.

Preparation For Childbirth, by Mabel Lum Fitzhugh, R.P.T., is available from Margaret B. Farley, R.P.T., 21 San Margarita Drive, San Rafael, Calif. 94901.

Rapid Post Natal Figure Recovery, by Constance Reed, is a booklet available from Ortho Pharmaceutical Corporation, Raritan, N.J. 08869.

Several books on yoga and pregnancy are available from the ICEA Bookcenter, P. O. Box 70258, Seattle, Wash. 98107.

Aids for Maternity Nurses

An Obstetrics/Gynecology Reference And Record Book, a handy reference for nurses, is published by Pfizer, Inc., Laboratories Division, 235 East 42nd Street, New York, N.Y. 10017.

A plastic "Cervical Dilatation" chart for hanging in labor and delivery areas as a ready reference is available from Ross Laboratories, Columbus, Ohio 43216.

A series of eight full-color booklets on "variations and minor departures in newborn infants," and a two-volume series on "Characteristics In Infant Development" are available from Mead Johnson Laboratories, Evansville, Ind. 47721, or your local Mead Johnson Medical Sales Representative.

Periodicals on Maternity Nursing

Birth And The Family Journal
110 El Camino Real
Berkeley, Calif. 94705

This is an interdisciplinary journal for health care professionals and consumers with informative articles on "the family in its childbearing years." It is published quarterly (Cost: $10/year, $12 for institutions and foreign).

Clinical Obstetrics And Gynecology
Harper and Row Publishers
2350 Virginia Avenue
Hagerstown, Md. 21740

This is a hard cover quarterly publication (Cost: $32.50/year).

The Federal Monitor
Ann C. Gray, Editor
710 Bulls Neck Road, Dr. Q
McLean, Va. 22101

This is a newsletter covering "legislation, regulation and court cases affecting the health care of women and children, with an emphasis on childbearing," published by the Maternal And Child Health Legislative Alert, Inc. (Cost: $8/year, and published at least eight times yearly).

JOGN Nursing (see information under Nurses' Association of the American College of Obstetricians and Gynecologists in section on "Nursing Organizations").

Journal Of Nurse-Midwifery (see information under American College of Nurse-Midwives in section on "Nursing Organizations").

Maternal-Child Nursing Journal
3505 Fifth Avenue
Pittsburgh, Pa. 15213

This quarterly journal is published by the graduate faculties of the Departments of Obstetrical and Pediatric Nursing at the University of Pittsburgh. It is geared toward clinical specialists in obstetrical and pediatric nursing (Cost: $8/year).

MCN, The American Journal of Maternal Child Nursing
The American Journal of Nursing Company
10 Columbus Circle
New York, N.Y. 10019

This magazine covering topics of interest to maternity nurses is published bimonthly (Cost: $15.00/year in U.S., $19.00/year foreign).

Obstetrics and Gynecology
Journal Of The American College of Obstetricians And Gynecologists

This monthly publication is aimed at physicians in the field of obstetrics and gynecology and is also of interest to nurses in this field. Available from Elsevier North-Holland (Cost: $35/year for individuals, $50/year for institutions).

The Practicing Midwife
156 Drakes Lane
Summertown, Tenn. 38483

This quarterly newsletter is put out by Ina Mae and the Farm midwives. It contains information of interest to midwives and nurses (Cost: $5 a year).

Perinatal Press
Division Of Continuing Education
University Of Tennessee
Center For The Health Sciences
800 Madison Avenue
Memphis, Tenn. 38163

This non-profit publication is published ten times/year for health professionals working with pregnant women and newborns (Cost: $15 a year).

Audiovisual Aids on Maternity Nursing

General Maternity Topics

Photoview Instructional Aids produces eight 35mm slide series covering newborns, breastfeeding, prenatal exercises, obstetrical anesthesia, labor and delivery, and infant care. Write for brochure describing each series.

"The Chicago Maternity Center Story" is a film about the struggle to keep open the maternity center which conducted home deliveries for over 75 years. Though the women's fight to keep the center open was unsuccessful, the film documents home deliveries as well as the injustices in the system of health care for profits. Available from Kartemquin/Haymarket Films.

"The Cesarean Birth Experience," "Bonding Birth Experience," "Breastfeeding Experience" and "Are You Ready For The Postpartum Experience?" are excellent films for expectant parents from Parenting Pictures.

The *ICEA Film Directory* is a 53-page catalog of films and demonstration aids of use in childbirth education and the sources from which they can be obtained. Available from the International Childbirth Education Association.

Patient Education films and videotapes on all aspects of pregnancy, labor and delivery, post partum adjustment and family planning are available from Professional Research, Inc.

"Emotional Aspects Of Pregnancy," "Nine Months In Motion" (about regular exercise for the pregnant woman), "A Baby Is Born," "Birth Of A Family," "Labor Of Love: Childbirth Without Violence" (a film on the Leboyer method of childbirth), and "The Bond Of Breastfeeding" are all films available from Perennial Education, Inc.

"Having A Section Is Having A Baby," "Not Me Alone," "Having Twins," "Talking About Breastfeeding," "Adapting To Parenthood," and "Pregnancy After 35" are excellent films for parent education from Polymorph Films.

Films on Birth

FOR GENERAL AUDIENCES (Expectant Parents' Classes, lay audiences, and health professionals):

"Birth Without Violence," a film demonstrating the Leboyer

method of childbirth, designed to lessen the trauma of birth for the infant, is available from New Yorker Films.

"The Birth Film" is available from New Yorker Films.

"Becoming," a 16mm color film on preparation for labor and delivery which shows a prepared delivery with the mother awake and the father present, is available from the Joseph T. Anzalone Foundation.

"Birth" is a film which discusses and criticizes traditional childbirth practices as "detached, often inhumane." From Films Incorporated.

"The Birth Of Paul," "a slide/cassette/guide series" on home delivery, discusses "safe, family-centered prepared childbirth." Gale D. Watkins, R.N., who holds the copyright on the film, says that "it is not anti-hospital, it is pro-family." From Childbirth Education Associates.

"Birth And Bonding," a slide/casette presentation including instructor's manual details early parent-infant contact. From Media For Childbirth Education.

"Nan's Class" is a film for expectant parents covering Lamaze preparation, the labors and deliveries of five couples and one single mother, from A.S.P.O.

"Five Women, Five Births," covers five births including hospital and home births, a cesarean birth, Leboyer birth, births with an obstetrician and with a midwife present. It shows the alternatives presently available in childbirth. From Suzanne Arms Productions.

"A Shared Beginning" is a film on Lamaze preparation, labor and delivery, from Keith-Merrill Associates.

"The Story Of Eric," a film on Lamaze prepared childbirth, available in English or Spanish, is available from Centre Films, Inc.

"Bernita's Film," about single parenthood, follows the Lamaze preparation, labor, delivery and post partum adjustment of a young woman. From Centre Films, Inc.

"Miracle Of Birth," a film showing three births, is available from Brigham Young University.

The Bay Area ASPO Slides produces programs consisting of slides plus cassettes for expectant parents, including "The

Childbirth Experience," "The Hospital Tour," "The Childbirth Adventure," and "Breastfeeding ... A Family Experience."

"Firstborn," a film for expectant parents and maternity care workers, emphasizes the mother's emotions during pregnancy and childbirth. From Occidental Publishing Co.

"Gentle Birth" is a film showing delivery by the Leboyer method, from Polymorph Films.

"Primum Non Nocere" and "Not By Chance" are films on home births with Dr. Mayer Eisenstein, M.D., of the American College of Home Obstetrics, in attendance. From Cinema Medica. Cinema Medica also has excellent films on family centered maternity care, including one on "Cesarean Childbirth," as well as books on related subjects.

"All My Babies," a marvelous classic film on "Miss Mary," a lay midwife in Georgia and her work with pregnant women and infants, which is an inspiration to nurses and midwives, is available from the University of California Extension Media Center.

"The Gentle Celebration Of Aaron Isaac's Birth" is a film on a home birth, from the Association For Childbirth At Home, International.

Films on birth and on the Newborn are available from EDC Distribution Center.

For Nurses and Allied Health Professionals

"Management Of Shoulder Dystocia" is available from Association-Sterling Films.

"Assessment Of Fetal Presentation and Position: Leopold's Maneuvers," is available from Health Sciences Communication Center.

"Human Birth Films" is a film of seven different birth presentations including a spontaneous vertex delivery and various complications, from Lippincott's Audiovisual Media.

"Emergency Childbirth" is a film from Professional Research, Inc.

"Anesthesia For Labor And Delivery" is a film from Lippincott's Audiovisual Media.

Several excellent films and videocassettes on complications

of pregnancy and normal pregnancy and birth, are available from the American Journal Of Nursing Company.

"Midwife" is a new film showing home births assisted by two nurse-midwives in the San Francisco area. It includes information on the training of nurse-midwives as well as how they function. Available from Michael Anderson, 402 San Francisco Blvd., San Anselmo, CA 94960.

"Intrapartum Fetal Monitoring," a film showing proper application of the monitor, is available from Corometrics Medical Systems, Inc.

Audiovisual Aids on Breast Feeding

"Breastfeeding: A Special Closeness," is available from Motion, Inc.

"Breast Feeding: Prenatal And Postpartal Preparation," teaches nurses and doctors how to assist and teach new mothers. Available from Health Sciences Communications Center.

"Breast Feeding: Nutrition, Nursing And The Working Mother," is available from Health Sciences Communications Center.

"Mother And Child" and "The Nursing Family," are two films on breast feeding made in conjunction with the La Leche League, from Mary Jane Company.

The La Leche League International has available for rental or purchase several films on breast feeding and natural childbirth. Write for complete listing.

"Thoroughly Modern Mom" is an educational slide film on breast feeding from Monterey Laboratories, Inc.

Audiovisual Materials on Cesarean Birth

"Cesarean Childbirth," a film for patients needing a cesarean section, is available from Jay Hathaway Production Services.

"A Shared Cesarean Beginning" is available from Keith Merrill Associates.

A series of cassette tapes from C/Sec, Inc. (Cesareans/Support Education and Concern), is available. The tapes include sessions on nutrition in pregnancy, breast feeding, exercises following cesarean birth, and other topics on cesarean sections. From Bauer Audio Video, Inc.

Audiovisual Aids on Fathering

"Pregnant Fathers" is a 16mm color film of a prepared childbirth emphasizing the father's experience and encouraging the participation of fathers, from Joseph T. Anzalone Foundation.

"The Nurturing Father" is a slide/cassette presentation for expectant fathers, from Media for Childbirth Education.

"Especially For Fathers" is a film on the father's role in childbirth from the University Of California Extension Media Center.

Audiovisual Aids on Infant Care

"Loving Hands," a film by Dr. Frederick Leboyer, shows an Indian mother relating lovingly to her infant through massage. From New Yorker Films.

"Bathing Your Baby" is a film from Bandera Enterprises.

"Baths And Babies" is a film with a bath demonstration for parents, from Johnson and Johnson.

"Mother Love" is a film on Dr. Harry Harlow's work with newborn rhesus monkeys showing the importance of holding and cuddling, from Carousel Films.

Audiovisual Aids on Neonatology

"Recognition Of Narcotic Withdrawal Symptoms In Newborn Infants," and "Resuscitation Of The Newborn" are available from Association-Sterling Films.

"Fetal Alcohol Syndrome" is available from Films Incorporated.

"The Amazing Newborn" is a film showing the behavior of three normal infants during the first week of life, and how this is important in the early communication between newborns and their parents. From Health Sciences Communication Center.

"The Dubowitz Assessment Of Newborn Gestational Age" demonstrates the method for this assessment, from Health Sciences Communication Center.

"Talking With Parents Of A Premature Infant," "A Discussion With Parents Of A Malformed Child," and "Death Of A Newborn" (dealing with a couple whose premature child died three weeks after birth, their grief, things that helped them and things that did not), are all available from Health Sciences Communication Center.

"Newborn Appraisal" is a slide/tape program for nurses on newborn assessment, from Audio Visual Service, College of Physicians & Surgeons, 630 West 168th St., New York, N.Y. 10032.

Audiovisual Aids on Pregnancy

"Fullness" is a film portraying the sexual activity of a couple when the woman is eight months pregnant. It is for use with pregnant couples to show the possibilities for sexual closeness during pregnancy. From Multi Media Resource Center.

"Early Abortion" is a simple and accurate description of atraumatic vacuum abortion procedures. The film is intended for women who are about to have this procedure, to alleviate fear and anxiety. From Perennial Education, Inc.

"Alcohol: Crisis For The Unborn," "Unfinished Child," and "Great Expectations" are a few of the films available for loan from the National Foundation/March Of Dimes. They deal with the need for proper nutrition and care during pregnancy to prevent birth defects.

A comprehensive series of films on medical genetics is available from Milner-Fenwick, Inc.

"Miracle Of Life," a film showing actual fertilization of the human egg and development of the embryo and fetus, and "Prenatal Care," a film on the needs of pregnancy, are available from Pyramid Films.

Schools with Educational Programs in Nurse-Midwifery

College of Medicine And Dentistry Of New Jersey
School Of Allied Health Professions
100 Bergen Street
Newark, N.J. 07103

Columbia University
School Of Nursing
630 West 168th Street
New York, N.Y. 10032

Emory University
School Of Nursing
Atlanta, Ga. 30322

Frontier Nursing Service
Hyden, Ky. 41749

Georgetown University
School Of Nursing
3700 Reservoir Road, N.W.
Washington, D.C. 20007

Johns Hopkins University
School Of Hygiene And Public Health
615 North Wolfe Street
Baltimore, Md. 21214

Medical University Of South Carolina
College Of Nursing
80 Barre Street
Charleston, S.C. 29401

Mehany Medical College
Department Of Nursing Education
Box 61-A
1005 18th Avenue, North
Nashville, Tenn. 37208

St. Louis University
Department Of Nursing
1310 South Grand Boulevard
St. Louis, Missouri 63104

SUNY Downstate Medical Center
Box 1216
450 Clarkson Avenue
Brooklyn, N.Y. 11203

University Of California At San Diego
Office Of Continuing Education And Health Sciences
School Of Medicine
La Jolla, Calif. 92093

University Of California At San Francisco
San Francisco General Hospital
Ward 25, Room 16
1001 Patrero Avenue
San Francisco, Calif. 94110

University District Hospital
Caparra Heights Station
Puerto Rico 00935

University Of Illinois
College Of Nursing
845 South Damen Avenue
Chicago, Ill. 60612

University Of Kentucky
College Of Nursing
Albert B. Chandler Medical Center
Lexington, Ky. 40506

University Of Miami
School Of Nursing, Building 49L
P. O. Box 248106
Coral Gables, Fla. 33124

University Of Minnesota
School Of Nursing
3313 Powell Hall
Minneapolis, Minn. 55455

University Of Mississippi Medical Center
265 Woodland Hills Building
Jackson, Miss. 39216

University Of Utah
College Of Nursing
25 South Medical Drive
Salt Lake City, Utah 84112

Yale University
School Of Nursing
38 South Street
New Haven, Conn. 06520

Adapted from *A Directory Of Expanded Role Programs For Registered Nurses*, 1979, Division of Nursing, Health Resources Administration, U.S. Department of H.E.W.

7 Nursing Care of Children

The nursing of children requires an understanding of normal growth and development and of the needs of the growing child as well as an ability to perceive the needs of the child's family in relation to his/her health care.

Information offered in this section includes guidelines for nurses both in the physical assessment and care of children and in providing teaching and support to the child and family.

The need for parental involvement in the care of hospitalized children is emphasized in the Policy Statement of the Association for the Care of Children in Hospitals and in the article on the parent to parent support group in the care of high-risk newborns. The promotion of parental involvement should be incorporated into the practice of nurses working with children in all settings.

The nurse's role in well-child care has been expanding rapidly as increasingly pediatric nurse practitioners are giving primary care to children and families in a variety of settings. A list of schools training pediatric nurse practitioners is included here for nurses interested in pursuing this field.

I. **Growth and Development**

    Developmental Patterns
    Essential Milestones
    Normal Development in the First Three Years
    Accidents Related to Developmental Levels

II. **Immunizations**

    Recommended Schedule for Active Immunization
    Contraindications to Immunization

III. **Common Infectious Diseases**

IV. **Preventive Dental Practices for Children**

V. **Children in Hospitals**

    Policy Statement of the Association for the Care of Children in Hospitals
    A Child's Letter
    Nursing Approaches by Level of Development
    Factors Affecting Adjustment to Hospitalization
    Effects of Chronic Hospitalization
    Intramuscular Injection Sites
      For Premature and Newborn Infants
      For Older Children
    Pediatric Psychological Checklist for Surgery
    Recommended Contents of Pediatric Resuscitation Kit
    Observations of the Neonate
    Normal Reflexes of the Neonate
    Comparison of Premature and Small-for-Dates Infants
    Postmaturity Syndrome
    Equipment for Neonatal Intensive Care
    Infant Suctioning Methods
    Respiratory Distress in the Neonate
    Cardiovascular Disorders in Infants
    Parent-Parent Support in the Care of High-Risk Infants
    Sudden Infant Death Syndrome—Counseling of Families
    Burns in Children—The "Rule of Fives"
    Pediatric I.V.'s

VI. *Home Care for the Dying Child*—A Review

VII. **The Disturbed Child's Family**

VIII. **Child Abuse—The Nurse's Role**

Growth and Development

Assessment of Developmental Patterns

Skill	Assessment Instrument
Motor (fine and gross)	Birth—6 months: Physical assessment
	6 months—6 years: Physical assessment augmented by direct developmental testing (e.g., Denver Developmental Screening Test) or indirect testing (e.g., Preschool Attainment Record).
	School-age to adult: Physical assessment augmented by direct developmental testing (e.g., Valett Psychoeducational Test) or indirect testing (e.g., Vineland Social Maturity Scale).
	Children with physical handicaps evaluated by observation and use of reinforcers to obtain maximum effort. Suspected perceptual motor difficulties may be screened by the Ayers Test (Southern California Test Battery) for ages 4–11.
Language	Same instruments as for fine and gross motor skills. Additionally, the Vocabulary Language Test helps pinpoint deficits in language development. After 8 years, articulation errors may be assessed with the Templin Darley Screening Test. Suspected childhood aphasia may be evaluated with the Eisenson Examining for Aphasia Test.
Social and emotional	Same instruments as for motor and language development. Presenting emotional problems may further be screened with the Devereaux Child Behavior Rating Scale. The nurse who holds clinical membership in transactional analysis may find script analysis useful with the adolescent.
Cognitive	Assessment of cognitive or intellectual development is seldom a screening procedure. When there is a question about the potential of the child of 3 to 18 years, the Peabody Picture Vocabulary is an excellent tool. The Wide Range Achievement Test will also give an indication of the level at which the child or adolescent is functioning academically.

Reprinted by permission of McGraw-Hill from *Comprehensive Pediatric Nursing*, Gladys Scipien, et al., McGraw-Hill, 1975.

Essential Milestones

Many milestones of development may be important, but the following are the essential milestones which anyone responsible for assessing babies needs to know:

Birth	Prone—pelvis high, knees under abdomen.
	Ventral suspension—elbows flex, hips partly extended.
4–6 weeks	Smiles at mother.
6 weeks	Prone—pelvis flat.
12–16 weeks	Turns head to sound.
	Holds object placed in hand.
12–20 weeks	Hand regard.
20 weeks	Goes for objects and gets them, without their being placed in the hand.
26 weeks	Transfers objects, one hand to another.
	Chews.
	Sits, hands forward for support.
	Supine—lifts head up spontaneously.
	Feeds self with biscuit.
9–10 months	Index finger approach.
	Finger thumb apposition.
	Creep.
	Patacake, byebye.
	Helps dress—holding arm out for coat, foot out for shoe, or transferring object from hand in order to insert hand in sleeve.
13 months	Casting (ceases by about 15 months).
	Walks, no help.
	2–3 single words.
15–18 months	Domestic mimicry.
15 months	Feeds self fully if given a chance, picking up a cup, drinking, putting it down without help.
	Casting stops. Mouthing stops.
18 months	Begins to tell mother about wetting.
21–24 months	Joins 2–3 words together spontaneously.
2 years	Mainly dry by day.
3 years	Mainly dry by night.
	Dresses self, except for buttons at back, if given a chance.
	Stands momentarily on one foot.

Reprinted by permission of Churchill Livingstone from *The Development of the Infant and Young Child*, 6th edition, R.S. Illingworth, Copyright 1975, Churchill Livingstone Publishers.

Summary of normal development in the first three years (based largely on Gesell).

Age*	Gross motor	Manipulation	General understanding	Speech	Sphincter control	Miscellaneous
4 weeks	Held in sitting position—may hold head up momentarily. Held in prone position with hand under abdomen, momentary tensing of neck muscles should be noted. Prone—momentarily holds chin off couch. Pulled to sit—almost complete head lag.		Watches the mother when she talks to him. Opens and closes mouth as she speaks, bobs his head, quiets. (In next two weeks or so, before smiling begins, note the duration and intensity of this reaction in assessing a child.) Supine position—regards dangling toy when it is brought into his line of vision and will follow it, but less than 90 degrees.			
6 weeks	Held in prone position with hand under abdomen—the head is held momentarily in line with the body. Prone—readily lifts chin off couch so that the plane of face is at angle of 45 degrees to couch. Pulled to sit from supine—head lag not quite complete.		Smiles momentarily when talked to by mother. (Smiling henceforward becomes more and more frequent. The frequency of smiling and the ease with which it is elicited should be noted. Supine—looks at dangling toy when it is in midline; follows it to midline when it is moved from the side. Beginning to follow moving persons with eyes.			
8 weeks	Held in sitting position—head is held up but recurrently bobs forward. Held in prone position with hand under abdomen—holds head up so that its plane is in line with that of the body. Prone—head no longer mainly turned to one side as in earlier weeks. Recurrently lifts chin off couch so that plane of face is at angle of 45 degrees to couch. Held in standing position—is able to hold head up more than momentarily.		Supine—follows dangling toy from side to point past midline. (Always note the promptness with which child sees the ring. At this age he does not usually see it immediately.)			Eyes show fixation, convergence, focussing.
12 weeks	Prone—holds chin and shoulders off couch prolongedly, so that plane of face is at angle of 45-90 degrees from couch. Bears weight on forearms. Pulled to sit from supine—only moderate head lag. Held in prone position with hand under abdomen—holds head up so that its plane is beyond that of the body.	Pulls at his dress. No more grasp reflex. Holds rattle voluntarily when it is placed in his hand; retains it more than a moment. Hands no longer tightly closed as in previous weeks, but mostly open. Desire to grasp objects seen (see next column).	Supine—follows dangling toy from one side to the other (180 degrees). Catches sight of it immediately. Not only smiles when spoken to but vocalizes with pleasure. Squeals of pleasure heard. (From now onwards it is essential to note the child's interest in what he sees. One must also note the obvious desire to grasp objects. This desire can be observed long before he can voluntarily go for them and get them. In another month his hands go forward for the object, but he misjudges the distance. By 5 months he can get the object.)			Supine—characteristically watches movements of own hands.

Continued on next page

Age*	Gross motor	Manipulation	General understanding	Speech	Sphincter control	Miscellaneous
16 weeks	Held in sitting position—holds head well up constantly. He looks actively around, but head still wobbles if examiner causes sudden movement of trunk. Curvature of back now only in lumbar region as compared with rounded back of earlier weeks. Prone—holds head and chest off couch so that plane of face is 90 degrees to couch. Weight still on forearms. Pulled to sit—only slight head lag in beginning of movement. Supine—head no longer rotated to one side as in earlier weeks.	Hands come together and he plays with his hands. He pulls his dress over his face in play. Approaches object with hands, but overshoots the mark and fails to reach it. Plays with rattle prolongedly when it is placed in his hand, and he shakes it.	General understanding becoming much more obvious. Excites when he sees toys. Shows considerable interest when he sees breast or bottle. Shows interest in strange room. Laughs aloud. Vocalizes pleasure when pulled to sitting position. Likes to be propped up in sitting position. Turns head towards a sound.			
20 weeks	Full head control. Held in sitting position—head stable when body is mildly rocked by examiner. Pulled to sit—no head lag.	Now able to grasp objects deliberately. He plays with his toys, splashes in the bath and crumples paper. (From this time onwards one must note the maturity of the grasp, the ease with which he is able to secure objects, the security with which he holds them and the size of the object which he is able to grasp. He cannot bring finger and thumb together to grasp a small object of the size of a thin piece of string till he is about 9 months old.)	Smiles at image of self in mirror. When he drops his rattle he looks to see where it has gone to.			
24 weeks	Prone—weight borne on hands with extended arms, the chest and upper part of abdomen therefore being off the couch. Pulled to sit—head lifted off couch when about to be pulled up. Hands are held out to be lifted. Sits (supported) in high chair for a few minutes. Rolls from prone to supine. Held in standing position—bears large fraction of weight.	He grasps his feet. Holds bottle. Supine—may take toes to mouth. If he has one cube in hand he drops it when second one is offered.	Smiles and vocalizes at his mirror image. When he drops the rattle he tries to recover it. May 'blow bubbles' or protrude tongue in imitation of adult. May show fear of strangers and be 'coy'. Laughs when head is hidden in towel in peep-bo game. Beginning to show likes and dislikes of foods.			
28 weeks	Prone—bears weight on one hand. Sits with hands forward for support. Rolls from supine to prone. Standing position—can maintain extension of hip and knees for short period when supported. He bounces with pleasure. (Previously he sagged at hip and knees.) Supine—spontaneously lifts head off couch.	If he has one cube in hand he retains it when second cube is offered. Transfers objects from one hand to the other. Bangs objects on the table. Now goes for objects with one hand instead of two, as he did previously. Takes all objects to mouth. Feeds self with biscuit. Loves to play with paper	Pats image of self in mirror. Responds to name. Tries to establish contact with person by cough or other noise. May imitate movement, such as tongue protrusion.	Says 'Da,' 'Ba,' 'Ka.'		Feeds well from cup. Chews and so can take solids.

Age*	Gross motor	Manipulation	General understanding	Speech	Sphincter control	Miscellaneous
32 weeks	Readily bears weight on legs when supported. Sits for a few moments unsupported.		Reaches persistently for toys out of reach. Responds to 'No.'	Combines syllables, 'Da-da,' 'Ba-ba.'		
36 weeks	Stands holding on to furniture. Sits steadily for 10 minutes. Leans forward and recovers balance. (Cannot lean sideways.) Prone—in trying to crawl may progress backwards. May progress by rolling.	Can pick up small object such as currant between finger and thumb. When he has two cubes he brings them together as if making visual comparison between them.	Puts arms in front of face to try to prevent mother washing his face. (From this age onwards note excitement when certain liked foodstuffs are seen. Note particularly degree and maintenance of concentration in getting objects and in playing with toys.)			Slobbering and mouthing beginning to decrease.
40 weeks	Pulls self to standing position. Pulls self to sitting position. Goes forward from sitting to prone, and from prone to sitting. Sits steadily without risk of falling over (except for occasional accident). Crawls, pulling self forward with hands, abdomen on couch.	Goes for objects with index finger. Beginning to release objects, letting them go deliberately instead of accidentally as before.	May pull clothes of another to attract attention. Plays 'Patacake' (clapping hands). Waves bye-bye. Pats the doll. Holds arm out for sleeve or holds foot up for sock in dressing. (From this age the understanding of words should be observed. The child can understand the meaning of perhaps a dozen words by the age of a year, though he is only able to say two or three words at that age. At 9 months he may respond to such questions as 'Where is Daddy?' 'Where is the cow?')			
44 weeks	Prone—creeps (abdomen off couch). When standing holding on he lifts and replaces one foot. Sitting—can lean over sideways.	Will place object into examiner's hand on request, but will not release it.	Covers own face with towel in peep-bo game. Drops objects deliberately in order that they will be picked up. Beginning to put objects in and out of containers. (The maturity of the release behaviour and the manipulative skill must be noted as he plays with his toys.)	Says one word with meaning.		
48 weeks	Walks sideways, holding on to furniture. Walks with two hands held. Sitting—can turn round to pick up object.	Rolls ball towards examiner. Gives and takes toy in play, releasing object into examiner's hand.	Repeats performance laughed at. Now likes repetitive play, putting one cube after another into basket, etc. Anticipates with bodily movement when nursery rhyme being told. Shows interest when shown simple pictures in book. (This interest should be carefully noted from now onwards.)			

Continued on next page

Age*	Gross motor	Manipulation	General understanding	Speech	Sphincter control	Miscellaneous
1 year	Walks with one hand held. Prone—walks on hands and feet like a bear. May shuffle on buttocks and hand.		May understand meaning of 'Where is your book?' 'Where is your shoe?' May kiss on request. (Such evidence of developing memory is important and must be noted.)	Says two or three words with meaning.		Apt to be shy. Very little mouthing of objects. Little slobbering except during concentration on an especially interesting toy.
13 months	Stands alone for a moment.	Can hold two cubes in one hand. Makes line or marks with pencil.	May kiss mirror image.			
15 months	Can get into standing position without support. Creeps upstairs. Walks without help with broad-base, high-stepping gait and steps of unequal length and direction. (The maturity of the gait must be noted from now onwards.)	Builds tower of two cubes. (This requires some accuracy in release.) Constantly throwing objects on to floor. Takes off shoes.	Asks for objects by pointing. Pats pictures and may kiss pictures of animals. Negativism beginning. Feeds self, managing cup.	Jargon.	Tells mother that he has wet pants. (First sign of sphincter control.)	
18 months	Climbs stairs unaided, holding rail. Runs. Seldom falls. No longer broad-base and high-stepping gait when walking. Seats self in chair, often by process of climbing up, standing, turning round and sitting down. Pulls toy as he walks. Throws ball without falling, as previously	Builds tower of three cubes. Manages spoon without rotating it near mouth as previously. Turns pages of book two or three at a time. Scribbles spontaneously. Takes off gloves, socks. Unzips fasteners.	Points to picture of car or dog in book. Picture Card† Points correctly to one when asked 'Where is the …?' Simple objects.‡ Names one. Points to nose, eye, hair on request. Copies mother in her domestic work— e.g. sweeping the floor, dusting. Carries out two simple orders.§		Clean and dry with only occasional accident.	Dawdling in feeding.
21 months	Walks backwards in imitation. Picks up object from floor without falling. Walks upstairs, two feet per step.	Builds towers of five or six cubes.	Pulls people to show them objects. Knows four parts of the body. Picture Card.† Points correctly to two when asked 'Where is the …?' Simple orders.§ Obeys three.	Joins two words together. Repeats things said. Asks for drink, toilet, food.		Sleeping difficulties common. Sleep rituals beginning.
2 years	Goes up and down stairs alone, two feet per step.	Builds tower of six or seven cubes. Turns pages of book singly. Turns door knobs, unscrews lid. Puts on shoes, socks, pants. Washes and dries hands.	Imitates train with cubes, without adding chimney. Imitates vertical stroke with pencil. Knows two common objects.‡ Obeys four simple orders.§ Parallel play—watches others play and plays near them, without playing with them.	Uses words. I, me, you. Talks incessantly.	Dry at night if lifted out late in evening.	

Age*	Gross motor	Manipulation	General understanding	Speech	Sphincter control	Miscellaneous
2½ years	Jumps with both feet. Walks on tiptoe when asked.	Builds tower of eight cubes. Holds pencil in hand instead of in fist.	Picture Cards.† Names three when asked 'What is this?' Identifies five when asked 'Where is the ....?' (Much can be learnt by noting the maturity of the play and the imaginativeness shown.) Imitates train with cubes, adding chimney. Imitates vertical and horizontal stroke with pencil. Repeats two digits (one out of three trials)—e.g. asked to say 'Eight—six'. Picture Cards.† Names five objects when asked 'What is this?' Identifies seven when asked 'Where is the ....?' Common objects.‡ Names three. Beginning to take interest in sex organs. Peak of negativism. Gives full name. Helps to put things away.		Attends to toilet without help, except for wiping. Climbs on to lavatory seat	Colour sense beginning.
3 years	Goes upstairs one foot per step, and downstairs two feet per step. (Goes downstairs with one foot per step at four years.) Jumps off bottom step. Stands on one foot for a few seconds. Rides tricycle.	Builds tower of nine cubes. Dresses and undresses self if helped with buttons, and advised occasionally about back and front and the right foot for the shoe. Unbuttons front buttons. Can be trusted to carry china and so to help to set the table.	Copies circle with pencil, imitates cross (copies cross at 3½, square at 4, diamond at 5.) Constantly asking questions. Knows own sex. Picture Card.† Names eight when asked 'What is this....?' (Names ten at 3½ years.) Repeats three digits (one out of three trials). (Repeats four digits in one out of three trials at 4½) Obeys two requests when asked. 'Put the ball under the chair, at the side of the chair, behind the chair, on the chair.' (Obeys four at 4 years.) Knows some nursery rhymes. May count up to 10. Now joins children in play. Dresses and undresses doll. Beginning to draw objects spontaneously (e.g. a man), or on request. Cubes. Imitates building bridge of three cubes.			

§ 'Take it to mother', 'Put it on the chair', 'Bring it to me', 'Put it on the table'. Copying a circle implies copying a representation of a circle on a card given by the examiner. When a child 'imitates' a circle he draws one after seeing the examiner do it.

* For mature babies; due allowance to be made for prematurity.
† Two cards showing dog, cup, house, shoe, flag, clock, star, leaf, basket, book.
‡ Penny, shoe, pencil, knife, ball.

Reprinted from *The Normal Child*, 6th edition, Ronald S. Illingworth, Copyright 1975, Churchill Livingstone.

LANGUAGE DEVELOPMENT

The methods by which a child learns to use language are very poorly understood; however, the sequence of language development and the relationship of cerebral hemispheric dominance to that development are well known. The table below lists the stages of language development along with corresponding central nervous system lateralization and maturation at those stages.

Language Development, CNS Maturation and Lateralization

AGE	USUAL LANGUAGE DEVELOPMENT	EFFECTS OF ACQUIRED, LATERALIZED LESIONS	PHYSICAL MATURATION OF CNS	LATERALIZATION OF FUNCTION	EQUIPOTENTIALITY OF HEMISPHERES	EXPLANATION
Months						
0–3	Emergence of cooing	No effect on onset of language in half of all cases; other half has delayed onset but normal development	About 60 to 70% of developmental course accomplished	None: symptoms and prognosis identical for either hemisphere	Perfect equipotentiality	Neuroanatomic and physiologic prerequisites become established
4–20	From babbling to words					
21–36	Acquisition of language	All language accomplishments disappear; language is reacquired with repetition of all stages	Rate of maturation slowed down	Hand preference emerges	Right hemisphere can easily adopt sole responsibility for language	Language appears to involve entire brain; little cortical specialization with regard to language, although left hemisphere beginning to become dominant toward end of this period
Years						
3–10	Some grammatical refinement; expansion of vocabulary	Emergence of aphasic symptoms; disorders tend to recover without residual language deficits (except in reading and writing).	Very slow completion of maturational processes	Cerebral dominance established between 3 and 5 years, but evidence that right hemisphere may often still be involved in	In cases where language is already predominantly localized in left hemisphere and aphasia ensues with left lesion, it is pos-	A process of physiologic organization takes place in which functional lateralization of language to left is predominant. "Physiologic redundancy"

	During recovery period, two processes active: diminishing aphasic interference and further acquisition of language		sible to reestablish language, presumably by reactivating language functions in right hemisphere
11–14	Accents characteristic to region or country emerge	Some aphasic symptoms become irreversible (particularly when acquired lesion was traumatic)	An asymptote is reached on almost all parameters. Exceptions are myelinization and EEG spectrum	speech and language functions. About one-fourth of early childhood aphasias due to right hemisphere lesions	Marked signs of reduction in equipotentiality	is gradually reduced, and polarization of activities between right and left hemisphere is established. As long as maturational processes have not stopped, reorganization is still possible
Midteens to Adulthood	Acquisition of second language becomes increasingly difficult	Symptoms present 3 to 5 months postinsult are irreversible	None	Apparently firmly established, but definitive statistics not available	None for language	Language markedly lateralized, and internal organization established irreversibly for life. Language-free parts of brain cannot take over except where lateralization is incomplete or had been blocked by pathologic conditions during childhood
				In about 97% of the entire population, language is definitely lateralized to the left		

Reprinted by permission of W.B. Saunders Co. from *The Whole Pediatrician Catalog*, McMillan, Nieburg and Oski, © 1977, W.B. Saunders Co.

Typical Accidents Related to Developmental Level

Behavioral characteristics	Type of accident	Preventive measures
Infant		
Increasing acquisition of mobility such as ability to squirm, roll over, creep, crawl, and pull self erect	Falls	Do not leave infant alone on tables, etc., from which the infant can fall
		Keep crib sides raised
		Keep stairs fenced
Exploration of environment with touch, movement (locomotion), taste	Aspiration or ingestion of foreign objects	Do not give small items to infant
		Check items carefully for removable parts
Oral stage of development; placing anything and everything in mouth	Poisoning	Do not feed small solid items, such as peanuts, whole-kernel corn, etc.
		Keep harmful substances out of reach
Reaching for items such as an appliance cord, table cover	Burns	Keep hot items out of reach
		Keep handles of pans on stove out of reach
Placing objects into openings		Cover electrical outlets
Helpless in water	Drowning	Do not leave alone in tub or water or near a pool, lake, or stream when able to crawl or creep
Toddler		
Increased mobility with upright posture	Falls	Provide adequate supervision
Unaware of danger	Burns	Place gate at head of stairs
Climbing with ease	Drowning	Place screens on windows
Navigation of stairways	Motor vehicle accidents	Keep in enclosed space when outdoors and/or not in company of adult
Curious	Pedestrian	
Imitative	Passenger	Place handles of pots and pans on stove out of reach and containers of hot foods away from table
Placing almost anything in mouth	Ingestion and/or aspiration of harmful substances or items	
Almost helpless in water		
Investigation of drawers and cupboards		Keep harmful substances (medicines, cleaners) and items (scissors) out of reach
	Suffocation	Avoid demonstrating unsafe behaviors
		Cover unused electrical outlets; keep cords out of reach
		Use safety belt or selected infant car seats
		Examine toys for presence of safety
		Protect from water in tub, pool, or other area
		Purchase fire-retardant clothing
		Make certain any enclosed container large enough to hold child has airway or is unable to be tightly closed (for example, discarded refrigerator)
Preschooler		
Ability to open doors	Falls	Keep doors locked if danger of falls
Running and climbing with ease	Drowning	Place screen guards on windows
Investigation of drawers, cupboards, closets	Ingestion or aspiration of harmful substances or items	Teach safety: watch out for automobiles in driveways and streets, play in approved areas
Riding tricycle		Keep harmful items (knifes, medicines, electrical equipment) out of reach
Playing with mechanical gadgets	Burns	
Ability to throw	Motor vehicle accidents	Teach swimming and water safety
	Pedestrian	Examine toys for safety
	Passenger	Keep firearms locked up
		Provide safe play equipment for use
		Caution against talking to strangers
		Teach safety with matches, lighters, etc.
School-age child		
Daring and adventurous	Falls	Teach safety rules for pedestrians, bicycles, skateboarding, and sports activities
Increased motor skills	Sports injuries	
Playing in hazardous places	Drowning	Encourage playing in safe places
Need for strenuous physical activity	Burns	Teach swimming and water safety
Need for peer approval	Motor vehicle accidents	Keep firearms safely locked up except during adult supervision
Attempting hazardous feats	Pedestrian	
Accompanying peers to hazardous facilities	Passenger	Teach safety with fires, matches, lighters, barbecues, bonfires
	Bicycle	
		Provide safe sports and other equipment and teach their proper use
		Provide facilities for supervised recreation

Behavioral characteristics	Type of accident	Preventive measures
Adolescent Strong need for peer approval may lead to attempting hazardous feats Increased strength and agility Age permitted to drive automobile	Motor vehicle accidents 　Pedestrian 　Passenger 　Driver Drowning Suicide Poisoning (drug abuse)	Teach motor vehicle safety; provide supervised instruction Provide safe recreational facilities Teach safe use of sports equipment Instruct in safe use of firearms Recognize signs of depression Educate regarding hazards of drug abuse

Reprinted by permission of The C.V. Mosby Co. from *Nursing Care of Infants and Children*, by Lucille Whaley and Donna Wong, © 1979, The C.V. Mosby Co., St. Louis.

Immunizations

RECOMMENDED SCHEDULE FOR ACTIVE IMMUNIZATION OF NORMAL INFANTS AND CHILDREN

2 mo	DTP[1]	TOPV[2]
4 mo	DTP	TOPV
6 mo	DTP	TOPV
1 yr	Measles[3] Rubella[3]	Tuberculin Test[4] (Mumps[3])
1½ yr	DTP	TOPV
4–6 yr	DTP	TOPV
14–16 yr	Td[5]	and thereafter every 10 years

[1] DTP. Diphtheria and tetanus toxoids conbined with pertussis vaccine.

[2] TOPV. Trivalent oral polio virus vaccine. This recommendation is suitable for breast-fed as well as bottle-fed infants.

[3] May be given at 1 year as measles-rubella or measles-mumps-rubella combined vaccines. See Rubella, p. 661, and Mumps, p. 681 for further discussion of age of administration.

[4] Frequency of repeated tuberculin tests depends on risk of exposure of the child and on the prevalence of tuberculosis in the population group. The initial one should be at the time of, or preceding, the measles immunization.

[5] Td. Combined tetanus and diphtheria toxoids (adult type) for those over 6 years of age in contrast to diphtheria and tetanus (DT) containing a larger amount of diphtheria antigen. Tetanus toxoid at time of injury: For clean, minor wounds, no booster dose is needed by a fully immunized child unless more than 10 years have elapsed since the last dose. For contaminated wounds, a booster dose should be given if more than 5 years have elapsed since the last dose.

Reprinted with permission from Vaughan and McKay, *Nelson Textbook of Pediatrics*, 10th edition, p. 211. © 1975, W.B. Saunders Company, Philadelphia.

Contraindications to Immunizations

Inactivated vaccines	Attenuated vaccines
Febrile illness	Febrile illness
Intercurrent infections	Intercurrent infections
Specific contraindication to pertussis and DPT	Eczema (e.g. smallpox, BCG)
	Immune deficiency
'Over-immunization' with tetanus toxoid	Corticosteroid and/or immunosuppressive therapy (e.g. drugs, radiotherapy)
Allergy to egg protein (e.g. influenza vaccine)	Malignant conditions such as leukaemia
	Pregnancy
	Allergy to egg protein (e.g. measles vaccine)
	BCG in tuberculin positive patients

Reprinted by permission of Churchill Livingstone from *Recent Advances in Paediatrics,* Number 5, David Hull, editor, Copyright 1976, Churchill Livingstone.

Incubation Period and Duration of Infectivity of Common Infectious Diseases

Disease	Incubation period (days)	Period of infectivity
Chickenpox	15–18	1 day before rash to 6 days after start of rash.
Diphtheria } Scarlet fever	2–5	Till swabs negative.
Enteric group	7–21 (especially 14)	2 days before symptoms, till stools and urine negative.
Measles	10–15	5–6 days before rash till 5 days after temperature becomes normal.
Mumps	12–26 (especially 18)	2 days before swelling, till swelling has subsided.
Poliomyelitis	4–30 (especially 7–14)	3 days before symptoms start to 2 weeks after onset if temperature is normal
Rubella	10–21 (especially 18)	1 day before rash till 2 days after start of rash.
Whooping cough	7–10	2 days before start, 5 weeks after start.
Glandular fever	33–49 days	Uncertain.

Reprinted by permission of Churchill Livingstone Publishers from *The Normal Child,* 6th edition, Ronald S. Illingworth, Copyright 1975, Churchill Livingstone Publishers.

Preventive Dental Practices for Children

Bethea Brost, R.N., B.S.N.

Despite efforts in the past two decades, tooth decay is still the most prevalent health problem in the United States. Preventive dental practices in the child population must be implemented in order to insure healthy adult dentition in the future. Although dental caries is not life threatening, the associated pain, infection, disfigurement, speech and mastication problems, and expense cannot be overlooked.

If prevention of dental disease in the child population is to be attained, oral health habits must start at birth through parent directives. To be effective teachers in this area, parents must be aware of the environmental protection, dietary control, and personal hygiene needs for healthy dentition. The nurse in any pediatric setting has the ideal opportunity to impart this preventive dental information to parents and children.

The Carious Process

Dental caries is a bacterial disease but is influenced by many factors. Calcified structures are broken down by organic acids released from microflora during the fermentation of carbohydrates. In order for caries to develop, the host, microflora, and substrate must all co-exist for a period of time (Keyes, P., 1968).

Prevention Of Dental Caries: Nutritional Aspects

The carious process requires the presence of carbohydrate substance on the enamel surface of the tooth. The frequency, rather than the quantity, of eating foods containing sugar, especially sucrose, has a bearing on tooth decay (Andlaw, 1977; Colman, 1976; Grenvy, 1976; Mizel, 1977).

The "nursing bottle syndrome" is a frequently observed problem in three- and four-year-old children who have used the bottle as a pacifier at bedtime. The pooling of the sweetened liquids from the bottle causes rapid decay of the upper deciduous teeth and lower molars. This painful and unattractive phenomenon can be prevented by simply making parents aware of the problem. Placque must be removed by gauze or toothbrush and only water should be offered in the bottle at bedtime.

Parental counseling by the nurse should point out the snack foods recommended by the American Dental Association, including fresh fruit, vegetables, nuts, cheese, popcorn, milk, sugarless candy and gum, and pretzels. Sweets should be limited to meal times, and, as previously mentioned, parents should be aware of the fact that the frequency of snacks is more destructive than the quantity. "Cleansing foods" such as raw fruits and vegetables should be encouraged because of the mechanical removal of foodstuffs and the stimulation of the saliva flow (Fomon and Wei, 1977; Moss, 1977; Nizel, 1977; Slattery, 1976).

Cleansing Infants' And Preschoolers' Teeth

Professional dental supervision should be implemented by eighteen months to three years of age and should be repeated at intervals of six months until adolescence (Hildes, 1967; Fomon et al, 1976; Moss, 1977; Slattery, 1976).

Dental hygiene should begin with the eruption of the first teeth. Soft cotton or gauze can be used initially to cleanse the teeth (Moss, 1977; Slattery, 1976). By about eighteen months of age, a soft or medium toothbrush can be introduced. Children should have the opportunity to brush their own teeth followed by parental inspection and brushing. The prime times for brushing should be after breakfast, before bedtime, and, if possible, following snacks (Moss, 1977).

Fluoride

The use of fluoride in the prevention of dental caries has proven to reduce such lesions by 40 to 80 percent (Grenby, 1976; Fomon et al, 1976; Hiles, 1976; Nizel, 1977). Fluoride supplements should be prescribed to families if their local water supply contains less than 1 ppm. This is very important during the first thirteen years to aid the enamel's resistance to caries (Nizel, 1977). Approximately 50 percent of the United States population still has non-fluoridated water. In such areas, a school-based fluoride mouthrinsing program has much potential (Leske, 1977), yet parents must be made aware of their children's fluoride needs prior to the school years.

In conclusion, the nurse caring for children in any setting must be aware of these preventive dental practices. They can be taught in both individual or group approaches. This practice will not only contribute to the overall effort to eradicate tooth decay, but will contribute to the comprehensive health care of the population.

Bibliography

Andlaw, R. Diet and dental caries ... a review. *Journal Of Human Nutrition,* 1977, 31, 45–52.

Fomon, S., and Wei, S. Prevention of dental caries. *Nutritional Disorders Of Children* (U.S. Public Health Service Publication No. 76-5612).

Grenby, T. Dental decay and sugary foods. *Nursing Mirror,* 1976, 143 (29), 46–51.

Hildes, L. Preventive dentistry and the child patient. *Preventive Medicine,* 1976, 5, 393–399.

Keyes, P. Etiologic factors of dental caries. *Medical Annual Of The District Of Columbia,* 1968, 34, 463–467.

Leske, G., and Ripa, L. Guidelines for establishing a fluoride mouthrinsing caries prevention program for school children. *Public Health Reports,* 1977, 92(3), 240–244.

Moss, S. *Your Child's Teeth,* Boston: Houghton Mifflin, 1977.

Nizel, A. Preventing dental caries: the nutritional factors. *Symposium On Nutrition In Pediatrics,* 1977, 24(1), 141–155.

Slattery, J., "Dental Health in Children" in *American Journal of Nursing,* July, 1976, Vol. 76, p. 1159–1161.

Children in Hospitals

Statements Of Policy For The Care Of Children And Familes In Health Care Settings

ASSOCIATION FOR THE CARE OF CHILDREN IN HOSPITALS

Preamble

Advancement of technology and medical science has permitted more children to live, to live longer and in most cases, to live more fully. In the process, other dangers to children's healthy development have arisen or come to

Continued on next page

light. These problems have in turn stimulated the current progress in the behavioral sciences.

Threats posed to the emotional security and development of many children and their families by serious illness, disability, disfigurement, treatment, interrupted human relationships and nonsupportive environments have been clearly demonstrated by worldwide research studies. The outcomes can range from temporary but frequently overwhelming anxiety and emotional suffering to long-standing or permanent developmental handicaps. Such interference with the fullest possible development and expression of individual potential is an unacceptable price to pay.

Closer contact with the emotional life of children, increased parent involvement and communication amongst professionals have also contributed to greater understanding as well as to improvements of care. Whereas there is still much to learn regarding the inter-relatedness of such factors as age, type of illness, length of hospitalization, critical developmental periods and vulnerability, sufficent knowledge now exists to direct action toward both minimizing and preventing such harm.

The Association for the Care of Children in Hospitals endorses the following policies:

All pediatric health care settings should:

1. Have a stated philosophy of care which is specific, easily understood by, and made available to patients and families, and which applies in a coordinated manner to all disciplines and departments.

2. Assist or provide programs of prevention and restorative care which respond to emotional, social and environmental causal factors of accidents and illness.

3. Create and maintain a social and physical environment which is as welcoming, unthreatening and supportive as possible, and which fosters open communication, encourages human relationships, and invites involvement of children, their families and the community in decisions affecting their care.

4. Avoid hospitalizing children whenever possible through the development of alternatives.

5. Develop and utilize ambulatory, day and home care programs which are financially and geographically accessible.

6. Minimize the duration of unavoidable hospital stays, while recognizing discharge planning needs.

7. Provide for and encourage the presence and participation in the hospital of persons most significant to the child, to approximate supportive home patterns of interactions and routines.

8. Provide consistent, emotionally supportive nurturing care for young children during the absence of their parents.

9. Respect the unique care-taking role of parents as well as their individual responses, and provide ongoing understandable information and support which will enable them to utilize their strengths in supporting their child.

10. Provide a milieu which is responsive to the uniqueness of each child and adolescent, their ethnic and cultural backgrounds and developmental needs.

11. Provide readily accessible, well designed space, equipment and programs for the wide range of play, educational and social activities which are essential to all children and adolescents, particularly those who have been deprived of normal opportunities for development.

12. Provide child care professionals who are skilled at assessing emotional, developmental and academic needs, communicating with and fostering the involvement of patients and their families in activities appropriate to their needs.

13. Ensure that children and their parents are informed, understand and are supported prior to, during, and following experiences which are potentially distressing.

14. Carefully select all staff and volunteers according to their commitment to the foregoing policies. Those in direct contact, however limited, with children, youth, and families should be sensitive, perceptive and compassionate. Professionals involved in more extended, intimate and responsible positions of child care should have special training in child development, family dynamics and the unique psychological needs of children when ill and under stress.

Continued on next page

15. Facilitate orientation, continued learning, and consultation in relation to all of the above, and provide support which recognizes the emotional demands on staff.

16. Encourage and foster the inclusion of the above educational focus in the basic curriculum and field experiences of the various professional and technical personnel preparing for careers in pediatric settings.

17. Support the evolvement of resources for early detection, and of attitudes and facilities for ongoing care of children with health and/or developmental problems.

18. Provide for ongoing evaluation of policies and programs by the recipients of care and staff at all levels.

19. Support and disseminate research which clarifies and pertains to the above.

20. Promote education within the community about the health and developmental needs of children.

Reprinted by permission of the Association for the Care of Children in Hospitals, 3615 Wisconsin Ave., N.W., Washington, D.C. 20016.

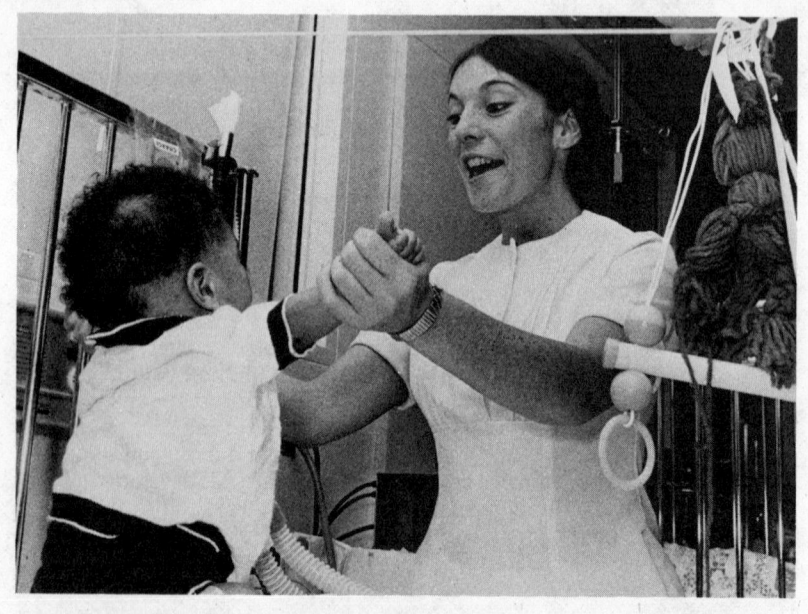

This picture is reprinted with permission of the publisher of *Pediatric Nursing*, Vol. 4, No. 5, September/October, 1978, from "Developmental Nursing Care: Infant Stimulation for High Risk Children," by Lynn Czarniecki, R.N., M.S.N.

A Child's Letter

The following letter serves as a poignant reminder of the needs and feelings of hospitalized children:

Dear Doctor:

Richard was a 10 year old leukemic child who died in April or May this year at the _____ hospital. I am estimating when I say that Richard lived one year after diagnosis and, again estimating, spent six months of that year hospitalized.

Richard was in a private room and everyone entering the room used masking precautions. His parents visited daily for most of the day. As far as I know there were no conversations with Richard or his parents and the nursing staff concerning his diagnosis or prognosis.

When Richard died, the nursing staff found the enclosed composition in his bedside stand. It has been very inspirational for the pediatric staff at our hospital.

Reasons Why You Should Send Me Home

1. I could get some sleep.
2. I could exercise more.
3. I would eat better.
4. I could go outside when I want to.
5. I'd be a lot happier.
6. I wouldn't be stuffed up in one room.
7. I could get better quicker.
8. I'd be comfortable.
9. I could help around the house.
10. I wouldn't be bored.
11. I'd make my mother happier by showing her I'm eating.
12. I'd be with my family.
13. I could get more fresh air.
14. It would be peaceful and quiet.
15. I wouldn't get any shots.
16. I could talk and see my mother and father before 11:00 A.M.
17. I could stay up later in the night.
18. I wouldn't be such a grouch.
19. I wouldn't be laying down all day.
20. I could go to sleep in *my own bed*.
21. I could build up my muscles.
22. I could get out of bed when I want to.
23. I wouldn't be in the hospital.
24. I could play all different games and stuff.
25. I could watch color TV instead of black and white TV.
26. It's Spring.

Ricky

Reprinted by permission of W.B. Saunders Co. from *The Whole Pediatrician Catalog*, McMillan, Nieburg and Oski, Copyright © 1977, W.B. Saunders Co.

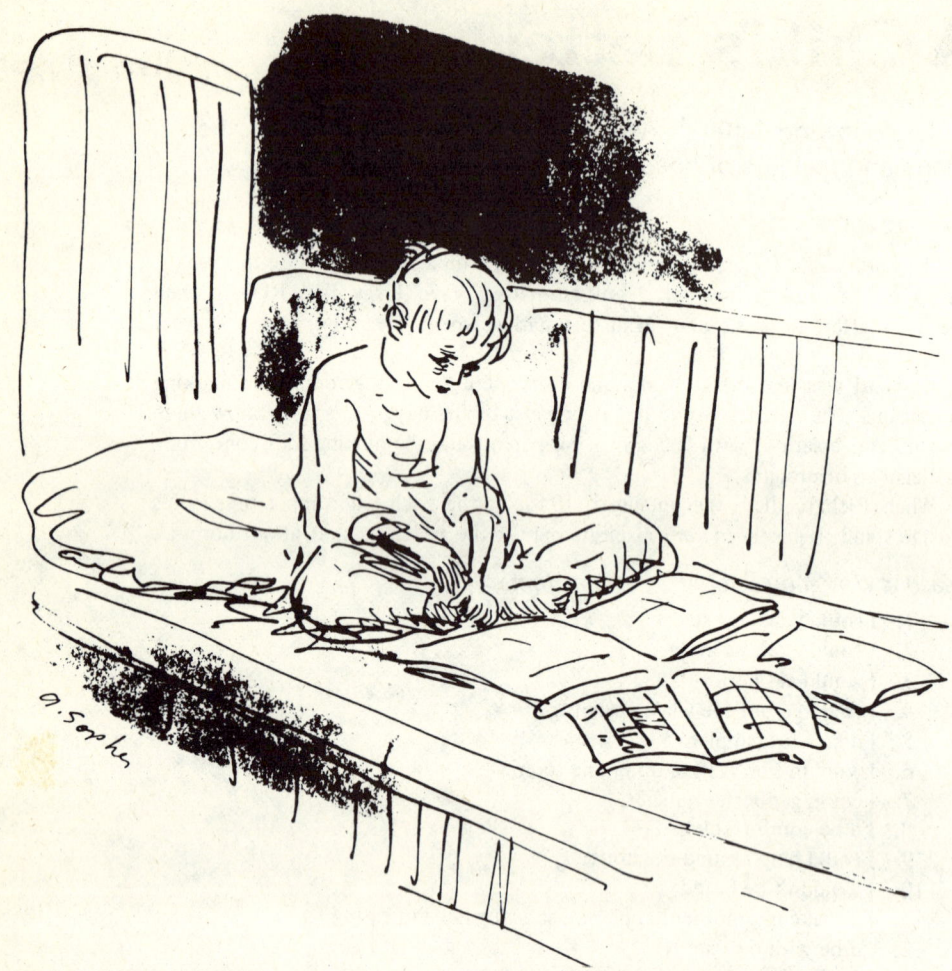

Reprinted by permission of The Johns Hopkins Press from *The Hospitalized Child and His Family* edited by J. Alex Haller, Jr., James L. Talbert, Robert H. Dombro, Copyright 1967, The Johns Hopkins Press, Baltimore.

A Guide to the Development of Nursing Approach

Level of Development	*Effect of Hospital Environment*	*Nursing Approach*
FIRST YEAR The infant is relaxed. He coos and smiles. Frustration initiates aggressive responses.	If the infant is improperly fed, restrained, or hurt, increasingly vigorous activity will be observed. If the nurse responds to the infant's aggressive action, no distress will result. However, if	Capacity for memory and anticipation begins in the first few months of life. Thus early experiences influence the reaction to later experiences and affect psychological growth and develop-

Level of Development	Effect of Hospital Environment	Nursing Approach
	frustration and tension continue and increase, behavior will take on a destructive quality. If the child is at an age where he cannot direct his aggression to solve his needs, aggression will be expressed internally and may be manifested by later psychological disturbances.	ment. The nursing approach should strive to reduce tensions in the infant to tolerable limits. Do not allow him to cry for prolonged periods of time, without providing comfort and attempting to meet his needs. The use of a pacifier may be one method of meeting the needs of a young infant on parenteral feedings.
The need for emotional satisfaction is present in every infant from birth.	During family separation it is essential that a mother-infant relationship be established and maintained. A mother-substitute should be provided when the natural mother cannot participate in the care of the child (especially if the child is on mechanical monitors).	Cuddling, rocking, handling, bathing, and talking to the infant are important aspects of nursing care. Using visiting hours constructively and including mothers in the nursing care plan for the infant can meet these needs.
The sense of trust must the mastered during this stage of development.	The infant should not be made to feel "abandoned" in the hospital setting.	The nurse should spend time with the child and develop rapport with him in situations other than therapeutic activities so that the child will not develop a feeling of abandonment or loneliness.
PRESCHOOL The child increases his ability to understand and exercise self-control. Play and trial-acting are forerunners of thinking. Value judgments of right and wrong begin to develop.	The small child needs repeated explanations of limits in his new environment in order to prevent accidents. Increased demands and restraints can precipitate anger, rebellion, and aggression.	The child should be allowed to accept some responsibility for his own care in order to give him a sense of accomplishment. Judicious use of approval and disapproval is essential. Many therapeutic procedures can be presented in the form of play. The child should be encouraged to "play-out" and express his reaction to his experiences.
SCHOOL AGE Maturation of the central nervous system increases the child's ability to coordinate movements. Male-female identity emerges. A greater intellectual capacity emerges.	The hospital environment may precipitate feelings of inadequacy. The child should be adequately prepared for therapeutic experiences in an honest and clear manner.	The child should be encouraged to carry out everyday activities and participate in the procedures necessary in his treatment. Questions should be elicited and answered honestly. Children of the same sex should be grouped together.
ADOLESCENT A change in body configuration occurs with appearance of secondary sexual characteristics. Capacity for abstract thinking and reasoning develops to a keen level.	The adolescent is easily frustrated in a restrictive hospital setting. Emotional instability which may be evidenced should invite understanding rather than punishment in the hospital setting. An adolescent should be placed near children of his own age whenever possible.	Privacy is essential for the adolescent patient. The adolescent should be given greater responsibility for his care, but too much should not be expected of him. Rebellious or aggressive outbursts should be constructively diverted. It is desirable to provide some occupational therapy.

Reprinted by permission of W.B. Saunders Co. from *Principles and Techniques in Pediatric Nursing*, 3rd ed., Gloria Leifer, © 1977, W.B. Saunders Co.

PREFERRED INTRAMUSCULAR INJECTION SITE
for older children

GLUTEUS MEDIUS

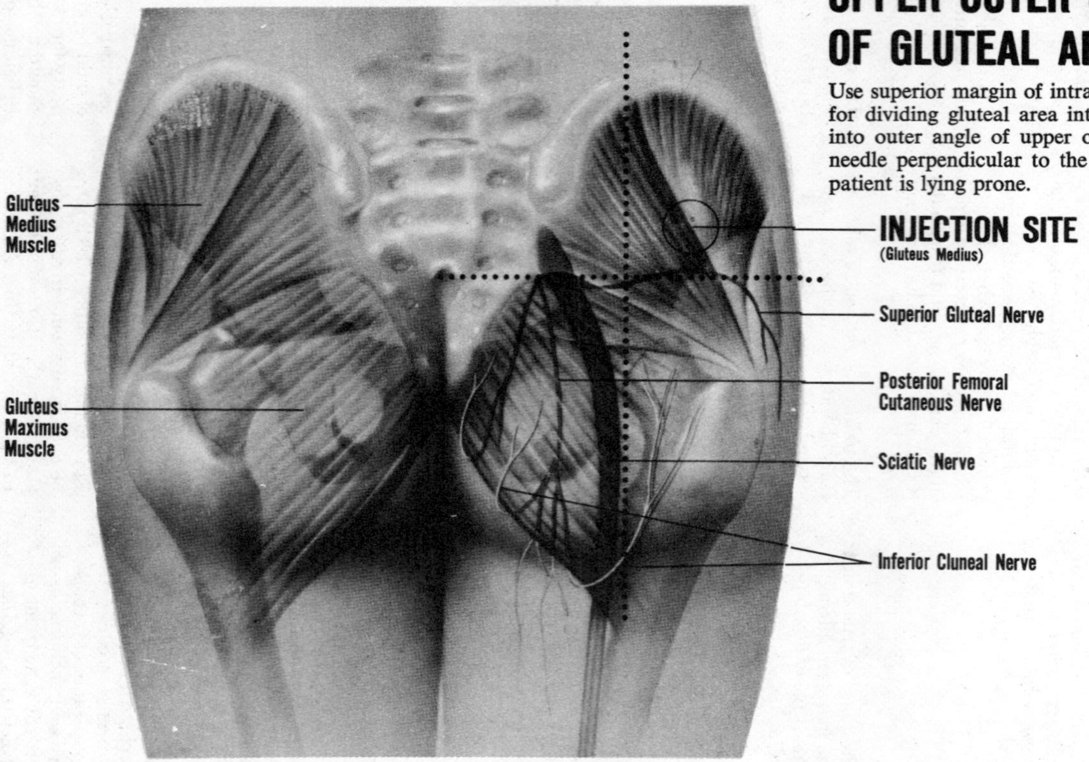

UPPER OUTER QUADRANT OF GLUTEAL AREA

Use superior margin of intragluteal fold as landmark for dividing gluteal area into four quadrants. Inject into outer angle of upper outer quadrant, directing needle perpendicular to the surface upon which the patient is lying prone.

- INJECTION SITE (Gluteus Medius)
- Superior Gluteal Nerve
- Posterior Femoral Cutaneous Nerve
- Sciatic Nerve
- Inferior Cluneal Nerve
- Gluteus Medius Muscle
- Gluteus Maximus Muscle

PREFERRED INTRAMUSCULAR INJECTION SITES
for premature and newborn infants

Midanterior Muscle of Thigh
Inject into middle 1/3 of anterior thigh.

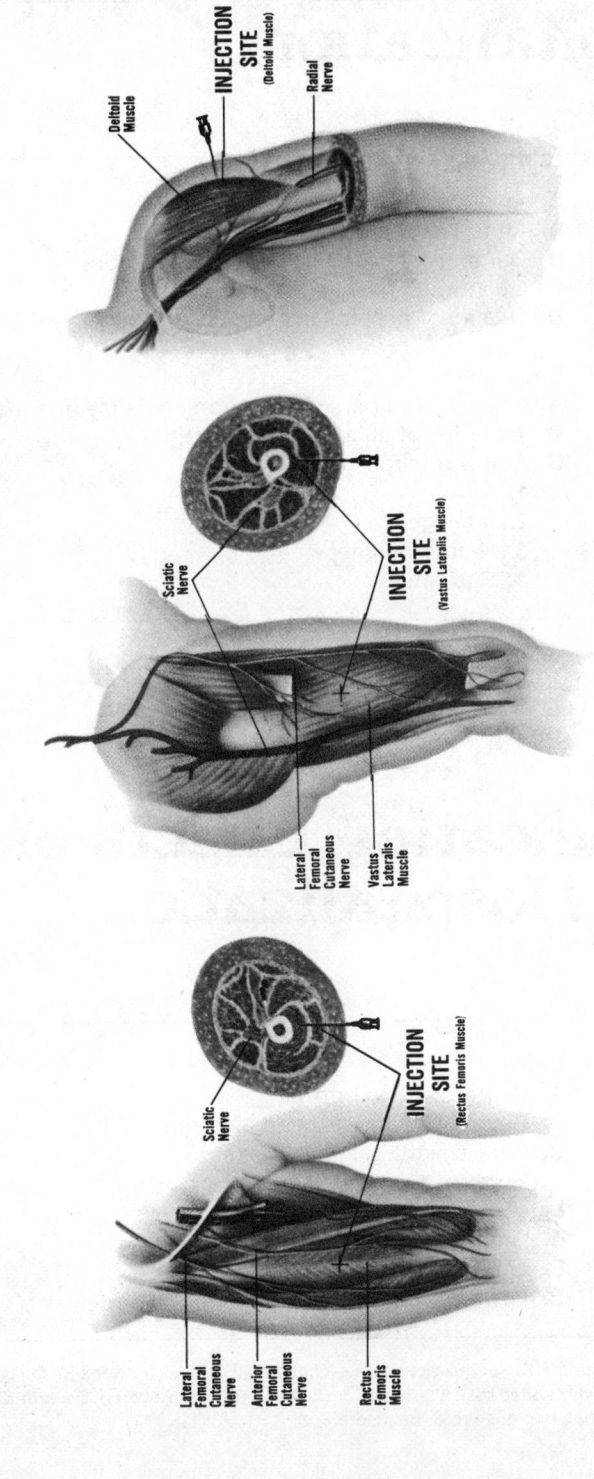

Midlateral Muscle of Thigh
Inject into middle 1/3 of lateral thigh, anterior to the femur.

Deltoid Muscle
Inject between the upper and lower portions of the deltoid muscle.

Nursing Inservice Aid, © 1965, Roso Laboratories, Columbus, Ohio, reprinted by permission.

Factors Affecting Adjustment (To Hospitalization)

> I. Exogenous
>   A. Attitudes of parents
>   B. Duration of hospitalization (deprivation)
>   C. Quantity of hospital experiences
>   D. Quality of hospital experiences
>
> II. Endogenous
>   A. Physical and personality characteristics (feedback)
>   B. Attitudes of child (preparation)
>   C. Ability to cope
>   1. Age
>   2. Intelligence
>   3. Nature of illness
>   4. Resilence

Signs Indicating Effects of Chronic Hospitalization

> I. Early
>   A. Depression, withdrawal
>   B. Repetitive activity (head banging, etc.)
>   C. Poor weight gain, listlessness
>
> II. Late
>   A. Limited affection
>   B. Limited abstract thinking(?)
>   C. Lowered I.Q.(?)

Reprinted by permission of The Johns Hopkins Press from *The Hospitalized Child and His Family* edited by J. Alex Haller, Jr., James L. Talbert, Robert H. Dombro, Copyright 1967, The Johns Hopkins Press, Baltimore.

Pediatric Psychological Checklist for Surgery	
Patient's Name: **Unit #:** **Rm #:** **Service:**	**Directions:** 1. The following items will be covered before surgery or procedures. 2. All explanations will include parents or some other responsible person(s). 3. All explanations will consider the child's developmental level.

ITEM	INITIAL
1. Explain operation or procedure. Have patient verbalize understanding.	
2. Explain and get return demonstration of coughing, deep breathing, and using blow bottles. Emphasize importance and rationale.	
3. Explain dietary limitations, if any.	
4. Explain postoperative use of equipment, bandages, tubes, restraints. Use pictures if they are necessary.	
5. Inform child of preoperative injections. Be honest. It will hurt.	
6. Explain about the "stretcher man" who wears green and will take the child to the operating room on a stretcher. Explain that O.R. personnel also wear green suits and that someone will be with the child at all times. Allow the child to play with O.R. hats, masks, gloves, etc.	
7. Let child know that parent will wait closeby for his return.	
8. Explain about the "special sleep" (anesthesia) for the operation or procedure and the method of inducing it. Emphasize that the doctor will wake the child up only when the operation is over. For those seven years old and younger anesthesia is administered via face mask. Let child play with demonstration mask. For those 8 years and older intravenous medication is used.	
9. Explain about the recovery room and how the child will stay there until awake. Emphasize that the child will be cared for by special nurses in green.	

Continued on next page

10. Allow child to select gift from the Toy Chest.	
11. Answer questions.	
Comments: _____ _____ _____	

Copyright 1978, Amer J Nursing Co., Reprinted with permission from "Pediatric Psychological Checklist for Surgery" by Dina Treloarn, in MCN, The American Journal of Maternal Child Nursing, Jan-Feb 1978, Vol 3, No. 1

Pediatric Resuscitation Kit: Recommended Contents

Airway equipment

1. Bag and masks (infant, child, adult) with nonrebreathing valve that has universal 15-mm female adaptor for male 15-mm endotracheal tube connectors
2. Oropharyngeal airways (Guedel sizes 0, 1, 2, 3, 4)
3. Orotracheal tubes (complete sterile set with connectors) (see Table 5–22)
4. Aspiration equipment:
   Metal tonsil suction tip
   Disposable sterile plastic suction catheters sizes (Fr.) 5, 8, 10, 14
5. Laryngoscope:
   Standard handle
   Blades: Miller—newborn
           Wis-Forreger—1½
           Flagg—child
           Macintosh—adult (no. 3)
   2 extra batteries
   1 extra light bulb for each blade

Drugs

Sodium bicarbonate	1 mEq/ml	4 50-ml vials
Epinephrine	1 mg/ml	4 1-ml vials
Isoproterenol	0.2 mg/ml	2 2-ml vials
Calcium chloride	100 mg/ml (10%)	2 10-ml vials
Dextrose	500 mg/ml (50%)	1 20-ml vial
Pentobarbital	50 mg/ml	1 30-ml vial
Heparin	1000 u/ml	1 10-ml vial
Saline (for dilution)	0.9%	2 30-ml vials

Miscellaneous

Intracardiac needles: 20- and 22-gauge, 6–8 cm. length
Syringes (plastic disposable): 2, 5, 10 ml, 2 each
Needles: 3 each, 18-, 20-, 22-, 25-gauge regular
        2 each, 19-, 21-, 23-, 25-gauge scalp vein

Other:

Tongue blades
Sterile 4 × 4 gauze sponges
Alcohol swabs (packaged individually)
Sterile hemostat
Sterile scissors

Reprinted by permission of W.B. Saunders Co. from *Nelson Textbook of Pediatrics*, 10th ed., Vaughan and McKay, © 1975, W.B. Saunders Co.

Observations of the Neonate

Optimal outcomes are basically dependent on constant scrutiny of infants by personnel rather than by gadgets. The crucial factors listed here are direct observations that can be made only by well-trained nurses. *None of them is detectable by monitors:*

1. Acceptance of feedings; course of weight gain
2. Early detection of regurgitation to prevent aspiration of vomitus
3. Abdominal distention; frequency and character of stools
4. Changes in activity (lethargy, convulsive phenomena, hyperactivity)
5. Jaundice
6. Pallor and early cyanosis
7. Skin lesions that indicate infection
8. Deviations from prescribed volumes of intravenous infusions
9. Edema
10. Respiratory distress characterized by tachypnea, retractions, flaring of alae nasi, and grunting
11. Quality of breath sounds
12. Character and location of heart sounds

From Korones, Sheldon B.: *High-risk newborn infants,* 2nd ed., St. Louis, 1976. The C.V. Mosby Co. Reprinted with permission.

Reflexes of Neonates

REFLEX	AGE AT WHICH REFLEX USUALLY APPEARS	AGE AT WHICH REFLEX IS NORMALLY NO LONGER OBTAINABLE
Moro	Birth	3 months
Stepping	Birth	6 weeks
Placing	Birth	6 weeks
Tonic neck	2 months	6 months
Neck righting	4–6 months	24 months
Landau	3 months	24 months
Parachute reaction	9 months	Persists
Sucking and rooting	Birth	4 months awake 7 months asleep
Palmar grasp	Birth	6 months
Plantar grasp	Birth	10 months
Adductor spread of knee jerk	Birth	7 months

Reprinted by permission of W.B. Saunders Co. from *Nelson Textbook of Pediatrics,* 10th edition, Vaughan and McKay, Copyright 1975, W.B. Saunders Co.

Physical Observation and Appraisal of the Newborn

Full-term Underweight Newborn

1. Infant appears long and skinny.
2. Head circumference is normal.
3. Each hair on head is distinct and separate.
4. Skin is dry, flaky, wrinkled.
5. Cartilage of external ear is rigid, less pliable.
6. Breast has palpable nodule, with erect nipple.
7. Lies with arms and legs drawn up to fetal position; elbows and knees elevated from mattress; head in line with trunk.
8. Testes descended; rugal folds and pigmentation of scrotal sac is present.
9. Labia major covers labia minora.

Premature Newborn

1. Infant has large trunk and short-appearing extremities.
2. Head circumference is less than normal.
3. Hair on head is fuzzy—tends to clump together.
4. Skin is transparent, less wrinkled.
5. Cartilage of external ear is soft, pliable.
6. No palpable nodule of breast tissue. Nipple is identifiable.
7. Lies flat in frog-like position with shoulders, elbows, and knees touching mattress and head turned to one side.
8. Testes undescended; rugal folds and pigmentation of scrotal sac are absent.
9. Labia major open and gaping.

Reprinted by permission of W.B. Saunders Co., from *Principles and Techniques in Pediatric Nursing,* 3rd edition, Gloria Leifer, Copyright © 1977, W.B. Saunders Co.

Comparison of the Two Major Groups of Low-Birth-Weight Infants

(Significance of the two conditions)

Premature	Small-for-Date
Higher neonatal mortality	Higher incidence of congenital anomalies

Continued on next page

Premature	Small-for-Date
Major regulatory problems: 　Frequent apneic spells 　Cardiac arrhythmias common 　Accentuated temperature fluctuations 　High incidence of hypoglycemia and hypocalcemia	Problems due to low energy reserves: 　High incidence of fetal distress and asphyxia neonatorum 　Hypothermia when energy stores are exhausted 　Higher incidence of hypoglycemia 　Hypocalcemia occurs postasphyxia
Marked initial weight loss	Initial weight loss less severe or prolonged
Major respiratory problem is hyaline membrane disease	Most frequent respiratory problem is meconium aspiration pneumonia
High incidence of intracranial hemorrhage	High incidence of pulmonary hemorrhage
Accentuated physiologic anemia	Polycythemia
Accentuated physiologic jaundice	Less frequent non-hemolytic jaundice
Low resistance to neonatal bacterial infections	Intrauterine infections frequent cause of growth retardation

Problems Encountered in the Newborn with Postmaturity Syndrome

1. Fetal and neonatal asphyxia or depression at birth.
2. Meconium aspiration.
3. Pulmonary air leak (pneumothorax, pneumomediastinum, pulmonary interstitial emphysema, etc.).
4. Respiratory failure due to any or all of the above.
5. Polycythemia and hyperviscosity syndrome.
6. Hyperbilirubinemia due to bruising and polycythemia.
7. Transient hypoglycemia.
8. Hypocalcemia if acidosis corrected with bicarbonate.
9. Double incidence of major congenital anomalies.

Reprinted by permission of F.A. Davis Company from *Childbearing: A Nursing Perspective*, 2nd edition, by Ann L. Clark, Dyanne Affonso, with Thomas Harris, Copyright 1979, F.A. Davis Company, Philadelphia.

Equipment Required for Neonatal Intensive Care

I. *Monitors*
   A. Respiration (apnea)
   B. Heart rate
   C. Blood pressure
   D. Temperature (rectal or skin probes), with or without controller
   E. Electrocardiogram (oscilloscopes, writers)
   F. Oxygen analyzers (ambient), with or without controllers

II. *Therapeutic equipment*
   A. Incubators, with servocontrolled temperature
   B. Infusion pumps for intravenous fluid administration
   C. Phototherapy lamps
   D. Radiant heaters over treatment tables

III. *Oxygen administration*
   A. Plastic head hoods
   B. Humidifier warmers, preferably with variable temperature control
   C. Repirators (positive pressure with pressure or volume limiters; negative pressure)
   D. CPAP apparatus

IV. *Resuscitation equipment*
   A. Insufflation bags with masks
   B. Endotracheal tubes and adapters
   C. Laryngoscopes with premature blades

From Korones, Sheldon, B.: *High-risk newborn infants,* 2nd ed., St. Louis, 1976, The C.V. Mosby Co. Reprinted with permission.

Infant Suctioning Methods

	Bulb Suction	**DeLee Mucus Trap**	**Mechanical Suction**
Use	Suction of mouth and nares Stimulation of respiration	Suction of oro- and nasopharynx, mouth, and nares Gastric suction	Suction of oro- and nasopharynx, mouth, and nares Gastric suction
Advantages	Small, easy to grasp and use Readily able to clear mouth of draining secretion Can be left next to infant for quick	Suction deep into throat and nasopharynx Suction tip can be easily directed Suction can be continued with-	Fewer maneuvers needed to obtain effective suction Suction can be maintained until mucus has been removed from mouth

	Bulb Suction	**DeLee Mucus Trap**	**Mechanical Suction**
	use	out removing tube (mucus collects in trap) Good control of suction with mouth Disposable trap available	Quick and easy to use in isolette A Y-connector or other finger control permits finger regulation of the suction
Disadvantages	Unable to reach far into throat without causing trauma Bulb must be squeezed, removed, and emptied during suctioning until mouth is clear Bulb left near infant and reused is source of contamination	Capacity of trap for mucus limited (rare problem) Awkward to use in isolette	Outside source of suction needed With excessive suction, catheter may adhere to mucosa and cause trauma as it is pulled away Prolonged suction (10 seconds or more) could deprive infant of oxygen
Precautions	Must not be forced into mouth to reach mucus further down in the throat An old soft bulb will not provide enough suction	Too deep suction can cause trauma to mucosa, laryngospasm, or vagal stimulation and bradycardia Suctioning should be limited to 10 seconds or less—prolonged suction may produce laryngeal spasm Disposable trap should be tightly attached to create suction Catheter should be rotated to prevent adherence	Same as for DeLee trap Only catheter with finger control attachment should be used Suction should be limited to the period of catheter withdrawal

Reprinted by permission of the American Journal of Nursing Co. from "Suctioning the Newborn" by Joyce E. Roberts in *American Journal of Nursing,* January, 1973, p. 64, © 1973, American Journal of Nursing Co.

Signs Indicative of Respiratory Distress in the Neonate

Clinical Data	*Rationale for Manifestation*
Tachypnea (respiratory rate greater than 60/minute)	Indicates stiffening of the lung or mild hypoxia, and represents an attempt by the baby

Continued on next page

Clinical Data	Rationale for Manifestation
	to move more air with less effort and increase the amount of oxygen being brought into the lungs.
Expiratory grunting (audible sound made by exhaling against a partially closed glottis)	Indicates hypoxia and a tendency for the alveoli to collapse, and represents an attempt by the baby to keep open his alveoli with back pressure until the very end of expiration and allow more oxygen exchange.
Retractions or depression of the sternum and sucking in of the suprasternal notch (space above the sternum), intercostal spaces (between the ribs) and subcostal margin (below the ribs) on each inspiration.	Retractions are indicative of decreased lung compliance (stiffness or difficulty expanding the lungs) and represent an increased effort by the baby to overcome this. The increased negative pressure thus generated in the intrathoracic space (between lung and chest wall) sucks in the tissues between and around the ribs.
Flaring of the alae nari (nostrils) on inspiration.	Attempt to allow more air flow into the lungs by widening the external passageways.
Cyanosis (dusky blue color of the skin)	Indicates desaturation of the hemoglobin (reduced amount of bound oxygen) in the presence of still adequate circulation.
Pallor (pale, clammy skin)	Pallor reflects poor circulation to the periphery, usually in conjunction with severe hypoxia and circulatory collapse.
Apneic spells (cessation of breathing with change of color and dropping heart rate)	Indicates an immature or depressed respiratory center unable to maintain spontaneous rhythmic respirations without additional stimulation or support.
Bradycardia (heart beats less than 100 times per minute)	Associated with apneic episodes and hypoxia leading to reduced cardiac activity.
Hypothermia (reduced body temperature)	Low body temperature reflecting inability to produce body heat by metabolic processes requiring oxygen.
Hypotonia and hyporeflexia (reduced muscle tone and weak reflex responses)	Indicates a depressed central nervous system from drugs, trauma, hypoxia or exhaustion.

Reprinted by permission of F.A. Davis Company from *Childbearing: A Nursing Perspective*, 2nd edition, by Ann L. Clark, Dyanne Affonso, with Thomas Harris, Copyright 1979, F.A. Davis Company, Philadelphia.

Signs and Symptoms of Cardiovascular Disorders in Infants

1. Cry: weak and muffled, loud and breathless.
2. Color:
   a. Cyanotic: usually generalized; increases in supine position; often unrelieved by oxygen *; usually deepens with crying; gray, dusky; mild, moderate, severe.
   b. Acyanotic: pale, with or without mottling with exertion.
3. Activity level:
   a. Restless.
   b. Lethargic.
   c. Unresponsive except to pain.
   d. Lack of movement of arms and legs when crying (severe distress).
   e. Arms become flaccid when eating.
4. Posturing:
   a. Hypotonic; flaccid even when sleeping.
   b. Hyperextension of neck.
   c. Opisthotonos.
   d. Dyspnea when supine.
   e. Favors knee-chest position.
5. Persistent bradycardia $\leq$120/min or persistent tachycardia $\geq$160/min.
6. Respirations: Count when neonate is sleeping to identify problem early.
   a. Tachypnea $\geq$60/min.
   b. Retractions with nasal flaring or tachypnea.
   c. Dyspnea with diaphoresis † or grunting.
   d. Gasping followed in 2 or 3 minutes by respiratory arrest if untreated promptly.
   e. Chronic cough (not often seen).
   f. Grunting with exertion such as crying or feeding by nipple.
7. Feeding behavior:
   a. Anorexic.
   b. Poor suck: from lack of energy or when unable to close mouth around nipple due to dyspnea.
   c. Difficulty coordinating suck, swallow, breathing; pulls away from nipple to take breath.

* *Suspect hematologic problem as well (e.g., methemoglobinemia).*
† *Diaphoresis: uncommon response in normal newborn.*

d. Slow, with pauses to rest.
e. Unable to feed by nipple.

Reprinted by permission of The C.V. Mosby Co. from *Maternity Care* by Margaret Duncan Jensen, Ralph C. Benson and Irene M. Bobak, © 1977, The C.V. Mosby Co., St. Louis.

Parent-Parent Support in the Care of High-Risk Newborns

Henry H. Mangurten, MD, Charlyn Slade, RNC, BSN, and Dana Fitzsimons, RN, BSN

Despite the expertise of professional personnel in supporting parents of high-risk infants, parents with similar previous experiences can play a strong adjunctive role also. One program in which these parents were used as the key resource is described, including organization, actual operation, results, and problems.

The past decade has been a profitable one for the high-risk newborn, who has become the recipient of improved nursing and medical care. In addition, the parents of the high-risk newborn have also been receiving increasing attention, as nursing and medical personnel recognize their important supportive roles. Despite the increasing sensitivity of nursery personnel toward these parents, many parents often seek non-professional support, e.g., relatives, friends, and neighbors. The information given by these sources may often confuse the parents and strain the relationship with the nursery personnel. However, these non-professional people may offer a form of support not usually rendered by professional personnel, e.g., concern about economic matters, concern over older siblings at home, and concern over other day-to-day problems such as getting to the hospital, baby sitters, excessive phone bills, etc. Although the supportive role of family, friends, and neighbors should not be minimized, these people generally will not have personally experienced the birth of a high-risk infant. Accordingly, they will not have the same sensitivity and comprehension of the problems facing parents of high-risk infants as will parents of similar infants.

We have always had an intense interest in the parents of high-risk infants and have worked closely with them. Accordingly, we were rather disappointed several years ago when we learned that two couples felt that something was lacking in the emotional support rendered to them during the long-term stay of their three infants in the high-risk nursery. (One couple had a tiny preterm infant who required three months of hospitalization, whereas the second couple had tiny preterm twins who required four and five months respectively in the high-risk nursery.) All three infants ultimately survived and were sent home in good condition. At the time of discharge, the parents expressed gratitude to the nursery staff for all of their support during the hospitalization of the infants. However, both sets of parents indicated that they might have benefited from support of other parents who had previously encountered similar medical problems in their infants. As a result of this suggestion, a meeting was held between these parents, the medical director of the unit, and a group of interested nurses. From this meeting was born the "Concerned Parents Organization" (CPO), a group of parents dedicated to the support of other parents with sick newborn infants.

Organization of the Parents' Group

Initially, five couples were involved. Although the fathers were extremely interested and supportive, the major efforts in organization and development were accomplished by the mothers. These initial five had expressed interest in such a group during the hospitalization of their infants. The expressed purpose of the group was three-fold: 1) to be a self-help group that would offer concern, listening, and general assistance in the everyday problems peculiar to the parents of high-risk newborns, e.g., concern over the baby's survival and future, method of transportation to the hospital, baby sitting, behavioral problems of the older siblings, etc.; 2) to act as liaison between new parents and the high-risk nursery staff, thus promoting trust and confidence in the high-risk nursery personnel; and 3) to assist each other in the long-term goals and care available for their infants, e.g., seeking early intervention support for their infants.

Actual Operation of the Parents' Group

The nursing staff started a logbook in which was listed the names of previous high-risk babies, as well as their problems and other relevant information, e.g., need for assisted ventilation, number of days on respirator, etc. When a new baby is admitted, the parents are introduced to the availability of the CPO; they are informed that this is an optional service which they may find supportive. If they do not see the need for this type of support, nothing more is said again unless they initiate the interest. However, if they show interest in the group, the nurses caring for the baby, in consultation with the neonatologist and one or two additional experienced staff nurses (or a nurse who has become close to the parents), select a veteran mother who matches up closest with the new mother in terms of the infant's gestational age, birth weight, disease process, personalities of parents, etc. If possible, geographical proximity between the parents is attempted.

The veteran mother is called by the nursing staff and apprised of the problems specific to the new infant and parents. The veteran mother then contacts the new mother by telephone. Depending on the response of the new mother to this call, the veteran mother decides the next step: this may be a personal visit to the hospital, an additional phone call, or simply waiting to hear from the new mother. The veteran mother calls the nursery as often as necessary for update reports on the baby in order to allow her to interact more appropriately with the new mother. The nursing staff has been instructed to share the problems and progress of the baby with the veteran mother.

The parents and the nursing staff have identified two especially critical periods: 1) the period immediately following birth, and 2) the period prior to and following discharge. Parents react quite differently during the days immediately following the birth of a high-risk infant. Some parents prefer to be left alone to deal with their problems and feelings; accordingly, the CPO is not imposed upon them. Other parents feel the value of the CPO immediately, and hence are immediately introduced to the program and to specific referral parents. The period related to the discharge is stressful and difficult for virtually all parents. In the situation where a positive, strong relationship has been established between the referral parents and the new parents, the former can play an extremely supportive role in reassuring the new parents about the many concerns related to discharge, e.g., will the baby survive through the night, is home monitoring necessary, will visitors be harmful, etc. The transition from hospital to home can be eased nicely by the reassuring words of parents who have experienced the same concerns and anxieties with their own infants.

In addition to the personal phone calls and/or visits, the parents hold a monthly group meeting where they share their experiences and problems. At several meetings throughout the year, the parents invite a speaker who may be able to help them deal with their referrals as well as their own families. For example, one mother was quite distressed when the baby of one of her referrals died. This mother expressed anxiety over how to approach the referral mother and what to say to her. Many mothers in the group had the same questions. Accordingly the group invited a chaplain especially interested in death and dying to speak at a monthly meeting. The session was extremely successful and supportive.

Results

To date, 150 referrals have been made. For the most part, these have been beneficial. As expected, the new mothers have obtained support which has aided them to better appreciate their own babies' problems. The veteran mothers have given hope to parents of babies requiring long-term ventilation, as well as babies with long-term nutritional problems that result in slow weight gain. In addition, the veteran parents have often assisted the nursery professional staff by instilling confidence in the new parents. This is particularly important in the parents whose baby has been transferred from a distant hospital. These parents often tend to regard the high-risk nursery staff as strange people in a strange hospital. The veteran parents play a significant role in diminishing the suspicion toward the high-risk nursery personnel.

Problems

A number of problems have emerged from this program. Occasionally, the veteran parent expresses information that is not entirely representative of the nursery staff's thoughts. In addition, on occasion there will be personality differences between parents which result in an unsatisfactory referral. An occasional veteran mother is hurt by the referral, e.g., she becomes attached to the new mother and baby, and feels the pain of the baby's death. Rarely, a veteran mother encounters a new mother who is not receptive or appreciative of the referral.

Conclusion

For the most part the program has worked to the advantage of most parents. The nursery nursing staff now knows that in an especially difficult situation, they can call on the parents' group for support. The parents' group has also broadened their interest, developing a number of related activities such as fund-raising, social events, etc. The highlights of the year are the Annual CPO Family Picnic and the Annual CPO Nurses' Tea. The picnic is a family affair attended by parents, other relatives, ex-patients of the high-risk nursery, their siblings, and the nursery professional staff. The picnic allows the parents to show off their babies and the progress that they have made. The Annual Nurses' Tea, held in the hospital, is intended to honor the nurses who give so much of themselves to the care of these infants. This provides still another opportunity for the parents to show off their babies.

The idea of parent-parent support is not a new one. Our experience indicates that this type of group may play a supportive role in intensive care nurseries throughout the country.

References

1. Warrick LH: Family-centered care in the premature nursery. Am J Nurs 71:2134, 1971
2. DuHamel TR, Lin S, Skelton A, Hantke C: Early parenteral perceptions and the high-risk neonate. Clin Pediatr 13:1052, 1974
3. Benfield DG, Leib SA, Reuter J: Grief response of parents after referral of the critically ill newborn to a regional center. N Engl J Med 294:975, 1976
4. Hallinan PM: Working with parents of handicapped children: The role of the medical profession. NZ Med J 84:322, 1976
5. Slade CI, Reidl CJ, Mangurten HH: Working with parents of high-risk newborns. JOGN Nurs 6:21, 1977
6. Farrell HM: Crisis intervention following the birth of a handicapped infant. J Psychiatr Nurs 15:32, 1977
7. Glass L, and Hickerson M: Dialysis and transplantation: A mothers' group. Soc Work Health Care 1:287, 1976

Address for correspondence: Henry H. Mangurten, MD, Director, High-Risk Nursery, Lutheran General Hospital, 1775 Dempster, Park Ridge, IL 60068.

Henry Mangurten, MD, is director of the high-risk nursery at Lutheran General Hospital in Park Ridge, Illinois, and associate professor of clinical pediatrics at the University of Illinois, Chicago. Dr. Mangurten received his MD from the University of Illinois, Chicago, and is certified by the Sub-Board of Neonatal-Perinatal Medicine of the American Board of Pediatrics. He is a fellow of the AAP.

Charlyn Slade is head nurse of the high-risk nursery at Lutheran General Hospital, Park Ridge, Illinois. She holds a BSN from the University of Illinois, Chicago, and is certified by the Sub-Board of Neonatal Midwifery. Ms. Slade is a member of NAACOG.

Dana FitzSimons received her BSN from the University of Iowa. She worked in the high-risk nursery at Lutheran General Hospital, Park Ridge, Illinois.

Reprinted by permission of Lippincott/Harper Company from *JOGN Nursing*, Sept./Oct., 1979, © 1979, Harper and Row Publishers.

The Counseling of Families in the Professional Management of Sudden Infant Death Syndrome

Introductory Material:

By definition, Sudden Infant Death Syndrome (SIDS) is the sudden death of any infant or young child, which is unexpected by history and in which a thorough postmortem examination fails to demonstrate an adequate cause of death. The history of an infant dying of SIDS is generally one of a child between the ages of one month and six months who succumbs during a normal sleeping period and who may have symptoms of a mild cold or sniffles.

While SIDS has probably been with us since biblical times, the term SIDS and acceptance of this entity as a disease was not established until 1969. The inclusion of SIDS in the classification of disease occurred in the United States in the fall of 1973. The medical and lay community frequently continue to refer to SIDS by the lay term, "crib death."

In early 1975, it was still correct to identify SIDS as a non-predictable, non-preventable disease whose exact cause is still unknown or unclear. Many theories about SIDS prevail with the majority disproven and the remainder awaiting or undergoing more careful scientific research and study.

The sudden, unexpected nature of SIDS places this disease within the medical-legal system. The vast majority of cases are within the jurisdiction of medical examiners and coroners. Because such deaths rarely occur within hospitals or other institutions, SIDS is isolated from the traditional patterns of medical professional disease management. As a consequence, a long period of time occurred where the majority of practising professionals had little practical and academic knowledge of SIDS.

The past lack of appropriate death certification, the lack of sound medical knowledge about this disease, the inclusion of SIDS in the medical-legal system and the emotional trauma of finding an apparently healthy baby dead, created a climate of extreme guilt and prolonged and abnormal grief reactions for many surviving families. Further mental health problems with such families were created in the areas of surviving siblings and subsequent children.

A survey was conducted in 1972 into the community management of SIDS. That survey, funded by the Department of Health, Education and Welfare, was conducted in representative communities in the Continental United States. The survey identified how SIDS was generally managed at that time and from those findings there emerged a definition of the role of the professional in the effective handling of SIDS. Since SIDS is not preventable, the professional role addressed itself to the preventive mental health aspects of the surviving families.

This program is designed to meet the criteria of one of the most important elements of the professional handling of SIDS—the counseling of the family soon after the death of the child. It has been accepted that such initial counseling should be done by a knowledgeable health professional from within the community.

The counseling visit is designed to reduce the number of extended grief reactions observed previously and to provide families with enough basic information about SIDS to avert unnecessary guilt reactions. The visit should support parental self-worth and productiveness without removing the necessary right to mourn the loss of a loved one. The visit also provides support in the area of grief, grief reactions and feelings about death. The counselor can be from any one of a number of professional categories: the physician, various nursing agencies, social workers, clergy, etc. For a variety of reasons, the public health nurse has been established as the most appropriate professional to render this counseling service to families in the majority of situations.

The Management Of SIDS

To be most effective, and for the counselor to gain the best appreciation of the role involved, the following is a brief explanation of the elements of a maximum SIDS management system.

1. Identification: The establishment of SIDS as a preliminary cause of death by means of autopsy and/or other acceptable standards. Such preliminary identification must be established as soon as possible and studies have shown the gross autopsy to be sufficiently accurate when correlated with later microscopic studies. Most jurisdictions can provide such preliminary identification within 24–48 hours.

2. Certification: The importance of using the term SIDS on preliminary and final death certificates, when applicable, has vast importance in the death acceptance and mental health aspects of the surviving family.

3. Notification: Observation of the cause of death to the family should be done by a recognized medical or jurisdictional authority as soon as identification is established. Notification can be done by telephone, letter, or both.

4. Information: The basic facts about SIDS should be provided to the family as soon as possible. This is especially important in areas where delays in providing the counseling visit cannot be avoided.

5. Professional and civic support, informed inhalator personnel, police, emergency medical personnel, clergy and funeral directors, are integral to the effective management of the SIDS family.

6. Counseling: The counseling visit should occur within two weeks following the death of the child. It is essentially a listening visit and consolidates any previous information or (misinformation that the family has encountered).

It also identifies any initial problems in the family's ability to understand the disease. The visit can take place in the home or any other area acceptable to the family and counselor. Because of the nature of the problems encountered with grief and subsequent reactions, the anticipation of a return counseling visit should be considered.

7. Referral or contact with voluntary agencies working with SIDS. (Contact on a one to one basis with another parent who has lost a child to SIDS, or group contact and efforts relating to the disease can provide an important support system and emotional outlet for families. It should be rec-

ognized by the professional that such contact is optional and voluntary agencies are primarily middle and upper middle class phenomenon. Referral to such groups is an individual consideration and is done at the request of the family.

The Counseling Visit

The counseling opportunity for the health professional is generally referred to as the "home visit." While the most valuable setting for assistance to the family is probably within the home setting, it should be recognized that other areas or settings can be utilized. Periodically, the telephone may be the only resource to reaching the family. The decision as to where the counseling visit should take place rests with the family and the counselor.

The counseling visit is an option for the family and may be refused by them. It is suggested that families in a period of grief do not always make appropriate decisions. Initial contact with the family in terms of determining a time and location should carry a positive and affirmative note from the counselor.

Whenever possible, the counseling session should include both parents or the persons primarily involved in caring for the infant. This is sometimes not possible nor practical. The tone of the visit is determined by the nurse or counselor but most families will take the lead without too much difficulty. The initial visit should be carefully managed so that the family can discuss the infant and the events surrounding his life and death without feeling interrogated or regarded with suspicion. The most frequent observation by personnel participating in such visits is that the family is grateful for someone who will listen and who is also capable of dispelling any potential guilt feelings.

While there are many similar patterns in SIDS families in terms of reactions and questions, each family must be considered unique in their appreciation of the event that has occurred. Different life styles and patterns provide any number of coping mechanisms and support systems. The counselor should be prepared to accept some unique attitudes that may not be within the counselor's personal attitudes or concepts.

Since SIDS occur primarily to young parents and families, the visit is also an opportunity for the public health professional to identify other living problems that may be intrinsically involved in the death of the child but not necessarily related to the cause of death. Marital problems, inadequate housing, financial problems, single parents, and other health and emotional problems will most likely be brought to the counselor's attention. The management and assistance of other problems should be handled in such a manner as to not potentially reinforce or provoke guilt feelings related to the child's death.

In addition to its original intent, the SIDS counseling visit can be a unique opportunity to assist families living in situations that might have otherwise been overlooked or ignored by the professional and the family.

Reprinted by permission of the National Sudden Infant Death Syndrome Foundation, 310 S. Michigan Ave., Chicago, Illinois, 60604, from the Foundation brochure prepared by Mrs. Carolyn Szybist, R.N., Executive Director, National SIDS Foundation.

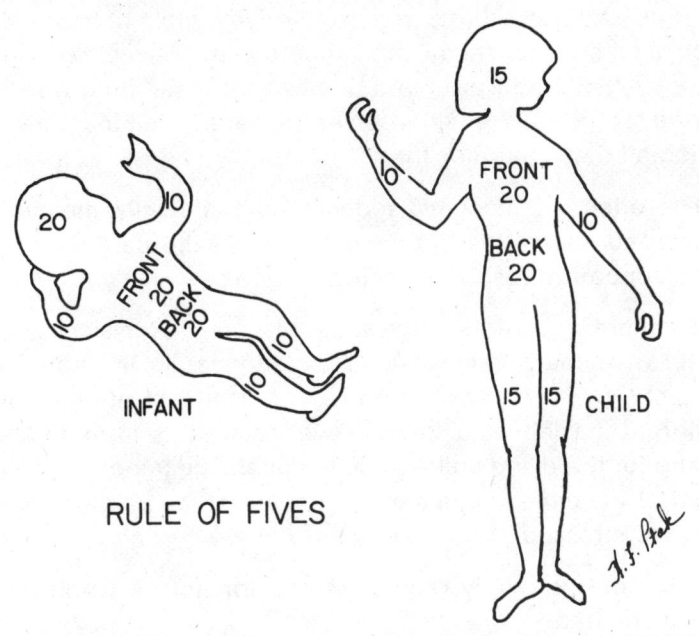

RULE OF FIVES

Courtesy, Appleton-Century-Crofts, Steele, Shirley, Edit., *Nursing Care of the Child With Long-Term Illness*, 2 ed., p. 418, fig. 2, © 1977, Appleton-Century-Crofts.

Pediatric I.V.'s

An excellent resource on Pediatric I.V.'s is the tear-out reminder on "Pediatric I.V.'s Nursing Implications at a Glance," *RN* Magazine, March, 1979, p. 44 and 45. It includes developmental information on the various age groups, sites for I.V. placement, information on preparing the child and family, nursing actions, protection of the I.V. site, how to enable the child to be mobile with the I.V. in place, and safety considerations. Any pediatric unit which utilizes I.V. therapy could benefit from posting this helpful guide.

Home Care for the Dying Child

In describing the University of Minnesota School Of Nursing's project on home care for dying children, this book is both moving and informative. The poignant personal experiences of the health care workers and family members involved with the project leave a lasting impression on the reader.

The project was established to provide nursing support to parents who wished to care for their dying child at home rather than add hospitalization (and thus separation) to the already traumatic situation of illness and fear of impending death. By caring for the children themselves the parents felt that they were doing all they could for them.

The effect of the child's death on the family members is discussed as well as the need for the health care workers to have support in resolving their own grief.

Chapters by parents, nurses, social workers, physicians and a chaplain recount each of their experiences in the home care project. There is a section on recent treatment of leukemia in children and lab data in leukemia, as well as information on caring for the dying child in the hospital. The importance of the relief of the child's pain and the impact of the pain on the parents are stressed.

This book is highly recommended for nurses working with dying children.

Ida Marie Martinson, Appleton-Century-Crofts, New York, 1976.

Nursing Diagnoses and Interventions: The Disturbed Child's Family

Nursing diagnosis	Intervention
Inability to handle feelings and attitudes about having a severely disturbed child in the family.	Parental counseling to establish an understanding of the child. Family meetings with those members having the most contact with the child. Serve as a therapeutic ally and advocate to the family.

Nursing diagnosis	Intervention
	Act as an information resource.
	Provide support by listening empathetically and clarifying feelings and conflicting values.
Dysfunctional parent or parent relationship that precipitates disturbed behaviors in child.	Assess dysfunctional dynamics and determine counseling or therapy needs.
	Explore problem areas that can be ameliorated by parent education, financial assistance, better decision making, and activities which will better meet needs of family members.
	Provide a role model for more effective behavior with child client.
	Serve as a role model for more effective communication patterns within family.
	Make appropriate referral for treatment unless nurse functions as a primary therapist and is available as a treatment agent for the family.
	If parenting process causes severe disorganization in the child, consider recommending removal of child to a foster or residential setting.
Inability to cope with or accept the idea of separation from a child who needs residential placement.	Provide a forum for family to discover and explore their feelings about placement.
	Arrange for family to have contact with their child in placement.
	Provide supportive counseling after placement to help with working through feelings of loss, guilt, and mourning.
	Provide any special assistance needed to help siblings and other family members deal with their particular grief reactions.
Excessive guilt, anger, and blaming within the family, centering around or precipitated by the presence of a disturbed child.	Help family to explore these attitudes by identifying the presumed source and providing an alternative point of view about the process.

Reproduced with permission of McGraw-Hill Book Co., from *Comprehensive Psychiatric Nursing*, by Haber, Leach, Schudy and Sideleau, © 1978, McGraw-Hill Book Company.

The Nurse and the Abused Child

by JOAN HOPKINS, R.N.*

When an injured or ill child comes to the attention of the medical profession, is the reaction the same as when the patient is an adult? Generally, it is not. Many adults admit that they become emotionally involved, and that caring for a sick or injured child is a difficult task. How then do these professionals react when they find that the child they are caring for has a condition that was caused by the abuse or neglect of that child's parents?

Continued on next page

The reaction we professionals generally communicate to the parents is one of accusation and hostility. It is a challenge to us to develop the ability to communicate to the family that finally they have found someone who understands and cares.

In order to develop a positive attitude toward the battering parent, the nurse should have a complete understanding of these parents, of the fact that they have been raised to come up to the expectations of their own parents and that they expect their children to meet these same expectations. One must also realize that most of these parents do love their children.

INVESTIGATING THE BACKGROUND AND CHARACTERISTICS OF THE ABUSING PARENT

A study of the battered child began at the University of Colorado Medical Center several years ago. Dr. C. Henry Kempe, Professor and Chairman of the Department of Pediatrics, requested that a psychiatric evaluation be done on a mother who had injured her child. The evaluation was done by Dr. Brandt Steele, Professor of Psychiatry and Chief of the Psychiatric Liaison Division at the Medical Center.

During the time that followed, more abusing parents were evaluated and Dr. Carl B. Pollock, Assistant Professor of Psychiatry, was called in to help in studying these families. In five and one-half years, 60 families were studied. These families were referred by other physicians or outside agencies and by self-referral.

A relationship with the parents was maintained by the psychiatrist, and a social worker was also utilized to make home visits. The families were encouraged to call their therapist day or night when they felt they had a need to talk with someone. Because of the close and continuing relationship with these abusing parents the group was able to formulate a description of the characteristics of the abusing parent.

An observer would find these people to be very much like any other group of parents. Although it might be expected that these parents would be very needy and poorly educated, this did not prove to be the case. All income levels and job types, including the proressional group, were represented. These people came from all religions. Some lived in

---

*Coordinator, Battered Child Team, University of Colorado Medical Center, Denver.

This study was supported by the Children's Bureau of the Department of Health, Education and Welfare, Project No. 12: HS, Project 218.

immaculate homes, while others lived in a filthy, cluttered environment.

The distinguishing features of the abusing parents were their attitudes toward discipline and child-rearing. The children of these families are expected to perform as adults. When asked about disciplining, these parents emphatically explain the requirements their children must meet.

An example of unrealistic expectations of the child is quite often found with toilet training. For example, Mrs. G. came to the clinic at the Medical Center for her prenatal care. Both she and her husband were quite excited over the coming birth of their new child. Mrs. G. often was accompanied to the clinic by her mother. On one occasion during prenatal classes Mrs. G. made the remark that she would have her child toilet-trained by one year of age, and her mother strongly reinforced this by proudly announcing that all of her children had been toilet-trained by one year of age.

Mrs. G. delivered a healthy little girl, and upon discharge a public health nurse referral was sent. The nurse visited when the baby was two weeks of age. She found the mother to be doing well with the newborn. She mentioned that the grandmother was present during the visit and both mother and grandmother were quite confident that the child would be toilet-trained by one year. No mention was made by either this nurse or the prenatal nurse as to whether they had tried to discourage such early toilet training.

At six months of age, the child was brought to the hospital with bruises over the entire back, buttocks, and legs. The mother later admitted she became uncontrollably angry with the child when she wet her pants after having sat on the "potty chair" for one hour.

Many parents expect their children to be happy, responsive little adults. The parents become frustrated when the child cries after he has been fed and his diapers have been changed. They feel the child does not love them or that he is accusing them of being bad parents.

It soon became evident that a significant pattern was presented by the abusing parents. These parents were raising their children in the same manner in which they themselves had been raised. Frequently the parents would deny knowing the cause of the injury to their child or even conjure up a story regarding the cause of the injury. However, after repeated visits they revealed their feeling that they had a right to discipline their children in a fashion that would teach them a lesson. They then explained that their parents had punished them in the same manner and it certainly had taught them a lesson.

Let us take for example Mr. P. His two sons were brought to the clinic for treatment of burns on their hands that had become infected. The physician was told by the boys that "daddy did it." Instead of lec-

Continued on next page

turing the parents on child-rearing practices, the physician informed the parents that the burns were badly infected and that hospital care would be necessary. During the evaluations done by social service and psychiatry, the father revealed that he felt quite justified in burning his sons' hands, since the two boys had been playing with fire, which is very dangerous. When Mr. P. was young, his father had burned his hands for playing with fire, and therefore he would teach his sons in the same manner.

The third characteristic that was prevalent among these parents was the relationship they had with others. They appeared to be very suspicious and were antagonistic toward everyone in the hospital. On closer contact, during home visits, these people appear to be leading very isolated lives. They frequently do not reach out to their neighbors, often their curtains are closed, and they have an unlisted telephone. Quite often their parents add to their insecurity by their constant criticism.

Some thought that the abusive parents would be found to be psychotic at the time of an attack. It was found by Steele and Pollock[1] that these people did have some emotional problems, but these problems could not be blamed for the abuse. Abuse occurs when the child do not shape up and meet the expectations of their parents.

THE APPEAL FOR HELP

The nurse, more than any other professional, is strategically placed to do case-finding and to listen to the plea for help these parents make. It is important for the nurse to recognize the symptoms that are predisposing to the battering. These symptoms may well be discovered in a prenatal clinic prior to the birth of the baby. It is not unusual for the public health nurse, on her home visit, to recognize a mother in extreme distress over the behavior of her child. The nurse in a pediatric clinic or doctor's office may hear a mother describe her frustration at her crying infant. The staff nurse in a hospital may be told by the mother of her patient how difficult this child is to care for.

How should a nurse react to these people? Should we quickly call for help, or can we listen to these people? In most cases of battering, one parent or the other has made a plea for help that was not heard. In retrospect this might have been very significant if the person who heard it could have interpreted its meaning and offered the parents the interest and attention they needed.

One common event that should be recognized as a plea for help is when a parent brings a child to the physician for "no reason at all." These office visits should not be passed off as unimportant. If there is nothing wrong with the child, then the nurse should see the visit for what it is. The mother may be trying to tell her "There is nothing wrong with my child, but take a look at me." The nurse might chat with the mother and obtain valuable information. What are her stresses? How is she holding up? Is the responsibility of wife, home, and newborn infant really overwhelming?

The nurse caring for a new mother and her infant should listen closely to see how that mother views her child. A mother displaying digust with her child's urine, feces, or vomitus should be evaluated further. If the crying infant brings on a great deal of anxiety or the mother cannot hold the child close to her, this too should be further investigated.

The one great plea for attention that many new mothers give is "I don't know how to put on diapers, will you show me?" Not only the nurse, but many others, quite dutifully show the anxious young mother the procedure. They even go so far as to offer possible methods of diaper folding, and then, very efficiently, they go on their way. Very few, if any, realize that if this mother does not know the first thing about putting on a diaper, it is likely that she hasn't the vaguest idea of what the art of mothering really includes.

It is notable that the preceding examples of case-finding have all dealt with very young infants. The mother of a young child is no doubt overwhelmed, even if she does not have the potential to be a battering mother. But listen closely to her. Are other adults in the family adding to her stress by criticism of her child-rearing practice? Does she expect her child to perform as an adult?

BECOMING INVOLVED

The ability to identify the parent who has battered or has the potential to batter brings up the question: Should I get involved? The paramedical staff frequently has difficulty suggesting to the physician that his patient could possibly be a battered child. Many physicians do not give consideration to the "battered child syndrome." The reluctance to "get involved" is usually attributed to not wanting to "get the law involved." Many simply state they do not want to go to court. Others feel that if they were to report the battering, the parents would go elsewhere, or perhaps even worse, would not see a physician at all.

Because of this reluctance and the difficulty in diagnosis, a team approach is beneficial. Information obtained by the nurses, social worker, psychiatrist, and physician may then be evaluated and the disposition decided on. The nurse is usually not seen as a suspicious or critical person. The parents will often talk with her as she cares

Continued on next page

for their child and become very open as to their feelings about their roles as parents. Many times they see their physician as a very busy person and state that they do not want to burden him with their problems. The social worker, on the other hand, may not be as readily available as the staff nurse.

To accuse a parent of battering is not an easy thing to do. This is a serious accusation. What if the parent becomes violent? What if it is not true? Will he take the child and run? The ability to interview effectively, and the art of expressing concern and interest, will be valuable to the nurse in this situation and will certainly help put the parent at ease.

It is interesting that the majority of people dealing with child abuse cases think only of the parents and of the legal entanglements they themselves may become involved in. Very few look at the child and feel obligated to speak up and defend him. Remember, the child cannot defend himself.

What about the child who is old enough to speak for himself? This is the group with which the school nurse must be concerned. If a child comes to school with strap marks on his back, with cigarette burns, or hungry, should one ask the child to tell what has happened?

As has been indicated, the abusing and neglecting parent has a fear of being made to look inadequate and quite often is surrounded by critical friends and relatives. If the child, when asked, tattles on his parents, he most likely will receive further abuse, so it is best to see the parent and inquire as to the needs of the family and how best they can be helped if they reveal their child is "hard to handle."

The technique used to interview the parents must serve to establish the interviewer as one who cares and understands. An understanding of the family stresses and behavior patterns of children in the particular age group is helpful.

One young child was brought to the Emergency Room by a baby-sitter. The child was covered with bruises from a beating. The baby-sitter stated that the mother worked, and had brought the child to her with a coat on. The coat had not been removed until after the mother had left. When questioned, the child told the baby-sitter that she had been spanked by her mother because she was naughty.

Since medical treatment cannot be given without parental consent, the mother was asked to come to the hospital. She became very suspicious and stated that she was too busy to come into the hospital, and that she was sure the child was not sick enough to be seen. She finally did consent to come in but wanted to take her child to her family physician for treatment. The physician was contacted and gave permission for the care of the child to be transferred to the Medical Center. The mother was given the physician's message, which appeared to cause her to panic.

The interviewer then confronted the mother with the fact that she appeared frightened, and suggested that it must be very difficult to have total care of the child and earn the family living also. The mother then explained how difficult it really was. Her work was very demanding and she was having a great deal of difficulty toilet training the little girl we were seeing. She also had a son five years of age; she had been called to school the day before because the teachers were having trouble disciplining him.

A concerned attitude and a promise to help get things organized were welcomed. The interviewer made the mother feel she understood the situation, whereas a detective technique of asking who, when, where, how, and why would have put the mother on the defensive and she would have felt that her ability as a parent was being criticized.

If the parents describe situations in which they were unable to deal with the child, a technique described by Pollock as "the rescue operation" is useful. Simply ask "whom have you turned to when the care of the child becomes most difficult?" If there is such a person available, the mother should be encouraged to turn to this person in times of stress.

Questions frequently asked to encourage these parents to describe their child's behavior patterns are:
1. When your child cries, what do you do?
2. If that does not work, what do you do?
3. What do you do if you are unable to stop the crying?
4. Does your child sleep well?
5. What do you do when he does not sleep?

It was found in the research study previously mentioned that parents who abuse their children often become anxious or even quite upset when they have to express their feelings about dealing with the child's behavior. Parents who have a plan for dealing with such situations are less likely to practice abuse.

TEACHING CHILD-REARING PRACTICES

Treatment of the abusive parent can be undertaken by many types of professionals. In many cases the ideal person for teaching child-rearing practices is the nurse. She has knowledge of the diagnosis and treatment of many minor ailments that the parent might be concerned

Continued on next page

with. She is also able to help the parents better understand their child's behavior at different age levels.

Jenny was described as being an impossible child. Her mother reported the daily antics of her two-year-old daughter to the public health nurse during a home visit. Jenny had dumped out oatmeal, covered the bathroom with cleansing powder, and displayed her artistic abilities all over her bedroom wall. Behavior such as this would be trying for any mother. The public health nurse sat down with the mother and talked about the child. They read pamphlets describing behavior patterns, cautions that must be taken, and constructive play the mother could use to keep the child occupied and out of trouble.

Let us go back to the mother of the newborn child who expected the child to be toilet-trained at one year of age. Nurses on the postpartum ward and the public health nurse should have talked with this mother about the reality of toilet training very young infants. Admittedly, it would have been a difficult task to compete with grandmother, but young mothers are quite open to suggestions on childrearing. The nurse may feel that all her teaching is falling on deaf ears, but when the mother starts to have difficulties with toilet training, she may then recall the teachings of her nurses.

TEACHING THE ART OF MOTHERING

In our society, it is assumed that if a woman is able to bear children she is capable of mothering. Obviously this is not true.

Modern woman is caught up in the educational world. She may attend classes for hair styling, cake decorating, interior design, sewing and cooking. There are no classes available that truly teach the art of mothering. Prospective mothers often search for suggestions on child-rearing in baby care books, magazines, and radio programs. The mother then becomes concerned with questions such as: Should she breast feed? Should the child start sleeping in a crib or should she use a bassinet? Should the child be allowed to have a pacifier? It is rare to find a mother who will go against the teachings of "the book." When things are not going well, she is usually unable to try anything new that might put her more at ease in her relationship with the child.

Since we are assuming that mothering is learned, what do we teach a woman in order that she may provide mothering for her children? Case workers and public health nurses frequently report an evaluation of their home visit such as, "The mother, children and home were very clean, the children were well behaved and there appears to be no problem with disciplining." Little, if any, mention is ever made of the type of mothering the worker has observed.

The mothering ability must necessarily be described in vague terms because it is not a tangible item about which we may gather information. The mothering instinct is certainly not confined to the biological mother, since the ability to mother can be found in the very young. Single men and women too are often found to have the ability to mother.

The fact has previously been established that battering parents love their children, therefore the presence of love does not guarantee mothering ability. The mechanical care a mother administers, such as diapering, bathing, and feeding, cannot be considered mothering. What, then, does this word connote?

When describing mothering, the attitude of the parent toward the child gives an indication of that parent's ability to mother. What is an attitude? Webster's Dictionary defines attitude as "a manner of acting, feeling or thinking that shows one's disposition or opinion." By observing the look on a woman's face while she is breast-feeding her infant, it is possible to obtain a clue as to that mother's attitude toward her child. The manner in which a parent disciplines a child may give the observer some understanding of the parental attitude about that child.

The parents can gradually learn the art of motherliness or fatherliness by an association with a mothering person. Very often the mother is the only member of the abusive family who is available. The relationship that is established with her should be one of giving and genuine concern. She must never feel that she is being criticized or dominated.

The experience of following an abusive family is very challenging. The social worker, nurse, or lay therapist must prove that she is available to reach out and offer comfort and concern even when it is not convenient to do so. She must offer the mother a chance to ventilate her feelings about her role as a woman, wife, and mother. Parents repeatedly question the therapist concerning her opinion as to whether they are good parents. The question "Do you think I am a bad mother?" is frequently asked. The therapist must communicate her faith in the patient's mothering ability. The manner in which this message is communicated depends on the personality of the therapist and the presenting circumstances.

Here we might mention some do's and don'ts that should be remembered when dealing with abusive parents.

Do Not: a. Criticize, dominate, or set limits.
          b. Criticize the handling of the child even if it appears abusive. At a suitable time discuss disciplining methods.
          c. Impart your values.
          d. Become "pushy" or expect rapid results.

Continued on next page

Do:
    a. Give assistance by working side by side to teach mothering abilities.
    b. Be tolerant of any anger the mother expresses.
    c. Obtain consultation frequently as to information communicated and goals to work for.

Gradually as the relationship between mother and therapist becomes more meaningful, the mother's ability to give to the husband and children should improve.

SUMMARY

The nursing profession must assume its role in the tremendous responsibility of case finding, prevention, and treatment of the abused and neglected child. No other profession has the opportunity to spend as much meaningful time with these patients and their families as does the nurse.

Nurses have been taught to observe symptoms. These parents, many times, makes an unconscious plea for help while they are pregnant or perhaps soon after delivery while recovering on the postpartum ward.

Utilization of the pediatric training that is a requirement for nurses is invaluable in the teaching that these parents so desperately need. If a young mother is taught what the normal behavior for her child should be and what she should expect of that child, then she will be better able to cope with the child's behavior.

We must be willing to accept the diagnosis of child abuse. If the nurse is comfortable with a patient, the patient will be more accepting of his problems. The ability to recognize the problem for what it is, by understanding the history, treatment, and prognosis of battering and neglectful parents, is important in developing a meaningful relationship with these families.

REFERENCE

1. Helfer, R. E., and Kempe, C. H., Eds.: The Battered Child. Chicago, University of Chicago Press, 1968.

Box 2751
University of Colorado Medical Center
Denver, Colorado 80220

Reference

Helfer, R. E., and Kempe, C. H., Eds.: *The Battered Child.* Chicago, University of Chicago Press, 1968. (2nd edition, 1974)

<small>Reprinted by permission from *The Nursing Clinics of North America*, Vol. 5, No. 4, December, 1970, © 1970, W. B. Saunders Co.</small>

Further References on Child Abuse and Neglect

Bernstein, Arthur H., "Hospital Liability for Battered Children," *Hospitals,* March, 1976, p. 95–97.

Chase, Naomi Feigelson, *A Child Is Being Beaten,* Holt, Rinehart and Winston, New York, 1975.

Children Today (Special child abuse issue), 4(3), May/June, 1975. DHEW Pub. No. (OHD) 75-14.

Court, Joan, and Anna Kerr, "The Battered Child Syndrome-2: A Preventable Disease?", *Nursing Times,* 67(23):695–7, June 10, 1971.

Helfer, Ray E., and C. Henry Kempe, eds., *Child Abuse and Neglect: Community Approach to Family Treatment,* Ballinger, Cambridge, 1976.

Kempe, C. Henry and Ray E. Helfer, Eds., *Helping the Battered Child and His Family,* J. B. Lippincott Co., Philadelphia, 1972.

Martin, Harold, ed., *The Abused Child: A Multidisciplinary Approach to Developmental Issues in Treatment,* Ballinger, Cambridge, 1976.

Newberger, Eli H., and James N. Hyde, "Child Abuse: Principles and Implications of Current Pediatric Practice," *Pediatric Clinics of North America,* 22(2), August, 1975.

Savino, Anne and Wyman Sanders, "Working With Abusive Parents: Group Therapy and Home Visits," *American Journal of Nursing,* 73(3), March, 1973, p. 482–4.

Schmitt, B. and C. Henry Kempe, "The Pediatrician's Role in Child Abuse and Neglect," *Current Problems in Pediatrics,* 5(5), March, 1975, p. 1–47.

Resources in Pediatric Nursing

General Resources

The American Academy Of Pediatrics
P. O. Box 1034
Evanston, Ill. 60204

The Academy publishes several manuals for health professionals, paperback books, booklets, reprints, and health education materials. Included are manuals on school health, infectious diseases, care of children in hospitals, pediatric nutrition, accident prevention, adolescence, asthma, child abuse, day care health recommendations, drugs, environmental concerns, learning disabilities, medical ethics, neonatal care, guidelines for pediatric care, screening, sudden infant death syndrome, and adoption. Write for "Publications List." The Academy also published *Pediatrics,* a monthly journal ($17 in U.S., $10 a year for medical students and residents).

Child, Inc. (Children's Holistic Institute for Life Development, Inc.)
172 W. 79th St.
New York, N.Y. 10024

Child, Inc. is a non-profit organization which promotes health practices and health education for children. It emphasizes holistic care and encourages self-help. For further information and for the newsletter, "The C.H.I.L.D. Report," contact the above address.

Coalition For Children and Youth
Bowen Building, Suite 600
815 15th Street, N.W.
Washington, D.C. 20005

This is an organization of national, state and local groups working together to improve conditions for children and youth. The Coalition acts "as an information center, forum for exchange of ideas, and a national voice for child advocates." Full voting membership is open only to organizations concerned with children and youth but individuals may join as associate members. Publications include *Focus On Children And Youth,* a monthly newsletter providing current information on issues involving children and youth.

Ross Laboratories
625 North Cleveland Avenue
Columbus, Ohio 43216

Ross Laboratories makes available several "Nursing Inservice Aids" including: "Observation Of Retractions" in the infant, "Apgar Scoring Chart," "Danger Signs In The Newborn," "Conversion Table For Newborn Weights," "Clinical Criteria For Gestational Assessment," "Common Variations In The Neonate," "Cleft Lip And Cleft Palate," "Abnormalities Of The Central Nervous System," and "Congenital Orthopedic Anomalies." All are appropriate for posting in the clinical setting to serve as easy reference guides.

Other Publications

Child Health Conference—Nurses' Resource Manual
Visiting Nurse Association Of New Haven, Connecticut
Published by National League For Nursing, 1975
The League Exchange No. 101
Pub. No. 21-1502, $4.95

This manual is a guide for nurses in child health conferences. It includes basic materials on schedules for well child visits, normal growth and development, interviewing and counseling parents, diagnostic tests, and immunization schedules and procedures. There are sections on nutrition and toys for children of various ages and a description of this agency's child abuse policy. The manual is a useful tool for nurses new to the child health conference setting and is a good review for nurses already practicing in this area.

Family Health Care, edited by Debra Hymoruch and Martha Underwood Barnard, McGraw-Hill Book Co., 1979, 394 pages, $8.95

This book consists of articles on working with families, written mostly by nurses. The articles deal with helping families adjust to change (such as parenthood) and crisis situations (birth of a handicapped child, for example). It is intended for professionals concerned with all aspects of family health care.

Resources On Parenting And Parent Education

Wheelock College
200 The Riverway
Boston, Mass. 02215

Wheelock College, through its Center For Parenting Studies, offers courses for professionals on the parenting experience and working with parents. The courses cover a variety of topics. Contact the Office Of Continuing Education at the above address for further information.

Gerber Products Co.
Medical Marketing Services Department
445 State Street
Fremont, Mich. 49412

Gerber products has available patient education booklets for pediatric offices covering pregnancy, child care, safety, and nutrition.

Growing Child/Growing Parent
22 North Second Street
Lafayette, Ind. 47902

This is a monthly newsletter for parents on growth and development at different ages. Teachers of expectant parents' classes can send in the names and addresses of their students to enable them to receive a four-months' subscription free of charge with no obligation for future subscriptions.

Practical Parenting
c/o Meadowbrook Press
16648 Meadowbrook Lane
Wayzata, Minn. 55391

Practical Parenting is "a bimonthly newsletter by parents and for parents," edited by Vicki Lansky. It is a forum for the sharing of ideas, experiences and problems among parents. It is a good resource for nurses to recommend to new parents (Cost: $5 a year for six issues, $6 in Canada). Meadowbrook Press also has several helpful books available for parents, including *Feed Me! I'm Yours* and *The Taming of the C.A.N.D.Y. Monster* by Vicki Lansky, and two new books, *Practical Parenting Tips* and *Free Stuff for Parents*.

Ourselves And Our Children, A Book By and For Parents
by the Boston Women's Health Book Collective
copyright 1978, Random House,
$12.95 cloth, $6.95 paperback

This book emphasizes the realities of parenthood and the need for parents to be fulfilled as individuals in order to be better parents. By focusing on the parents, this book can stimulate parents to think more about their roles and themselves as persons. It is a useful tool for nurses themselves and for recommending to parents.

Growing Parents' Groups

Segregated parties—where men huddle up to discuss important business, leaving women to chit-chat about the "insignificant" concerns of childrearing and family life—are becoming a thing of the past. For one thing, the he-works/she-mothers split is softening as women take on outside jobs and men become actively involved in raising their children. It's a new art with its own name—PARENTING. The "business" of parenting is also becoming more businesslike, complete with its own conferences, books, manuals, courses, centers—even *newsletters*. And the status of the business of parenting is on the rise!

For the most part, this new parenting activism is a grass roots movement. Countless local groups and programs are independent and largely unaware of one another's existence. They are being formed by individuals and through Ys, churches, Junior League chapters, adult vo-tech programs and even neighborhood elementary schools.

The Parent Place in Seattle is a drop-in store front agency that offers counseling, classes and a place parents can "just run away to." Some other programs are Bananas, in Oakland, CA; BYOB (Bring Your Own Baby), in Portage, IN; and C.O.P.E. (Coping with Overall Pregnancy/Parenting Experiences) in Boston, MA.

Many groups are outgrowths of classes in prepared childbirth, natural extensions for new parents who have actively participated in the deliveries of their children. One such group is the Parents and Childbirth Education Society (PACES), in Western Springs, IL. Eight years ago, PACES started a post-partum Mother's Help Line, a telephone support service, with a handful of volunteers. Today it provides workshops, seminars, a speakers' bureau and other services for a 400-family membership.

Diane Mason, Gayle Jensen and Carolyn Ryzewicz, mothers who were

Continued on next page

officers in PACES parents' group early years, have committed their experiences to paper. The aim of their book, HOW TO GROW A PARENTS GROUP, is to help others avoid their pitfalls and provide helpful ideas for setting up a new group or rejuvenating an established one.

One ambitious and innovative program begun in Minnesota which now has offshoots across the country is MELD (Minnesota Early Learning Design). MELD grew out of a year-long research and planning grant by Ann Ellwood, an early childhood specialist. Her study indicated that the best way to strengthen the family is to provide timely information coupled with peer support.

MELD is a program for first-time parents who meet regularly in small neighborhood self-help groups from the time of pregnancy until their children are 2. The groups are led by other, specially trained parents called facilitators.

"Support in the beginning," said one young mother, "is coming into a room where everyone else is pregnant." Other key words that come from MELD parents, besides "support," are "timely advice," "exchange of ideas," "extended family" and "you're not alone."

Today six MELD groups are active in Minneapolis alone, and others have been formed in Milwaukee, Albuquerque and Boston. The staff at MELD is happy to share their format and get other groups started, including direction toward private funding from one's local resources.

Besides meeting and talking with parents, mothers and fathers today are reading. They're reading books by other parents, such as THE MOTHER'S ALMANAC and OURSELVES AND OUR CHILDREN, which now sit on bookshelves next to the books by the "experts." Parents thrive on the humor of other parents who have "been there" —Erma Bombeck, Lynn Johnston, Judith Viorst. And parents are writing information of current and daily interest for one another in such periodicals as the magazine NEW YORK PARENT in New York City and the tabloid monthly newspaper SEATTLE'S CHILD in Washington. Both are well done and feature calendars of local events as well as interesting articles on parenting. These are only two of many such publications, and more, we are sure, are being born each month.

In short, the family unit is alive and well, and those who talk of it as dying are not looking at what parents today are doing for themselves and for one another!

★★★★★★

HOW TO GROW A PARENTS GROUP, by D. Mason, G. Jensen and C. Ryzewicz. To order, send $5.95 (ppd) to CDG Enterprises, PO Box 97, Western Springs, IL 60558. The authors are also available to speak to groups.

MELD, 123 East Grant Street, Minneapolis, MN 55403.

The Parent Place, 1608 E. 150th Street, Seattle, WA 98155.

★★★★★★

Reprinted by permission of Meadowbrook Press, Inc., from *Practical Parenting*, Vicki Lansky, ed. March/April, 1980, Vol. 2, © 1980, Meadowbrook Press, Inc.

Resources On Developmental Testing

Ladoca
Project And Publishing Foundation
East 51st Avenue and Lincoln Street
Denver, Colo. 80216

Ladoca supplies materials for developmental screening of infants and preschoolers. These include materials for conducting the widely used DDST (Denver Development Screening Test): the DDST kit, reference manual, test forms (manual and test forms are available in English and Spanish), and the "DDST Training Film." Materials are also available for the Denver Articulation Screening Exam (DASE) for ages 2½ to 7, the Denver Eye Screening Test (DEST) for children six months and older, and the Denver Audiometric Screening Test (DAST) for children three and older. "Introduction To Pediatric Screening," a slide/tape program for health professionals, can also be obtained from Ladoca.

Neonatal Behavioral Assessment Scale
by T. Berry Brazelton, M.D.
Spastics International Medical Publications
in association with J. B. Lippincott Co., Philadelphia, and William Heinemann Medical Books, LTD., London, 1973.

This book describes in detail Dr. Brazelton's method of studying the behavior of newborns and making assessments based on these observations. It is a valuable tool for nurses working with newborns.

Resources On First Aid And Safety

Prudential Insurance Co.
5 Prudential Plaza
Newark, N.J. 07101

Prudential has available "First Aid Guide," a guide for the home, and "Child Safety Is No Accident," a pamphlet for parents.

Council On Family Health
633 Third Avenue
New York, N.Y. 10017

The Council produces a wall chart, *First Aid In The Home.*

Scott Paper Company
P. O. Box 4260
Chester, Pa. 19016

Scott has available a pamphlet on infant safety, "The Gentle Art Of Babyproofing."

Safety Now Company
P. O. Box Drawer 567
Jenkintown, Pa. 19046

A free *Child Safety Catalog* may be obtained from Safety Now. (This listing is adapted from *Medical Self Care, Access To Medical Tools*, #5, 1978.)

Dunn and Reidman
1027 Kagama Street
Pacific Palisades, Calif. 90272

Dunn and Reidman publishes a handy home guide on poison antidotes and emergency procedures, "Poison Antidote Slide Guide," available for $1.98 each, with reduced rates for bulk orders.

Juvenile Products Manufacturers Association, Inc.
66 East Main Street
Moorestown, N.J. 08057

"Sitting Pretty . . . But Is She Sitting Safe?" is a brochure on high chair safety which can be obtained from Juvenile Products.

Physicians For Automotive Safety
50 Union Avenue
Irvington, N.J. 07111

This group of concerned Physicians publishes "Don't Risk Your Child's Life," a brochure on the importance of infant car seats and a list of the seats which are considered the safest. It is an excellent guide for nurses to distribute to expectant and new parents. For nurses interested in parent education on infant car protection there is also an in-hospital program which includes a teaching manual, film and hand out literature. For details contact Dr. and Mrs. Arnold Constad, A Safe Ride For Every Child, Inc., 16 Hobart Gap Road, Short Hills, N.J. 07078.

U.S. Consumer Product Safety Commission
Washington, D.C. 20207

This U.S. Consumer Product Safety Commission has available, on request, materials on child safety including children's furniture and equipment and preventing falls.

Resources On Adolescence

Families Anonymous
P. O. Box 344
Torrance, Calif. 90501

This is a support group for relatives and friends of teenagers who are troubled due to drug abuse or other problems. The local groups meet weekly, allowing parents and other concerned relatives and friends to air their frustrations and discuss ways of dealing with them. Though aimed at the families of troubled teenagers, Families Anonymous can indirectly affect the teenagers themselves by changing family attitudes. Publications available include information on starting a Families Anonymous group and literature directed at concerned families.

Society For Adolescent Medicine
P. O. Box 3462
Granada Hills, Calif. 91344

This professional organization is "open to health care professionals throughout the world who are involved in health service, teaching, or research that is concerned with the welfare of adolescents." The Society publishes information related to adolescent medicine and conducts scientific meetings twice a year on this topic.

Common Focus
The Center For Early Adolescence
Peabody Hall 037A
University Of North Carolina at Chapel Hill
Chapel Hill, N.C. 27514

The Center publishes *Common Focus: An Exchange Of Information On Early Adolescence,* a newletter which is distributed free of charge to professionals working with adolescents.

Publications

"Very Personally Yours," "The Miracle Of You," and "Your New Self-Discovery," are pamphlets for pre and early adolescent girls on menstruation and their developing bodies. From Kimberly-Clark Corporation, The Life Cycle Center, Neenah, Wisc. 54956.

Several books on sex education for parents, professionals, adolescents and younger children are available from Ed-U-Press, 760 Ostrom Avenue, Syracuse, N.Y. 13210. Write for complete listing.

Audiovisual Aids For And About Adolescents

"Growing Pains," a film on the difficulties of growing up, is available from American Educational Films.

"Puberty In Boys" discusses changes of puberty, from Films Incorporated.

"Female Cycle" is an animated portrayal of menstruation, from Films Incorporated.

"Human Development: The Adolescent Years, 12 to 16" and "Human Development: Dilemmas of Six Adolescents" are filmstrips and sound cassettes for adolescents or professionals working with adolescents, from Concept Media.

"Are You Ready For Sex," a film for facilitating open discussion among teenagers, from Perennial Education, Inc.

"Your Changing Body For Blind Children And Others" is a kit of two cassettes with a written guide for parents or teachers. It instructs the blind teenager in exploring his or her body with touch in order to learn about "Sexuality And 'Growing Up.'" From Perennial Education, Inc.

"Conflict And Awareness: A Film Series on Human Values" is a series of 35 films for teenagers or those working with them, on adjustments in adolescence. From McGraw-Hill Films.

"Thirteenth Place" is a film for professionals working with teenagers, dealing with why runaways leave home and methods of helping them deal with their problems. From the American National Red Cross.

"Who Will Come To My Party?" is a film on teenage acne, from Westwood Pharmaceuticals, Inc.

"You Can Do Something About Acne!" is a film from Syntex Laboratories, Inc.

Audiovisual Aids On Teenage Pregnancy

"Lucy" is a film dealing with teenage pregnancy from Pictura.

"And Baby Makes Two," on teenage pregnancies, is available from Films Incorporated.

"The Beat Of A Different Drummer" is a film showing the feelings of a group of black teenagers in South Carolina on their pregnancies, abortion, marriage, birth control, and other related topics. It is a sensitive film, beautifully done. From Nurse Midwife Program, Medical University Of South Carolina.

Audiovisual Aids On Adolescent Drug Abuse

"Focus On Drugs Series" is a series of five films on different addictive drugs, describing their effects, available in English and Spanish from American Educational Films.

"Students Look At Drugs" is a film of high school students discussing their experiences with drugs, from Eli Lilly Company.

"Reading, Writing And Reefer" is a film on marijuana usage of teenagers, from Films Incorporated.

"It's Only Booze" is a film for teenagers and parents on the problem of teenage drinking, from Films Incorporated.

"Short Distance Runner" is a film on problems of teenagers, including alcohol and drug use, from Narcotics Education, Inc.

"We Have An Addict In The House" is a film showing the effects of drugs on young people, from Narcotics Education, Inc.

A series of filmstrips and cassettes/records on drug education is available from Marshfilm. Filmstrips are available for primary, intermediate and junior high school students. They are particularly useful for school nurses.

Resources On Child Abuse And Neglect

American Humane Association
5351 S. Roslyn Street
Englewood, Colo. 80111

This non-profit organization is involved in the prevention of child abuse. Consultation is provided to improve child protection services and surveys are conducted on the availability of such services. Publications include books and pamphlets on child protection and a quarterly newsletter.

CALM
Child Abuse Listening Mediation, Inc.
P. O. Box 718
Santa Barbara, Calif. 93102

This largely volunteer organization was founded by a nurse, Claire Miles. The main function is prevention of child abuse. A 24-hour hotline is provided which offers listening, caring, and referrals; family aides are available for direct service; and community education on child abuse is offered. CALM has a list of pamphlets and reprints on child abuse which are available for purchase, and the organization publishes a newsletter.

National Center On Child Abuse And Neglect
Children's Bureau
Administration For Children, Youth And Families
P. O. Box 1182
Washington, D.C. 20013

The Center provides publications and posters on child abuse and neglect, including diagnosing and treating the problem, public education on abuse and neglect, information on H.E.W. regional programs on abuse and neglect, and annotated bibliographies.

National Center For The Prevention And Treatment Of Child Abuse And Neglect
1205 Oneida Street
Denver, Colo. 80220

As a regional demonstration resource, this Center provides workshops on child abuse in the Denver area. It also conducts research into the causes and prevention of abuse. Publications include *The National Child Protection Newsletter,* published quarterly; reprints of articles by the staff of the Center; bibliographies on child abuse and neglect; and videotapes and slides for training professionals working in this field (a free catalog is available on request).

National Committee For Prevention Of Child Abuse
111 East Wacker Drive, Suite 510
Chicago, Ill. 60601

A national organization for the prevention of child abuse, this group has several publications available, including booklets and pamphlets, *The National Directory Of Child Abuse Services and Information* (a listing of treatment and prevention agencies across the U.S.) a newsletter, *Caring,* and a medical bibliography. Write for complete publications listing.

Parents Anonymous (P.A.)
National Office
22330 Hawthorne Boulevard, Suite 208
Torrance, Calif. 90505

Toll-free numbers: within California: 800-352-0386
outside California: 800-421-0353

Parents Anonymous is a self-help group for parents with child abuse problems. There are nationwide local chapters which meet to talk about the members' relationships with their children, and any abuse they received as children. Parents help each other learn to control their anger and to avoid taking it out on their children. Publications include *P.A. Frontiers,* a newsletter; "Child Abuse Is Scary" and "Now You've Done It' ("A Handbook for New Mothers"); as well as literature on setting up a local P.A. chapter. This is an excellent resource for nurses to refer parents to.

"How To Start A Parental Stress Hotline" is a booklet available from Parental Stress Hot Line, P. O. Box 285, Palo Alto, Calif. 94302 (Cost: $2).

Resources On Communicable Diseases
Publications

"Childhood Diseases" is a pamphlet for parents from Prudential Insurance Co., 5 Prudential Plaza, Newark, N.J. 07101.

"A Parent's Guide To Childhood Immunization" is available from Consumer Information Center, General Services Administration, Pueblo, Colo. 81009.

"Family Immunization Record" cards for parents can be obtained from Metropolitan Life, 1 Madison Avenue, New York, N.Y. 10010.

"Recommended School Control Measures For Communicable Diseases," a poster-type publication giving pertinent data on communicable diseases for public health and school nurses, is available from the Bureau Of Communicable Disease Control, Division Of Public Health Services, New Hampshire State Department Of Health And Welfare, Health And Welfare Building, Hazen Drive, Concord, N.H. 03301.

"Scabies, Anyone Can Get It," "About Head Lice," "Questions And Answers About Head Lice," and "Lice and Scabies: From Infestation to Disinfestation," are educational materials available from Reed and Carnrick Pharmaceuticals, 30 Boright Avenue, Kenilworth, N.J. 07033.

Audiovisual Aids On Communicable Diseases

"Immunization Now" is a film on the importance of immunization, from American Educational Films.

"Communicable Diseases," a film emphasizing prevention and symptoms of communicable diseases, is available from American Educational Films.

"Immunization Against Infectious Diseases," a film for health professionals which shows the methods of immunizing against several infectious diseases, is available from Lederle Laboratories.

Resources On Genetic Disorders And Birth Defects

Cystic Fibrosis Foundation
3379 Peachtree Road, N.E.
Atlanta, Ga. 30326

The Foundation is concerned with research into cystic fibrosis and providing education on the disease for professionals and the general public. It has several centers throughout the country involved in diagnosing and treating cystic fibrosis and related diseases. Publications include "Cystic Fibrosis—A Nurse's Viewpoint," "Cystic Fibrosis: Guidelines for Health Personnel," *Sourcebook In Pediatric Pulmonary Disease,* and several other booklets, most of which are available free of charge. Also available is a teaching film, "Diagnosis And Management Of Cystic Fibrosis."

The National Foundation/March Of Dimes
1275 Mamaroneck Avenue
White Plains, N.Y. 10605

A national organization for the prevention of birth defects, the March Of Dimes has programs available in research, education, medical service and genetic counseling. It makes grants available to schools of nursing, particularly for training nurse-clinicians and nurse-midwives involved in preventing birth defects. The organization sponsors conferences and workshops for nurses and other health professionals. Publications available include *The Birth Defects Compendium,* a complete summary of known data on birth defects, revised in 1979; the *Original Article Series,* articles on birth defect research; *Reprint Series,* articles reprinted from journals; *International Directory Of Genetic Services,* a reference guide to facilities for genetic studies; Educational Modules for nurses on perinatal care (including "The First Six Hours Of Life," "Prenatal Care" and "Intrapartal Care"); and a large variety of literature for patient education on preventing birth defects, genetic counseling, nutrition in pregnancy, teenage pregnancy, V.D., and drug and alcohol use in pregnancy.

National Hemophilia Foundation, Inc.
25 West 39th Street
New York, N.Y. 10018

This national organization with over 50 chapters helps hemophiliacs lead normal lives by promoting the development of treatment centers for hemophiliacs, by supporting research into the disease, seeking funds for patients, promoting summer camps for hemophiliacs, working towards making blood more available, and providing educational materials. Write for list of publications and audio-visual aids on hemophilia.

National Tay/Sachs And Allied Diseases Association, Inc.
122 East 42nd Street
New York, N.Y. 10017

The Tay/Sachs Association provides education on Tay-Sachs and related diseases, referral services for genetic counseling, medical treatment, psychological counseling and peer support for families of afflicted children. "What You Should Know About Tay-Sachs Disease... And How To Protect Against This Fatal Illness" is an educational brochure available from the Association.

Spina Bifida Association Of America
343 S. Dearborn Street
Chicago, Ill. 60604

This non-profit, advocacy organization for persons with spina bifida provides current information on spina bifida and promotes legislation which assists the handicapped. There are local chapters and parent group affiliates located throughout the country. Publications include a bi-monthly newsletter, *Pipeline* ($6 a year), literature on spina bifida for children, parents, and teachers, and a slide presentation on spina bifida.

"The Road To Normalcy" is a booklet for parent education on cleft lip and cleft palate, from Mead Johnson and Company, Evansville, Ind. 47721.

Resources On Handicapped Children

American Association On Mental Deficiency (AAMD)
5101 Wisconsin Avenue, N.W.
Washington, D.C. 20016

This is an interdisciplinary professional and scientific organization on mental retardation. Members work together to provide education and research and to enhance the services available to the mentally retarded and their families. There is a Nursing subdivision of the organization. Publications include the *American Journal Of Mental Deficiency* (published six times a year), *Mental Retardation* (also published six times a year), and an AAMD Monograph Series on topics related to mental retardation.

Association For Children With Learning Disabilities
4156 Library Road
Pittsburgh, Pa. 15234

This is an organization with over 765 state and local affiliates whose purpose is to aid children with learning disabilities, both in their education and in their feelings about themselves. Parents and professionals working with learning disabled children may join by contacting local affiliates or becoming general members of the national organization. Publications include a monthly newsletter and an extensive list of literature in the field.

Closer Look
P. O. Box 1492
Washington, D.C. 20013

Closer Look is a "national information center for parents of children with handicaps." It offers education for parents and professionals and information on services available both nationally and locally. Any nurse working with handicapped children and their families would do them a great service by referring them to Closer Look.

Closer Look has available lists of books recommended for children and parents and professionals working with them. The following is a partial listing of the books recommended:

The Disabled And Their Parents: A Counseling Challenge by Leo Buscaglia, 1975, Charles B. Slack, Inc. (for professionals working with the disabled).

Don't Feel Sorry For Paul by Bernard Wolf, 1975, J. B. Lippincott Co. (A book for children, parents and professionals about a seven-year-old boy who is physically handicapped.)

The Exceptional Parent
Exceptional Parent Magazine
P. O. Box 641
Penacook, N.H. 03301
(A magazine for parents of disabled children, Cost: $10 a year.)

You Are Not Alone by Clara Claiborne Park with Leon N. Shapiro, M.D., 1976, Little Brown and Company (a book for people wanting information on "emotional problems, mental illness, and how to get professional help").

The Council For Exceptional Children (CEC)
1920 Association Drive
Reston, Va. 22091

CEC "is a professional organization which promotes the advancement and education of all exceptional children" through dissemination of information, training and educational workshops, and by promoting legislation. Publications include *Exceptional Children,* a periodical, and *Update,* a quarterly newspaper. The Council has subdivisions within it on particular categories of exceptional children, such as the Council For Children With Behavioral Disorders, the Division On Mental Retardation, Division For Children With Communication Disorders, The Association For The Gifted, and others,

Federation For Children With Special Needs
Suite 338
120 Boylston Street
Boston, Mass. 02116

This Federation consists of parent groups representing children with many disabilities. It serves parents, parent groups and professionals working with children with special needs, by providing information, referrals, speakers and parent training. Publications include *Newsline*, a newsletter.

Muscular Dystrophy Association (MDA)
810 Seventh Avenue
New York, N.Y. 10019

This voluntary health organization supports research and patient care in neuromuscular diseases. It has several local chapters providing medical services and public health and professional education. Through the chapters the Association provides orthopedic aids prescribed by a doctor, respiratory equipment and limited physical therapy, occupational therapy and respiratory therapy. Transportation of patients for medical and related visits can be arranged and many chapters provide recreational camps. For a list of the MDA clinics and further information on services provided, contact the association.

National Association For Retarded Citizens (NARC)
2709 Avenue E, East
Arlington, Tex. 76001

This voluntary organization works to improve the status of all mentally retarded children and adults. The emphasis is on providing services at the local level and NARC has listings of addresses for State Associations For Retarded Citizens. The Association provides support for retarded persons and their families, education to professional and lay people, works for the rights of retarded citizens, and conducts a research institute which works toward preventing retardation and improving the lives of the retarded. Publications include *Mental Retardation News,* a newspaper published six times a year; *Action Together/ Information Exchange,* a monthly newsletter; *Government Report,* by NARC, a monthly report on legislation affecting retarded citizens; and information on research, residential services, vocational rehabilitation, prevention, and education of the retarded.

**The National Easter Seal Society
For Crippled Children And Adults
2023 West Ogden Avenue
Chicago, Ill. 60612**

The Easter Seal Society is a national organization with local affiliates which provides educational materials, consultation services, professional staff training, research, public education and scholarship programs to help serve the needs of the handicapped. Easter Seal Societies also have rehabilitation programs and serve as advocates for the rights of the handicapped. Publications include *Rehabilitation Literature,* a professional journal published ten times a year (Cost: $15 in the U.S.; $16 in Canada; $17 in other countries; $12 for students), extensive bibliographies on the handicapped, posters and other literature. *Let's Play Games* by Croke and Fairchild is a 61-page illustrated book on games for physically handicapped children ($1.25 plus 75¢ postage for single copy, lower rates for bulk orders). *The Art And Science Of Parenting The Disabled Child,* a collection of talks from a 1976 symposium exploring the roles and needs of parents of handicapped children, is available ($1.25), as well as the *Easter Seal Directory Of Resident Camps For Persons With Special Needs,* which lists over 225 camps by state ($2 a copy plus $1 postage and handling).

**United Cerebral Palsy Associations, Inc.
66 East 34th Street
New York, N.Y. 10016**

This Association has extensive literature for parents and professionals, including *Handling The Young Cerebral Palsied Child At Home,* a paperback book and *A Developmental Approach To Casefinding* by Una Haynes, an excellent booklet for nurses on identifying children with cerebral palsy and other developmental disorders. This book includes a "Wheel Of Developmental Milestones" which serves as a handy pocket reference.

Publications

Growing Up Handicapped: A Guide to Helping the Exceptional Child, by Evelyn West Ayrault, © 1977, The Seabury Press, 815 Second Ave., New York, N.Y. 10017.

This book by a clinical psychologist who was born with cerebral palsy is an excellent resource for parents and professionals working with physically handicapped children. The book describes in depth the problems and needs of the handicapped, and equally important it contains an extensive resource section which includes addresses for organizations serving the handicapped; sources for aids to daily living and an extensive description of some of the aids available such as aids for self-feeding, for homemaking, etc.; a listing of State Offices for Occupational Therapy, Physical Therapy and Speech Pathology and Audiology; and a "Directory of Colleges and Universities With Facilities for Handicapped Students."

Growing Up Handicapped is highly recommended to any individual or agency working with handicapped children and their families and is also a good resource to recommend to parents.

Helping the Severely Handicapped Child: A Guide for Parents and Teachers, by Phyllis Doyle, John Goodman, Jeffery Grotsky and Lester Mann, illustrated by Joseph Connolly, © 1979, Thomas Y. Crowell Publishers, New York.

This is another helpful guide for parents and professionals.

A bibliography of "Recommended Reading in Developmental Medicine" by Nancy Bender and Leonard Bender, is available from the American Academy for Cerebral Palsy and Developmental Medicine, 1255 New Hampshire Avenue, N.W., Suite 1030, Washington, D.C. 20036.

"Plain Talk About Learning Disabilities" is a pamphlet for parents from Consumer Information Center, General Services Administration, Pueblo, Colo. 81009.

Yes You Can, a 25-page booklet for children with learning disabilities is available from the National Easter Seal Society, 2023 West Ogden Avenue, Chicago, Ill. 60612. (Cost: 50¢ plus 25¢ for postage and handling.)

Resources On Hospital Care Of Children

Association For The Care Of Children In Hospitals
3615 Wisconsin Avenue, N.W.
Washington, D.C. 20016

This is a multidisciplinary organization with regional affiliates, which promotes "humanizing health care for children and their families" through education, research and interdisciplinary communication. Anyone interested in pediatric care may become a member of the Association (individual membership: $30 a year; student membership: $15 a year). Publications include a bimonthly newsletter and a quarterly journal, *Journal Of The Association For The Care Of Children In Hospitals,* from Charles B. Slack, Inc., Publishers. An annual conference is held on concerns related to hospitalization of children.

Children In Hospitals, Inc. (CIH)
31 Wilshire Park
Needham, Mass. 02192

Children in Hospitals is an organization of parents and health care workers which promotes rooming in of parents with hospitalized children and lenient visiting hours for parents. The group encourages preparing children for hospitalization by use of films, literature, and toy hospital sets (a list of such materials and their sources is available from CIH). Publications include a newsletter with information on organizations throughout the country concerned about children in hospitals, educational information, and letters from parents sharing their experiences.

Publications

The following publications are available from the U.S. Government Printing Office, Superintendent of Documents, Washington, D.C. 20402:

Books That Help Children Deal With A Hospital Experience, prepared by Anne Altshuler (50¢).

"When Your Child Goes To The Hospital," Department of H.E.W., Pub. No. (OHD) 76-30092 (85¢).

Resources On Juvenile Diabetes

The Juvenile Diabetes Foundation (JDF)
23 East 26th Street
New York, N.Y. 10010

This is a "national, non-profit, voluntary agency" for research in preventing complications of diabetes and curing the disease. The Foundation has educational programs for diabetic children and their familes and for the community. JDF publishes several brochures for parents and children, including, "Diabetes: There Is Hardly A Family It Doesn't Touch," "Parent To Parent: Babies With Diabetes," "What You Should Know About The Student With Diabetes," "What You Should Know About Insulin," and the Foundation's newsletter, "Dimensions In Diabetes."

Resources on Life-Threatening Illnesses in the Child

The Candlelighters Foundation
123 C Street, S.E.
Washington, D.C. 20003

The Candlelighters is an international organization of parent groups for parents of children who have or have had cancer. Local groups provide support through self-help groups, 24-hour hotlines, social functions, exchanging information, and easing fears and frustrations through the sharing of experiences. Membership is open to professionals working with children who have cancer as well as to parents. The national organization supplies bibliographies on childhood cancer, including books for children and parents. Information is also available on local resources for parents. The Candlelighters also publishes a quarterly magazine, a bimonthly newsletter (with information of interest to nurses on what families experience and their needs when they have a child with cancer), and the "Candlelighters Handbook."

Center for Attitudinal Healing
19 Main Street
Tiburon, Calif. 94920

This Center provides a means of support for children with catastrophic illnesses and their families. The emphasis is on allaying fear in an attempt to foster peace of mind. The Center compiles a Pen Pal-Phone Pal exchange for children and parents to keep in touch with others in similar situations, and it offers workshops for people interested in starting similar centers in other areas. The Center offers special groups for children with catastrophic illnesses, for mothers, fathers, and siblings.

Publications available include: *There Is A Rainbow Behind Every Dark Cloud*, a book by and about some of the children helped by the Center, written for other children with catastrophic illnesses; *How To Start A Group For Children With Catastrophic Illnesses;* and *Peer And Self-Healing In Children With Catastrophic Illnesses.* Write for complete list of educational materials.

The Compassionate Friends, Inc.
National Headquarters
P. O. Box 1347
Oak Brook, Ill. 60521

This is "a self-help organization offering friendship and understanding to bereaved parents." There are many local chapters in the United States, The United Kingdom, and Canada, offering support to parents who have recently experienced the death of a child. Anyone interested in starting a local chapter should contact the national headquarters.

National Sudden Infant Death Syndrome Foundation
310 S. Michigan Avenue
Chicago, Ill. 60604

The Foundation is a non-profit organization which promotes research into the cause and prevention of S.I.D.S., provides support and information to families of infants afflicted with S.I.D.S., and educates the lay public and health professionals on this condition. It makes available, for a small fee, several excellent publications for parents ("Facts About Sudden Infant Death," "The Subsequent Child," a publication of the U.S. Department of H.E.W., "How Shall We Tell The Children," and others), and for health professionals ("The Counseling Of Families In The Professional Management Of S.I.D.S." and "Preparing For A Nurse's Visit To S.I.D.S Families"). Also available from the Foundation are three films by the U.S. Department of H.E.W. on S.I.D.S., "You Are Not Alone" (for parents), "After Our Baby Died" (for parents and counselors), and "A Call For Help" (for Emergency Medical Workers, "on the importance of sensitivity to the family's feelings and needs").

Parent Involvement

Vancouver General Hospital in Vancouver, British Columbia, has an Oncology Center which encourages parental involvement. Parents are given educational material on their children's illnesses, and informal discussions are held to discuss concerns about the children. Pam Kundareurich, of the hospital, is compiling written stories of patients' experiences with Hodgkins disease, brain tumors, Wilm's tumors and neuroblastomas. She is seeking stories of "Living With" the diseases to share with parents. Anyone with such stories is urged to send them to: Pam Kundareurich, Health Centre for Children, Social Service Department, Vancouver General Hospital, 855 West 12th Ave., Vancouver, B.C. Canada V5z1M9.

This material is adapted from *Candlelighters National Newsletter,* Winter, 1980, Vol. 111, No. 4, p. 6, published and distributed by the American Cancer Society, Inc.

A Story About Cancer and *A Story About Leukemia,* by J. Dobos and P.Thorp, 1978, are two children's coloring books for use in teaching children about these diseases and their treatments. They are available from University Hospitals Cancer Center, At-Home Rehabilitation Program, 2074 Abington Rd., Cleveland, Ohio, 44106. Also available are "Pediatric Oncology Resource Guide," edited by Marjorie B. Sachs, an excellent guide for nurses, patients and their families in the local Cleveland area but of use to those in other areas as well, and "Pediatric Oncology Bibliography," compiled by Marjorie Sachs and Paulette Thorp, January, 1980, an extensive bibliography for patients, their families and health professionals. The bibliography includes references on general pediatric oncology; audiovisual aids; cancer information resources; hospitalization of children; nutrition; child development; activities and play therapy; schools, camps and employment; books for children on illness and death; and general books on death, dying and the grieving process.

Resources in Perinatology

Institutes In Perinatology For Nurses
The New York Hospital-Cornell Medical Center
525 East 68th Street
New York, N.Y. 10021

The New York Hospital-Cornell Medical Center, sponsored by the New York State Department Of Health and the U.S. Department of H.E.W., offers three-week institutes for training nurses in up-to-date practices in perinatology. They are open to nurses currently working with high-risk infants. Write for applications.

"Narcotic Addiction In The Newborn: Programmed Instruction" is an educational tool for nurses prepared by Johnson and Johnson Co., 1972, from Johnson and Johnson, New Brunswick, N.J. 08903.

Periodicals on Pediatric Nursing

American Journal Of Diseases Of Children, a monthly journal published by the American Medical Association (see address under Index of Publishers). (Cost: $18 a year, U.S., $28 Foreign.)

Children Today, a journal published six times a year by the Children's Bureau, Administration for Children, Youth and Families, U.S. Department of H.E.W., it contains articles of interest to those working with children and their families. Available from the Superintendent of Documents (See address under Index of Publishers).

Issues In Comprehensive Pediatric Nursing, a bimonthly journal available from McGraw-Hill Book Company ($17 a year).

The Journal Of Pediatrics, a monthly publication of The C. V. Mosby Co., is geared to physicians but also of use to nurses and allied health professionals ($24 a year).

Pediatric Clinics Of North America, a quarterly publication of W. B. Saunders Co. ($21 a year).

Pediatric Nursing, the official journal of NAPNAP (see: Nurses' Association Of Pediatric Nurse Associates And Practitioners, under "Nursing Organizations.")

Audiovisual Aids for Pediatric Nursing

"Growth And Development: A Chronicle Of Four Children," a series of films which follows the development of four children from infancy to four years old, is available from Lippincott's Audiovisual Media.

"Human Development: First 2½ Years" and "Human Development: 2½ to 6 Years" are series of filmstrips and sound cassettes from Concept Media.

Parents' Magazine Films, Inc. produces several films on "child development," "parent education," "family relationships" and "caring for children." Write for current catalog.

"How Babies Learn" is a film on development in the first year of life, from University Of California Extension Media Center.

"Car Safety: Don't Risk Your Child's Life," a film on the need for car seats for infants, excellent for showing to expectant and new parents, is available from Physicians For Automotive Safety.

"The Pediatric Examination: Art And Process" is a series of five films or videocassettes showing the techniques for a complete physical exam of children from birth through school-age. From Lippincott's Audiovisual Media.

"Resuscitation Of The Newborn," a film demonstrating procedures, is available from the American Heart Association.

"Examining The Well Child" is a film from International Film Bureau, Inc.

"The Brazelton Neonatal Assessment Scale: An Introduction" and "The Brazelton Neonatal Assessment Scale: Variations In Normal Behavior" are two films demonstrating this assessment method, from EDC Distribution Center.

"Appraisal Of The Infant," a film to instruct nurses in identifying developmental problems, and "Nursing Appraisal Of Neurological Development at 3, 6, and 12 Months Of Age," are available from the United Cerebral Palsy Associations, Inc., as are many other films and audiotapes on developmental disabilities.

Cassette tapes on all aspects of child care and welfare, taken from conferences and workshops given by authorities in child care, are available from the Child Care Information Center. Of particular interest to nurses are tapes made in conjunction with the Children's Rehabilitation Center, University Of Virginia Medical Center at their various conferences. Topics from these include "Spinal Cord Injuries In Children And Adolescents," "Scoliosis" (with tapes on screening and treatment), "Treatment Of The High Risk Infant" and "Ethical Issues In Decision Making In The Care Of The Handicapped Child." For complete catalog contact the Child Care Information Center. The Center also conducts bibliographic searches for children's institutions and individuals on request.

"Ethan Has An Operation," a film story of a seven-year-old boy hospitalized for a hernia operation, told in his own words, is available from Health Sciences Communication Center. It is useful in preparing children for surgery and for hospital staff, as an aid to better understanding of children's feelings.

"When A Child Enters The Hospital," a film on the feelings of children and the importance of the participation of parents in the child's hospital care. From Polymorph Films.

"Children In The Hospital," a film on the emotional reactions of children to hospitalization, is available from International Film Bureau, Inc.

"We Won't Leave You," a film showing parents' participation in the hospitalization of a child to help reduce the child's fears, and "Care Through Parents: Creating A New Space In Pediatrics," on the benefits of parent participation, are available from the University Of California Extension Media Center.

"Just Awful" is a film on one child's visit to the school nurse, intended to teach children and allay their fears. From Paramount Communications.

"Child's Visit To The Hospital," a sound filmstrip program for preparing children for a hospital stay, is available from Robert J. Brady Co.

"My Friend, Edi" is an animated film for juvenile diabetics and their parents on diabetes and how to control it, from Eli Lilly and Co.

"Low Blood Sugar Emergencies In The Diabetic Child," a film for teaching lay people and professionals who come in contact with diabetic children, is available from the Juvenile Diabetes Foundation, Greater Washington Area Chapter.

"Handicapped By Fate" is a film for health professionals showing the treatment of a child with harelip and cleft palate, from Hoechst.

"PKU Mental Deficiency Can Be Prevented" is a film from Ames Company.

"The Handicapped Child: Infancy Through Preschool" is a series of eight filmstrips and sound cassettes from Concept Media.

"Congenital Malformations Of The Heart" is a film available from the American Heart Association.

"The Public Health Nurse And The Mentally Retarded Child" is a film for public health nurses, from International Film Bureau, Inc.

"Special Children, Special Needs," a film on adapting the environment to meet the educational needs of handicapped children, available from University Of California Extension Media Center.

"Kelly," a film about a child with cerebral palsy, "Somewhere To Go," on a study of children with Down's Syndrome, and "Sara Has Down's Syndrome" are all available from EDC Distribution Center.

"A Minority Of One," a film on autism and the use of behavior modification to treat it, is available from Films Incorporated.

"A Boy Named Terry Egan," a film about a nine-year-old autistic boy and his family, is available from Carousel Films.

Films on child abuse and family violence for professionals are available from Motorola Teleprograms, Inc.

An extensive catalog of audiovisual materials on child abuse and neglect is available from the National Center On Child Abuse and Neglect, D.H.E.W. Publication No. (OHDS) 78-30127.

"Child Molestation: When To Say No," a film for children on dealing with being approached by child molesters, is available from Aims Instructional Media, Inc.

"Child Abuse—Don't Hide The Hurt," a film for school-age children on the importance of reporting an incident of child abuse to an adult who can help them. From Aims Instructional Media, Inc.

"The Nurse In Child Abuse Prevention" is a film from the American Journal Of Nursing Co.

"Battered Child," is a film on child abuse, the causes and effects of it, from University Of California Extension Media Center.

"Children's Conceptions Of Death" is a film on how children perceive death at different ages, from the University Of Wisconsin-Milwaukee, Media, School Of Nursing.

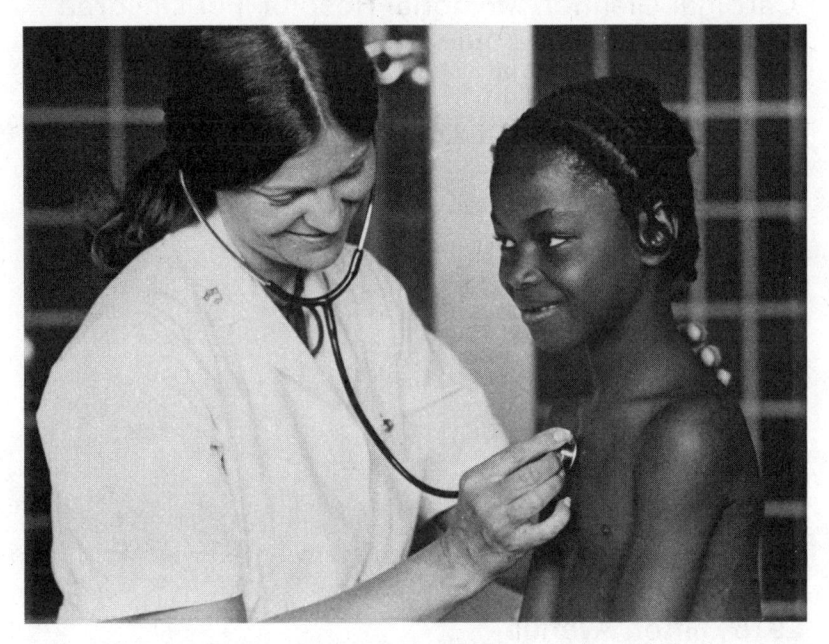

Reproduced with permission of the publisher of Pediatric Nursing, Vol. 4, No. 5, September/October, 1978, from "The ABC's: 3 R's and H," by Phyllis Nichols, RN, MPH, PNP.

Schools with Educational Programs for Pediatric Nurse Practitioners, Associates, and Clinical Specialists

Albert Einstein College Of Medicine
1300 Morris Park Avenue
Bronx, N.Y. 10461

Bronx Municipal Hospital Center
Pelham Parkway and Eastchester Road
Bronx, N.Y. 10461

California State University At Fresno
Valley Medical Center
445 South Cedar Avenue
Fresno, Calif. 93740

California State University At Long Beach
School Of Applied Arts And Sciences
1250 Bellflower Boulevard
Long Beach, Calif. 90840

Cardinal Glennon Memorial Hospital For Children
1465 South Grant Boulevard
St. Louis, Mo. 63104

Catholic University Of America
School Of Nursing
Washington, D.C. 20064

Columbia University
School Of Nursing
630 W. 168th Street
New York, N.Y. 10032

East Carolina University
School Of Nursing
Greenville, N.C. 27834

Good Samaritan Hospital
O'Connell Unit
2915 Clifton Avenue
Cincinnati, Ohio 45220

Indiana University
School Of Nursing
1100 West Michigan Street
Indianapolis, Ind. 46202

Loma Linda University
School Of Nursing
Loma Linda, Calif. 92354

Meharry Medical College
Department Of Nursing Education
Box 61-A
1005 18th Avenue, North
Nashville, Tenn. 37208

Northeastern University
College Of Nursing
11 Leon Street
Boston, Mass. 02115

Rush-Presbyterian-St. Luke's Medical Center
1753 West Congress Parkway
Chicago, Ill. 60612

Seton Hall University
College Of Nursing
400 South Orange Avenue
South Orange, N.J. 07079

SUNY At Buffalo
School Of Nursing
3435 Main Street
Buffalo, N.Y. 14214

SUNY Upstate Medical Center
College Of Health Related Professions
750 East Adams Street
Syracuse, N.Y. 13210

University Of Alabama In Birmingham
School Of Nursing
University Station
Birmingham, Ala. 35294

University Of Arkansas For Medical Sciences
College Of Nursing
4301 West Markham Street
Little Rock, Ark. 72201

University Of California At Los Angeles
School Of Nursing
10833 Le Conte Avenue
Los Angeles, Calif. 90024

University Of California At San Diego
Office Of Continuing Education and
Health Sciences
School Of Medicine
La Jolla, Calif. 92093

University Of California At San Francisco
Department Of Family Health Care
Nursing N411Y
San Francisco, Calif. 94143

University Of Colorado
School Of Nursing
4200 East Ninth Avenue, C287
Denver, Colo. 80262

University Of Iowa
College Of Nursing
Iowa City, Iowa 52242

University Of Miami
School Of Nursing
Sewell Building D-2-5
Miami, Fla. 33152

University Of Michigan
School Of Nursing
1355 Catherine Street
Ann Arbor, Mich. 48109

University Of Minnesota
School Of Public Health
1325 Mayo
Minneapolis, Minn. 55455

University Of Mississippi
School Of Nursing
2500 North State Street

University Of Missouri At Kansas City
Nursing Education
Health Sciences Building
2220 Holmes Street
Kansas City, Missouri 64108

University Of Oregon
School Of Nursing
Health Sciences Center
3181 S.W. Jackson Park Road
Portland, Ore. 97201

University Of Pittsburgh
School Of Nursing
Victoria Building
Pittsburgh, Pa. 15261

University Of Texas
School Of Nursing
Galveston, Tex. 77550

University Of Virginia
School Of Nursing
McLeod Hall
Charlottesville, Va. 22903

University Of Washington
School Of Nursing SM24
Seattle, Wash. 98195

University Of Wisconsin-Madison
School Of Nursing
1402 University Avenue
Madison, Wisc. 53706

Virginia Commonwealth University
School Of Nursing
Medical College Of Virginia Station
Richmond, Va. 23298

Washington University
School Of Medicine
Division Of Health Care Research
St. Louis, Mo. 63110

Yale University
School Of Nursing
38 South Street
New Haven, Conn. 06520

Adapted from *A Directory Of Expanded Role Programs For Registered Nurses,* 1979, Division Of Nursing, Health Resources Administration, U. S. Department Of H.E.W.

8 Gerontological Nursing

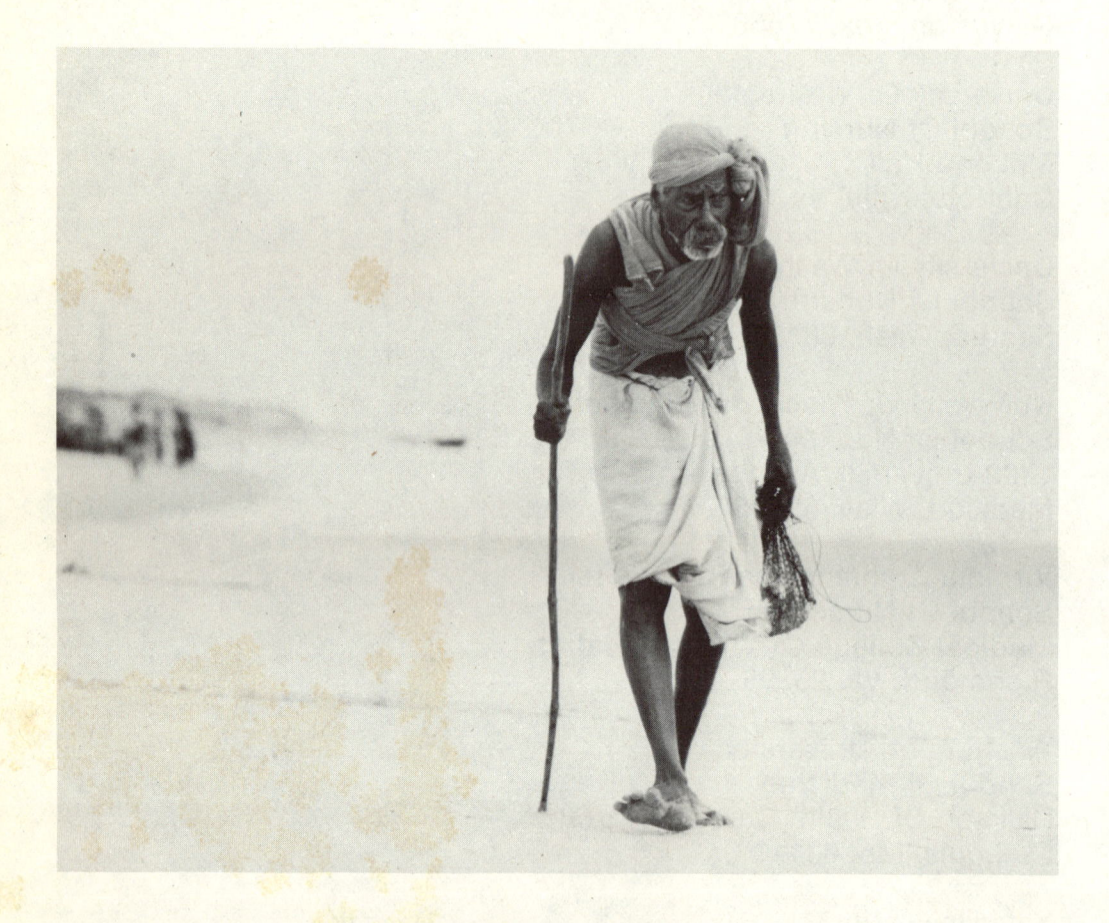

Cover photograph of *New Yorker Films Educational Catalogue*, 1978–1979, taken from their film, "Phantom India." Reprinted by permission of New Yorker Films.

In recent years care of the elderly has become a nursing specialty, due in part to increased knowledge of the needs of the elderly, and to the fact that more people are living to the age of 65 and older. Many innovations in geriatric care are currently being practiced. Four examples of these follow. They are reprinted from *Analysis and Planning for Improved Distribution of Nursing Personnel and Services,* ed. by Sheila Kodadek, 1976,

Division of Nursing, Health Resources Administration, U.S. Department of H.E.W.

Also included is a list of educational programs in this field, and a description of changes of aging which predispose the elderly to falling.

I. Aging Changes
II. Innovations in Geriatric Nursing
III. Resources in Geriatrics
   Organizations
   Publications
   Audiovisual Materials
   Schools for Geriatric Nursing

Aging Changes

Changes occurring with age as a result of diminished functioning of the circulatory, nervous, and musculoskeletal systems that predispose the elderly to falling and to serious complications from falls.

- decreased circulation in brain, causing vertigo, dizziness, fainting
- mechanical obstruction of vertebral arteries in brain by crushed osteoporotic vertebrae
- decreased auditory acuity
- decreased night vision, color vision, visual acuity
- cataracts, glaucoma
- inner ear canal problems
- arteriosclerosis
- orthostatic hypotension
- loss of sense of position
- diminished space perception
- decreased muscle mass, strength, coordination
- decreased ability to balance

drop attacks

osteoporosis and increased stress on weight-bearing areas

alteration in gait

susceptibility to fractures

foot abnormalities

diminished muscular activity necessary for adequate venous return

decreased capacity of blood vessels

slowed nervous system response

osteoarthritis and other arthritic conditions

parachute reflex (spreading arms for balance)

Reprinted from "Why The Elderly Fall" by Natalie Slocumb Witte in *The American Journal of Nursing*, November, 1979, Vol. 79, No. 11, p. 1951. © 1979. The American Journal of Nursing Co.

An excellent guide on "The Aging Process" for use in teaching family members involved in home care of the elderly is available in *Family Health and Home Nursing*, © 1979 by the American National Red Cross, pages 185–193.

Innovations

Nursing Home Telemedicine Program
Boston City Hospital
Boston, Massachusetts

Purpose: There are about one million Americans in 23,000 nursing homes in the United States, and the numbers are growing. Medical care for this population, which in the past has been considered a secondary priority to busy private practitioners, is overdue for major improvement.

At Boston City Hospital, appropriate use of nurse practitioner-physician teams has provided an infusion of quality care that is so obviously needed. The Nursing Home Telemedicine Program was established in 1972 at Boston City Hospital to study a method of improving the quality and accessibility of primary medical care to nursing home patients. The target population is residents of 13 Boston nursing homes.

Nursing Role: The health team is composed of one hospital-based internist and four nurse practitioners who provide primary care to the 349 patients currently in the system, which has a planned capacity of 500. The four nurses are each assigned to four to six nursing homes, generally working in teams of two in each home. The average caseload is 90, with the ideal estimated to be 125. The team provides coverage 24 hours a day, seven days a week. Within 24 hours after discharge from a hospital, the patient is seen by the nurse practitioner. She performs a complete patient work-up, including history, family interview, physical examination, and hospital chart review, and she reviews the hospital orders with the nursing home staff. Within a few days, the team physician examines the patient and reviews the nurse practitioner work-up. The nurse practitioner has considerable responsibility for the medical management of her patients. She is responsible for performing all scheduled follow-up assessments, which include interval history, limited physical examination, and the ordering of necessary laboratory work. She also develops individualized flow charts to facilitate record-keeping and chart review. She is responsible for the initial evaluation of a new problem or emergency. In some cases, the nurse practitioner may deal with the problems without direct physician consultation; in others, a physician consultation is requested via telephone or in person.

In the event of transfer from the nursing home, the team will act as patient advocate with a hospital staff, a consultant, or community agencies. The role of the nurse practitioner is modified to some extent by the special characteristics and problems of the geriatric nursing home resident. These residents typically have multiple medical problems, usually of a chronic, degenerative nature, requiring careful and consistent monitoring of clinical status. In addition, nursing home residents characteristically have many psychosocial needs relating to their chronic disease, their institutionalization, and, in some cases, their impending death. The nurse's previous education and experience is particularly important in dealing with these problems. The nurse practitioner assesses the rehabilitation potential of the residents and applies or facilitates expert nursing techniques to optimize each resident's potential for independent living. She also coordinates the services of other professionals, including occupational therapists, dentists, dieticians, and podiatrists.

Another responsibility of the nurse practitioner is to relate effectively with the nursing home staff, from nursing directors to nurse's aides. Inservice education is one contribution. Finally, the nurse is responsible for working with terminally ill residents, their families, and the staff of the nursing home.

Cost: The initial funding for this program was through the RANN Program of the National Science Foundation. During the 1975–76 year, the Nursing Home Telemedicine Program was funded by direct payment from Medicaid. An annually renewable contract was arranged with the Nursing Home Telemedicine Program as a pilot project, guaranteeing $20 per every nurse charge allowed for the general physician coverage, which is paid only for a single illness visit per month.

Based on preliminary estimates, the expected cost of the nurse practitioner-physician visits is comparable to the existing fee schedules of the visiting nurses' association or a visit to a neighborhood health center. Further information will be available with more study.

Evaluation: The preliminary findings, based on a fraction of the patient population (200 study/200 control clients), suggest the following. The nurse practitioner sees an average of nine patients per day, with an average visit length of 36 minutes. The initial work-up lasts 83 minutes, and the follow-up visits last 27 minutes. Eighty percent of the visits do not require physician consultation. Fifty-seven percent of the average day is spent in patient visits and related paperwork. The average number of days between visits is 16, compared to a 30-day interval for patients receiving traditional care. Hospitalization rate per 100 patient-months is three days, compared to four days for nursing home patients receiving traditional care. Mortality rate per 1,000 patient-months is nine, compared to 14 for nursing home patients receiving traditional care. Further information will be available as the statistical data are reviewed.

Contact for Further Information:
Anne A. Ripley, RN
Clinical Director of Nursing for Ambulatory Services

Beth Israel Hospital
330 Brookline Avenue
Boston, Massachusetts, 02215

Sunset Park Senior Health Assessment and Preventive Education Demonstration Project
Visiting Nurse Association of the Denver Area, Inc.
Denver, Colorado

Purpose: Between October and November 1974, the Sunset Park Residence participated in a demonstration project with the Denver Visiting Nurse Service in a nurse-run health-assessment clinic. Sunset Park is a rent-subsidized high-rise apartment complex with an estimated 300 residents. It is operated by the Volunteers of America. The program offered physical assessment of individuals by a nurse practitioner, with group health-teaching sessions conducted by the district public-health nurse.

Nursing Role: The nurse practitioner spent six hours per week at the facility to provide individual physical assessment to residents and nonresidents on request. In addition, she provided counseling, screening, teaching, and referral services when necessary. The public-health nurse spent two hours per week conducting health-education and health-screening sessions. Topics included diabetes and stroke, blood pressure, cardiac disease, arthritis, mental health, and defensive living. The latter dealt with an elderly person living in the city and included ideas for self-defense.

Cost: The project was supported by contract money. A cost-effectiveness study was not provided.

Evaluation: A general evaluation of the project was conducted, and several recommendations were made for future work. The suggestions included emphasizing health screening in the education sessions and charging a nominal fee. Informa-

Contact for Further Information:
Dolora Cotter, RN, MS
Administrative Associate Director
Visiting Nurse Association of the Denver Area, Inc.
605 Bannock Street
Denver, Colorado 80204

Smiley Point Clinic
Minneapolis, Minnesota

Purpose: The Smiley Point Clinic delivers primary health care to elderly clients of four high-rise buildings. The clinic provides experience in geriatric health care for family practice residents and for nursing students from St. Olaf College, Northfield, Minnesota.

Nursing Role: The geriatric nurse practitioner works closely with the elderly client and the family practice residents to provide coordinated, comprehensive health care. Her responsibilities include case finding, data base development of individual clients, and referrals to the family practice residents for differential diagnoses when needed. She collaborates with residents to design and implement plans for client care and provides follow-up, health education, and counseling. She makes hospital rounds and nursing home visits to Smiley Point Clinic clients.

Contact for Further Information:
Beryl Westphal, RN
Nurse Practitioner, Smiley Point Clinic
2200 Riverside Avenue South
Minneapolis, Minnesota 55404

Iowa's Well Elderly Clinics
Iowa State Department of Health
Des Moines, Iowa

Purpose: A major goal of the Iowa State Department of Health is to make health services available and accessible to every citizen. In the predominantly rural areas of Iowa, the physician often is the only medical resource available; prevention, supervision, and education generally are not provided unless the patient receives the services of a public-health nurse. These nurses are beginning to provide expanded health-care services by assuming more responsibilities for health screening through the Well Elderly Clinics. These clinics deliver health-supervision services on a demonstration basis to well persons 60 years of age or older in five areas of the state, two of which are rural. The health-screening clinics were established between October 1975 and March 1976. About 100 public-health nurses have been trained in short-term programs to conduct these clinics. Each of the designated areas contracts with two certified family nurse practitioners for consultation and staff development.

Nursing Role: Public-health nurses in the well elderly clinics are responsible for taking health histories of individuals and families and conducting comprehensive appraisals of an individual's health status, including physical assessment, coping ability, and emotional and social well-being. They are trained to discriminate between normal and abnormal findings and between normal variations of development and abnormal deviations. They assist families through health education and counseling, delegate appropriate health-care activities to assisting personnel, collaborate with physicians and other health professionals in devising ways to deliver primary care, help families and individuals use appropriate community resources, and coordinate those resources when necessary. Seventy-four percent of the nurses employed as county public-health nurses in Iowa are diploma-school graduates.

Evaluation: Health problems have been assessed with clients at clinic settings and in the client's home, with follow-up by the public-health nurse. The 70 county public-health nursing agencies certified for the Health Insurance Benefits Program in Iowa do a time study and cost analysis annually. The nursing section of the Iowa State Department of Health will share information.

Contact for Further Information:
Darleen Sickert, RN, MPH
Assistant Director
Iowa State Department of Health
Division of Community Health Nursing Section
Des Moines, Iowa 50319

Resources on Geriatrics

Administraiton on Aging
DHEW
Washington, D.C. 20201

This is a clearinghouse and source for educational materials on aging. Publications include a monthly newsmagazine, AGING; "Facts About Older Americans 1978" (U.S. Dept. of H.E.W. Publication Number OHDS 79-20006), a brochure with statistics on the elderly; "To Find the Way to Opportunities and Sources for Older Americans," a booklet (Dept of H.E.W. Pub. No. OHD 75-20807); and several other booklets and pamphlets.

American Health Care Association
1200 Fifteenth St., N.W.
Washington, D.C. 20005

This is an organization made up of long-term health care institutions which promotes good health care for people with chronic illnesses. Publications available include materials on management of long-term facilities (especially nursing homes), training manuals for personnel in these facilities, materials for family members of people in nursing homes, materials on aging and related topics.

National Council of Senior Citizens, Inc.
1511 K St., N.W.
Washington, D.C. 20005

This national non-profit organization has over 3000 local club affiliates throughout the country. It promotes political and legislative concerns of the aging and provides social and recreational activities for members. Benefits to members include savings on prescriptions, a health insurance plan to supplement medicare at group rates, travel discounts, discounts on books, and the monthly *Senior Citizen News.*

National Council on the Aging
1828 L St., N.W. Suite 504
Washington, D.C. 20036

This is a non-profit resource agency focusing on concerns of the elderly. Several publications on aging can be obtained from the Council, including *Fact Book on Aging: A Profile of America's Older Population,* several books, pamphlets, tapes and films.

Publications on Geriatrics

Journal of Gerontological Nursing. This is a bimonthly specialty journal with information on nursing care of the elderly, from Charles B. Slack, Inc. ($10.00/year).

Audiovisual Materials on Geriatrics

"The Instructor" is an audiovisual program for nursing home employees and new residents. It includes a projector as well as film and sound cartridge. Available from American Health Care Association/Peshak Films.

"Nobody Ever Died of Old Age," a film on the plight of the elderly in our society, is available from Films, Incorporated.

"Perspectives on Aging" is a series of 5 filmstrips and sound cassettes from Concept Media.

"Crime: Senior Alert" is a film for senior citizens on ways to avoid being crime victims, from Aims Instructional Media, Inc.

"Aging: A Fact of Life" consists of 2 filmstrips and cassettes appropriate for nurses and patients, from Eye Gate Media.

"Rescue From Isolation" is a film on the use of day hospitals for the elderly as a possible solution to isolation problems, from Polymorph Films.

"The Rights of Age" and "The Steps of Age" are 2 films on adjustments to aging from International Film Bureau, Inc.

A series of videotape/film classes on gerontological nursing is available from the American Journal of Nursing Company. Titles include "Aging: Who Is Listening?," "Aging: An Individual Matter," "Aging: The Losses," and "Aging: Slowing Down."

"56½ Howard St." and "Older and Bolder" are 2 films on aging from EDC Distribution Center.

Schools Having Educational Programs in Geriatric Nursing

Boston University
School of Nursing
635 Commonwealth Ave.
Boston, Mass. 02215

Case-Western Reserve University
School of Nursing
2121 Abington Rd.
Cleveland, Ohio 44106

College of Nursing
University of Arizona
Tucson, Arizona 85724

Columbia University
School of Nursing
630 West 168th St.
New York, N.Y. 10032

Cornell University—N.Y. Hospital
School of Nursing
515 East 71st St.
New York, N.Y. 10021

Emory University
Nel Hodgson Woodruff School of Nursing
Atlanta, Georgia 30322

School of Nursing
University of Wisconsin
1402 University Ave.
Madison, Wisconsin 53706

Seton Hall University
College of Nursing
400 South Orange Ave.
South Orange, N.J. 07079

SUNY Upstate Medical Center
College of Health Related Professions
750 East Adams St.
Syracuse, N.Y. 13210

University of California at Davis
Department of Family Practice
Davis, Ca. 95616

University of Colorado
School of Nursing
4200 East 9th Ave., C287
Denver, Co. 80262

University of Kansas
School of Nursing
39th and Rainbow Boulevard
Kansas City, Kansas 66103

University of Lowell
Graduate School and College of Health Professions
Nursing Division
1 University Ave.
Lowell, Mass. 01854

University of Miami
School of Nursing
Sewell Building D-2-5
Miami, Florida 33152

University of Minnesota
School of Public Health
1325 Mayo
Minneapolis, Minn. 55455

University of Pittsburgh
School of Nursing
Victoria Building
Pittsburgh, Pa. 15261

University of Utah
College of Nursing
25 South Medical Dr.
Salt Lake City, Utah 84112

Adapted from *A Directory of Expanded Role Programs for Registered Nurses*, 1979, Division of Nursing, Health Resources Administration, U.S. Department of H.E.W.

9 Death and Dying

The following information includes a sampling of the vast amount of material available on death and working with the dying and their families. These topics have been receiving much attention in the nursing literature as nurses have become aware of the special needs of the dying and how our own feelings about and fears of death affect the way we relate to these patients and their families.

I. The Dying Person's Bill of Rights
II. Nurse Specialists For The Dying
III. Stages in the Acceptance of Death
IV. Death—A Part of Living
V. Separation and Loss
VI. GRAMP—A Review
VII. "Extraordinary Life-Support Measures"
VIII. Resources on Death and Dying
Rights of the Dying
Support for the Dying
Support for the Bereaved
Hospices
Publications
Audiovisual Materials

The Dying Person's Bill of Rights *

I have the right to be treated as a living human being until I die.

I have the right to maintain a sense of hopefulness however changing its focus may be.

I have the right to be cared for by those who can maintain a sense of hopefulness, however changing this might be.

I have the right to express my feelings and emotions about my ap-

Continued on next page

proaching death in my own way.

I have the right to expect continuing medical and nursing attention even though "cure" goals must be changed to "comfort" goals.

I have the right not to die alone.

I have the right to be free from pain.

I have the right to have my questions answered honestly.

I have the right not to be deceived.

I have the right to have help from and for my family in accepting my death.

I have the right to die in peace and dignity.

I have the right to retain my individuality and not be judged for my decisions which may be contrary to beliefs of others.

I have the right to discuss and enlarge my religious and/or spiritual experiences, whatever these may mean to others.

I have the right to expect that the sanctity of the human body will be respected after death.

I have the right to be cared for by caring, sensitive, knowledgeable people who will attempt to understand my needs and will be able to gain some satisfaction in helping me face my death.

Reprinted with permission of Appleton-Century-Crofts, from *Cancer Care Nursing* by Donovan and Pierce, © 1976, by Appleton-Century-Crofts.

Nurse Specialists for the Dying

Due to the recognition of the needs of the dying and their families, a new specialty in nursing has developed, "the nurse specialist for the dying." The functions of nurses in this field are detailed below:

"The Nurse Specialist for the Dying

...*formulates* a patient group through personal observation or rounds, or referrals from nursing staff, medical staff, or social service

... **assists** nursing staff to plan and implement with the patient's participation, a care regimen, suitable to the patient's needs

... **gives** total patient nursing care on a selected basis to formulate a basis for future interaction

... **assesses** terminally ill patients to determine their perception of illness

... **intercedes** for patient with staff, family, or friends as the patient sees this need

... **functions** as a team member with social service and pastoral care on behalf of these patients

... **teaches** hospital personnel the dynamics of thanatology

... **learns** the dying process, not only from literature, seminars, and conferences, but especially from dying patients—Joy Ufema"

Reprinted from "Dare to Care For the Dying" by Joy K. Ufema in *American Journal of Nursing*, January, 1976, © Copyright American Journal of Nursing Company, 1976.

Stages in the Acceptance of Death

The dying patient has to pass through many stages in his struggle to come to grips with his illness and his ultimate death. He may deny the bad news for a while and continue to work "as if he were as well and strong as before." He may desperately visit one physician after the other in the hope that the diagnosis was not correct. He may wish to shield his family (or his family may want to shield him) from the truth.

Sooner or later he will have to face the grim reality, and he often reacts with an angry "why me" to his illness. If we learn to assist this angry patient rather than to judge him—if we learn not to take his anguish as a personal insult—he will then be able to pass to the third stage, the stage of bargaining. He may bargain with God for an extension of life, or he may promise good behavior and religious dedication if he is spared more suffering. He will try to "put his house in order" and "finish unfinished business" before he really admits, "This is happening to me."

In the depression stage he mourns past losses first and then begins to lose interest in the outside world. He reduces his interests in people and affairs, wishes to see fewer and fewer people and silently passes through preparatory grief. If he is allowed to grieve, if his life is not artificially prolonged and if his family has learned "to let go," he will be able to die with peace and in a stage of acceptance.

Reprinted by permission of Macmillan Publishing Company from *Questions and Answers On Death and Dying*, Elisabeth Kübler/Ross, © 1974, by Ross Medical Associates S.C.

"I believe death is difficult if we haven't lived. Patients express to me their remorse when they are suddenly terminally ill and realize that, for them, life has been meaningless. It's too late then for them to make up for all the wasted time.

"And so, what can you do about it? How? I think nurses are fortunate in that, while giving, we receive. In giving to the dying, the living find reward. *Care* about the man with carcinoma. Talk to him, openly and sincerely.

"If you dare to become so involved with a dying person that you even cry, don't be afraid. Perhaps some day, someone will cry at your passing."

Reprinted from "Dare to Care for the Dying" by Joy K. Ufema in *American Journal of Nursing*, January, 1976, © Copyright American Journal of Nursing Company, 1976.

Separation and Loss

THE CRISIS OF SEPARATION AND LOSS

The crisis of separation and loss can be either developmental or situational in origin, and both kinds of losses may occur simultaneously.

Continued on next page

Life—A Series of Losses

Loss and the universal reaction to loss, grief and mourning, are experienced by everyone at some time in their lives, and you are frequently the one most involved with and available to the person who is experiencing loss.

As one's interdependence with others grows, the likelihood increases that separation, loss of something valuable, or death of a loved one will induce a crisis. The capacity to have warm and loving relationships also leaves one vulnerable to sadness, despair, and grief. The more one has emotionally invested in that which is lost, the greater the threat felt to the self.

Every person is also subjected to separations or losses that are subtle and may not be recognized. Any crisis, developmental or situational, involves some degree of loss. If nothing else, there is a loss through change in old behavior patterns and the addition of different coping mechanisms. The process of achieving independence in psychosocial development in the course of normal upbringing involves a whole series of separations. The way these early separations are dealt with affects how later separations and loss, including death, will be resolved.

Nursing Process for the Person Experiencing Loss

The nurse's role with the person experiencing any kind of significant loss is essentially the same as with the person and family experiencing the greatest loss, death. For a thorough account of these nursing measures, see Murray and Zentner's chapter on death as the last developmental stage.[60,]

Reactions to loss are not always obvious. In assessing the patient who is admitted for a medical or surgical illness following a serious loss, direct your assessment and intervention to the mourning process as well as to the illness. Recognize the necessity of grief work for this patient if he is to achieve an optimum level of wellness.

The principles of crisis intervention described earlier and the concepts of primary, secondary, and tertiary prevention are applicable to the person experiencing loss.

You can help the person finish the mourning process by supporting him as he disengages himself from the significant object and seeks new and rewarding relationships and patterns of living. The person cannot be hurried through mourning to resolution of the crisis. He will need encouragement as well as a time and place to talk, weep, and resolve grief. He will need help in developing a philosophy about life to the point where he can again tolerate stress, changing his behavior to meet the situation rather than using behavioral mechanisms excessively to protect himself from reality. Encourage the person to do what he can for himself. Help him experiment with new modes of living and behaving and with new relationships. At times you may be a source of anxiety to this person as you attempt to encourage change and growth, but your simultaneous support will aid his resolution.

The person who has been in mourning for some time may exhibit inappropriate behavior. Denial, feelings of emptiness, self-depreciation, anger at self and others, self-pity, somatic complaints, hopelessness, and helplessness may be expressed. Although such behavior may be disturbing, this person needs respect and acceptance from you and others before he can again respect himself and accept his life situation.

Reprinted by permission of Prentice-Hall, Inc., from *Nursing Concepts for Health Promotion*, 2nd edition, by Ruth Beckmann Murray and Judith Proctor Zentner, © 1979, Prentice-Hall, Inc.

In *Journal of Psychiatric Nursing*, May, 1979 (p. 16), Baker and Lynn describe a method which one hospital employed, of utilizing a psychiatric nurse consultant to help nurses cope with their feelings about the deaths of their patients. The psychiatric nurse conducts an inservice program for medical-surgical and community health nurses which consists of five meetings for lectures and group discussions on death.

This program recognizes the need for health care workers to have help in coping with their own grief.

Gramp
by Mark Jury and Dan Jury
Grossman Publishers, A Division of The Viking Press
New York, 1976.

A moving photographic essay on aging and death, this book portrays the last three years in the life of Frank Tugend, a retired

Pennsylvania miner. Written and photographed by his two grandsons, it is a strikingly realistic portrayal of death.

Mr. Tugend died at home after his body and mind had gradually deteriorated by arteriosclerosis. The changes that his illness caused in him and the difficulties these caused for himself and his family are discussed and photographed.

The family chooses to respect Mr. Tugend's wishes to die at home and he is not hospitalized for I.V. infusions when, in the end, he refuses to eat. Rather, he is allowed to die in familiar surroundings with his family present.

The pain inflicted on the family members by being witnesses to the decline of this once independent, active man, is made very clear. But the overall impression of the book is of the naturalness of death, that it is a part of life and need not be separated from our experience. There is beauty in this family's love of Mr. Tugend and in their acceptance, however painful, of his decline and death.

The book can be a source of inspiration to nurses working with dying patients and to families experiencing the death of a loved one.

For further information on home care for the dying, see "Hospice Home Care Program," by Barbara J. Ward, in *Nursing Outlook,* October, 1978, pg. 646–649.

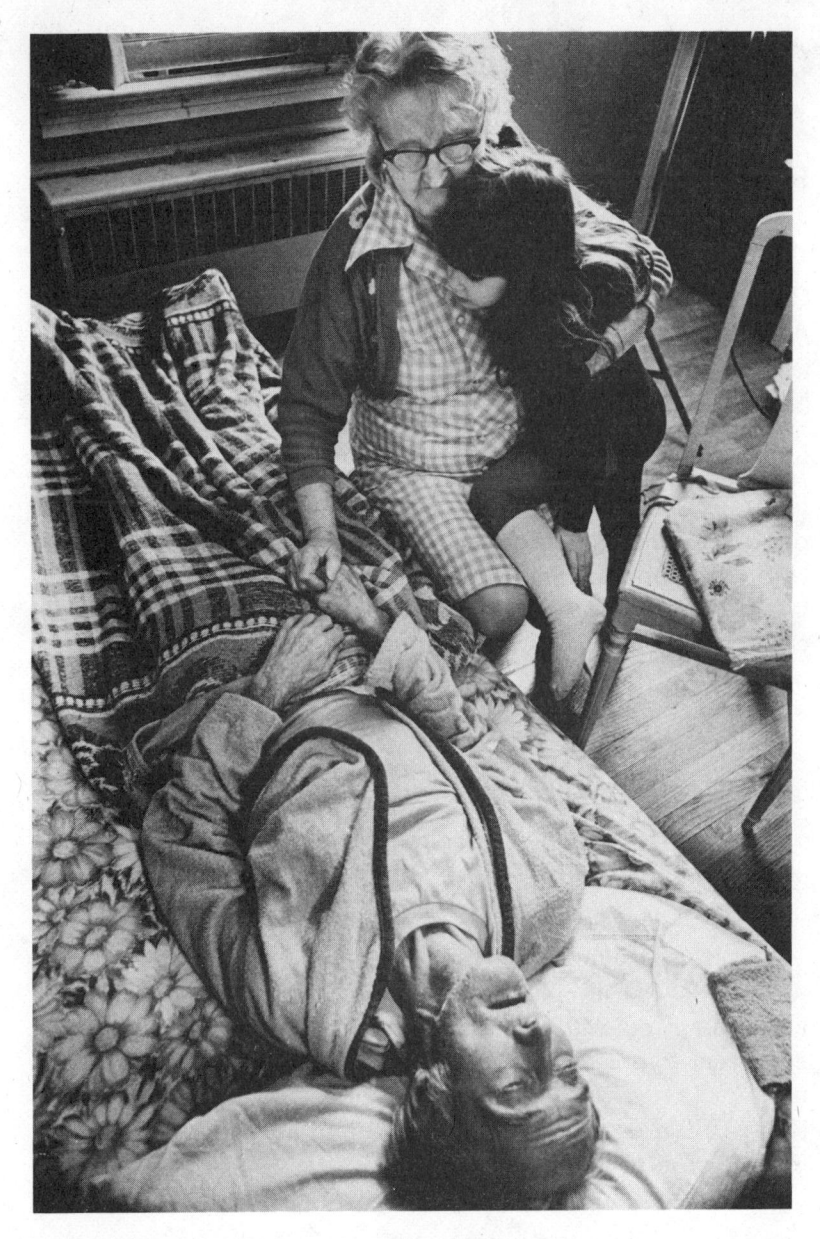

Reproduced with permission of The Viking Press from *Gramp* by Mark Jury and Dan Jury, Grossman Publishers, A Division of the Viking Press, New York, 1976.

"What Gramp did want was somebody to be with him all the time. His bony but still strong fingers clutched the hand of whoever was with him. Once, while I was with Gramp, it seemed as if he were oblivious to the fact that I was in the room, and I tried to move my hand from his. But the wiry fingers instantly closed down on my hand."

Resources on Death and Dying

Rights Of The Dying

Concern For Dying
An Educational Council
250 W. 57th Street
New York, N.Y. 10019

The Concern For Dying organization fosters the rights of the terminally ill to have a say in their treatment and opposes painful prolongation of the dying process. It sponsors conferences and workshops on the care of the terminally ill and provides educational materials to lay people and health care workers on euthanasia, the living will, and publishes a quarterly newsletter on developments in the area of death and dying.

Society For The Right To Die, Inc.
250 W. 57th Street
New York, N.Y. 10019

This is an organization which supports "legislation for death with dignity." The Society publishes a "Legislative Newsletter," an annual *Legislative Manual* on bills proposed and passed each year to protect the rights of the dying ($3 a copy), "Summary of Model Bill With Personal Directive," a "Bibliography: Right-To-Die Law Journal Articles," and a *Handbook: Enacted Right-To-Die Laws* ($3 a copy).

Support for the Dying

Make Today Count
514 Tama Building, Box 303
Burlington, Iowa 52601

This is an organization founded by a cancer victim "to improve the quality of life for patients and their families facing life-threatening illnesses and to assist health care providers in caring for seriously ill patients." (Quoted from a letter from the organization.)

Support groups are available on a local basis which enable people to share their problems. The national group publishes a newsletter ($10 a year) and provides information on establishing local Make Today Count chapters.

Shanti Project
c/o Dr. Charles A. Garfield, Ph.D.
106 Evergreen Lane
Berkeley, CA 94705

Founded by Dr. Garfield, the Shanti Project is a "volunteer counseling service" which provides support to the terminally ill and their families. It runs a 24-hour hotline with follow-up and referrals available as necessary.

The Shanti Project also provides training for professionals and lay people and serves as a model for other groups wishing to establish this kind of service. Contact Dr. Garfield at the above address for information on training programs or establishing a similar service. Dr. Garfield has edited two important resource books in this field: *Psychological Care of the Dying Patient,* Charles A. Garfield, © 1978, McGraw-Hill Book Co., and *Stress and Survival: the Emotional Realities of Life Threatening Illness,* Charles A. Garfield, © 1979, The C. V. Mosby Co. They are both very useful and are recommended required reading to all professionals and lay people working with the terminally ill.

This material is adapted from *Stress and Survival: The Emotional Realities of Life Threatening Illness,* © 1979, The C. V. Mosby Co.

Support for the Bereaved

The Naim Conference
721 N. LaSalle Street
Chicago, Ill. 60610

Post-Cana
Family Life Movement
1200 17th Street, N.W.
Washington, D.C.

Both of the above groups are local Catholic support groups for widows and widowers which function in their respective areas to aid people in the adjustment to loss of a spouse. Though the groups function locally and are of a Catholic orientation, they can serve as models to other areas for both Catholics and non-Catholics, on the needs of the newly bereaved and ways of helping them cope with their loss.

Hospices

"A hospice is a program which provides palliative and supportive care for terminally ill patients and their families. Originally a medieval name for a way station for pilgrims and travelers where they could be refreshed, replenished and cared for, the term is now applied to an organized program of care for people going through life's last station. The whole family is considered the unit of care and hospice help extends through the bereavement period. Emphasis is placed on symptom control and support before and after death. A hospice makes available the services of an inter-disciplinary team, twenty-four hours a day, seven days a week." (From: Introductory letter from Dennis Rezendes, Executive Secretary, National Hospice Organization, reprinted with permission.)

National Hospice Organization
765 Prospect Street
New Haven, Conn. 06511

A national organization for hospices and individuals involved with them, this group provides a means of communication between hospice groups, education to health professionals, and assistance and information to new hospices. Publications include, the "National Hospice Organization Directory Of Developing Hospices," The *NHO Newsletter,* and the *International Journal Of Hospice Care.*

Suggested References on Death and Dying

Books

Bluebond-Langner, Myra, *The Private Worlds Of Dying Children.* Princeton University Press, 1978.

Epstein, Charlotte, *Nursing The Dying Patient.* Reston Publishing Co., Prentice-Hall Company, 1975.

Hamilton, Michael and Helen Reid, ed., *A Hospice Handbook.* Wm. B. Eerdmans Publishing Co., Grand Rapids, Michigan, 1980.

Kübler-Ross, Elisabeth, *Death—The Final Stage Of Growth.* Prentice-Hall, 1975.

Kübler-Ross, Elisabeth, *On Death And Dying.* Macmillan, 1969.

Kübler-Ross, Elisabeth, *Questions And Answers On Death And Dying.* Macmillan, 1974.

Kübler-Ross, Elisabeth, *To Live Until We Say Good-bye.* Prentice-Hall, 1978.

Martinson, Ida Marie, *Home Care For The Dying Child.* Appleton-Century-Crofts, 1976.

Sell, I., *Dying and Death: An Annotated Bibliography,* The Tiresias Press, New York, 1977.

In the past several years several articles on death and dying have appeared in professional journals. The following articles are just a sample of the many articles available on this topic. Another excellent source for information on all aspects of death is *Death Education,* a periodical published by the Hemisphere Publishing Corporation, 1025 Vermont Ave., N.W., Washington, D.C. 20005.

Periodicals

Baker, B. S. et al., "Psychiatric Nursing Consultation: The Use of an Inservice Model to Assist Nurses in the Grief Process," *Journal of Psychiatric Nursing,* May, 1979, 17:15–19.

Baqui, M. A., "Muslim Teaching Concerning Death," *Nursing Times,* April 5, 1979, 75:43–4.

Benollel, J. Q. et al., "A Holistic Approach to Terminal Illness," *Cancer Nursing,* April, 1978, 1:143–9.

Berg, D. L. et al., "The Right to Die Dilemma. Where Do You Fit In?," *RN,* August, 1977, 40:48–54.

Boccuzzi, N. K., "Humanistic Supervision for Terminal Care," *Supervisor Nurse,* August, 1977, 8:26–7.

Branson, H. K., "Grieving . . . and Growing," *Journal of Practical Nursing,* December, 1976, 26:34.

Brimigion, J., "Living With Dying," *Nursing '78,* Sept., 1978, p. 76–9.

Burgess, K. E., "The Influence of Will on Life and Death," *Nursing Forum,* March, 1976, 15:238–58.

Clark, L., "Terminal Illness: Time to Be Home With the Family," *Nursing Mirror,* March 1, 1979, 148:36–7.

Deni, L., "Death and Nursing Care," *Journal of Nursing Care,* Sept., 1978, 11:20–3.

Denton, J. A. et al., "Death Experience and Death Anxiety Among Nurses and Nursing Students," *Nursing Research,* Jan/Feb, 1977, 26:61–4.

Formby, J., "Christian Teaching Concerning Death. A Roman Catholic Approach, An Anglican Approach, A Nonconformist Approach," *Nursing Times,* May 25, 1978, 74:58–60.

Goffnett, Carol, "Your Patient's Dying. Now What?", *Nursing '79,* November, 1979, p. 27–33.

Groliman, E. A., "Explaining Death to Children," *Journal of School Health,* June, 1977, 47:336–9.

Grosso, P., "Death, Dying and Decision-making," *Imprint,* December, 1977, 24:33–5.

Harper, B. C., "Death and Dying. Death: The Coping Mechanism of the Health Professional," *American Health Care Association Journal,* May, 1977, 3:42–4.

Hopping, B. L., "Nursing Students' Attitudes Toward Death," *Nursing Research,* Nov/Dec, 1977, 26:443–7.

Hornby, A., "Death, Dying and Bereavement," *Nursing Mirror,* Feb 16, 1978, 146:18.

Keeling, B., "Giving and Getting the Courage to Face Death," *Nursing '78,* November, 1978, 8:38–41.

Kerr, J. C., "Dying In Hospital," *Canadian Nurse,* November, 1978, 74:17–9.

Koch, J., "When Children Meet Death," *Psychology Today,* August, 1977, 11:64–6.

Kübler-Ross, Elisabeth, "What Is It Like To Be Dying?", *American Journal of Nursing,* January, 1971, 71:54.

Lamerton, R., "Going Deeper Into Care of the Dying," *Nursing Mirror,* March 3, 1977, 144:64–5.

Lannie, V. J., "The Joy of Caring for the Dying," *Supervisor Nurse,* May, 1978, 9:66.

Le Roux, R. S., "Communicating With the Dying Person," *Nursing Forum,* #2, 1977, 16:144–55.

Levenstein, M. et al., "Jewish Teaching Concerning Death," *Nursing Times,* March 23, 1978, 74:35–6.

McEver, D. H., "Death Education: An Inservice Program," *Nurse Educator,* Nov/Dec, 1977, 2:7–8.

McLaughlin, M. F., "Encounters With Grief: Who Helps the Living?", *American Journal of Nursing,* March, 1978, 78:422–3.

Mills, G. C., "Nurses Discuss Dying: A Simulation Experience—Southeast Virginia," *Journal of Continuing Education in Nursing,* Sept/Oct, 1977, 8:35–40.

Murphy, Joan C., "Communicating With the Dying Patient," *American Journal of Nursing,* June, 1979, 79:1084.

Nuttall, D., "Attitudes to Dying and the Bereaved," *Nursing Times,* October 13, 1977, 73:1605–6.

Pennington, E. A., "Postmortem Care: More Than Ritual," *American Journal of Nursing,* May, 1978, 78:846–7.

Raines, F., "The Dying Patient: Can You Help When You Care Too Much?", *Nursing '77,* March, 1977, 7:40–3.

Schultz, C. A., "Cultural Aspects of Death and Dying," *Journal of Emergency Nursing,* Jan/Feb, 1979, 5:24–7.

Sharpe, G., "Listening for the Death-bells," *Canadian Nurse,* January, 1978, 74:20–3.

Shivnan, J. et al., "The Dark Side of Nursing . . . Death," *Nursing Mirror,* April 5, 1979, 148:14–20.

Simms, L. M., "Dignified Death: A Right Not A Privilege," *Journal of Gerontological Nursing,* Nov/Dec, 1975, 1:21–5.

Stanley, Sr. A. T., "Is It Ethical to Give Hope to a Dying Person?", *Nursing Clinics of North America,* March, 1979, 14:69–80.

Ufema, Joy, "Do You Have What it Takes to Be A Nurse Thanatologist?", *Nursing '77,* May, 1977, 7:96.

Willis, R. W., "Bereavement Management in the Emergency Department," *Journal of Emergency Nursing,* March/April, 1977, 3:35–9.

Winder, A. E., et al., "Therapist for the Cancer Patient's Family," A New Role for the Nurse," *Journal of Psychiatric Nursing,* October, 1978, 16:22–7.

Audiovisual Materials on Death and Dying

"On Death And Dying," a filmed interview with Dr. Elisabeth Kübler-Ross. From Films Incorporated.

"Until I Die," a film featuring Dr. Elisabeth Kübler-Ross and her work with the dying as well as an interview with a 60-year-old cancer victim. From American Journal Of Nursing Co.

"What Man Shall Live And Not See Death?", a film on the need to talk openly of death, from Films Incorporated.

"Loss And Grief," a series of seven filmstrips and sound cassettes, from Concept Media.

"Perspectives On Dying," a series of filmstrips and sound cassettes, from Concept Media.

"A Dose Of Reality," a film on a special program in a Pennsylvania hospital for working with the terminally ill and their families, and "Grief Therapy," a film on a doctor's intensive therapy used in treating grief, are both available from Carousel Films.

"Death: A Natural Part Of Living," a filmstrip with cassette or record, portraying death factually and naturally for young people. From Marshfilm.

"Death," a study of one man facing death and the reactions of those around him, and "Death," a "cross-cultural study" of death, are available from the University Of California Extension Media Center.

"Coping," a film on a young leukemia patient's adjustment to the fact of impending death and the importance of family support. From the University Of California Extension Media Center.

"Though I Walk Through The Valley," a film on the last months of a cancer patient, portraying his and his family's reactions to impending death. From Pyramid Films, Inc.

"The Right To Die," a film on euthanasia including interviews with patients, doctors, lawyers and clergymen who have varied opinions on the subject. From the University Of California Extension Media Center.

10 Mental Health and Psychiatric Nursing

The role of the nurse in mental health has changed in the past several years from one of custodial care-giver to one of much more responsibility. The nurse in some cases is the primary therapist a client sees.

The articles in this section discuss three key roles nurses are filling in psychiatric care: psychiatric liaison nurse; private, independent practitioner; and group therapist. They point out some of the opportunities currently open to nurses in this field and suggest how nurses are functioning in these roles.

There is a need for the psychiatric nurse to be well versed in developmental theory and therapeutic techniques, because of these increased responsibilities. The tables and resource information following the articles are intended as guides to be referred to as needed.

Nurses in all fields of nursing must consider the emotional and psychiatric aspects of a patient's health status, so the following material is applicable not only for psychiatric nurses but for nurses in other fields as well.

An index of schools for psychiatric nurse practitioners is included for nurses interested in pursuing further study in this field.

I. Psychiatric Liaison Nurse

II. Private Practice of Psychotherapy in Psychiatric Nursing

III. Group Work Theory and Practice

IV. Self Acceptance

V. Erikson's Theory of Growth and Development

VI. Ego Defense Mechanisms

VII. Assessing Suicide Potential

VIII. The Professional Client

IX. Sexual Myths

X. Treating Sexual Dysfunction

XI. Gay Rights in the Hospital

XII. Adolescent Drug Use
Comparison of Experimental and Dysfunctional Use of Drugs
Terms of the Drug User

XIII. COMPREHENSIVE PSYCHIATRIC NURSING—A Review

XIV. Resources
General Mental Health Resources
Resources in Alcohol and Drug Abuse
Resources in Suicide and Suicide Prevention
Psychiatric Nursing Education
Publications and Audiovisual Aids on Mental Health and Psychiatric Nursing

The Psychiatric Liaison Nurse in the General Hospital
Three Models of Practice

Marie Berarducci, M.S., R.N.
Psychiatric Clinical Specialist
Beth Israel Hospital, Boston, Massachusetts

Kathleen Blandford, M.S., R.N.
Clinical Coordinator of Psychiatric Nursing
Mount Auburn Hospital, Cambridge, Massachusetts

Carol A. Garant, C.F., M.S.N., R.N.
Nurse Clinical Specialist
New England Deaconess Hospital, Boston, Massachusetts

Abstract: *The creation and implementation of the role of the psychiatric liaison nurse in three general hospitals are described. The historical evolution and theoretical bases of the role are reviewed, as well as the specific reasons for creation of such a role in each of the three hospitals. Three typical patient consultations by liaison nurses illustrate the need for provision of such services within the general hospital. Similarities in the implementation of the role of liaison nurse in the three hospitals are discussed.*

The history of the development of consultation-liaison psychiatry as a subspecialty has been marked by the opening of the first general hospital psychiatry unit in 1902, the emergence of psychosomatic medicine in the 1920s, the creation of small consultation-liaison services in the 1930s, and the recent expansion in the number of general hospital inpatient units (1). As knowledge has been derived from research on the interface between psychosocial stress and illness onset, increasing emphasis has been placed on the socioemotional components of patient care. A theoretical framework for consultation-liaison psychiatry has been developed (2–5), and the role of the mental health consultant in illness prevention has evolved (6).

In the last decade, the nurse has begun to play an important role in the consultation-liaison team (7). Since the early 1960s, when Dr. Lisa Robinson, a pioneer nurse clinician and researcher in the field of psychiatric liaison nursing, established a clinical practice as well as a graduate program in liaison nursing, more and more nurses have been seeking out and creating psychiatric liaison positions (8). The nurse has naturally evolved as the most appropriate health care professional to assume this liaison role because of the large number of nurses who provide direct patient care in nonpsychiatric settings and require assistance in meeting the psychological needs of patients (9).

Although descriptions of current practice of liaison nurses are available (10–22), as well as a review of the role from a historical perspective (23), there is little in the literature to assist a liaison nurse newly establishing a role. Specific functions, supervision, accountability, and peer support are all issues that need to be addressed. In this paper the authors describe the mechanics of establishing such a role, provide some insight into a typical patient consultation, and discuss specifically the varied functions of a liaison nurse.

Definition of the Liaison Nurse Role

Although the liaison nurse's title may vary, her responsibilities always include minimizing the amount of anxiety the patient must tolerate during hospitalization and assisting the staff in dealing effectively with both those patients with a mental disturbance who have been hospitalized with physical illness and those who find the experience of illness and hospitalization threatening to their usual style of coping with stress (24).

The liaison nurse is a masters-prepared nurse with a specialty in psychiatric or mental health nursing. It is strongly recommended that she have medical–surgical as well as psychiatric nursing experience and a knowledge of general hospital systems. Her work with patients and staff is founded on an understanding of personality structures, defense mechanisms, and interpersonal and environmental relationships. She must be able to utilize short-term treatment interventions which minimize transference and maximize coping abilities. She must also be sensitive to current nursing practice and its implementation in her particular institution and be capable of facilitating psychosocial interventions in the often frantically paced acute-care setting.

Models of Role Implementation

The authors, as newly appointed liaison nurses in three different general hospitals in the Greater Boston area, began to meet on a regular basis primarily for peer support. Although each liaison position had been established to help nurses understand more about the intersect between psychosocial and physiological aspects of patient care, the implementation of each role varied greatly in each institution, as illustrated in the following models.

Model 1: Psychiatric Clinical Specialist

The first hospital chose to place its Psychiatric Clinical Specialist in a staff position, under the umbrella of Nursing Education and Research, consulting primarily with nursing staff about their interactions with patients. Because there was a preexisting psychiatric consultation-liaison group composed of 2 staff psychiatrists and psychiatric residents, as well as a psychologically oriented social service department, the need for individual diagnostic assessment and psychotherapeutic intervention was already being addressed. Nursing staff, however, needed assistance in understanding the dynamics of patients' behavior and the nursing approach required.

Only about one-third of the clinical specialist's time was spent in direct consultation, usually when staff were unable to clearly identify the problem, when the patient presented such behavior that staff largely avoided him, or when the patient was not already being actively followed by psychiatry or social service. It should be noted that fully 50% of the patient-centered referrals had already been evaluated by psychiatric consultation.

Intervention by the Clinical Specialist was primarily crisis oriented because of her educational responsibilities; patients who needed to be followed over a long period would be referred to preexisting services.

In the first 12-month period, a total of 99 requests for assistance was made. Regularly scheduled patient care conferences, didactic conferences on individual units, program participation in department workshops, as well as informal contacts with nursing staff and other professionals accounted for much of the clinical specialist's time. In addition to exploring feelings and reactions of nursing staff toward patients individually and in groups, time was also utilized to develop specific nursing actions for incorporation in the overall nursing care plan and to follow up with individual staff and patients to determine efficacy of planned actions.

The Clinical Specialist often participated as a faculty member in workshops offered by Nursing Education and Research, presented programs with an audiovisual component on broad mental health concepts to the nursing service as a whole, and consulted with such individuals as clinical directors of nursing and with a multidisciplinary group providing a diversional therapy program.

The primary support group for this nurse was

Continued on next page

composed of the 3 other clinical specialists in the institution as well as the large Department of Nursing Education and Research.

Model 2: Clinical Coordinator of Psychiatric Nursing

In contrast, the role of the second liaison nurse included administrative supervisory responsibility for a specific nursing division in the hospital in addition to clinical participation on an existing liaison team. The position, requested jointly by nursing administration and psychiatry, was to be accountable to the Director of Nursing and work in collaboration with the Department of Psychiatry.

Initially, a major area of responsibility was planning for, staffing and supervising a new 16-bed, inpatient psychiatric unit. In addition, the nurse worked with the psychiatrist, who provided a well-utilized consultation service to the medical staff and was responsible for developing a liaison service to the nursing staff in medical-surgical areas of the hospital.

She began work as a liaison team member by making rounds with the psychiatrist, who was instrumental in introducing her to medical staff as well as to nursing personnel. Although initially the nurse and psychiatrist would jointly see patients referred by medical staff for psychiatric consultation, staff gradually began to accept consultations done solely by the nurse. A patient interview, written consultation note, including an assessment of the problem and recommendation for intervention, and discussion with the referring physician were required by the consultation protocol. If the liaison nurse or referring physician believed that the psychiatrist's assessment was necessary (for example, medications or a difficult diagnosis), they would then request the psychiatrist's involvement.

Nursing staff often became a part of the consultation procedure if a patient was presenting nursing care problems. Despite her attempts to discuss the patient with nursing staff, the liaison nurse often had to rely on the chart's consultation progress notes as her primary mode of communication. As relationships developed with various head nurses and staff nurses, they began to request patient conferences focused upon either a particular "difficult patient" or general psychosocial issues. The frequency of such requests varied greatly, depending on the energy the nursing staff had available to devote to the "luxury" of conferences. Because a rather threatening hospital-wide nursing service reorganization was occurring, units were short staffed due to a high turnover, and participation in organizational change often took priority over such patient conferences. But the visibility of the liaison nurse through individual consultations did result in her being approached by individual staff nurses with questions about patients.

In addition to working with nursing and medical staffs, the liaison nurse established good relationships with the Social Service and Occupational Therapy Departments, offering them both informal consultation and formal presentations. Her collegial relationship with the psychiatrist provided a superb role model for both nursing and medical staff.

Weekly liaison rounds were begun to address the problem of apparent duplication of effort resulting from two main sources: a highly active Social Service Department and insistence by some physicians that the psychiatrist reevaluate patients seen by the liaison nurse. These meetings included psychiatrist, liaison nurse, social workers, and occupational therapists, who attempted better coordination of their efforts. Assignment of specific patient units to the psychiatrist and liaison nurse involved them in weekly patient care conferences in which they were able to participate in planning with nurses, social workers, physical and occupational therapists, dieticians, continuing care coordinator, and, occasionally, house staff. Such exposure in routine unit activities was seen as a primary means of expanding the liaison component in the general hospital setting.

Model 3: Nurse Clinical Specialist

The third hospital developed its psychiatric liaison nurse position, as a staff position within the Nursing Service Department, in response to requests for assistance in meeting the psychosocial needs of patients from all levels of nursing personnel. Because the department had already employed 3 other nurses with various clinical specialties, it had set a precedent for independent nursing consultations that did not require a doctor's order or permission, and both medical and nursing staff were familiar with utilizing their services.

Careful planning was necessary in establishing the role of a Clinical Specialist in Psychiatric Nursing. Announcements about the position were sent out to all the patient care units. When the nurse arrived, she made a point of personally meeting with the nursing staff of each floor in the hospital as well as with department heads and informally building relationships with members of the nursing and medical staffs. Planned exposure at orientation classes, nursing service council, and committees all seemed to provide opportunities to obtain patient referrals.

The Nurse Clinical Specialist provided consultation in a variety of ways. At times she saw patients directly and then gave recommendations to the nursing and medical staff regarding appropriate intervention. These consultations often included making differential diagnoses, implementing referrals, and advising medical house staff on appropriate use of psychotropic medication. Besides making recommendations for staff to carry out, she also carried a caseload of patients in short-term treatment.

In addition to client-centered case consultation, this nurse provided conferences in which nursing personnel could assess their own responses to patients as well as developing an increased understanding of patients' emotional responses to illness and hospitalization. Finally, the nurse initiated and conducted formal continuing education workshops, which focused on various psychosocial topics.

Although some private psychiatrists on the hospital staff did occasional consultations, the Nurse Clinical Specialist was the only full-time mental health professional hired for this purpose. Her primary support group was a psychiatrist with whom she had supervision. psychiatric liaison nurses from other hospitals, and, at times, the clinical specialists in her own hospital.

During the first year of work, a total of 164 patient care consultations were done for a monthly average of 13.6 consults. During the second year there were 123 patient care consultations for a monthly total of 10.25, a decrease due to increased consultation time requested by the hospital's inpatient psychiatric unit.

Liaison Nursing Interventions

The following cases are provided to illustrate typical liaison nurse interventions and the benefits for patient and staff alike.

Case 1

This consultation, done by the Psychiatric Clinical Specialist, was initiated at a scheduled weekly conference on a surgical unit, when the nursing staff requested assistance in dealing with a patient with an already established diagnosis of chronic depression.

The patient, Mr. R, was a 76-year old Jewish man hospitalized with a leg abscess secondary to peripheral vascular disease, necessitating first a guillotine procedure and later a standard below-the-knee amputation. The patient also had congestive heart failure and diabetes mellitus, and had suffered a CVA 30 years ago, which had resulted in some nominal aphasia complicated by a preference for speaking Yiddish.

The patient's previous psychiatric history included three hospitalizations. Before admission, he had been living alone, relying upon a male friend his age for social contact. At the time of referral, Mr. R was withdrawn and uncommunicative but followed directions and complied in his treatment regimen. Although he had submitted to his initial surgery, staff feared that the loss of his leg would increase his depression and thus affect his ability to participate in rehabilitation.

After a review of the patient's record in staff conference, the Clinical Specialist determined that the patient could indeed communicate verbally and adequately in English and that he had sufficient physical functioning to learn the use of a prosthesis. After a discussion of the dynamics, symptoms, and treatment of depression with the staff, the major difficulty was identified as staff avoidance of the patient, who seemed unable to respond positively to their efforts.

At the end of the conference, the following plans had been made:

1. One consistent nurse would be assigned to the patient.
2. Other staff would stop in to see the patient several times per shift to prevent further isolation.
3. The surgical team would be contacted to obtain information about further surgical plans and the process of prosthesis fitting and rehabilitation.
4. Nursing staff would request that patient's previously prescribed Elavil[1] be restarted, as it had been discontinued postoperatively.
5. The clinical specialist would obtain further information from the psychiatric consultant and the psychiatric unit nursing staff to determine what interventions they had found helpful when they treated Mr. R.

Follow-up by the Clinical Specialist took place every few days. The psychiatric nursing staff shared their impression that Mr. R, although a fiercely independent man, responded well to someone sitting with him and holding his hand while waiting for him to answer. Because the patient had very few social contacts, members of the psychiatric nursing staff were asked to visit with Mr. R. His animated response to these visits encouraged the surgical nursing staff to realize that, with patience, he would also respond to them.

---

[1]Amitriptyline.

Continued on next page

Despite a necessary second surgical procedure, the below-the-knee amputation, Mr. R did very well. Once he was able to sit in a wheelchair, staff involved him in the weekly diversional therapy group, continued frequent contact, actively discussed his loss with him, and focused on mobilizing him to return home. Eventually nursing staff learned, through active participation in developing and implementing a plan of care, that they did have a real impact upon the patient. Through the actual experience of working with Mr. R, the staff learned more effectively than through a didactic presentation the difficulty of working with a depressed patient.

The joint efforts mentioned above were coordinated by the Clinical Specialist, who maintained close contact with nursing staff, reinforcing the importance of small gains in the overall picture. Here, the clinical specialist's role clearly was more appropriately to intervene indirectly with nursing staff. Although the patient had received psychiatric evaluation and treatment, unless staff that cared for him on a daily basis could effectively deal with his isolation and withdrawal, his rehabilitation might have been grossly impaired.

Case 2

As a result of her weekly visits to the coronary care unit, the Clinical Coordinator of Psychiatric Nursing was asked to see Mr. D, a 58-year old engineer admitted with an acute myocardial infarction. Because Mr. D had been given "a clean bill of health" by his doctor 3 days prior to admission, he and his family were quite alarmed when he developed chest pain. In the hospital, Mr. D experienced severe angina. It was difficult to differentiate between pain due to severe coronary artery disease (CAD) and that intensified by severe anxiety. Mr. D saw himself as a man who habitually used physical activity to cope with stress. The loss of this defense made it impossible for him to deal with his fears.

An intelligent man whose work involved designing sophisticated machines in hospital laboratories, Mr. D was unable to comprehend explanations of his illness because of his severe anxiety. Staff then tended to become irritated when he "forgot" what he had been told. His family was also extremely anxious; they spent a great deal of time hovering over the patient, repeatedly asking questions, and protecting one another as a way of dealing with their own fears.

First, determining that the patient was already receiving an antianxiety medication, the liaison nurse spent time with the patient and his family, allowing them to talk about the shock of Mr. D's illness and its meaning to them. She also discussed with nursing staff how anxiety can affect an individual's comprehension and perception of the environment. The nurse also met with the patient's physician, explaining the need for a great deal of input and for opportunities for discussion.

Because of the severity of the patient's CAD, a coronary artery bypass graft was done within 1 week of his admission. Although there was little time to prepare him for surgery, the coronary care nurses were able to alert staff of the intensive care unit (ICU), to which Mr. D had been transferred, of the need for frequent family meetings, and the liaison nurse continued to follow the patient throughout this time.

Unfortunately, Mr. D had a psychotic episode the second night after his transfer from the ICU. The liaison nurse was able to alert the psychiatrist who was already involved, and appropriate medications were quickly prescribed. For a few days, Mr. D showed evidence of organic psychosis, which gradually resolved. During this period, the liaison nurse worked with the patient and family and met daily with nursing staff to review the patient's condition and to plan such interventions as frequent contact with the patient to orient him, reality testing, use of night lights and calendars, and continued emphasis on explanations of all procedures.

A conference including nursing staff, the liaison nurse, and ICU and post-ICU area coordinators was held to discuss postoperative psychosis, early detection, and intervention. Nursing staff found it helpful to discuss their reactions to Mr. D and to apply what they had learned to planning preventive measures for future patients.

Mr. D still has some difficulty with anxiety about his condition; the liaison nurse and his primary physician still meet periodically with him to discuss the treatment.

Case 3

The third patient was referred to the Nurse Clinical Specialist by her physician, who described the patient as a 54-year old, single, female executive, now bedridden, aware of the diagnosis of metastatic carcinoma of the breast but with a strong desire for denial of her prognosis.

Nursing staff and members of the dietary department on the floor, however, provided additional information necessary for the effectiveness of the consultation. Although the main purpose of the consultation was to provide supportive psychotherapy to a terminally ill, middle-aged woman, the other issues that needed to be addressed were the patient's behavior and attitude towards the nursing and dietary staff and management of her nursing care.

On interview, the patient presented as an attractive, middle-aged, slender, dashing, social woman. Her first words to the Clinical Specialist were, "I've been unhappy, unloved and unappreciated all my life." She was verbal and able to associate her feelings and behavior. She feared total immobility, loneliness, pain, and her own death. As the therapeutic relationship progressed, much anger, bargaining, and intellectualization were expressed by the patient. Under the polished exterior and the controlled, intelligent, inquiring mind was much infantile narcissism, rage, and condescending behavior, which she displayed to nursing and dietary staffs. Part of the challenge for the liaison nurse was to help the staff express their angry and frustrated feelings toward the patient and to convert that energy into a workable care plan as well as to confront the patient with her behavior and try to modify it.

After several conferences in which the attending physician and nursing and dietary staffs had expressed their feelings, a contract was made with them: Over the patient's initial objections (and with the assistance of the booking office), we moved the patient to a room closer to the nursing station and social center of the floor. Much role playing was done to help staff provide appropriate feedback to the patient about her behavior. For example, when the patient had previously thrown dishes or banged plates if she didn't like a particular item on the menu, the staff had meekly gone about their business to clean it up and left the room as quickly as possible. Now they were more apt to say, "You really must be quite angry to do that, but you are making me so angry that it's hard for me to want to help you or even stay to chat with you." Limits were set.

Staff refused to be manipulated. If the patient began to talk about another member of the nursing staff, the nurse would reply, "It sounds like you have an issue to talk about with Mary. Why don't you take it up with her, not me?" After a few weeks, nursing staff really began to see the patient as a person and most would stop in "just to chat." One day a week, as the liaison nurse had suggested, they took her out—to the coffee shop, the hairdresser's, or even out of the hospital for lunch. This proved successful. The fights ceased; the dishes were broken no more. In several close relationships, the patient was able to vent her feelings and be supported, knowing the staff cared.

When the patient left to go home, she was made "an honorary member of the nursing staff" and invited to the head nurse's retirement luncheon. When she was told, she beamed, a changed person from the self-centered individual the staff had met a few weeks earlier.

Similarities in Role Implementation

All three nurses had as an ultimate goal minimization of the stress of hospitalization and illness for patients by educating staff about the interplay between physiological and psychological aspects of patient care. Although the amount of time spent giving direct patient care varied, each nurse continued to utilize and share her skills in patient assessment and care planning. All 3 nurses found it helpful to spend time meeting with other clinical specialists to define areas of overlap and to plan joint interventions. They all utilized introductory sessions with head nurses in each area as a way of gaining entry into the nursing units. Staff meetings that centered on patient care seemed to be more effective and readily received than those meetings that focused on the interpersonal issues and group dynamics of the nursing staffs, but each nurse was available to do either. Patient care conferences that included the liaison nurse were conducted "prn" on some units, and other units scheduled weekly case conferences.

At times, the liaison nurses were utilized by head nurses or supervisors as consultants for dealing with difficult staff issues. Two of the nurses used the ongoing hospital orientations as a means of educating new staff about the role of the liaison nurse, and the third nurse found this to be a useful suggestion. Although the degree of involvement with the Departments of Psychiatry and Social Service varied, all three nurses found it essential to have good communication with these departments.

The role of the liaison nurse can be fulfilled in many ways—as clinical coordinator with administrative duties, as nurse–educator with primarily educational responsibilities to nursing staff, and as clinical specialist in a setting in which specialists have already achieved autonomy. Although each liaison nurse worked in a different organizational structure and had different kinds of responsibilities, it was possible to provide psychiatric teaching and consultation in any of these systems. The important factors in effective implementation of this role seemed to be possession of some medical–surgical experience in addition to psychiatric experience, development of a good understanding of the nursing system operant in the

Continued on next page

hospital, maintenance of a high degree of visibility and feasibility and discovery of some kind of support group. It is important that nursing administration value the concept and goals of this kind of position so that nursing staff will be encouraged to understand that meeting the psychosocial needs of patients is not just something one does when one has "extra" time, but that it is standard care for which the Department is providing expert assistance.

References

1. Lipowski ZJ: Consultation-liaison psychiatry: an overview. Am J Psychiatry 131:623, 1974
2. Lipowski ZJ: Review of consultation psychiatry and psychosomatic medicine I: General principles. Psychosom Med 29:153–171, 1967
3. Lipowski ZJ: Review of consultation psychiatry and psychosomatic medicine II: Clinical aspects. Psychosom Med 29:201–224, 1967
4. Lipowski ZJ: Review of consultation psychiatry and psychosomatic medicine III: Theoretical issues. Psychosom Med 30:395–422, 1968
5. Kimball CP: Conceptual developments in psychosomatic medicine: 1939–1969. Ann Int Med 73:307–316, 1970
6. Caplan G: Principles of Preventative Psychiatry. New York, Basic Books, Inc., 1964, p. 214
7. Wise T: Utilization of a nurse consultant in teaching liaison psychiatry. J Med Educ 49:1067–1068, 1974
8. Garant C: Psychiatric liaison nursing: an interpretation of the role. Supervisor Nurse, April:75–78, 1977
9. Pranulis M: Liaison psychiatry: by whom? Unpublished manuscript presented at the American Psychosomatic Society Annual Meeting, April 14, 1972
10. Barton D, Kelso M: The nurse as a psychiatric team member. Int Psychiatry Med 2:108–115, 1971
11. Burch J, Mededith J: Nurses as the core of a psychiatric team. Am J Nursing 74:2037–2038, 1974
12. Davidson S, Noyes R: Psychiatric nursing consultation in a burn unit. Am J Nursing 73:1715–1718, 1973
13. Garant C: Psychiatric liaison nursing: an interpretation of the role. Supervisor Nurse April:75–78, 1977
14. Grace Mary Jo: The psychiatric nurse specialist and medical–surgical patients. Am J Nursing 74:481–483, 1974
15. Holstein S, Schwab J: A coordinated consultation program for nurses and psychiatrists. JAMA 194:163–165, 1965
16. Jackson H: The psychiatric nurse as a mental health consultant in a general hospital. Nurs Clin North America 4:527–540, 1969
17. Johnson BS: Psychiatric nurse consultant in a general hospital. Nurs Outlook II:728–729, 1963
18. Robinson L: Liaison Nursing: Psychological Approach to Patient Care. Philadelphia, F. A. Davis Co., 1974
19. Peplau H: Psychiatric nursing skills and the general hospital patient. Nurs Forum 3:28–37, 1964
20. Peterson S: The psychiatric nurse specialist in a general hospital. Nurs Outlook 17:56–58, 1969
21. Robinson L: Liaison psychiatric nursing. Perspect Psychiatr Care 6:87–93, 1968
22. Severin N, Beker R: Nurses as psychiatric consultants in a general hospital emergency room. Community Mental Health 10:261–267, 1974
23. Nelson J, Schilke D: The evolution of psychiatric liaison nursing. Perspect Psychiatr Care XIV:61–65, 1976
24. Robinson L: Liaison Nursing: Psychological Approach to Patient Care. Philadelphia, F. A. Davis Co., 1974, p. ix

The Private Practice of Psychotherapy in Psychiatric Nursing

Marie M. Smith, M.A., R.N.

Overview

From the mid 1960's to the present, we have seen a shift in the delivery of mental health services from the "institution" to the "community." During the same time, we have seen an expansive growth in nursing science whereby nursing's concern for man is not merely his illness, rather nursing's concern for man is at *all* levels of health and wellness. It naturally follows that nursing services are now provided in a variety of settings outside the hospital. There is not a segment of any population or geographic area where people do not question their mental health in the context of changing life situations, or perhaps the stagnation of *unchanging* life situations amidst chaotic social change. In either event, more people are aware of varying degrees of unhappiness in their lives. Most psychiatric nurses would agree that their skills must be made available to the client wherever he or she may be. While many practitioners prefer to give service in more or less traditional settings, i.e., clinics, hospitals, etc., an ever increasing number have chosen the private practice of psychotherapy in psychiatric nursing.

Visibility of Practice as Prerequisite to Keeping a Practice Going

One who wishes to start and maintain a private practice must first make visible the professional practice and expertise. There are a variety of places in which one finds ample opportunity to show oneself as an expert. First, the professional community of nurses is exposed to the clinician who teaches in the academic setting. It is here where knowledge and experience become evident to learners who then may make referrals and seek consultation. Second, other disicplines such as medicine, social work and psychology are exposed to the clinician in the multidisciplinary treatment teams of most mental health agencies. This author has experienced some physician support for the private practice of psychiatric nursing. Most commonly, clients have been referred by internists. Through collaboration in the treatment of such clients, referrals continue, especially when the sound medical assessment reveals depression with somatic symptoms. Social workers and psychologists are less reluctant than in past years to make referrals to nurses, especially since they find nurses more adept at treating clients who present symptoms of regression, chronicity, and require supervision of self-administered medication. Within nursing, the psychiatric nurse maintains alliances with all nursing groups through the contribution of research findings and the elevation of standards. Particular emphasis is placed upon peer group activities. The practitioner's specialty, such as adolescent treatment, becomes known to peers who readily make referrals. Proficiency and innovative approaches evolve as the nurse maintains practice. It is essential that the practitioner share these with the professional community through the publication of clinical papers; the presentation of papers to specific groups; and public speaking to community groups about mental health issues dear to the hearts of its members. For example, one might speak to a group such as the American Cancer Society, or, one might deliver a speech about the problems of growing children to a local Parent-Teacher Association. The practitioner's largest support system for the maintenance of referrals is the client. It is in the treatment where the client and nurse experience a certain degree of success through the collaborative process of psychotherapy. Some colleagues report that up to 80 percent of their referrals come from clients.

The Question of Certification

The psychiatric nurse clinician, sometimes called "Clinical Specialist," is well aware of the need to maintain competence and develop proficiency. This is accomplished first through practice with ongoing supervision. Second, through continuing education and certification by the professional organization. The certification process is the non-statutory issue of a certificate which verifies *proficiency* of practice which is above the minimum requirement for the Master's Degree. The reference to certification here is to the New York State Nurses' Association and the New Jersey State Nurses' Association Societies of Certified Clinical Specialists in Psychiatric Nursing. This author's certification included:

1. Education at the Master's level with a clinical minor.
2. Written examination.
3. Eighteen months of supervised practice.

4. Oral examination.
5. New York State licensure.
6. Membership in the professional organization.

While certification is not required in New York State, or any other state, certification sets the proficient practitioner apart from the competent one. The American Nurses' Association has developed a certification process similar to New York and New Jersey State affiliates which certifies practitioners at different levels of competence and proficiency. It is this author's belief that participation in certification, whether state or national, is essential when one considers the diversity of nursing education programs. There currently exists varying degrees of emphasis on the preparation of clinicians. For example: some graduate programs prepare generalists; others, educators; and others, administrators. Certification requirements, when met, assure expertise in the clinical area.

Liability Insurance

Most nurses are now aware of the need for liability insurance. The private practitioner is acutely aware of this need since the practice does not fall under the illusional protective umbrella of an agency. Maximum liability limits are usually maintained in addition to a consultation with a legal authority on malpractice. Liability for practice and laws determining malpractice differ from state to state.

Third Party Payment

Until recently, the client's access to nursing services has been limited due to a lack of statutory provision for third party payment. While the professional organization has a state and national legislative lobby for third party payment, the legislation for such payment does not yet exist. Third Party payment must be legislated, if the viability of nursing practice is to continue. This author has applied for payment from one insurance company, but not without requests for documentation of qualifications and practice. One must be willing to continue correspondence with insurance companies for purposes of education about the practice which then complements the political activities of our professional organization.

Marie M. Smith, M.A., R.N., is certified by the New York State Nurses' Association to practice Adult Mental Health Therapy. She was a clinical specialist and clinical supervisor and is now education coordinator at New York Hospital, Cornell Medical Center, Westchester Division. She is also in private psychotherapy practice.

Group Work Theory and Practice

Suzanne Lego, Ph.D., R.N.

Nurses have been acting as group leaders and publishing papers about their work for about 20 years. In 1963 Armstrong and Rouslin[1] published the first book of group psychotherapy by nurses. In the past decade it has been made possible for nurses who qualify, to become members of the American Group Psychotherapy Association.* Nurses have discussed through publications their work with groups of children, adolescents, chronic mental patients, acute hospitalized mental patients, out-patients, geriatric patients, and others. This is done in a variety of settings ranging from large public mental hospitals, to mental health centers, to clinics, schools, and so forth. In the area of primary prevention nurses have worked with groups of teachers, policemen, new parents, bereaved parents, families of alcoholics, and others.

Because many nurses will be involved in groups as leaders at one time or another, and all nurses will be group members at some time, it is important that we understand small group theory and that we know how groups work.

Theoretical Concepts of Group Work

Leadership

The leader sets the pace for what will happen in the group. The leader must be aware of the goals of the group without leading in a directive way. The natural process of the group's own development must be allowed to occur in its own way. Geller [25] has categorized three types of leaders, and described their effect on group development. These are the boss, the guide, and the stimulator. They operate as follows:

1. The *boss* plans, controls, directs, and decides autocratically what will occur in a group. The group submits and conforms. This group is often not very productive.
2. The *guide* plans and controls but less directly. The group then may register differences, complaints, make requests, and have some small influence. This group's productivity is limited to the leader's capacity.

* Further information may be obtained by writing to the AGPA at: 1995 Broadway, New York, New York. Phone (212) 787-2618.

3. The *stimulator* educates, facilitates production and communication, balances group forces, and shares leadership. The group may then generate ideas and methods which lead to healthy productivity beyond even the leader's own capacity.

There is a Chinese poem which captures well the spirit which a group leader should have:

A leader is best
When people barely know that he exists,
Not so good when they obey and acclaim him,
Worse when they despise him.
"Fail to honor people,
they fail to honor you";
But of a good leader, who talks little,
When his work is done, his aim fulfilled,
They will all say, "We did this ourselves."[25]

In addition to the assigned leader, two kinds of leaders emerge from the group itself. The first is the "task" leader who helps to move the group along toward its goals. The second is the "social" leader who becomes popular in the group due to an ability to ease tension among members.

Content and Process

An extremely important concept of group theory is the interweaving of group content and process. The content is what is *said* in the group. The process is what is *done.* When the group is allowed to progress in its own natural way, the members will begin to *do* what they are talking about. For example, a patient in a therapy group came to the session and reported that he had lost his job teaching a course to stockbrokers and didn't quite understand why. The other members began to ask him about the experience in an attempt to understand what went wrong. As they questioned him he became pompous and pedantic often putting down the questions until people became angry and frustrated with him. The longer this went on, the angrier the others became until it was clear that he had just *done* what the others had *said* he often did. He showed them through process what had only been talked about before. In this way it became clear why he'd lost his job.

There are two more examples, I have described elsewhere [25] and used frequently in lectures. Mary is accused in the group of constantly defending and speaking for her friend Ann. She replies, "Ann needs no defending!" She has just *done* what was *said*. Later group members accuse her of being too sweet and cheerful when it is unwarranted. She replies, "Thank you. That is very helpful to me!" The concept of observing "process" is important in all aspects of nursing. Clients often tell us more by what they "do" than what they "say." For example, a client may state that she is often pushed around by people and seldom given "respect." She then proceeds to act with the nurse in a subservient, masochistic way which demonstrated her part in the total problem.

Attractiveness and Approachability

Another concept common in small groups has been described by Blau.[4] This is the tendency for members to first appear attractive to one another, by "putting on a good face." This behavior is designed to impress the others. However, instead it leads to group competition, tension, and competitiveness, as all the members try to appear on top of things. This does not last for long, for the tension is too great. If left alone, finally one member will reveal a problem or weakness, a chink in the armor. After this, others will gratefully join in, and group tension decreases. The other members become "approachable," too, and a common bond develops. For example, in a group of cancer patients, early sessions may be devoted to members pointing out how well they are coping with their disease. Finally, someone will bring up a trying or anxiety-filled situation, others will identify with this, and social integration will begin.

Rank, Status, and Role

Three group concepts often discussed together are rank, status, and role. Rank has to do with the position each member has in the group vis à vis the others, in any given sphere. For example, a group member may rank high in relation to the others in the area of humor or intelligence. Where a person ranks in certain areas affects the degree to which he participates in the group.

Status has been called "a collection of rights and duties."[21] Members may either bring status into the group or earn it through group interaction. For example, in a group of head nurses, the one who has been in the agency longest, brings status to the group, and has certain rights and duties. If she also is sensitive and humorous, she may earn status in the group and more rights and duties.

Role is the dynamic aspect of status. When the group member

has earned status and uses it, a role is enacted. For example, the member may have the role of "trouble-maker." Part of the group process is to deal with this member in a way most beneficial to the person and to the group.

Norms

Norms are ideas in the minds of members which specify what the members should do, ought to do or are expected to do under given circumstances. This is not to be confused with the goal of the group, which may be determined in advance. The norms are developed as the group progresses and have to do more with group process than content. For example, in a sensitivity group the stated goal may be to be open and honest about feelings. However, the group may form implicit and unspoken norms about how far this openness should go. It might be a norm of the group that feelings about the leader are never stated openly.

Subgrouping

In most groups, smaller subgroups occur when group members are drawn to one another. Members of subgroups see themselves as better than other subgroups, and may be competitive with the leader. This is sometimes threatening to the group. It is important to realize that subgrouping is a normal part of group development.

Cohesiveness

This concept has been defined as "the resultant of all forces acting on members to remain in the group."[25] These forces may come from the group itself or from outside. When members meet over time a sense of "belonging" develops which causes all the members to want to continue in the group. This pull toward the group is useful in its growth as well as in the members' growth.

Before a group becomes cohesive, certain behaviors must occur. Members must be able to express both negative and positive feelings toward one another. Sometimes a leader who fears anger may prevent it from being expressed, thus thwarting true cohesiveness, and instead producing a kind of pseudocohesiveness based on mutual positive feelings alone. Cohesiveness cannot be rushed, but will develop naturally.

For the purpose of clarity, the remainder of this chapter will be divided into discussion of two categories of groups. The first is the discussion group, and the second is the specific task group.

Discussion Groups

Discussion groups are meant here to include any group which meets on a regular basis for the purpose of discussing issues of common interest, with a goal of self-growth or improvement. These might include psychotherapy groups,* parent-effectiveness groups, T-groups, consciousness-raising groups, as well as highly specialized groups such as those including dialysis patients, and recovering alcoholics.

Since the goal is self-growth, rather than completion of a specific task, the leader must help to maximize the potential of each member and the group as a whole by acting as a stimulator. Some experiences which prove helpful to these leaders are: (1) personal group experience (as a member), (2) didactic preparation in group theory, and (3) supervision of group leadership over an extended time period.

The group should consist of 6 to 10 members. If more than 12 members attend, there is a tendency for subdivision and more than one discussion at a time. If five or less members attend, participation drops off.

The leader should not set up rigid rules but should expect that participants will (1) attend every session or call if unable to come, (2) be as open as possible, (3) won't discuss with outsiders what others say in the group, (4) won't meet outside the group. All of the above factors affect the group's production. If problems occur in relation to any of these areas, the leader must bring this up in the group.

In self-growth discussion groups, most of the growth takes place as a result of learning how we behave with others. When we are anxious, we behave in defensive ways which are indicative of our inner worlds. Exploring these characteristic ways of responding to others can lead to personal growth. For example, the father in a parent-effectiveness group who bullies other group members, probably bullies his children. Because of the importance of examining these behaviors, the leader should help to *maintain* a low level of tension in the group. This is done in a number of ways. First, no table is used to "hide behind." If all members view one another fully, there is a tension created by the "exposure." The leader should change seats each week, again to throw things off balance. The group should not be prepared in advance for new members, for the spontaneous reaction of members toward one another is useful.

* For a more comprehensive view of intensive group therapy see Lego, S. "Group Dynamic Theory and Application" in Comprehensive Psychiatric Nursing (Haber, et al., editors). N.Y.: McGraw-Hill, 1978.

The first session sets the stage for what will follow in the group. The leader should be accepting, and non-directive, avoiding an "I am the expert" attitude. The leader must keep stirring up the dust to see how it settles, by commenting on what is happening in the group. However, comments should be limited to those things which other members cannot or will not say. Nothing should be done for the group which they can do for themselves. For example, in the case of the bully mentioned above, the leader might start the ball rolling by saying, "You seem to need to run things here, does that happen at home?" The leader must make what is covert, overt. For example, if one members seems particularly intimidated by the bully, the leader might say, "Does X scare you?" Most of all, the leader keeps track of content and process, pointing out process when necessary.

Contrary to what others have found, I have not found closure or "summing up" to be useful in these groups. There are several reasons. First, it suggests that there are "final solutions" to these problems, when there are only individual and often temporary resolutions. In other words, there is no "true truth." Second, this closure often stops exploration in these areas, as it suggests an "end to the chapter." Third, it gives the summing-up person too much power. Lastly, it reduces the tension of the group, when it is better to allow it to exist between sessions as well as during sessions.

Specific Task Groups

Specific task groups are meant here to include any group which meets on a regular basis for the purpose of accomplishing a task. The task may be worked on in the group, or it may be discussed in the group and then worked on between meetings. At any rate, self-growth is not a goal, though it may well occur. Examples of specific task groups are committees, staff groups, and head nurse groups.

In the case of committees, the leader is often in a position to choose the members. As mentioned earlier, it is helpful to have a "task leader" and a "social leader." Because votes must often be taken, the number of members should be uneven. Five has been found to be an ideal number for a committee.[2] No more than seven people should serve. Robert Bales, a researcher in small group behavior, has offered other suggestions in forming committees. Members should represent a gradient of participation. Not too many high or low participators should belong. If a person known to be a troublemaker must be included for reasons beyond the leader's control, then this member should be surrounded by constructive members.

As opposed to a discussion group where the leader lets the group take its own course, in a task group, the leader sets a general course. According to Bales, the procedure should follow these lines:

1. What are the facts?
2. What do we feel?
3. What shall we do?

A certain amount of time should be allowed for each step. When the discussion becomes either circular or bogged down, it may be time for the leader to move the group on to the next step. Sometimes it is best after sufficient discussion to take a vote or a poll of what the majority feeling is, and then move on.

Just as in discussion groups, the leader must look beyond what is overt, to what is covert. It is often the experiences of the members which matter, rather than the words. The skillful leader will pick up on these experiences and attempt to use these rather than act strictly on what is being said. Bales also suggests that the leader look at all members when they speak, not just those who express opinions similar to the leaders. Along these lines, the leader must bear in mind that leading a committee involves helping the group to decide how *it* wants to carry out a task. In this way, the leader is the servant of the group, and not the master. While it is often hard not to have personal opinions about how things should be done, the wise leader does not impose these opinions on the group.

In task groups which consist of members who work together day in and day out, unique problems exist for the leader. In this kind of group, conflict is unavoidable. In fact, a certain amount of conflict within a group is indicative of a healthy, productive group. The problem is that when people work together closely in a group that is not self-selected, and when the situation is inherently stressful (as in life-and-death hospital situations), the conflict can become destructive to group and individual functioning. This occurs when a competitive process is set in motion. Deutsch[10] has described the competitive process which perpetuates conflict. Its features are as follows:

1. Communication between the conflicting parties is unreliable and impoverished, and is used to mislead or intimidate one another. This leads to an inability to notice and respond to one

another's shifts away from a win-lose orientation.

2. It seems that conflict can only be solved through superior force, deception, and cleverness. The enhancement of one's own power and the decrease of the others become the objectives. The initial issue is forgotten and conflict over power becomes primary.

3. This leads to a suspicious, hostile attitude that increases the sensitivity to differences and threats while minimizing the awareness of similarities. The usual norms of conduct and morality seem less applicable. Each side becomes more outrageous and the conflict escalates.

Under these conditions of conflict and competition, perceptual distortions occur. Actions tend to be perceived as "black or white," and time perception is even distorted. Fear or hope-inciting rumors increase and people are more susceptible to them. Intellectual reasoning is decreased and alternatives are limited to victory versus defeat. Once immersed in this kind of conflict, we tend to stay in it to justify our original commitment.

In reading Deutsch's excellent description, we are probably all reminded of work situations where we have seen or been involved in this destructive kind of group conflict. I am reminded of competitive situations between shifts (days versus evening) which escalated to these proportions. In these situations group members often forgot the group goal (i.e., to care for patients) in light of the "larger" issue of power. While members often used the rationalization that the other group neglected patients, the truth was that each group wanted to control the other by the time the conflict had escalated.

This kind of group conflict can only be solved through what Deutsch calls the "cooperative process." This occurs when the individuals join in open and honest communication of relevant information. Sometimes this is best achieved by having a group leader who is not involved in the immediate situation sit down with both groups together. If information is shared openly, the leader can help the members to go beneath the manifest to the underlying issues. This decreases misunderstanding, confusion, and mistrust. It encourages the recognition of the legitimacy of the others' interests and the need to search for a solution that is responsive to the needs of each side. It limits the scope of conflicting interests and thus decreases defensiveness. Members can approach the problem with their own special talents, and decrease duplication of effort. The goal then becomes the enhancement of mutual resources and mutual power. According to Deutsch, this leads to a trusting, friendly attitude which increases sensitivity to similarities and common interests and decreases differences.

References

1. Armstrong, Shirley and Rouslin, Sheila. *Group Psychotherapy in Nursing Practice.* New York: The Macmillan Company, 1963.
2. Bales, Robert F. "In Conference," in *Basic Readings in Interpersonal Communication* (Griffin, K. and Patton, B., Editors). New York: Harper and Row, 1971.
3. Bell, Ruth W. "Activity as a Tool in Group Therapy," *Persp. in Psychiatric Care.* Vol. 8, No. 2, 1970.
4. Blau, Peter. "A Theory of Social Integration," *The American Journal of Sociology,* Vol. 45, May, 1960.
5. Cartwright, Dorwin and Zander, Alvin. *Group Dynamics Research and Theory.* New York: Harper and Row. 1968.
6. Chisham, Sr. Margaret and Danielson, Sharon. "An Experience with Group Orientation Sessions," *Persp. in Psychiatric Care,* Vol. 3, No. 2, 1965.
7. Coe, William, et al. "A Method of Group Therapy Training for Nurses in Psychiatric Hospitals," *Persp. in Psychiatric Care,* Vol. 5, No. 5, 1967.
8. Cohen, Roberta. "Cognitive Orientation for Patients in Group Psychotherapy," *Persp. in Psychiatric Care,* Vol. 7, No. 2, 1969.
9. Curry, Andrew. "Meditations on Group Psychotherapy and the Role of the Psychiatric Nurse," *Persp. in Psychiatric Care,* Vol. 2, No. 4, 1964.
10. Deutsch, Morton. *The Resolution of Conflict.* New Haven: Yale University Press, 1973.
11. Eddy, Frances, et al. "Group Work on a Long-term Psychiatric Service," *Persp. in Psychiatric Care,* Vol. 6, No. 1, 1968.
12. Eisenberg, Joan and Abbott, Ruth. "The Monopolizing Patient in Group Therapy," *Persp. in Psychiatric Care,* Vol. 6, No. 2, 1968.
13. Frost, Barbara E. "The 'Active Leader' in Group Therapy for Chronic Schizophrenic Patients," *Persp. in Psychiatric Care,* Vol. 8, No. 6, 1970.
14. Gauron, Eugene, et al. "Group Therapy Training: A Multidisciplinary Approach," *Persp. in Psychiatric Care,* Vol. 8, No. 6, 1970.

15. Gauron, Eugene, et al. "The Orientation Group in Pre-Therapy Training," *Persp. in Psychiatric Care,* Vol. 15, No. 1, 1977.
16. Goodson, Mary. "Group Therapy with Regressed Patients," *Persp. in Psychiatric Care,* Vol. 2, No. 4, 1964.
17. Greenfield, Rochelle Chernoff. "Trial by Fire: Rites of Passage into Psychotherapy Groups," *Persp. in Psychiatric Care,* Vol. 12, No. 4, 1974.
18. Heckel, Robert. "The Nurse as Co-therapist in Group Psychotherapy," *Persp. in Psychiatric Care,* Vol. 2, No. 4, 1964.
19. Hedman, Lorraine. "More than Custodial Care: Experience in Group Therapy in Five State Mental Institutions," *Persp. in Psychiatric Care,* Vol. 4, No. 5, 1966.
20. Holmes, M. et al. "Creative Nursing in Day and Night Care Centers," *Am. J. Nurs.,* Vol. 62, 1962.
21. Homans, George. *The Human Group.* New York: Harcourt, Brace, & World, 1950.
22. Horowitz, June A. "Sexual Difficulties as Indicators of Broader Personal and Interpersonal Problems (as reflected in the psychotherapy group)," *Persp. in Psychiatric Care,* Vol. 16, No. 2, 1978.
23. Joyce, Carol. "The Religious as Group Therapists: Attitudes and Conflicts," *Persp. in Psychiatric Care,* Vol. 15, No. 3, 1977.
24. Lego, Suzanne. "Five Functions of the Group Therapist—Twenty Sessions Later," *Am. J. of Nurs.,* Vol. 66, 1966.
25. Lego, Suzanne. "Group Dynamic Theory and Application," in *Comprehensive Psychiatric Nursing* (Haber, et al., editors). New York: McGraw-Hill, 1978.
26. Light, Nada. "The 'Chronic Helper' in Group Therapy," *Persp. in Psychiatric Care,* Vol. 12, No. 3, 1974.
27. Loomis, *Group Process For Nurses.* St. Louis: C. V. Mosby Company, 1979.
28. Lyon, Glee G. "Trust in the Nonhospitalized Group," *Persp. in Psychiatric Care,* Vol. 8, No. 2, 1970.
29. Marram, Gwen. *The Group Approach in Nursing Practice.* St. Louis: C. V. Mosby Company, 1973.
30. Maurin, Judith. "Regressed Patients in Group Therapy," *Persp. in Psychiatric Care,* Vol. 8, No. 3, 1970.
31. Mealey, Anne R. "Sculpting as a Group Technique for Increasing Awareness," *Persp. in Psychiatric Care,* Vol. 15, No. 3, 1977.
32. Pothier, Patricia. "Marathon Encounter Groups: Rationale, Techniques, and Crucial Issues," *Persp. in Psychiatric Care,* Vol. 8, No. 4, 1970.

33. Pratt, Sandra and Fischer, Joel. "Behavior Modification: Changing Hyperactive Behavior in a Children's Group" *Persp. in Psychiatric Care,* Vol. 13, No. 1, 1975.

34. Ramshorn, Mary. "The Group as a Therapeutic Tool," *Persp. in Psychiatric Care,* Vol. 7, No. 3, 1969.

35. Randell, Brooke P. "Short-term Group Therapy with the Adolescent Drug Offender," *Persp. in Psychiatric Care,* Vol. 9, No. 3, 1971.

36. Rawlings, Edna and Gauron, Eugene. "Responders and Nonresponders to an Accelerated Time-limited Group," *Persp. in Psychiatric Care,* Vol. 11, No. 2, 1973.

37. Rouslin, Sheila. "Relatedness in Group Psychotherapy," *Persp. in Psychiatric Care,* Vol. 11, No. 4, 1973.

38. Ruffin, Janice. "Racism as Countertransference in Psychotherapy Groups," *Persp. in Psychiatric Care,* Vol. 11, No. 4, 1973.

39. Schuurmans, Marilyn. "Five Functions of the Group Therapist," *Am. J. of Nurs.,* Vol. 64, 1964.

40. Smith, Adrienne. "A Manual for the Training of Psychiatric Nursing Personnel in Group Psychotherapy" *Persp. in Psychiatric Care,* Vol. 8, No. 3, 1970.

41. Smith, E. Frances Blackwell. "Teaching Group Therapy in an Undergraduate Curriculum," *Persp. in Psychiatric Care,* Vol. 11, No. 2, 1973.

42. Swanson, Mary. "A Checklist of Group Leaders," *Persp. in Psychiatric Care,* Vol. 7, No. 3, 1969.

43. Ward, Judy Trowbridge. "The Sounds of Silence: Group Psychotherapy with Non-verbal patients" *Persp. in Psychiatric Care,* Vol. 12, No. 1, 1974.

44. Werner, Jean A. "Relating Group Therapy in Nursing Practice" *Persp. in Psychiatric Care,* Vol. 8, No. 6, 1970.

Self Acceptance

Professional workers in training are much more likely to make progress toward their goals if they can begin with an honest acceptance of themselves where they are. An attitude of acceptance is a major characteristic of adequate personalities. It is also a basic requirement for the helping relationship. An effective helper is one who has learned how to use himself effectively and efficiently to carry out his own and society's purposes. The problem of becoming an effective professional worker, then, is not a question of trading one's old self in for a new one. Rather, it is a matter of learning how to use the self one has and how to improve it slowly over a period of time. A very good place for the professional worker, then, to start his professional growth is by applying the principle of acceptance to himself, to begin his growth with the declaration, "It's all right to be me!"

Reprinted with permission of Allyn and Bacon, Inc., from *Helping Relationships, Basic Concepts For the Helping Professions* by Arthur Combs, Donald Avila, and William Purkey, Allyn and Bacon, Inc., 1971, Boston, Mass.

Erikson's Theory of Social Growth and Development

Stage of development	Time frame	Developmental tasks	Examples
Sensory	Birth to 18 months	Trust vs. mistrust	Experiences with the nurturing person are the foundations of the level of trust a person will develop.
Muscular	1 to 3 years	Autonomy vs. shame and doubt	The toddler learns the extent to which the environment can be influenced by direct manipulation.
Locomotor	3 to 6 years	Initiative vs. guilt	The child learns the extent to which being assertive will influence environment. If important others disapprove of beginning assertiveness, the child will experience guilt.
Latency	6 to 12 years	Industry vs. inferiority	The child either learns to utilize energies to create, develop, and manipulate, or the child learns to shy away from industry, feeling inadequate to the task.
Adolescent	12 to 20 years	Identity vs. role diffusion	The adolescent either integrates all life experiences into a coherent sense of self or is unable to integrate these experiences and feels lost and confused.
Young adulthood	18 to 25 years	Intimacy vs. isolation	The young adult is primarily concerned with developing an intimate relationship with another person.
Adulthood	21 to 45 years	Generativity vs. stagnation	The adult is primarily concerned with establishing a family and guiding the next generation.
Maturity	45 years to death	Integrity vs. despair	The life-style gives life meaning and the person must come to accept his or her life as fulfilling and meaningful. The lack of ego integration results in fear of death.

Reproduced with permission of McGraw-Hill Co., from *Comprehensive Psychiatric Nursing*, by Haber, Leach, Schudy and Sideleau, © 1978, McGraw-Hill Publishers.

Ego Defense Mechanisms

Defense mechanism	Example
Repression: A widely used unconscious mechanism. Painful experiences, disagreeable memories, unacceptable thoughts and impulses are barred from consciousness. Selfish, hostile, and sexual impulses are also usually repressed. It takes a constant expenditure of energy to keep repressed material out of awareness. Consequently, less energy is available for constructive activity.	Mrs. S does not remember having spent 6 months in a body cast at age 7. Mr. Z does not remember having sexually exposed himself on a subway train.
Regression: The ego returns to an earlier stage of development in thought, feeling, or behavior. Regression is a normal component of our developmental sequence and appears transiently during times of stress, when it is utilized as a retreat from anxiety and conflict.	Mr. B, an adult, has temper tantrums (child behavior) when frustrated. Tim, a 4-year old, is confronted with the birth of a new sister. He is toilet-trained and articulate but responds to the birth of the new baby by regressing to nighttime bed-wetting, daytime soiling, and baby talk. All this stems from his effort to regain his old unchallenged position with his mother.
Identification: A person becomes like something or someone else in one or several aspects of thought or behavior. This contributes to ego development but does not replace the person's own ego. The personality consists of multiple identifications that have been tested for their ability to reduce anxiety.	Mr. K, a young man whose father has recently died, begins to talk and act like the father. Miss Thomas, who is studying nursing, incorporates into her personality the assertiveness she admires in one of her instructors.
Introjection: A form of identification which is a symbolic taking in or incorporation of a loved or hated object or person into the individual's own ego structure. Introjection is important in the development of the superego when the child incorporates the parents' instructions, rewards, and punishments.	Paul, a 5-year-old boy tells his 2-year-old brother, "Look both ways when you cross the street."
Reaction Formation: Occurs when an individual expresses an attitude that is directly opposite to unconscious feelings and wishes.	Mr. J has unconscious feelings of hate and anger toward his boss; he covers them up by being excessively polite. Johnny, a teen-ager, has an unconscious desire to be dependent and cared for; this is masked by his independent attitudes.
Undoing: Closely related to reaction formation. A person negates an act by behavior which is the opposite of what was done before.	Miss M crosses her fingers while telling a white lie. Little Peter, who has just told his mother that he hates her, goes over to her and hugs and kisses her.
Isolation: The exclusion from awareness of the feelings connected to a thought, memory, or experience. The person remembers the experience or thought but does not reexperience the emotion that originally accompanied it.	Mrs. James, an obsessive client, relates her repeated thoughts of having thrown her baby out of the window. As the woman speaks, she conveys no affective response to the content of this frightening thought.
Displacement: The discharge of emotions feelings, or ideas upon a subject other than the one to which the feelings rightly belong. This is a security operation in which the feelings are discharged away from the actual source of the emotion because it is not considered safe to express them directly.	Mrs. Green has had a difficult day at the office. A project she had worked hard on was rejected by her boss. When she comes home from work, she begins yelling at her husband and children, displacing the anger felt toward the boss onto her family.
Projection: The attribution of one's feelings, impulses, thoughts, and wishes to others or the environment in an effort to deny their existence in the self. Projection is used in a wide variety of normal situations. It is used excessively by clients with paranoid thought patterns.	David, a freshman, has failed an exam. He blames the instructor for having made a poor choice of questions on the exam. Miss K, a suspicious, paranoid client, projects hostile, aggressive feelings that are part of the self onto others when stating "I can't eat, the food is poisoned," and "I can't go to sleep, they're just waiting to kill me."

Defense mechanism	Example
Rationalization: A coping mechanism that is universally employed. It is an attempt to make one's behavior appear to be the result of logical thinking rather than of unconscious impulses or desires. It is utilized when a person has a sense of guilt or uncertainty about something that has been done. It is a face-saving device that may or may not deal with the truth. It relieves anxiety temporarily.	Mary S, a sophomore, fails a course and says that the teacher was ineffective. Mr. W has no friends; he says people do not appreciate his efforts at friendship. Miss B says she wants to get married but has trouble with dating. Every time she goes out with a man, she refuses a second date, saying, "He's not my intellectual equal." In doing this she is probably rationalizing deep fears of sexuality.
Denial: The total failure to acknowledge the existence of an affect, experience, idea, or memory. The person simply pretends that what is painful, anxiety-provoking, or threatening does not exist.	Mr. L, who has cancer, was told that he was terminally ill and had approximately a month to live. Later in the day, the nurse hears him talking to his travel agent. He is planning a trip to Europe next summer.
Substitution: The replacement of a highly valued, unacceptable object with a less valued one which is acceptable.	Mr. E wants to marry Miss L, probably because she looks quite a bit like his mother.
Sublimation: Transformation of psychic energy associated with unwanted sexual or aggressive drives into socially acceptable pursuits. The activity or its object is changed, but the energy is discharged.	After Bobby's father forbade him to use the family car, Bobby spent a half hour punching a punching bag. Eleanor's boyfriend has left her to pursue a career as a rock musician. Now she spends much of her time writing love poems.

Reproduced with permission of McGraw-Hill Co. from *Comprehensive Psychiatric Nursing*, by Haber, Leach, Schudy, and Sideleau, © 1978, McGraw-Hill Co.

Assessing Suicide Potential

Assessing a Person's Suicide Potential

"I'm at the end of my rope and I'm going to commit suicide," is the tone of the message spoken by many people who phone "hot lines" such as the National Save-a-Life League and other suicide prevention centers throughout the country.

To assess both the seriousness of the situation and the type of intervention required, the people who answer such phone calls often use a suicide potential scale which is based on some of the following criteria. A "yes" to every question listed does not mean that the caller will definitely commit suicide, nor does a "no" answer guarantee that he will not. But studies of suicidal individuals show that a high "yes" score is closely correlated with a high risk of attempted suicide.

1. **Suicide plan.**
   Has the person chosen a time, place and method? Is the method lethal? Is the plan well-organized, well-detailed and feasible?
   The person with a definite, well-organized suicide plan that includes a lethal method of suicide is at high risk for carrying out suicidal wishes. Careful attention should, therefore, be given to any at-risk person's actual suicide plan.

Continued on next page

2. **Age and sex.**
Is the potentially suicidal person a male? Is he over fifty?
While women attempt suicide more often than men, men are much more successful at carrying out a suicide threat. The likelihood of a successful attempt is greater if the person is over fifty, although in recent years the suicide rate among young people is increasing.
3. **Stress.**
Has the person just suffered through a serious illness? Death of a loved one? Loss of a job?
Periods of great stress increase the risk of suicide.
4. **Medical problems.**
Is the person suffering from a chronic, debilitating illness?
5. **Prior attempts**
Has the person previously threatened or actually attempted to commit suicide?
A pattern of suicidal behavior increases the risk of a fatal suicide attempt.
6. **Significant Others.**
Does the person have family or friends? Is it difficult for him to communicate with them? Are they unwilling to help? Are their reactions defensive, punishing or rejecting? Do they deny that the person needs help?
Significant others may be unable to face the reality of a potential suicide. They may also have been alienated by the behavior of the suicidal person. Their rejection can reinforce the low self-esteem the person is already feeling and thus increase the risk of suicide.
7. **Additional risk factors**
Is the person an alcoholic? Does he have trouble sleeping? Does he show feelings of hopelessness and/or loneliness? Is he a rigid person? Is he unusually impulsive?
8. **Duration of risk factors.**
Did these occur suddenly? Were they long-standing, but recently increased significantly? Are they reoccurrences of prior problems?

Reprinted by permission from *Journal of Practical Nursing*, January, 1979, page 20, Copyright 1979, *JPN*.

The Professional Client

It is often difficult for nurses to assume the role of patient and for nurse-colleagues to relate to the nurse-patient. The following chart points out a few helpful suggestions to aid nurses working with nurses (or doctors) who are also clients.

Nursing diagnoses	Goals	Approaches
Professional identity threatened by client role, therefore does not relinquish professional role and is unable to become engaged in the therapeutic alliance.	Client discusses feelings about change in status (from professional to client), is receptive to the treatment regime.	Deliberately bring up the topic for discussion. Example: "Sometimes it is difficult to be the client after being the nurse (doctor)."
Fears of loss of control over emotions, body functions, day-to-day regulation of life.	Client expresses fears.	Emphasize client's right to have ordinary needs and feelings. Encourage activities which are of interest and meet client's needs for control.
Staff feel that their professional integrity is threatened by an ill colleague.	Staff identify and verbalize own feelings of vulnerability, anger, etc., toward ill colleague.	Discuss: Own experiences as a client. Meaning of illness (i.e., failure). Career choice (i.e., physician or nurse as healer). Feelings relating to caring for a professional peer.
Staff feel threatened when providing care to a peer, i.e., that peer will be evaluating them and will be critical.	Staff identify and verbalize fear of failure and inadequacy precipitated by these clients.	

Reproduced by permission of McGraw-Hill Publishing Co., from *Comprehensive Psychiatric Nursing* by Haber, Leach, Schudy and Sideleau, © 1978, McGraw-Hill Book Company.

Sexual Myths and Facts to Refute Them

Sexual myths and facts to refute them

MYTHS (OR COMMON MISCONCEPTIONS)	FACTS (BASED UPON RESULTS OF CURRENT RESEARCH)
The sex drive or "libido" is of primary importance in early development and behavior in infancy.	The bases for one's developing sexuality are established during the first five years of life as a result of learning, mainly through nonverbal channels. The self-gratifying behavior and pleasure-seeking activities of the infant are not "sexual" in the adult sense of the word, for sex as such, is rarely a human need prior to adolescence.
Each person is endowed with a finite amount of sexual drive which is overdrawn in youth or in young adult life leaves little reserve for the later years.	Actually the correlation between sexual activity and length of time it persists throughout life is just the opposite. The more sexually active a person is, the longer it continues into the later years of life.
The need for expressing one's sexuality becomes less important in the latter half of one's life.	Physiologically, sexual desire and ability do not decrease markedly after middle age. The expression of one's sexuality, as an integral part of development, follows the overall pattern of health and physical performance.
Sexual abstinence is necessary in training for the devel-	While there is great variation in sexual activity, physiologically the achievement of orgasm is rarely more demanding than most

Continued on next page

opment of optimum physical performance in sports, dance, or other strenuous activities.	activities encountered in daily life. The desire for sleep which often follows is most commonly due to factors other than physical exhaustion from sexual activities. Orgasm may bring a relief of sexual tension with a feeling of relaxation and a readiness for sleep. A sense of weariness is more likely due to related activities resulting in improper eating, sleeping, drinking, or feelings of guilt.
Excessive sexual activity can lead to mental breakdown.	The biological significance of man's sexuality is of no greater impact on his total development than any other necessary biological function. Most behavioral scientists do not regard sex as *the* prevailing instinct in man so that his sex life must be paramount in his emotional development. There is no scientific basis for believing that one will develop a mental or physical illness unless one's sex needs are satisfied.
Nocturnal emissions (wet dreams) are indicators of sexual disorders.	Erotic dreams that culminate in orgasms are common physiological phenomena in at least 85 percent of all men. They occur at any age, beginning in the teens when the maturing sex organs exert a new primacy in masculine development. The phenomenon is also common among females, who report in clinical studies, that their sexual dreams culminated in orgasm. In women, this practice is believed to increase with advancing age.
Because of the anatomical nature of the sex organs, the female is inherently passive and the male inherently aggressive.	Physiological studies disprove this myth by showing the woman to be far from passive. Maximum gratification requires each partner to be *both* passive and aggressive in participating mutually and cooperatively.
It is "unnatural" for a woman to have as strong a desire for sex as a man—for women normally do not enjoy sex as much as men.	These myths have been reinforced by a society which has traditionally taught women that they are to suppress sexual desires to gain love, security, and society's respect—based on the assumption that it is the "basic nature" of women to be submissive, dependent, and subordinate. Physiological studies indicate that, in some respects, the woman's sex drive is not only as strong but may be even stronger than that of the male.
Women who have multiple orgasms or who readily come to climax are actually nymphomaniacs.	Physiological studies at this time suggest that we do not know women's sexual potential—but indicate that there is a wide range of intensity and duration of orgastic experience—and the potential for multiple (or frequent orgasms within a brief period of time) is not at all uncommon. Therefore, women have greater orgastic capacity than men with regard to duration and frequency of orgasm.
There is a difference between vaginal and clitoral orgasm. The former being the more "mature" according to Freudian theory; the latter indicating signs of narcissism or inadequacy.	Physiological misunderstanding has produced the myth of separate clitoral and vaginal orgasms rather than their interrelationships. Female orgasm is normally initiated by clitoral stimulation, but since it is a total body response there are marked variations in intensity and timing. There is no reason to believe that the quantitative differences in the female response to the sex act are due to vaginal rather than a clitoral orgasm.
A mature sexual relationship requires the male and female to achieve simultaneous orgasm.	While simultaneous orgasm may be desirable it is an unrealistic goal in view of the complexity of human sexuality. Often it is possible only under the most ideal circumstances and is not a determinant of sexual achievement or of satisfaction (except to someone who accepts this as dogma).

It is dangerous to have intercourse during menstruation.	Since the source of the menstrual flow is from the uterus rather than the vagina, there is no basis for concern about tissue damage to the vagina nor is there any reason for the woman's sexual drive to diminish during the menstrual period. There is no physiological basis for abstinence during the menses.
The larger penis has greater possibilities for pleasurable stimulation or for producing orgasm in the female.	Physiologically, there is practically no relationship between the size of the penis and a man's ability to satisfy a woman sexually. Furthermore, there is very little correlation between penile size and body size and their relationship to sexual potency.
The face-to-face coital position is the proper, moral and healthy one for it is this position that distinguishes the sexual activity of man from the remainder of the animal kingdom.	Recent knowledge of human sexual practices dispel this myth with the recognition that there is no *normal* or *single most acceptable* sexual position. Whatever position offers the most pleasure and is acceptable to both partners is correct for them. Any variation is normal, healthy, and proper if it satisfies both partners.
The ability to achieve orgasm is an indicator of an individual's sexual responsiveness.	Achievement of a satisfactory sexual response is the result of the successful interaction of numerous physical, psychological, and cultural influences. Too often the physical fact of orgasm (or lack or orgasm) is taken to be symbolic of sexual responsiveness and seen out of context of the entire relationship between man and woman. Such distortions add to the tension and anxiety of those who strive to attain this singular goal—contributing to conditions of impotence and frigidity.

Reprinted by permission of J. B. Lippincott Co. from *Fundamentals of Nursing*, 6th edition, by LuVerne Wolff, Marlene Weitzel, and Elinor Fuerst, © 1979, J. B. Lippincott Co.

A Comparison of Approaches to Treating Sexual Dysfunction

	Intrapsychic	Dyadic	Behavioral-learning
Therapeutic focus	Intrapersonal conflicts	The relationship	The problem or symptom, specific and modifiable mechanisms of behavior
Theoretical base	Psychoanalytic theory	Systems theory	Social learning theory Behavior theory
Who is the client?	The individual	The couple, the relationship	The individual or the couple
Must both partners be involved in therapy? (if there is a partner)	No	Yes	No

What concepts form the basis for therapy?	1. Concept of unconscious motivation, repression, resistance to treatment
	2. Influence of childhood experiences in shaping adult destiny
	3. Role of Oedipus conflict in production of sexual conflict
		1. Partner rejection, acceptance
		2. Communication problems
		3. Marital discord causes including:
		  a. Transfer of feelings to partner from parents
		  b. Lack of trust
		  c. Power struggles
			1. Behaviors are conditioned
			2. When certain contingencies are present, certain behaviors occur; behaviors that are reinforced persist
			3. Behaviors, thoughts, and feelings become associated with negative labels

Continued on next page

	Intrapsychic	Dyadic	Behavioral-learning

		d. Contractual disappointments
		e. Sexual sabotage such as:
		  (1) Using pressure and censure
		  (2) Using sabotaging timing
		  (3) Making oneself repulsive
		  (4) Frustrating the partner's sexual desires and preferences
			4. Part of therapy is changing labels from negative to neutral or positive ones, or interrupting the connections between thoughts, feelings, behaviors, and negative labels

What points would be emphasized in the sexual history?	Sources of conflicts, for example, experiences as a younger child Developmental history emphasized	The developmental aspects are important for each partner, but more important is how they *together* come to have the sexual problem	1. Description of current problem 2. Onset and course, contingencies 3. Client's concept of cause and maintenance of the problem 4. Past treatments and outcomes 5. Current goals and expectations
What role does the therapist play?	Analyst of behavior	Counselor for relationship	Analyst of problem and its contingencies; teacher of new behaviors; can include 1. Giving permission 2. Providing limited information 3. Giving specific suggestions 4. Providing intensive therapy
How does therapy proceed?	1. Superficial conflict is dealt with via the use of techniques to attain symptom relief. The conflict is not necessarily eliminated by experientially oriented techniques, but these approaches may be more efficient than exclusive reliance on cognitive insight methods. Conflict is not ignored, but the focus is on modifying the immediately operating results of the conflict. *If necessary*, the therapist may interpret and work with the patients' unconscious Oedipal material. 2. Many patients respond well to intervention in the level of specific conflict alone. Others need additional conflict resolution. 3. Experiential techniques (structured sexual tasks) are used to foster conflict resolution by exposing the patient to feelings and aspects of self that have been avoided. 4. An attempt is made to help the partners understand their problems intellectually, emotionally, and experientially. 5. A combination of experiential and psychoanalytic techniques (free association) is used.	1. Although primary emphasis is on sexual difficulties, this approach also focuses on pathogenic transactional dynamics. 2. Intervention focuses on modifying specific sexual interactions and communications. 3. Sometimes treatment of the sexual problem can bypass marital obstacles. In other cases, basic resolution of the interactional problem must be effected first. 4. Changing the sexual ambience to one of nondemand and low pressure is often an essential first step.	1. Assessment of each sexual symptom and its contingencies 2. Plan for reinforcement or extinction contingencies 3. Use strategies to remove rewards from a sexual symptom, to punish the undesired sexual reaction, or to extinguish fear
What assumptions are basic to the method?	The patients' sexual symptoms are expressions of deeper conflicts that derive from childhood; sexual pleasure becomes associated with guilt as a result of child-rearing practices and constrictive upbringing.	Sexual difficulties spring directly from the destructive sexual system.	Sexual symptoms occur because of reinforcing or negative contingencies. Sexual symptoms are learned inhibitions.

Reprinted by permission of The C. V. Mosby Company from *Human Sexuality in Health and Illness*, 2nd edition, by Nancy Fugate Woods, Copyright 1979, The C. V. Mosby Company.

Acceptance of the Client's Differences

Psychiatric nurses require a special sensitivity to and acceptance of the differences in people and the wide range of "normal" behavior. The following article illustrates the importance of this acceptance, for nurses in other fields of practice as well as psychiatric nurses.

Gay rights in the hospital

Are homosexual patients in your hospital being denied their right to total, high quality nursing care? Here are some guidelines to help you insure the rights of the homosexual patient, and to avoid unnecessary conflict between patient and staff.

QUESTIONS
—to ask yourself,
or to present at a patient care conference:
• Is the patient really homosexual?
On what basis has this been determined? His or her own statement? The doctor's say-so? Some kind of written record? Is homosexuality being assumed on the basis of the patient's behavior, or association with other people who appear to be homosexual? Is it merely a rumor?
• Who knows the patient is homosexual? The staff? The other patients?
• How is the information communicated? By gossip? By the patient? By the physician?

ANSWERS
—to some questions
about homosexuality:
• *Is homosexuality a mental illness?*
The American Psychiatric Association removed homosexuality from its list of diagnostic categories in 1973. There is no valid research that provides evidence that homosexuality is a mental illness.
• *How widespread is homosexuality?*
It's estimated that there are at least 20 million homosexuals in the U.S.
• *How can you tell if someone is homosexual?*
You can't. While a few homosexuals may be "overt" in their behavior, and while others may seek to raise public consciousness by "coming out" themselves, most homosexuals probably prefer to keep their sexual preference a private matter, to avoid censure. The vast majority of homosexuals, male or female, live rather ordinary lives, often as

Continued on next page

- What are the attitudes toward this patient's homosexuality?
Is the staff upset by it? . . . allowing it to interfere with caring for the patient? . . . accepting of it? Are the other patients, especially the patient's roommate, uncomfortable being around the patient? . . . unconcerned about it? Does the patient seem to be at ease with his or her sexual orientation? . . . talk about it? . . . make it obvious? . . . maintain reserve?
- Is the patient's behavior being attributed to his or her homosexuality, rather than to general personality traits?
- Are attitudes toward the patient negatively influencing the therapeutic environment?
- What does the staff know, and think about homosexuality in general?
- Is the staff treating for homosexuality, rather than the admitting diagnosis?

couples or in communal situations. They are not distinguishable from heterosexuals in dress, speech, mannerisms, professional performance, or social behavior. To quote John Lawrence, RN, MS, "Committed homosexual relationships receive no societal affirmation, recognition or support . . . Homosexuals are not socialized to share or celebrate their relationships, but rather to take care to hide them . . . This holds true especially in public places, including the hospital. Few homosexuals fit our usual stereotype, while some heterosexuals may seem to. So it's important to avoid jumping to conclusions.
- *What are a homosexual patient's rights?*
Homosexual patients have a right to the same quality of nursing care as any other patient. They and their associates should be accorded the same consideration extended to any person faced with serious illness.

Reprinted by permission from "The Gay Patient: What Not to Do" by Elaine Pogoncheff, R.N., in *RN Magazine*, April, 1979, Copyright 1979, Litton Industries.

Comparison of Experimental and Dysfunctional Use of Drugs (In Adolescents)

Overt and Covert Reasons for Drug Use	Socialization Factor	Behavior Patterns
Experimental		
Recreational Use	individually/group	Drugs are sought as a means of achieving a relaxed state. Usually this entails weekend or intermittent use, sometimes on a regularly planned basis.
Personal Growth	group	Often the adolescent who wishes to achieve a mystical experience will experiment with the so-called psychedelic drugs. Be-

		cause of their systemic effects it is important to try to obtain as accurate a picture of the pattern of use as possible.
Social Influences	group	The adolescent is particularly vulnerable to group pressures. The use of drugs is limited to group experiences and the adolescent rarely if ever uses drugs when alone. Drug use may be quite frequent and regular in the pattern of group association.
Rebellion/ Self-Assertiveness	group	The classic adolescent stance—self assertion—is at the very least a sign of hostility. Impulsive acts against the family and family values are part of this necessary but painful stage of normal development.
Dysfunctional		
Escapism	alone	The social history of the adolescent may have a theme of loss, deprivation, or abandonment. The use of drugs indicates a need to ignore the pain of day-to-day living, and may or may not be incapacitating.
Dependency	alone or group	The most obvious feature of this group of adolescent clients is their mixed emotions regarding the endless need for support from their environment. Often this client is "lost in the crowd."
Personality Disorder	alone in a group	While there is not a single personality type which can be characterized as typically drug dependent, drugs are often used to alleviate the ever present anxiety in a variety of emotional disturbances, interfering with the individual's ability to respond to life crises.

Continued on next page

Overt and Covert Reasons for Drug Use	Socialization Factor	Behavior Patterns
	Dysfunctional	
Self-Medication for Psychosis	alone in a group	This group of clients presents a chaotic thought process and uses drugs to reduce the stress of the psychosis. Their association with the group is only for drug use and conversely drug use enables them to tolerate the group.

Reprinted by permission of McGraw-Hill Book Co. from "Interventions with the Adolescent Drug User and the Family" by Victoria Palmer-Erbs and Virginia DeForge in *Issues in Comprehensive Pediatric Nursing*, Nov., 1978, Vol. III, No. 5, © 1978, McGraw-Hill Book Company.

Commonly Used Terms of the Drug User

Colloquial terms	Definitions
Drugs	
(1) Reds (2) Rainbows (3) Yellow Jackets (4) Blue heavens (5) Goof balls (6) Pink lady	"Reds" are secobarbital sodium (Seconal); "yellow jackets" are pentobarbital sodium (Nembutal); numbers 1 through 6 are all barbiturates.
(7) Snow (8) Stuff (9) H (10) Junk (11) Smack	Numbers 7 through 11 all represent heroin.
(12) Bennies (13) Pep pills (14) Footballs (15) Whites (16) Hearts (17) Copilots	Numbers 12 through 17 all represent amphetamines. "Bennies" are specifically benzedrine.
(18) Snow (19) The Leaf (20) Speed ball	Numbers 18 through 20 denote cocaine; "speed ball" specifically denotes cocaine mixed with heroin.

(21) Joints
(22) Sticks
(23) Reefers
(24) Weed   } Numbers 21 through 27 are all familiar names for marijuana.
(25) Grass
(26) Pot
(27) Mary Jane
(28) LSD
(29) Acid
(30) Mescaline } Numbers 28 through 32 are common names for hallucinogens.
(31) STP
(32) DMT

Drug amounts
(1) Nickel bag — Five dollars worth of drugs. Formerly, this was 50 tablets, when used in reference to methamphetamine. Inflation has reduced the "nickel bag" to 30 or 40 tablets.
(2) Dime bag — Ten dollars worth of drugs.
(3) Jar — One thousand "whites" or "reds."
(4) Pillow — One hundred "jars."
(5) Spoon — A measurement of powdered drugs.
(6) Tabs — Tablets.
(7) Caps — Capsules.
(8) Lid — One ounce of marijuana.

Other terms
(1) Score — Succeed in buying drugs.
(2) Busted — Arrested.
(3) Burn out — Lose desire for the drug.
(4) Freak — Drug user.
(5) Freaked out — Irrational on drugs.
(6) Blowing it — Becoming irrational on drugs; "freaking out."
(7) Stoned — In a stupor with drugs.
(8) Loaded — "Stoned."
(9) Out-to-lunch — "Super-stoned."
(10) Trip — Experience with LSD or other psycheledic drug or amphetamine.
(11) Crash — Sleep.
(12) Party — Get loaded with other drug users.
(13) Come down — Wear off the effect of a drug.
(14) Step on (a drug) — To cut a drug with some other substance, to dilute it.
(15) Strung out — Addicted.
(16) Cold turkey — Kicking a drug habit by total abstinence.

Reprinted by permission of J. B. Lippincott Co. from *The Practice of Emergency Nursing* by James Cosgriff and Diann Anderson, Copyright © 1975, J. B. Lippincott Co.

Comprehensive Psychiatric Nursing

Comprehensive Psychiatric Nursing
Judith Haber, Anita M. Leach, Sylvia M. Schudy, Barbara Flynn Sideleau
Copyright 1978, McGraw-Hill, Inc.
Reviewed by Marie M. Smith, M.A., R.N.

The "publication explosion" in nursing has brought forth a multitude of books and articles, many of which are long overdue and others which are "more of the same." One happy exception to the latter is *Comprehensive Psychiatric Nursing*. While its value would seem to fall into the realm of psychiatric practice, which it does, the reader would be mistaken to view it simply as that "branch" of nursing, for *Comprehensive Psychiatric Nursing* utilizes a theoretical matrix based upon a holistic approach to client care. There are significant contributions having application "wherever nursing takes place." It is a text designed for nurses who practice in many specialty areas because it integrates psychiatric concepts and interventions throughout the life cycle of a client in a variety of health-illness situations. For example, topics such as death and dying, group and family dynamics, depression, terminally ill children, the aged, use of medical technology and many others are addressed. Problems that were previously considered strictly "psychiatric" in nature are reframed in this text from the point of view of psychologic, social and biologic dysfunction.

The second most noteworthy overall contribution of the text is the consistent use and application of the nursing process. This sometimes nebulous concept appears in most literature. Here it is clearly exemplified in operational form with the nursing diagnosis. This approach, as opposed to the mere descriptive, is thought-provoking, informative, and more importantly, operationalizes, for the reader, processes that occur between the helper and the client. As the processes in a number of chapters are described, interventions are enumerated. Rationale for interventions flow clearly from the operationalized processes. Clinical examples illustrate for the reader the manner in which nursing actions are conducted.

Commendation is due the authors for pointing out the fact that clients generate broad categories of feeling states in helpers. For example, one chapter, "The Client Who Generates Anger," implies that the client is angry and that he/she makes others angry. We all know that many nursing care situations make people angry. The adolescent, the sociopath, the organically impaired, the addicted and the schizophrenic are all capable of becoming angry and of evoking anger in others.

The book incorporates the use of research and current literature appropriately into each chapter. It is apparent that regardless of subject matter, the authors have creatively provided a comprehensive nursing text which has something unique in it for everyone, student and practitioner of nursing.

Resources in Mental Health and Psychiatric Nursing

Organizations

American Art Therapy Association, Inc. (AATA)
Business Office
428 E. Preston St.
Baltimore, MD 21202

This is a professional organization for Art Therapists (therapists involved with the use of art for communicating and resolving emotional conflicts). The AATA promotes research into this field, sets standards of practice and training for art therapists, and provides education on art therapy. The Association has available a list of schools offering courses in art therapy. Active membership is open to art therapists and associate membership is open to other interested individuals. Publications of the organization include the *AATA Newsletter* (published six times/year, $6.00), the *American Journal of Art Therapy* (published quarterly, $10.00/year), and a bibliography of literature on art therapy.

American Dance Therapy Association, Inc.
2000 Century Plaza
Columbia, Maryland 21044

An organization open to individuals trained in dance therapy; "the psychotherapeutic use of movement as a process which furthers the emotional and physical integration of the individual" (quoted from A.D.T.A. brochure). The association establishes standards for the education and certification of dance therapists and publishes "ADTA Newsletter," the *Journal of Dance Therapy,* and bibliographies and abstracts from conferences.

American Psychological Association
1200 Seventeenth St., N.W.
Washington, D.C. 20036

This is the national organization for psychologists. It functions to promote psychological research and foster high standards of practice. Publications of the APA which are of interest to nurses in the mental health field include: *Contemporary Psychology,* a monthly journal ($30.00/year), *Journal of Abnormal Psychology,* published bimonthly ($28.00/year), *Journal of Counseling Psychology,* published bimonthly ($24.00/year), *The Psychology of Adult Development and Aging* (a book by Carl Eisdorfer and M. Powell Lawton, 1973, $11.00), *Rehabilitation Psychology* (a book by Walter Neff, 1972, $7.00), and many other journals and books.

American Society of Group Psychotherapy and Psychodrama
39 East 20th Street, 8th Floor
New York, New York 10003

A multidisciplinary organization for mental health professionals which conducts training workshops in the field of psychotherapy and psychodrama.

Anorexia Nervosa and Associated Disorders (ANAD)
Suite 2020, 550 Frontage Road
Northfield, Illinois 60093

"A national non-profit educational and self-help organization" for anorectics and their families, ANAD provides "counseling, information and referrals, self-help groups for both victims and parents, educational programs, and a listing of therapists, hospitals and clinics teaching anorectics. The group also encourages research." (Quoted from letter from Vivian Meehan, President, ANAD.) ANAD has available literature on starting local self-help groups, on therapies used in anorexia nervosa, bibliographies and posters.

Association for Humanistic Psychology
325 Ninth Street
San Francisco, California 94103

An association founded in 1961 by Abraham Maslow and fellow psychologists, as a forum for sharing of ideas, education and research into humanistic psychology. Membership is open to anyone supporting the work of the association.

Publications include: *The Journal of Humanistic Psychology,* a quarterly journal; *AHP Newsletter,* published monthly; *Together,* a semi-annual publication on humanistic education; "Women: A Bibliography" by Lucinda Cisler, 1970; and "Women: A Bibliography" by Karen Kaiser, 1977; and lists of schools in Humanistic Psychology and growth centers.

National Association for Mental Health, Inc.
1800 North Kent Street
Arlington, Virginia 22209

A non-governmental organization for research into prevention and treatment of mental illness, promotion of mental health, social action for humane treatment of the mentally ill, and public and professional education. The association functions on the national, state and local levels, largely through the work of volunteers. An extensive list of publications of interest to nurses in the mental health field is available. Write for catalog.

National Association for Music Therapy, Inc.
901 Kentucky, Suite 206
P. O. Box 610
Lawrence, Kansas 66044

This organization promotes music therapy (the use of music to help people with emotional or physical problems) through literature on music therapy, approving schools in the field, and sponsoring workshops and conferences.

Publications include: *The Journal Of Music Therapy,* a quarterly publication ($12.00/year); *Membership Directory,* printed yearly, listing registered music therapists and their locations; and several pamphlets on music therapy.

National Council on Family Relations
1219 University Avenue
Minneapolis, Minnesota 55414

This is an interdisciplinary forum for professionals working in family counseling, education or research.

Publications include: *Journal Of Marriage And The Family,* a quarterly journal ($20.00/year to individuals); *The Family Coordinator,* a quarterly journal aimed at professionals working with families ($15.00/year to individuals); and cassette tapes on topics of interest to those working with families. Write for complete listing of publications.

National Institute of Mental Health
Public Inquiries Section
5600 Fishers Lane
Rockville, Maryland 20857

The National Institute of Mental Health has available several publications of interest to nurses working in mental health. Write for complete listing.

Neurotics Anonymous International Liaison, Inc.
Room 304, Colorado Building
1341 G. Street, N.W.
Washington, D.C. 20005

A group which functions like Alcoholics Anonymous to help individuals with mental and emotional problems. There are many local groups where people get together to share their experiences and provide mutual support.

Publications include: Literature on Neurotics and Mental Health; *Journal of Mental Health.*

Psychiatric Nurses Association of Canada
871 Notre Dame Avenue
Winnipeg, Manitoba
Canada
R3E OM4

An organization of psychiatric nurses all across Canada, with a membership of about 5,000 men and women. Nurses join their local province association.

Publications include: "Psychiatric Nursing ... A Worthwhile Career For Men And Women" (which includes a list of Canadian schools for training psychiatric nurses and addresses for the provincial associations); *Canadian Journal Of Psychiatric Nursing,* published bi-monthly.

Resources in Alcohol and Drug Abuse

Alcoholics Anonymous, Inc.
P. O. Box 459
Grand Central Station
New York, New York 10017

Alcoholics Anonymous is a group of people who share their experiences with alcoholism and provide support to each other in overcoming alcoholism. Literature is available on A.A. and how it functions and of particular interest to nurses are two pamphlets: "If You Are A Professional A.A. Wants To Work With You" and "Alcoholics Anonymous And The Medical Profession."

Al-Anon Family Group Headquarters
P. O. Box 182
Madison Square Garden
New York, New York 10010

Al-Anon is a resource for relatives and friends of alcoholics. It provides support and information to family members through local meetings, whether or not the alcoholic seeks help. The group includes "Alateen," a group for teen-aged children of alcoholics. An outgrowth of Alcoholics Anonymous, the group functions separately of it. Al-Anon publishes several pamphlets, books, and a monthly newsletter, *Forum*. Write for complete catalog of available materials.

Do It Now Foundation
P. O. Box 5115
Phoenix, Arizona 85010

This organization has a variety of pamphlets, books and booklets, posters, monographs and cassette tapes available on alcohol and drug abuse topics. Write for catalog.

National Clearinghouse for Alcohol Information
P. O. Box 2345
Rockville, Maryland 20852

A branch of the National Institute on Alcohol Abuse and Alcoholism, the Clearinghouse makes available current information on alcohol use and abuse. Materials are aimed both toward professionals and the general public. The Clearinghouse will conduct computerized searches for specific materials, provide bibliographies, referrals to local alcohol abuse programs, notification of new articles or books, and has available several pamphlets and books on alcohol and related topics (for example, a 26-page guide, "Alcohol Programs For Women, Issues, Strategies and Resources").

National Clearinghouse for Drug Abuse Information (NCDAI)
P. O. Box 1909
Rockville, Maryland 20850

This clearinghouse publishes several educational materials, reports of research, posters, bibliographies and technical papers. Single copies may be obtained by writing the NCDAI.

National Council on Alcoholism, Inc.
733 Third Avenue
New York, New York 10017

A national voluntary health organization for fighting alcoholism, comprised of state and local affiliates and the American Medical Society on Alcoholism, The National Nurses Society On Alcoholism (see below) and the Research Society On Alcoholism. The Council publishes several books and pamphlets including specific information for nurses on alcoholism. Write for *Catalog Of Publications.*

National Nurses Society on Alcoholism
733 Third Avenue
New York, New York 10017

A division of the National Council on Alcoholism, NNSA is an organization for nurses interested in the field of alcoholism. It supports programs to improve care and treatment of alcoholics and to educate nurses and the public on alcoholism. Members receive the *NNSA Newsletter,* quarterly. (Membership fee: $35.00.)

Narcotics Education Inc.
P. O. Box 4390
6830 Laurel Street, N.W.
Washington, D.C. 20012

An educational organization for the prevention of addictions. Write for Catalog of "Educational Tools and Aids That Train For A Life Without Drugs," full of excellent resources in this field.

Books and Articles
Loosening The Grip
A Handbook Of Alcohol Information
by Jean Kinney, M.S.W. and Gwen Leaton
The C. V. Mosby Co., St. Louis, Mo. (1978)

This is a resource book for those working with alcoholics, particularly counselors of alcoholics. The authors are both affiliated with the Alcohol Counselor Training Program, Dartmouth Medical School, Hanover, N.H.

"Helping the Nurse Who Misuses Drugs" by Elaine B., Clare M., June S. and Janet A., in *American Journal of Nursing,* September, 1974, pp. 1655–1671.

"The Alcoholic Nurse: What We Try to Deny" by Charlotte Isler, in *RN,* July, 1978, pp. 48–55.

Films and Audiovisual Resources on Alcohol and Drug Addiction

"Alcoholism—Disease In Disguise," from Ayerst Laboratories.
"Soft Is The Heart Of A Child," the effects of an alcoholic parent on a child, from Modern Talking Picture Service.

"If You Loved Me," the effects of alcoholism on the whole family, from Modern Talking Picture Service.

"Drinking," "Just One," "About Addiction," "Psychoactive," "Tomorrow Is Cancelled," all available from Narcotics Education Inc.

"The Secret Love of Sandra Blain," a film about a woman's experience with alcoholism, from Aims Instructional Media, Inc.

"Narcotics—Why Not?", a film showing residents of a California Rehabilitation Center discussing their addiction to drugs. Available in Spanish and English from Aims Instructional Media, Inc.

"New Beginnings: Women, Alcohol And Recovery," a film about three women's recoveries from alcoholism, from Aims Instructional Media, Inc.

"Junkies Are People," a film on different methods of treating the drug addicted, from the University of California Extension Media Center.

"Alcoholism: A Family Crisis," sound/slides and sound/filmstrips for the families of alcoholics from Robert J. Brady Co.

"Alcohol: A New Focus," especially for young people, available in English and Spanish from American Educational Films.

The National Institute on Drug Abuse has available several tapes, films, and records on all aspects of drug and alcohol abuse. Contact NIDA Resource Center for their audiovisual catalog.

An audiovisual catalog of drug abuse is available from the National Clearinghouse For Drug Abuse Information (NCDAI).

Several films and filmstrips on alcohol and drugs are available from Narcotics Education, Inc.

The American Hospital Association has available several films on alcohol and drug abuse.

In Focus: Alcohol And Alcoholism Media, a catalog of audiovisual materials on alcoholism, is available from the National Institute on Alcohol Abuse and Alcoholism. Ask for Department of H.E.W. Pub. No. (ADM) 77-32.

Resources In Suicide And Suicide Prevention

American Association of Suicidology
P. O. Box 3264
Houston, Texas 77001

A multidisciplinary organization of professionals and lay people concerned with preventing suicide. AAS sponsors annual meetings and publishes a quarterly journal, *Suicide And Life-Threatening Behavior,* a newsletter, *Newslink,* and a *Directory Of Suicide Prevention Centers,* as well as several pamphlets on suicide.

International Association for Suicide Prevention
Central Administrative Office
Attention: Dr. F. Wera Aigner
Psychiatrische Universitatsklinik
Spitalgasse 23
A-1090 Vienna, Austria

An international forum for sharing of knowledge and literature on suicide prevention. International conferences are held every two years for the discussion of scientific papers and the Association conducts worldwide studies on suicide and suicide prevention.

National Save-A-Life League
815 Second Avenue
New York, New York 10017

An organization which works toward the prevention of suicides through a central crisis center in New York City which works closely with crisis centers throughout the country. The league also provides public speakers and education on preventing suicide.

Merck, Sharp and Dohme
Division of Merck and Co., Inc.
West Point, Pennsylvania 19486

"Before It's Too Late," by Jan Fawcett, M.D., a pamphlet on suicide for family and friends of people who attempt suicide, is available from this company.

Films And Audiovisuals On Suicide

"Suicide," from Films Incorporated.

"Identification Of The Suicidal Individual" is a cassette tape by Tom Yarnell, Ph.D., from Communication Enterprises, Inc.

Psychiatric Nursing Education

Grants for psychiatric nursing education are available to universities, hospitals, laboratories and state and local governments from the Psychiatric Nursing Education Branch Of The Department Of Health, Education and Welfare. Grants are for education of psychiatric nurses and for continuing education in mental health and are given particularly to train nurses to work with specified priority groups, including the minorities, children and the elderly. The grants are for institutions, not individuals. Those interested in further information on the terms of the grants and the application procedure should contact: Dr. Jeanette G. Chamberlain, Acting Chief, Psychiatric Nursing Education Branch, Division Of Manpower And Training Programs, 5600 Fishers Lane, Room 9-C-24, Rockville, Maryland 20857.

Schools with Educational Programs for Psychiatric-Mental Health Nurse Practitioners

Columbia University
School of Nursing
630 W. 168th St.
New York, N.Y. 10032

Harlem Valley Psychiatric Center
Wingdale, N.Y. 12594

Meharry Medical College
Department of Nursing Education
Box 61-A
1005 18th Ave., North
Nashville, Tenn. 37208

Syracuse University
School of Nursing
426 Ostrom Ave.
Syracuse, N.Y. 13210

University of Arkansas for Medical Sciences
College of Nursing
4301 West Markham St.
Little Rock, Arkansas 72201

University of Minnesota
School of Nursing
3313 Powell Hall
Minneapolis, Minnesota 55455

University of Utah
College of Nursing
25 South Medical Drive
Salt Lake City, Utah 84112

Yale University
School of Nursing
38 South St.
New Haven, Conn. 06520

Adapted from *A Directory of Expanded Role Programs For Registered Nurses*, 1979, Division of Nursing, Health Resources Administration, Department of H.E.W.

Publications and Educational Materials on Mental Health

Several publications on mental health are available from the:

Mental Health Association
1800 North Kent St.
Arlington, Va. 22209

A series of five educational pamphlets for family members of the mentally ill is available from:

Dome Division, Miles Laboratories
400 Morgan Lane
West Haven, Conn. 06516

"This Question of Coping," a professional educational series of 14 brochures on coping, "Psychological Stress and the Postoperative Patient," "Stress and the Middle Years," and "Anxiety: Day-to-Day Stressors vs. Past Traumatic Events" (all booklets) are available from:

Roche Laboratories
Professional Services Department
Nutley, N.J. 07110

Periodicals

American Journal of Orthopsychiatry
1775 Broadway
New York, N.Y. 10019

This is the official journal of the American Orthopsychiatric Association, Inc., and is directed at all those working in mental health and human development. It is published quarterly. (Cost: $20.00/year, $14.00 for students.)

American Journal of Psychiatry
1700 Eighteenth St., N.W.
Washington, D.C. 20009

This is the official Journal of the American Psychiatric Association, published monthly, for psychiatrists and other mental health care workers. (Cost: $18.00/year, U.S.) Other publications of the Association include: *Psychiatric News,* a newspaper ($6.00/year), *Hospital and Community Psychiatry,* a monthly journal aimed at staff members of mental health agencies ($18.00/year), appointment books, and several books and pamphlets prepared by the Association.

Archives of General Psychiatry
535 North Dearborn St.,
Chicago, Ill. 60610

This is a monthly publication of the American Medical Association (Cost: $18.00/year, U.S.; $28.00, foreign.)

Art Psychotherapy

This is a quarterly journal from Pergamon Press, Maxwell House, Fairview Park, Elmsford, N.Y. 10523.

Behavioral Counseling Quarterly

This quarterly journal contains information on techniques and practices in behavior counseling. It is published by Human Sciences Press (Cost: $18/year).

Child Psychiatry and Human Development

A quarterly journal published by Human Sciences Press (Cost: $20.00/year).

Community Mental Health Journal

This is a quarterly journal "sponsored by the National Council of Community Mental Health Centers, Inc.," published by Human Sciences Press (Cost: $18.00/year).

Family and Child Mental Health Journal

A quarterly journal "sponsored by the Jewish Board of Family and Children's Services, Inc.," published by Human Sciences Press (Cost: $10.00/year).

General Hospital Psychiatry

This is a new quarterly journal focusing on the interrelationships between "Psychiatry, Medicine, and Primary Care." Topics considered include the use of psychiatric consultants to treat medical patients and the psychological components of disease states. This magazine is useful to nurses in medical-surgical nursing as well as those in mental health nursing. Available from Elsevier North Holland (Cost: $30.00/year).

Group

The Journal of the Eastern Group Psychotherapy Society

This is a quarterly publication from Human Sciences Press (Cost: $18.00/year).

Infant Mental Health Journal

The "Official Publication of the Michigan Association for Infant Mental Health," this journal deals with the social and psychological development of young children. It is published quarterly by the Human Sciences Press (Cost: $18.00/year).

International Journal of Family Therapy

A quarterly publication of Human Sciences Press (Cost: $18.00).

Issues in Mental Health Nursing

This is a quarterly journal from McGraw-Hill Book Company (Cost: $20.00/year).

Journal of Contemporary Psychotherapy

A semi-annual publication of Human Sciences Press (Cost: $10.00/year).

Journal of Psychiatric Nursing and Mental Health Services

A monthly publication from Charles B. Slack, Inc. (Cost: $14.00/year).

Journal of School Psychology

A quarterly publication of Human Sciences Press (Cost: $16.00/year).

Journal of Sex and Marital Therapy

A quarterly publication of Human Sciences Press (Cost: $20.00/year).

Perspectives in Psychiatric Care
Nursing Publications, Inc.
Park Ridge, N.J. 07656

A professional journal for psychiatric nurses, *Perspectives* is published bimonthly and contains articles by experts in the field (Cost: $15.00/year).

Psychiatric Quarterly

A publication "sponsored by the New York School of Psychiatry" and published by Human Sciences Press (Cost: $20.00/year).

The Psychoanalytic Review

The official journal of the National Psychological Association for Psychoanalysis, Inc., this is a quarterly publication from Human Sciences Press (Cost: $20.00/year).

Psychology of Women Quarterly

A quarterly journal "sponsored by the Division of the Psychology of Women, American Psychological Assocation," and published by Human Sciences Press (Cost: $20.00/year).

Psychosomatic Medicine
Journal of the American Psychosomatic Society

This journal contains articles on psychosomatic medicine and related topics and is published 8 times/year by Elsevier North-Holland (Cost: $35.00/year).

Mental Health Films

"Depression: Blahs, Blues, Better Days" discusses causes of depression and ways of dealing with it. American Educational Films.

"Stress: Dealing Positively With A Negative," American Educational Films.

"Escape From Madness," a study on patients discharged as cured from mental hospitals. From Films Incorporated.

"The Gestalt Series," a series of 8 films dealing with Gestalt therapy and its applications. Includes 2 films on dreams. Films Incorporated.

"Psychiatric Nursing: The Nurse-Patient Relationship," Association-Sterling Films.

"Here I Am" deals with Utah State Hospital's program of giving responsibility to "dangerous mental patients" to care for each other. Brigham Young University.

"Looking For Me," a film on the use of "body language" to reach the psychotic. Multi Media Resource Center.

"The Schizophrenic Patient: Recognition and Management," a series of sound-filmstrips from Eye Gate Media.

"Community Mental Health," a film on how a community started a mental health center to meet its needs. From International Film Bureau, Inc.

"Psychotherapeutic Interview," "The Long-Term Psychiatric Patient," "Psychogeriatrics," and "Psychiatric Emergencies" are among the film titles for psychiatric nurses from the American Journal of Nursing Co.

"The Abnormal Psychology Series," "The B. F. Skinner Film Series" and "The Developmental Psychology Today Film Series" are examples of the many films on psychology and mental health available from McGraw-Hill Films.

"Mental Patients' Association," a film on a group of former mental health patients who organized a self-help group for people newly discharged from mental institutions, to aid in the adjustment period. National Film Board of Canada.

"Hurry Tomorrow" is an shocking exposé on the treatment of mental patients that goes on today in some institutions. Tricontinental Film Center.

"Titicut Follies" is another shocking exposé on the treatment of patients in a mental institution. The Supreme Court of Massachusetts has ruled that this film may be shown only to those working in the social sciences or involved with custodial care of the mentally ill, or students in these fields. From Zipporah Films.

"On Becoming A Nurse-Psychotherapist," a film documenting a student nurse's relationship with her client and her instructor. Includes techniques in psychotherapy. University of California Extension Media Center.

Several films on the works of leaders in the field of psychology/psychotherapy, including B. F. Skinner, Erik Erikson, Carl Jung, Fritz Perls, Erich Fromm, Carl Rogers, Jean Piaget, R. D. Laing, and others, are available from the University of California Extension Media Center.

"Child at the Gate," a filmstrip with tape cassette on the use of music, poetry and art therapies with a schizophrenic woman, helping her to relate to the outside world, and "Moving True," a film of a session of dance therapy, are available from the Music Therapy Center.

A Comprehensive Resource Guide to 16MM Mental Health Films, a 120-page book with 1300 listings of films useful for mental health education, and *An Evaluative Guide to 16 MM Mental Health Films,* a 65-page book of 350 listings of films recommended by the Mental Health Association, are both available from the Mental Health Media Evaluation Project.

11 Public-Health Nursing

The phrase "public health nurse" has traditionally conjured up images of a nurse dressed in navy blue, carrying a black bag, and traveling around communities working in health education and disease prevention, especially in the area of communicable diseases.

This traditional image of the public health nurse has been changing rapidly. A nurse involved in public health today has many roles including home care of the sick and teaching home care to families, the traditional communicable disease follow-up, well child clinics, serving as community consultant on health care, teaching classes on preparation for childbirth and parenting, and many others.

The following 5 examples of innovations in public health nursing point out the diversity of this field. They are all excerpted from *Analysis and Planning for Improved Distribution of Nursing Personnel and Services, Inventory of Innovations in Nursing*, edited by Sheila Kodadek, and published by the Division of Nursing, Health Resources Administration, U.S. Department of H.E.W. These innovations are reprinted here to stimulate interest in the possibilities open to public health agencies and nurses.

Extended Role of the Public-Health Nurse: A Statement of Policy

Commonwealth of Virginia, Department of Health
Richmond, Virginia

Background: Many public-health nurses are practicing at their highest level of competence; others are not. Some need on-the-job training to enable them to carry out functions that extend beyond the usual skills of the public-health nurse. The staff of the Bureau of Public-Health Nursing, Virginia State Health Department, believe that in addition to confidence in her or his ability to perform at the highest level of competence, the public-health nurse needs a statement of policy that approves extending the scope of public-health nursing practice.

Purpose: The specific purpose of the statement of policy is to provide additional content for the *Public-Health Nursing Guide,* a manual used by public-health nurses in Virginia to help them function in the extended role. Objectives are to enable the public-health nurse to perform effectively in the extended role, to increase the delivery of quality health services to all families, and to interpret the role and functions of the public-health nurse in the extended role to clients, health colleagues, and to the public.

Nursing Role: The public-health nurse is seen as a primary health-care provider in rural and underserved areas. It is believed that the nurse will be responsible for assessing client/family health needs, determining nurse or physician responsibility, and carrying out activity components defined by the policies for the extended public-health-nursing role. This includes history taking, physical examination, family and group processes, process assessment, behavior-modification techniques, and genetic counseling. The statement of policy about the extended role of the public-health nurse provides the nurse policies in four major areas: nursing intervention, nursing assessment, laboratory, and treatment.

Contact For Further Information:
Sarah E. Sayres, RN, MPH
Director, Bureau of Public-Health Nursing
State Health Department
Commonwealth of Virginia
Richmond, Virginia 23219

Specialization of Public-Health Nurses

South Carolina Department of Health
and Environmental Control
Columbia, South Carolina

Purpose: The nursing staff of the South Carolina Department of Health and Environmental Control has chosen to focus on nursing specializations. This replaces the traditional pattern of generalized staff nursing, with limited specialized consultant nurse services from the state office. The change was made to enable each of the nurses to become more knowledgeable and self-confident in a specialty area.

South Carolina is divided into 12 health districts, with two to six counties in each district. Within each health district, there is a district director of public-health nursing who has overall responsibility for the quality of nursing care. The director has at least one nurse specialist assigned to manage a specialty program, such as home health, adult health, child health, maternity, and family planning. This specialist also gives clinical supervision to that program's nursing staff. Each nurse specialist has at least one team leader under her direction. Teams usually consist of a registered nurse leader, another registered nurse, a licensed practical nurse, and a nursing aide.

Each district staff is beginning to add clinical-nursing specialists with master's degrees and technically prepared nurse practitioners who provide some direct primary care and screening services. The clinical specialist devotes at least 50 percent of her or his time to direct nursing care of patients and families with highly complex health problems. The remainder of the clinical specialist's time is devoted to inservice education for all nurses and clinical supervision of the nurse practitioners.

Cost: No specific cost information was provided. Specific desired outcomes and personnel time are accounted for in the framework of each program's budget. Information is available on request.

Evaluation: One of the outcomes has been to reduce problems for nurses faced with the conflicting, simultaneous demands of several programs. Another has been the increase in the expertise of public-health nurses in specific areas. Larger numbers of patients are served in each program than has been the case with the generalized structure. An unintended outcome of this specialist system has been a deterioration in holistic family treatment. The problem is being studied with the intention of designing a modification to allow the best of both systems, with the expertise and accountability possible within a specialist system without the fragmentation that seems to accompany it.

Contact for Further Information:
Virginia C. Phillips, RN
State Director of Public Health Nursing
South Carolina Department of Health and Environmental Control
J. Marion Sims Building
2600 Bull Street
Columbia, South Carolina 29201

A Visiting Nurse Association's Affiliation with Group Physician Practices

Burlington, Vermont

Background: Nurses in a home-health agency traditionally have had to communicate with a number of physicians, and physicians have had to relate to several nurses who care for their patients. This has led to difficulties in communication and has not fostered a trusting, team approach to patient care. In an attempt to remedy this, the Visiting Nurse Association assigned one or two nurses to group physician practices and, in two situations, merged patient records.

Purpose: The purpose was to strengthen the team approach and promote continuity of care for the home-bound, chronically, acutely, and terminally ill patient. The target consumer population consists of patients of physicians in selected group practices.

Nursing Role: The nurses work in a collegial relationship with the physicians in planning home care for the patients. The nurses meet regularly with the physicians and have immediate access to physician consultation. The physicians make more appropriate use of the nurses' services as they become more aware of the skill level of the nurses. In two situations, the RNs had the responsibility of merging the two record systems needed to meet legal and certification requirements. This was possible where the physician practice was also using the problem-oriented record system. The RN has become a community resource for the practice. In one situation, the RN provides care in the practice setting.

Cost: This effort has not resulted in a cost increase for home visits.

Evaluation: Evaluation has been done only on a subjective basis, with these findings: 1) improved efficiency in transfer of patient information—the RN has access to physician records, 2) more appropriate utilization of RN skills, and 3) improved continuity of care for the patient marked by earlier intervention in potential crises. Patients identify the nurse and physician as a team.

Contact for Further Information:
Elizabeth J. Davis
Executive Director
Visiting Nurse Association, Inc.
260 College Street
Burlington, Vermont 05401

State of Connecticut
Department of Health
Hartford, Connecticut

Background: In the last decade, large institutions for the mentally ill have been moving toward more individualized care. One way of providing individualized care is through geographic decentralization and the use of existing community resources, thus allowing patients to remain with their families or in the area. Public-health nursing agencies have worked with mentally ill patients, but often they do not have the benefit of structured referral and reporting relationships with hospitals and agencies specifically designed to care for the mentally ill. The resulting lack of information exchange was detrimental to the patient.

Purpose: A formal contractual relationship was established between Connecticut Valley Hospital, a decentralized state institution for the mentally ill, and three public-health nursing associations. The goals were to extend hospital services into the community, to enlarge the therapeutic team by using nurses who are community experts and skilled in psychiatric nursing, and to close the psychological gap between the hospital and patients' homes. The target consumer population is selected patients of the Connecticut Valley Hospital system. Selection is made by hospital staff and public-health nurses, based on criteria established through experience and study.

Nursing Role: To accomplish the objectives of the program, liaison nurses, who have dual appointments with public-health agencies and the Connecticut Valley Hospital system, provide continuity of care and communication between the hospital and community. The liaison nurse's primary function is to ensure that nursing services are available for those patients and families who can benefit from them. In doing so, she becomes an expert in the needs of hospital-based patients from her work with the institution, her work with community resources, and her work with community agencies and public-health nurses in the field.

The liaison nurse's work includes attendance at all hospital meetings, where various treatment modalities are designed and planning for discharge is done. In addition, she is free to make her own ward rounds and to establish relationships with patients, relationships that can be transferred later to district nurses when the patient is discharged. Her relationship with the staff makes it possible to assist them in understanding family situations and possible alternatives to institutionalization.

When patients are admitted, there generally is a disruptive home situation. The liaison nurse contacts the district nurses and informs them of the situation. When a district nurse receives the referral, she makes every effort to visit within 48 hours. Often she finds a crisis situation. Her initial work with the family can lay the groundwork for later support when the patient comes home. Through the liaison nurse, the district nurse provides information about the family situation to the hospital staff. The public-health nurse functions as a coordinator and expediter and often the primary therapeutic agent.

Evaluation: With the public-health nursing followup, only one in eight first-admission patients is readmitted to institutions. Without public-health nursing follow-up, four in eight first-admission patients are readmitted. There are cost implications in this as well as indications of success. Currently, about 35 percent of the hospital population is being seen by the three participating agencies. All referrals are planned with the patient's participation, so there are no losses in the form of "not located" or "refused service." Additional information about evaluation results and statistical follow-up is available on request.

Contact for Further Information:
Nancy Stoppleworth, RN, MSN
Mental Health Nurse Consultant
Public Health Nursing Division, State of Connecticut,
State Department of Health
79 Elm Street
Hartford, Connecticut 06115
(203) 566-2547

Public-Health Nurse in Mental Health Follow-Up Care

Alaska Department of Health and Social Services
Ketchikan, Alaska

Purpose: The Section of Nursing, Division of Public Health, Alaska Department of Health and Social Services, provides community-health nursing services to all Alaska towns and villages except those in the Anchorage Borough, which is served on an advisory basis. Nursing services are a part of a public-health program directed to raising the current health status of the people of Alaska. The public-health nurse is the primary field representative, and through her, most public-health programs are implemented and services furnished. She participates in community programs of health promotion and rehabilitation, including those designed to prevent, detect, treat, and control illness. She helps families and individuals recognize their own health needs and assists them in working out appropriate solutions.

Nursing services are brought to remote areas by itinerant public-health nurses who travel to the villages by plane, boat, and, on occasion, snowmobile or dog team. In urban areas, public-health nurses, registered nurses, practical nurses, and community-health aides work out of local health centers.

Nursing Role: Public-health nurses participate in communicable-disease control through general preventive measures, early identification of disease, provision of care, and supervision to reduce effects of disease. They provide services to families during the maternity cycle, supplementing those received from physicians or clinics. Public-health nurses assist parents in keeping children healthy by means of individual counseling in home settings, child-health conferences, group instruction, and school-health services. They help locate handicapped individuals and assist them to procure treatment and rehabilitative services. They work with individuals and families with mental distress or disorders, alcoholism, or drug abuse, and support and actively engage in community programs directed to preventing those behavioral health problems. The public-health nurses are responsible for local home-care programs that provide skilled nursing and other therapeutic services in the home. The nurses are the primary health-care deliverers; they work primarily on a one-to-one basis and help detect individuals with acute conditions. In the absence of immediate medical care in villages, they treat minor illnesses and injuries according to medical orders. When additional medical recommendations are indicated, these are obtained from the responsible physician by telephone or radio. For the most part, these physicians are located in the Public Health Service, Alaska Area Native Health Service field hospitals. People in need of additional care are transported to the closest medical facility.

Contact for Further Information:
Mildred Manty, RN
Prince of Wales Itinerant Public Health Nurse III
Room 204, State Office Building
Ketchikan, Alaska 99901

Resources in Public Health

National Council for Homemaker
Home Health Aide Services, Inc.
67 Irving Place
New York, N.Y. 10003

This organization sets the standards for homemaker-home health aide services throughout the country. The Council makes available a directory on where these services are located and literature on them; including information on establishing homemaker-home health aide services.

Society for Public Health Education, Inc.
703 Market Street, Suite 535
San Francisco, Calif. 94103

The Society is a national interdisciplinary organization for those involved with health education. It promotes professional development and continuing education for health educators, encourages research in this field, and sets standards for quality health education. Publications include *Health Education Monographs,* a quarterly journal, and *SOPHE News and Views,* a bimonthly newsletter.

World Health Organization (WHO)
1211 Geneva 27
Switzerland

or

P. O. Box 5284
Church Street Station
New York, N.Y. 10249

WHO is the United Nations agency concerned with improving health and health care on a world-wide basis. WHO conducts research and provides education in its attempt to prevent and control disease. A large variety of publications are available from WHO, including the periodicals, *Bulletin Of The World Health Organization* (published six times a year), the monthly *WHO Chronicle,* the quarterly *International Digest Of Health Legislation,* and many reports on studies conducted by the WHO. Write for *World Health Organization Publications* catalog.

Periodicals on Public Health

Journal Of Prevention is a quarterly journal with articles and research on the health care specialty of prevention, published by the Human Sciences Press (Cost: $18 a year for individuals).

Public Health Reports is a bimonthly journal, published by the Public Health Service of the Department of H.E.W. and available from the Superintendent Of Documents. Articles deal with concerns of public health and community medicine (Cost: $10.35 a year in U.S., Canada and Mexico; $12.95 a year in most foreign countries).

12 Holistic Health

I. **Description of Holistic Health**
II. **Therapeutic Touch**
III. **Mind-Body Relatedness**
IV. **Resources in Holistic Health**

Holistic Health

Holistic health ... focuses on development of the joyful expression of good health, not on the achievement of normalcy or balance. A holistic system may include identification and treatment of disease, as one possible choice among many, but it does not focus on problems and errors.... It focuses, instead, on clarity of intention, development of wellbeing, and enjoyment of life in a system of self-responsibility.

This holistic-health system consists essentially of enabling good health to emerge from within the person who recognizes and acts upon life stresses, and undertakes a commitment to maintain self-expression in an environment of goodwill. Disease is seen as an important feedback message, to be dealt with consciously as part of the life process, not as a victimization by a hostile nature. The holistic assumption is that the body knows how to heal itself, is a natural "healing system" intent on good health, and that we must learn how to get our stresses and misunderstandings out of its way.

The Holistic Health Handbook © Copyright, 1978, Bauman, Piper, Brint and Wright All rights reserved. Published by: And/Or Press, P.O. Box 2246, Berkeley, Ca. 94702. Used by permission.

The Holistic Nurse

What makes a holistic nurse different? She is a nurturing, caring individual who incorporates concepts of mind-body-spirit into interactions with people. The Renaissance nurse is conscious of the total person; I stress the spiritual component because I believe that this important aspect has been overlooked in our efforts to emphasize bodily aspects. We have all dealt with people who have lost their will to live and laid down to die. Likewise, we've worked with infants labeled "failure to thrive," which is, in my estimation, a conscious decision not to mature normally because of a lack of nurturing. We've also worked with people who have defied their medical diagnosis and obstinately lived well beyond their medically calculated date of expiration.

As nurses, our awareness of this important component allows us to work in infinitely creative ways, as well as to view ourselves very differently. The role of the healer is expanding rapidly, and we must remain aware of our responsibility. Healing, as is stressed frequently by Dolores Krieger, is a volitional act, involving *intent* of the healer to heal. Dr. Krieger is teaching thousands of nurses across the U.S. to use Therapeutic Touch in their work with patients in multitudinous situations; as a result, many nurses are tuning in to the fact that we are channels for healing energy.

The Holistic Health Handbook © Copyright, 1978, Bauman, Piper, Brint and Wright All rights reserved. Published by: And/Or Press, P.O. Box 2246, Berkeley, Ca. 94602. Used by permission.

Therapeutic Touch in Practice
By Janet Macrae

Therapeutic touch is a treatment modality based on an exchange of energy between healer and patient. I look upon this technique as an extension of nursing practice since nursing traditionally has included touch as an aspect of patient care.

I learned therapeutic touch from Ms. Dora Kunz and Dr. Dolores Krieger. As a staff nurse in pediatrics, I have explored and developed various ways of integrating this technique with my other nursing skills. I would like to share some of these experiences, because I have found that therapeutic touch holds its own in the midst of sophisticated technology and offers a new dimension to modern nursing.

Basic to therapeutic touch is the concept that a human being is a highly complex field, or continuum, of various life energies. The physical body can be looked upon as the denser, or more compacted, aspect of the field. In a state of health, all the individual's energies are in harmony, or dynamic balance. Disease, within this framework, is a manifestation of disequilibrium, blockage, and/or deficits in the human energy flow. When using therapeutic touch, we sensitize our hands to the energy field and assess its condition. Then we knowledgeably help the patient to repattern his or her energies in a healthier way.

Before using therapeutic touch, I first practiced various methods of centering. This is the act of consciously putting myself in a very calm, alert state of being, of integrating myself in the here and now. Centering is important because, when I use therapeutic touch, the only tool I have is myself. If my thoughts are scattered, or if I am emotionally upset or irritated, the healing process is not facilitated at all. Since there is often quite a bit of tension on a busy hospital floor, and since many of our nursing actions are fragmented, I always take a moment to center, to feel my *wholeness,* before giving therapeutic touch to a patient.

I have found that there are no basic differences between treating children and treating adults with therapeutic touch. However, children's systems are very sensitive, and as with medication, therapeutic touch must be given in smaller, more gentle doses. Too much or incorrect repatterning can cause discomfort, so it is extremely important to be sensitive to the patients' responses.

In general, children in pain respond very well to therapeutic touch. The following example illustrates one way in which I have used this technique to help relieve pain.

Chris, a four-year-old boy who was two hours postop, complained of pain at his incision site. I ran my hands through his energy field—about four to six inches beyond the surface of his physical body. I literally found the pain, in a manner that I will explain, and directed it out of his field, using a stroking motion. The little boy stopped crying and fell asleep after about three to four minutes of therapeutic touch.

Practitioners of therapeutic touch generally work in the finer aspect of the individual's energy field, which is beyond the surface of the body. Although it is possible to do therapeutic touch using actual body contact, the area above the surface is usually preferred because it is less compacted. Dysrhythmias are more easily perceptible here, and the healing process proceeds more quickly. A casual observer might think we are dealing with nothing. However, if this observer took some time to practice, she would soon find her hands becoming sensitive to these finer energies.

I sensed the little boy's pain as an area of heat in his energy field. Another might have sensed it as tingling or pressure. Since we use ourselves as tools, we have to become aware of our own styles and to discern individually how we feel the various dysrhythmias such as pain, congestion, and anxiety. This is done through much practice, supervision, and patient feedback. I have found it helpful to keep a record of my experiences; this also gives isolated events a meaningful context.

It is important to realize that the energy field is a continuum; therefore, whatever we do to one aspect will have an effect on the whole. This concept of the wholeness of the individual is crucial when one is using therapeutic touch, as one can see from the following example.

A 10-year-old boy named Paul, who had leukemia, was suffering from jaw pain secondary to one of the chemotherapeutic agents. Analgesics were not completely effective in relieving it.

One day I asked him if I could put my hands on the place where it hurt. He said yes, so I centered myself quickly and passed my hands through his field. Above the right side of his jaw I felt a fine tingling sensation. I brushed it away. However, it reappeared above the left side of his jaw. I then cleared off both sides simultaneously, and Paul informed me that his jaw was fine but that his upper chest had begun to hurt. I put my hands over his chest and the pain went back to his right jaw. At that point I stopped to reevaluate the situation. I realized that I was not treating the patient's energy field as a whole, so I changed my method. I put my left hand over his jaw where the pain was, and with my right hand, I directed the area of tingling through his whole field and out past his feet.

Paul, on his own accord, told me that he had felt the pain go through his chest and into his abdomen, then move down his legs and go out his feet. So the energy field, as seen in this example, is a continuum that transcends definite organ systems. It can be, and must be, treated holistically.

I have also used therapeutic touch in the care of children with lung congestion. When treating these children, I center myself, find the areas within their fields where congestion has localized, and I then try to direct this congestion out of their energy fields, usually down through their feet.

Here again, the concept of wholeness is extremely important. Under repeated observation, it seems that when congestion is cleared out of the lung area, it can become established somewhere else in the field, causing discomfort. This also seems to happen with pain, as I described. So when using therapeutic touch, I always direct the energies bound up in pain and congestion out of the entire field.

One day I used therapeutic touch to help a little girl with cystic fibrosis clear her lungs. When the treatment was over, I listened to her chest with a stethoscope and, to my disappointment, found no improvement. Later, however, when her father was leaving, he told me that she "ate like a horse" that evening for the first time in weeks.

This incident and others similar to it have taught me to try to put my personal expectations, my own ego needs, out of the situation. I assess and treat as knowledgeably as possible, and then let the patient respond in his or her own way.

Since I do not like to work in secret, I generally explain the technique to the children and ask their permission before proceeding. The explanation, of course, will vary according to the situation. I might ask a four- or five-year-old if I could try to "brush the pain away." Nine- and ten-year-olds are generally fascinated by the idea of being an energy field. One little girl, in a very superior tone, told a friend of hers, "You just don't stop at your skin, you know!"

If a child is too little to talk, I explain therapeutic touch to the parents. I usually say that this technique is derived from an ancient practice of laying on of hands and that it is now being taught in some nursing schools.

If I am teaching a patient and another staff member enters the room, I briefly explain what I am doing and why I believe therapeutic touch is appropriate to this particular patient. In this way, the hospital staff is gradually becoming acquainted with therapeutic touch, a nursing modality.

Although it looks very simple, therapeutic touch is, in reality, a highly complex technique. What I have shared are some of its most basic principles and some of the ways I have used them in a clinical setting.

Janet Macrae, R.N., M.A., is a doctoral candidate at NYU and has been working with therapeutic touch for the past four years.

Reprinted with permission of the American Journal of Nursing Company, from "Therapeutic Touch In Practice" by Janet Macrae, in *American Journal of Nursing*, April, 1979, © American Journal of Nursing Company.

For more detailed information on Therapeutic Touch see *The Therapeutic Touch* by Dolores Krieger, Ph.D., R.N., published by Prentice-Hall, Inc., 1979. It is an excellent resource for nurses interested in pursuing this field.

Mind-Body Relatedness
by Susan J. MacKenzie

A healthy person is in a state of dynamic equilibrium of both mind and body. Illness occurs when part of the total system is upset. Returning to a healthy state usually includes a readiness to be well again, be it faith in a medication, in one's physician, or even faith in the powers of one's own body.

Much recent medical literature considers the mind factor in physical illness. Emotions and stress are proving to have a direct bearing on a person's physical status. Particular personality types are being coupled with disease states for which they may have a special affinity. *Type A Behavior and Your Heart* by Friedman and Roseman implicates prolonged stress and personality characteristics as causal factors in coronary disease. Dr. O. C. Simonton and S. Matthews Simonton, authors of *Getting Well Again,* propose that cancer victims also have a certain personality type in common, a feeling of basic rejection being one of the underlying factors. Their work encourages a change in a diseased person's life history pattern, which they feel could alter the course of the disease process. The Simontons ask their patients to take personal responsibility in regaining and maintaining their health.

Such practices as biofeedback and meditation are being taught to patients to help them have some control over their own state of health. The principles of biofeedback have been gaining in acceptance. Voluntary regulation of the autonomic nervous system was once considered impossible. Now many researchers find it very feasible. An individual with the volition and training to do so can alter various autonomic functions such as heart rate, muscle tension, body temperature and stomach acidity levels. One of the principal advantages of biofeedback training is that it may trigger a recognition in a patient that he/she is responsible for his/her own wellness-illness continuum, again stressing the concept of the mind-body as a unit.

Meditation is a practice dating back thousands of years. It utilizes the learned process of relaxation and although there is no concentrated focus on physiologic function, it does have the outcome of stress release and a general slowing down of metabolism, reflecting this in a physiologic lowering of blood pressure, pulse and respiration.

As health teachers we are able to introduce to our patients the concept of mind-body control. This introduction might be as simple as having a patient visualize himself walking to the bathroom after confinement in bed. It could also be incorporated into the birthing process by helping a woman focus on her body and the physiologic changes that happen in labor, such as dilatation of the cervix, movement of the infant through the birth canal, and involution of the uterus. On a more sophisticated level the teaching of mind-body control can be done by learned practitioners like the Simontons who guide their patients through meditation and visual imagery in an effort to alter the disease process of cancer.

Bibliography on the Emotional and Mental Aspects of Cancer

Cantor, Robert Chernin, *And A Time to Live, Toward Emotional Well-Being During the Crisis of Cancer,* Harper and Row Publishers, 1978.

Cousins, Norman, "The Mysterious Placebo, How Mind Helps Medicine Work" in *Saturday Review,* October 1, 1977, p. 9–16.

Fiore, Neil, "Fighting Cancer—One Patient's Perspective" in *The New England Journal of Medicine,* February 8, 1979, l. 284-9.

Frank, Jerome D., "The Medical Power of Faith" in *Human Nature,* August, 1978, p. 40–7.

Le Shan, Lawrence, *You Can Fight for Your Life: Emotional Factors in the Causation of Cancer,* M. Evans and Co., Inc., 1977, distributed in the U.S. by J. B. Lippincott.

O'Donnell, Walter, "The Will to Live" in *Woman's Day,* June 28, 1977, p. 50.

Simonton, O. Carl, and Stephanie Matthews-Simonton, James Creighton, J. P. Thatcher, *Getting Well Again,* 1978, distributed by St. Martin Press.

Simonton, O. Carl, "Management of the Emotional Aspects of Malignancy" in *Newsletter* of the International Association of Cancer Victors and Friends, Inc., P.O. Box 1541, Mesa, Arizona, 85201.

Wixen, Joan Saunders, "Cancer and the Mind" in *Modern Maturity,* December-January, 1978-1979, p. 46–8.

Resources in Holistic Health

Academy of Holistic Medicine, Inc.
11373 Willow Creek Road
Paicines, California 95043

This is an organization of health care workers from various disciplines who share an interest in holistic health care. Lifetime membership costs $60.00 and is open to anyone involved in health care. Publications include the *A.H.M. Newsletter.*

Association for Holistic Health
P. O. Box 33202
San Diego, California 92103

This is a non-profit organization which promotes holistic health by offering training programs, conferences, workshops, and serving as an information network.

Publications include: *Holistic Health Focus,* a newsletter; *The Journal of Holistic Health;* and pamphlets on holistic health.

Biofeedback Society of America
U.C.M.C C268
4200 East Ninth Avenue
Denver, Colorado 80262

The Biofeedback Society "is an open forum for the exchange of ideas, methods and results of biofeedback and related studies." (Quoted from the Society's brochure.) Membership is open to professionals involved in biofeedback. The Society offers workshops in biofeedback and conducts an annual scientific meeting.

Publications include: *Biofeedback And Self-Regulation,* the journal of the Society; *Biofeedback,* a quarterly newsletter; abstracts of the proceedings of the annual meetings; bibliographies; and a membership directory.

Center for Chinese Medicine
230 South Garfield Avenue, Suite 202
Monterey Park, California 91754

The center is a non-profit organization which provides educational programs and referrals for professionals and the general public in the field of Chinese medicine. Topics covered include: Acupuncture, Acupressure, Chinese eating habits which foster weight control, and related topics.

Center for Inner Motivation and Awareness
P. O. Box 3561
San Diego, California 92103

This "is a non-profit teaching and learning center which gathers and disseminates proven, easy-to-use practices and techniques that enhance the physical, emotional, mental and spiritual well-being of the participants." (Quoted from CIMA "Information Sheet.") The Center holds both local, national and international conferences and workshops on a large variety of topics including: "Integrative Healing"; "Natural Birth Control"; "Stress Management"; "Touch Therapy"; and many others. It is also involved in research projects. Workshops are approved by the California Board of Registered Nursing for Continuing Education credits.

East West Academy Of Healing Arts (EWAHA)
P. O. Box 31211
San Francisco, Calif. 94131

This is a "non-profit organization dedicated to holistic health research, education and care." Of special interest to nurses is the EWAHA's International Council Of Nurse Healers, a division of the Academy for nurses involved in holistic health care research, education or practice.

The EWAHA, in conjunction with the University Of California San Francisco Extension, offers a program in "Holistic Health and System of Chinese Healing Touch/Acupressure." It also offers consultation to educational institutions desiring to set up similar courses in holistic health training.

The organization also has available a variety of printed material and cassette tapes on Holistic Health. Write for complete listing.

Holistic Life University *
1627 Tenth Avenue
San Francisco, California 94122

This is a non-profit educational organization with courses and fields of study in holistic health, holistic childbirth and life-death transitions. It prepares counselors and educators in these fields. The faculty is composed of health professionals from all disciplines, including nursing. Special workshops in continuing education for nurses are offered and classes are approved by the State of California Board Of Registered Nursing for continuing education credits.

The Holistic Life University also has a referral service to help people find resources in holistic health both locally and across the country.

In affiliation with the Holistic Life University is Holistic Life Seminars, a series of workshops on various aspects of holistic health held at the Feathered Pipe Ranch, Box 1682, Helena, Montana, 59601. Write for information on upcoming seminars.

The following material is adapted from the Holistic Life University Catalog. *Write for the catalog for further information.*

National Council on Wholistic Therapeutics and Medicine
P. O. Box 15859
Philadelphia, Pennsylvania 19103

The Council is an organization of "groups dedicated to an integrated system of healing," and serves as a forum for exchange between the groups, promoting education on preventive and holistic medicine. Any group interested in being included in the Council's Guide to resources in Holistic Health should send information on its activities and publications to the Council.

The Council was founded by Leslie Kaslof, author of *Wholistic Dimensions In Healing, A Resource Guide,* published by Doubleday Dolphin and available from United Communications,* Box 320, Woodmere, New York 11598 (cost: $7.95 plus $1.50 for postage and handling). It includes articles on holistic health as well as extensive listings of names, addresses and descriptions of resources in holistic healing.

Also available from United Communications is an "Herb and Ailment Cross Reference Chart," a resource guide to the medicinal use of plants. It is 30" by 40", suitable for wall hanging, and costs $6.00 or $10.00 ($10.00 for a beautiful parchment version.)

Northeast Invitational Healers' Workshop
Pumpkin Hollow Farm
Box 135, RFD #1
Craryville, New York 12521
or

Northwest Invitational Healers' Workshop
Orcas Island Foundation
Box 86, Route 1
East Sound, Washington 98245

Contact the above addresses for information on Healers' Workshops given by Dora Kunz, National President Of Theosophical Society, and Dolores Krieger, Ph.D., R.N., author of *The Therapeutic Touch*.

The Mandala Society
P. O. Box 1233
Del Mar, California 92014

The Mandala Society functions as "administrative headquarters" for the yearly "Holistic Health Conference for Health Professionals" held every September in San Diego. Information and applications are available by contacting the Society.

Omega Institute for Holistic Studies
P.O. Box 396
New Lebanon, N.Y. 12125

The Omega Institute offers weekend seminars and 5-day programs in Holistic Health and in the Arts. It is open to all health professionals. Courses of particular interest to those in the health professions include "Holistic Health," "Herbology," "Homeopathy," "Acupuncture," "Hypnosis and Biofeedback," "Life, Death and Transitions," and others. Academic and continuing education credits are available. Write for catalog.

Wellness Resource Center
42 Miller Avenue
Mill Valley, California 94941

This is a center for the promotion of "wellness" rather than the treatment of disease conditions, where clients are members of the health team and take responsibility for their own state of health. Conferences and seminars are available for health professionals on the concept of "wellness" and how to promote it in themselves and their clients.

Publications include: *The Wellness Workbook For Health Professionals,* a manual on how to evaluate a person's state of wellness and on promoting wellness, including information on resources in holistic and wellness practices.

Periodicals in Holistic Health

Health Values: Achieving High Level Wellness is a bimonthly publication for health professionals interested in preventive health care, health promotion, health education, and helping people achieve a state of wellness. Available from Charles B. Slack, Inc. (Cost: $10 a year).

Holistic Health Review
P. O. Box 166
Berkeley, California 94701

This is a journal published quarterly by the Holistic Health Organizing Committee, a non-profit organization promoting holistic health. (Cost: $15.00 to individuals.)

Prevention (Emmaus, Pa. 18049) is a health magazine, published by the Rodale Press, and is aimed at the general public, with emphasis on preventive medicine, nutrition, self-help and natural healing (Cost: $9 a year for 12 issues).

Films on Holistic Health and Related Topics

"Introduction To Holistic Health" is a tape cassette by James Fadiman, Ph.D., available from Communication Enterprises, Inc.

"White Bird: An Alternative," a film on a healthcare program in Eugene, Oregon, which utilizes a holistic approach. From American Journal Of Nursing Company.

"The Therapeutic Touch: Healing In The New Age," a film on research on therapeutic touch, especially on the work of Dr. Dolores Krieger, showing her techniques. From Hartley Productions.

"Biofeedback: The Yoga Of The West," a film from Hartley Productions.

"Holistic Health: The New Medicine," a film showing the work of several doctors in the area of holistic medicine. From Hartley Productions.

"Introduction To Acupuncture," a film on the history and clinical application of acupuncture, showing line treatment with it, from Pyramid Films.

"Holistic Health," a series of four sound/slides or sound/filmstrips on aspects of holistic health, from Robert J. Brady Company.

A series of 15 tape cassettes on various aspects of Holistic Health is available from Association For Holistic Health.

13 Primary Nursing

I. Definition of Primary Nursing
II. Instituting Primary Nursing
III. Resources in Primary Nursing

Definition of Primary Nursing*

Primary nursing is a philosophy and a modality of humanistic health care delivery in which the client becomes a contributor to as well as a recipient of his plan of care. The client is assigned a professional nurse who cares for him utilizing the nursing process and scientific inquiry. The primary nurse has authority, autonomy and is accountable and directly available to the client. This modality may be applied in a variety of settings. The following concepts are considered as integral to a working definition of primary nursing:

1. Philosophy
2. Humanistic-holistic approach
3. Nursing process—scientific inquiry
4. Client involvement
5. Client—nurse autonomy
6. Health-illness continuum
7. Collaboration
8. Multi-setting applicability.

Reprinted with permission of National League For Nursing from *Primary Nursing, One Nurse, One Client, Planning Care Together,* © Copyright 1977, National League For Nursing, New York.

If You Are Instituting Primary Nursing

It has taken me eight years of intimate involvement in the implementation of primary nursing to reach one simple, basic conclusion: You can't do it by management edict.

* *Developed during the Primary Nursing Care Workshop.*

In my capacity as nursing administrator, I've participated in implementing primary nursing in three hospitals and I've observed its practice as a consultant in other hospitals throughout the country. I've seen what happens when it is implemented without staff involvement in the decision to do so. The effect is devastating—people are suffering tremendously under the imposition of a system of nursing that they were not involved in selecting. Morale can deteriorate to a point where people are no longer talking to each other about their patients' care. When that happens, when patient care is being given in isolation, the result can only be worse patient care.

Two or three times, I have advised *un*implementing primary nursing, going back to something like a case method rather than continuing to force down people's throats something that they're not ready to accept.

The decision to go into primary nursing requires a personal commitment by the individual nurses who are working as a group, a commitment to become involved with patients, a commitment to put oneself in a therapeutic relationship with patients. This is not something that should be decided by one person for another.

The trick is to introduce it in a way that enhances the ability of the group of nurses to work together to provide excellent patient care, and that minimizes the risk of separating or dividing the group so that its members can't work together. If, for instance, I mandated that primary nursing be established on a unit and decided for the group how they should organize themselves at the station level, I would be denying them the opportunity to learn the one fundamental thing necessary for them to become successful primary nurses, and that is how to be decision makers.

For primary nursing to succeed it has to be done in an atmosphere where risk taking and judgment making are supported, where everything isn't done according to rules and regulations, but where a nurse is expected to use clinical judgment in this or that precise situation. Now that is the tough part in implementing primary nursing.

It simply does not follow that a nurse can be expected to accept such responsibility by a decision to do so from on high. Just look at what is involved: responsibility for 24-hour nursing of a patient rests with the primary nurse; the nursing of that patient is based on decisions made by the primary nurse, who must communicate her decisions to the nurses who follow her;

the primary nurse plans for the discharge of the patient safely and effectively. She may accompany the patient home to see that he or she gets the specific clinical care needed. The primary nurse is care giver and care planner who must see to it that her decisions are initiated and followed by the nurses on each shift.

The role of the head nurse in primary nursing becomes that of teacher, resource person, validator of decision making, and quality-control agent. She is responsible for assigning the best qualified nurse to the most acutely ill patients.

Is it any wonder that primary nursing by fiat so often fails? I find it extraordinarily important that I not make these decisions for other people. I can make sure that everyone has an opportunity to understand the concept of primary nursing, and I can provide an atmosphere of support, without pressure, that enables them to implement primary nursing at their own rate, when and if they decide to do so.

I think it is time that we let our staff grow up and really take responsibility for their decisions, for the consequences of their own acts, because they're the ones who live with them.—Marie Manthey, *vice-president, Patient Services, Yale-New Haven Hospital, Conn.*

Copyright © 1978, American Journal of Nursing Company. Reproduced with permission from *American Journal of Nursing,* March, 1978, Vol. 78, No. 3.

Resources in Primary Nursing

Primary Nursing Development
1708 W. County Rd. F
Arden Hills, Minnesota 55112

Established in 1973 by Karen Ciske, R.N., M.S., Primary Nursing Development is "an independent consultation service" in primary nursing. Ms. Ciske is a clinical specialist, consultant, educator and researcher and author of several articles on primary nursing. She travels across the country to conduct workshops and conferences in primary nursing and to help nursing departments institute primary nursing, and evaluate it once it is in effect.

Nursing administrators, educators, and others interested in her service should contact Ms. Ciske at the above address. Each job she does is individualized to meet the specific needs of the hospital or agency.

Primary Nursing, One Nurse, One Client, Planning Care Together
Copyright 1977, National League For Nursing, Publ. No. 52-1695, Cost $4.95, National League for Nursing, 10 Columbus Circle, New York, N.Y. 10019.

This book is an excellent resource for information on primary nursing. Along with helpful articles on the subject there are also extensive bibliographies for further readings.

Primary Care, a quarterly publication available from W. B. Saunders Co. (Cost: $21.00/year).

The Nurse Practitioner
The American Journal of Primary Health Care
Health Sciences Media and Research Services, Inc.
3845 42nd Ave., N.E.
Seattle. WA 98105

This is a bimonthly journal of special interest to nurse-practitioners in primary care. ($19.00/year in U.S., $20.50,

Nurse Faculty Fellowships

Vanderbilt University
Nashville, Tennessee 37240

The Nurse Faculty Fellowships in Primary Care is a program of the Robert Wood Johnson Foundation set up to run from 1977 through 1982, with 20 Fellows taking part each year. These Fellows are nursing faculty who are selected to become teachers of primary clinical care. The aim of the program is to further clinical primary care as a specialty in nursing education.

The program is administered by the School of Nursing, Vanderbilt University, but the Fellowships are offered at the following four nursing schools (each school takes five Fellows a year): University of Colorado, Denver; Indiana University, Indianapolis; University of Maryland, Baltimore; University of Rochester, Rochester, New York.

Write Vanderbilt University for eligibility requirements and further information.

14 Resources in Women's Health

Boston Women's Health Book Collective
Box 192
West Somerville, Mass. 02144

This collective consists of the 11 women who co-authored *Our Bodies, Ourselves* (Simon and Schuster, 1973, 1976, Spanish version now available) and *Ourselves And Our Children* (Random House, 1978). *Our Bodies, Ourselves* is a medically accurate book which provides information on women's health care, with an emphasis on preventing illness. It is a good resource for nurses and clients alike. *Ourselves And Our Children* follows the precedent setting style of the collective's earlier book, focusing on various aspects of parenthood. Along with authoring these two books, the Health Book Collective is very active in promoting good health care for women through many projects and other publications. It is a prime source for information on women and women's health issues.

Coalition For The Medical Rights Of Women
4079A 24th Street
San Francisco, Calif. 94114

The Coalition is a non-profit organization for consumers and providers of women's health care, fostering quality health care for women. Within the Coalition are committees on reproductive rights, sterilization abuse, DES action, occupational health and pap smears (working for better quality laboratories for reading pap smears). A bimonthly newsletter, the *Coalition News,* is available for $6 a year, and the Coalition publishes educational pamphlets. Membership is open to anyone who wants to support the Coalition and work towards its goals. ($10–$25 a year for individual membership and $25–$50 for organization membership.)

Healthright
Women's Health Forum
41 Union Square, Room 206-8
New York, N.Y. 10003

This is a non-profit organization for "women's health education and consumer advocacy." Publications include a quarterly newsletter, "Healthright," several pamphlets on women's health issues (including breast cancer, menopause, vaginal infections, abortions, etc.) and books on women's health care. Healthright also gives courses and provides speakers on women's health.

National Women's Health Network
Parklane Building
Suite 105
2025 I Street, N.W.
Washington, D.C. 20006

This is a non-profit organization devoted to dispersing information on a national level on women and health care issues. The Network publishes a bimonthly newsletter, "Network News," which contains up-to-date information including current legislation in Congress which directly affects women's health, reviews of books in this field, and listings of conferences of relevance to the reader. The Women's Health Network also publishes *Health Resource Guides,* booklets on menopause, childbirth, hysterectomy, breast cancer, family planning, DES, self-help, abortion and sterilization ($3 each for non-members, $2 for members). The Network conducts conferences and supplies information on local and national contacts for women's health issues. Regular membership is $25 a year with special rates for the unemployed or low-income members. Group or institutional membership is also available.

Type II Association
P. O. Box 14
North Sydney, N.S.W. 2060
Australia

This is an association for people with Herpes Simplex Virus Type II. It was formed to dispense information on this disease to lay people and the medical profession, to promote research into it, and to provide moral support to the victims of it.

Publications on Women's Health

Books

Corea, Gena, *The Hidden Malpractice,* subtitled, "How American Medicine Treats Women As Patients And Professionals." Chapters such as "How Women Have Been Barred From Healing," "How The Male Domination Of Medicine Affects The Health Care Women Receive," and "The Women's Health Movement," provide a self-explanatory description of this gripping and scholarly work. Recommended for all nurses. William Morrow and Company, Inc., New York, 1977.

Cowan, Belita, *Women's Health Care: Resources, Writings, Bibliographies.* Ms. Cowan has done an excellent job of compiling information on the health care of women. This resource book contains brief discussions of topics including women health care workers, self-help, childbirth, breast cancer, sexuality, rape, DES and others. Each discussion is followed by an extensive reading list. The last 12 pages consist of lists of "Recommended Publications and Films" and a "Directory of Organizations" in the women's health field. This useful resource book is of interest to women and men seeking a background in women and health care and to nurses involved in any aspect of the health care of women. It is a good resource to recommend to clients. From Anshen Publishing, 382 T Street, N.W., Washington, D.C. 20007, second printing, 1978. ($4 per copy, 20% discount for 10 or more copies.)

Ehrenreich, Barbara and English, Deirdre, *Complaints And Disorders, Nurses, Witches And Midwives,* and *For Her Own Good,* are three works by these feminist historians who give an excellent perspective on the subject of women as healers and women as "good patients." The Feminist Press, New York, 1971, 1973 and 1978.

Frankfort, Ellen, *Vaginal Politics,* Bantam Books, New York, 1973.

Gardiner, Shirley, and Torge, Janet, *A Book About Sexual Assault,* 1979, Montreal Health Press, Inc., P. O. Box 1000, Station G, Montreal, Quebec, H2W 2N1, Canada. This is a 48-page booklet on all aspects of rape. It is useful to nurses and clients alike. Copies are available for the cost of postage and handling.

Jameson, Dee Dee, and Schwalb, Roberta, *Every Woman's Guide To Hysterectomy, Taking Charge Of Your Own Body,* Prentice-Hall, 1978. A good resource for clients about to undergo hysterectomy.

Kleiber, Nancy and Light, Linda, *Caring For Ourselves: An Alternative Structure For Health Care,* a report on the Vancouver Women's Health Collective, 1978. The Vancouver Women's Health Collective is a feminist organization which provides health education and preventive care to women. This report is a description and evaluation of the structure and services of the organization.

The report deals extensively with the Collective's non-hierarchical structure, feminist politics and its emphasis on self-help and the participation of lay women in the delivery of care. The group's services—a health information phone line, community education program, women's self-help clinic, doctor directory, abortion counseling service, and diaphragm clinic—are all discussed in detail. The report also contains a discussion of theoretical and methodological issues which have arisen from the research. The report includes profiles of Collective members and of those who use the Collective's services. Evaluation focuses primarily on members' and clients' satisfaction with their participation in Collective activities.

The conclusions and recommendations drawn from this research experience are not limited to either a feminist or a health care context, but are applicable in a wide range of other organizational settings.

This report is available free from: School Of Nursing, University Of British Columbia, 2075 Wesbrook Place, Vancouver, B.C., Canada, V6T 1W5.

This material is reproduced with permission from the Vancouver Women's Health Collective; the research project was supported under National Health Research and Development Project 610-1020A of Health and Welfare, Canada.

Llwellyn-Jones, Derek, *Everywoman: A Gynecological Guide For Life,* Faber and Faber, 1978, second edition.

Rennie, Susan, and Grimstead, Kirsten, eds., *The New Woman's Survival Sourcebook,* Alfred A. Knopf, New York, 1975.

Seaman, Barbara, *Free And Female,* Fawcett Publications, Inc., 1972.

Seaman, Barbara, and Seaman, Gideon, *Women And The Crisis In Sex Hormones.* This is the first exposé of the hazards of ingesting oral contraceptives and/or synthetic estrogen at menopause. Nurses must be aware of the pharmacological effects of taking synthetic hormones. Viable alternatives are offered. Rawson Associates Publishers, Inc., New York, 1977.

The Diagram Group, *Woman's Body, An Owner's Manual,* a largely diagrammatic book for lay people on the "functions and changes" of a woman's body. Paddington Press, Ltd., 1977.

Pamphlets and Periodicals

Hysterectomy, by Susanne Morgan, a 20-page booklet, is an excellent resource for women having this surgery. Available for

$1 plus 25¢ postage from: Susanne Morgan, 2921 Walnut Ave., Manhattan Beach, Calif. 90266 or from Healthright (41 Union Square, Rm. 206-8, New York, N.Y. 10003).

Issues in Health Care Of Women, a journal published six times a year is directed at providers of health care to women. Each issue deals in depth with a single topic in this field. From McGraw-Hill Book Co. ($20 per year.)

Menopause And Aging, U.S. Department Of H.E.W., Publication No. (NIH) 73-319, available from the Department of H.E.W., National Institute Of Child Health And Human Development, 9000 Rockville Pike, Bethesda, Md. 20014.

"More Than A Choice," a 24-page pamphlet on women's right to choose whether to have children, by the Abortion Action Coalition, available from the New England Free Press, 60 Union Square, Somerville, Mass. 02143. ($1 per copy with bulk rates available.)

"Type Of Vaginitis," a wall-chart guide to differential diagnosis and treatment, is available from Ortho Pharmaceuticals.

"Urinary Tract Infection In The Adult Female," a series of two monographs by Allan R. Ronald, M.D., from Roche Laboratories.

"Women And Health," a booklet, available from the Council on Family Health, 633 Third Avenue, New York, N.Y. 10017.

Women And Health, a journal, The Haworth Press, 149 Fifth Avenue, New York, N.Y. 10010. ($20 a year for an individual subscription.)

"Women's Bill Of Health Rights," an all-inclusive bill of rights for women's health care, may be obtained from M. Monique Harriton, 2413 Ronda Vista Drive, Los Angeles, Calif. 90027.

Audiovisual Materials on Women's Health

"Women's Health: A Question Of Survival," a film which questions the health care given to women. McGraw-Hill Films.

"The Inner Woman Series" is a series of six films to educate women about their bodies and body images. McGraw-Hill Films.

"Healthcaring From Our End Of The Speculum," a film which helps women feel good about their bodies and teaches what they have a right to expect from the health care system. Includes a discussion guide. From Women Make Movies, Inc.

"Understanding Vaginal Hysterectomy" and "Understanding Abdominal Hysterectomy" are two sound filmstrips from Robert J. Brady Co.

"Breast Self-Examination: How To Do It," a sound filmstrip, from Robert J. Brady Co.

"Your Pelvic And Breast Examination" is a film to relieve the anxiety of these exams, recommended for women of high school age and older. Perennial Education, Inc.

"Common Sense, Self-Defense," a film discussing ways of avoiding danger and defending one's self when faced with it. American Educational Films.

"Rape Alert" and "Rape—The Right To Resist," two films on preventing the possibility of rape and ways of dealing with it when faced with threat of rape. From Aims Instructional Media, Inc.

"No Tears For Rachel," a film on the emotional and legal aspects of rape, contains interviews with two rape victims, one victim's psychiatrist and the other victim's husband. Also featured is a program in Denver where nurses provide assistance to rape victims. From University Of California Extension Media Center.

15 Resources in Male Health Care

An excellent resource in male health (and there are far too few to date) is *Medical Self-Care* Number 5, Copyright 1978 by *Medical Self-Care Magazine.* This issue deals with "Stress/Unstress" and includes "A Field Guide to Men's Reproductive Health." Books which are resources in the health care of men are listed and reviewed and a guide for male self-exam is included. The issue may be purchased for $2.50 from *Medical Self-Care,* P.O. Box 717, Inverness, CA 94937.

The Men's Reproductive Health Clinic

The Men's Clinic is a free general health clinic for men with an emphasis on reproductive health, contraception, and sexuality. It is operated by the San Francisco Department of Public Health. The Men's Clinic provides free physical check-ups, testing and treatment for sexually-transmitted infections, premarital blood tests, birth control counseling and methods, and sexual and relationship counseling. With a family physician and a staff of five counselors, it operates two evenings a week and provides services to about thirty-five men weekly. Now in its third year of operation, it is one of a small but growing number of men's health/family planning facilities. The Men's Clinic has prepared an information packet on its operations and health care perspectives. The packet includes a program brochure, medical history forms, a detailed fact sheet on the clinic's history and operation, a statistical summary of its patients, and funding suggestions for other health agencies interested in programs for men. The packet is available on request from the Men's Reproductive Health Clinic, Room 310, 1490 Mason Street, San Francisco, CA 94133; or call (415) 558-2544.

Reprinted with permission from Castleman, Michael, in *Medical Self-Care,* Number 5, © 1978, Medical Self-Care Magazine.

Audiovisual Materials on Men and Male Health

"A Man," a "film about men and mourning," discusses feelings about being a male, available from Michael Chait.

"To Ourselves, Our Sons, Our Fathers" discusses the male role in our society, available from Michael Chait.

"Counseling the Vasectomy Patient," "Vasectomy Operative Procedures," "The Prostate: A Patient's View," and "Self Examination of the Testes" are patient education films from Norwich-Eaton Pharmaceuticals.

"Vasectomy" is a film on this surgery with a discussion of feelings and fears regarding it. From Churchill Films.

16 Family Planning and Infertility

I. **Oral Contraceptives**

   Contraindications to Estrogen-Containing Pills
   Pill Side Effects

II. **Contraindications to IUD Insertion**

III. **Resources**

   Organizations
   Publications
   Audiovisual Aids

Oral Contraceptives

Listed below are some of the contraindications to Pill use. When considering use of the Pill for women with strong relative contraindications, it is extremely important to weigh the risks and benefits of the Pill. Moreover, alternatives to the Pill must be seriously considered by both clinician *and patient*. In settings where abortion is available as a backup, use of methods like foam, diaphragm, or progestin-only Pills (Mini-Pills) should be considered carefully, as any of these methods with early abortion is an extremely safe and effective approach to birth control.

CONTRAINDICATIONS TO ESTROGEN-CONTAINING BIRTH CONTROL PILLS

Absolute Contraindications:
1. Thromboembolic disorder (or history thereof)
2. Cerebrovascular accident (or history thereof)
3. Impaired liver function
4. Coronary artery disease (or history thereof)
5. Hepatic adenoma (or history thereof)
6. Malignancy of breast or reproductive system (or history thereof)
7. Pregnancy (known or suspected)

Strong Relative Contraindications:

8. Termination of term pregnancy within past 10-14 days
9. Severe vascular or migraine headaches
10. Hypertension with resting diastolic BP of 110 or greater
11. Diabetes, prediabetes, or a strong family history of diabetes
12. Gallbladder disease, including cholecystectomy (or history thereof)

Continued on next page

13. Previous cholestasis during pregnancy
14. Mononucleosis, acute phase
15. Sickle cell disease or sickle C disease
16. Undiagnosed, abnormal vaginal bleeding*
17. Elective surgery planned in next 4 weeks (e.g., hysterectomy, exploratory laparotomy, or elective orthopedic procedures)
18. Long-leg casts or major injury to lower leg
19. Over 35-40 (risk is even greater if obese, hypertensive, heavy smoker, diabetic, or if patient has high cholesterol levels)
20. Fibrocystic breast disease and breast fibroadenomas

Other Relative Contraindications:

A. May contraindicate initiation of Pills:

21. Failure to have established regular menstrual cycles
22. Cardiac or renal disease (or history thereof)
23. History of heavy smoking
24. Conditions likely to make patient unreliable at following Pill instructions, such as mental retardation, major psychiatric problems, history of alcoholism, history of repeatedly taking Pills incorrectly, or being a young teenager.
25. Lactation (oral contraceptives may be initiated as weaning begins and may be an aid in decreasing the flow of milk)
26. Patient with profile suggestive of anovulation and infertility problems: late onset of menses and very irregular, painless menses

B. May initiate Pills for women with these problems and observe very carefully for worsening (or improvement) of the problem:

27. Depression
28. Hypertension with resting diastolic BP of 90-100
29. Chloasma or hair loss related to pregnancy (or history thereof)
30. Asthma
31. Epilepsy
32. Uterine fibromyomata
33. Acne
34. Varicose veins
35. History of hepatitis but now normal liver function tests

---

*Several reviewers of this book strongly feel this should be listed as an absolute contraindication to Pill use. It remains here since we cannot in a simple, straightforward manner define "abnormal." The authors would definitely concur that if you, the clinician, feel that the patient's bleeding pattern is "abnormal," do *not* provide her with birth control pills.

Reprinted by permission from *Contraceptive Technology, 1978–1979*, 9th revised edition, Robert Hatcher, et al., Copyright 1978, Irvington Publishers Inc., New York.

Pill Side Effects: A Time Framework

Worse in First 3 Months	Over Time: Steady-Constant	Worse Over Time	Worse Post-Discontinuation
1. Nausea plus dizziness	1. Headaches during 3 weeks that Pills are being taken	1. Headaches during week Pills are not taken	1. [b] Infertility, amenorrhea; hypothalamic and endometrial suppression, and miscalculation of the expected date of confinement
2. Thrombophlebitis (venous) Leg veins [a] Pulmonary emboli [a] Pelvic vein thrombosis [a] Retinal vein thrombosis	2. [a] Arterial thromboembolic events, blurred, vision, stroke	2. Weight gain	2. One form of acne
3. Cyclic weight gain edema	3. Anxiety, fatigue, depression	3. Monilial vaginitis	3. Hair loss — alopecia
4. Breast fullness, tenderness	4. Thyroid function studies Elevated PBI Depressed T3 resin uptake	4. Periodic missed menses while on oral contraceptives	
5. Breakthrough bleeding	5. Susceptibility to amenorrhea post-Pill discontinuation	5. [a] Chloasma	
6. [a] Elevated serum lipid levels even to the extent of pancreatitis	6. Change in cervical secretions — mucorrhea	6. [a] Myocardial infarction	
7. [a] Abnormal glucose tolerance test	7. Decrease in libido	7. Spider angiomata	
8. Contact lenses fail to fit because of fluid retention	8. Autophonia, chronic dilatation of Eustachian tubes rather than cyclic opening and closing	8. Growth of myoma	
9. Abdominal cramping	9. Acne	9. Predisposition to gallbladder disease	
10. Suppression of lactation		10. Hirsutism	
11. Failure to understand correct use of oral contraceptives; pregnancy		11. Decreased menstrual flow	
		12. Small uterus, pelvic relaxation, cystocele, rectocele, atropic vaginitis	
		13. Cystic breast changes	
		14. Photodermatitis — sunlight sensitivity with hypo-pigmentation	
		15. One form of hair loss — alopecia	
		16. Hypertension	
		17. Focal hyperplasia of liver and hepatic adenomas	

[a] May be irreversible or produce permanent damage.
[b] N.B. To avoid this complication in many patients, advise women desiring to become pregnant to discontinue Pills 3-6 months prior to desired pregnancy.

Reprinted by permission from *Contraceptive Technology, 1978–1979*, 9th revised edition, Hatcher, Robert, et al., Copyright 1978, Irvington Publishers Inc., New York.

Pill Side Effects: Hormone Etiology

Estrogen Excess	Progestin Excess	Androgen Excess	Estrogen Deficiency	Progestin Deficiency
1. Nausea, dizziness	1. Increased appetite and weight gain (non-cyclic)	1. Increased appetite and weight gain	1. Irritability, nervousness	1. Late break-through bleeding
2. Edema and abdominal or leg pain with cyclic weight gain	2. Tiredness and fatigue and feeling weak	2. Hirsutism	2. Hot flushes	2. Heavy menstrual flow and clots
3. Leukorrhea	3. Depression and decrease in libido	3. Acne	3. Uterine prolapse	3. Delayed onset of menses following last Pill
4. Increase in leiomyoma size	4. Oily scalp, acne	4. Oily skin, rash	4. Early and midcycle spotting	
5. Chloasma	5. Loss of hair	5. Increased libido	5. Decreased amount of menstrual flow	
6. Uterine cramps	6. Cholestatic jaundice	6. Cholestic jaundice	6. No withdrawal bleeding	
7. Irritability	7. Decreased length of menstrual flow	7. Prueitis	7. Decreased libido	
8. Increase female fat disposition	8. Hypertension (?)		8. Diminished breast size	
9. Cervical exotrophia	9. Headaches between Pill packages		9. Dry vaginal mucosa and dyspareunia	
10. Contact lenses don't fit	10. Monilia vaginitis cervicitis		10. Headaches	
11. Telangiectasia	11. Increase in breast size (aleolar tissue)		11. Depression	
12. Vascular type headache	12. Breast tenderness without fluid retention			
13. Hypertension(?)	13. Decreased carbohydrate tolerance			
14. Lactation suppression				
15. Headaches while taking Pills				
16. Cystic breast changes				
17. Breast tenderness with fluid retention				
18. Thrombophlebitis				
20. Cerebrovascular accidents				
21. Hepatic adenoma				

Reprinted by permission from *Contraceptive Technology, 1978–1979,* 9th revised edition, Hatcher, Robert, et al., Copyright 1978, Irvington Publishers Inc., New York.

Contraindications to IUD Insertion

Absolute Contraindications:

    Active pelvic infection (acute or subacute)
    Pregnancy

Relative Contraindications:

Infectious Problems

Recurrent pelvic infection
Acute cervicitis
History of ectopic pregnancy
Valvular heart disease (potentially making patient susceptible to subacute bacterial endocarditis)
Single episode of pelvic infection if patient desires subsequent pregnancy
Abnormal Pap smear

Uterine Abnormalities:

Cervical stenosis
Small uterus (see Table 9)
Endometriosis
Endometrial polyps
Bicornuate uterus
Severe dysmenorrhea (may not contraindicate Progestasert T)

Prolonged or heavy menstrual bleeding
Abnormal uterine bleeding
Uterine myomata
Endometrial hyperplasia

Other:

    Known or suspected allergy to copper
    Anemia

Reprinted by permission from *Contraceptive Technology, 1978–1979*, 9th revised edition, Hatcher, Robert, et al., Copyright 1978, Irvington Publishers Inc., New York.

Resources in Family Planning and Infertility

(The) Alan Guttmacher Institute
515 Madison Avenue
New York, N.Y. 10022

This is an agency for "research, political analysis and public education" in the field of family planning. Publications available from the Institute include: *Family Planning Perspectives,* a bimonthly journal; *Family Planning/Population Reporter,* a bimonthly report on current laws and court decisions concerned with family planning; *Planned Parenthood-World Population Washington Memo,* an up-to-date news report published at least 20 times yearly on family planning and related concerns in Congress, the White House and government agencies; and directories of family planning and abortion providers and services.

Association For Voluntary Sterilization, Inc.
708 Third Avenue
New York, N.Y. 10017

This non-profit organization publishes educational pamphlets on sterilization in both English and Spanish. All are free for single copies with a small fee for bulk orders.

Emory University—Grady Memorial Hospital
Family Planning Program
80 Butler Street, S.E.
Atlanta, Ga. 30303

The Family Planning Program prints a variety of excellent materials for patient and staff education. Patient materials include *The Joy Of Birth Control, The View From Our Side* (a magazine for men on family planning and sexuality), *Your Monthly Cycle And Birth Control,* a wall chart, instruction booklets for each type of birth control, and a comprehensive course for teaching women about reproduction, sexuality and birth control which includes slides, literature and samples of contraceptive methods. Materials for health professionals include *Contraceptive Technology,* an excellent family planning training manual, *Nurses In Family Planning,* a 150-page manual, and posters on birth control pills and I.U.D.'s. Write for complete listing and current prices.

(The) Human Life And Natural Family Planning Foundation
1151 K Street, N.W.
Washington, D.C. 20005

This foundation has available an instructional series on natural family planning which includes booklets, flip-charts, and slides on "fertility awareness," "ovulation method" and "sympto-thermal method."

Planned Parenthood Federation Of America, Inc.
810 Seventh Avenue
New York, N.Y. 10019

Planned Parenthood provides family planning services, educational programs, and programs for infertility, pregnancy counseling, abortion and sterilization. It publishes several educational pamphlets on types of birth control (some available in Spanish), DES, sickle cell anemia, marriage and family life, mental health and family planning, sexuality; and materials for training family planning staff and for use in family planning clinics; a flip chart on the methods of contraception (in English and Spanish); and family planning posters and buttons.

(The) Population Council, Inc.
One Dag Hammarskjold Plaza
New York, N.Y. 10017

The Population Council publishes works on population issues, supports research into population and contraception, and awards grants and fellowships for professionals working in the area of population. One of its publications is a book entitled *Contraceptives And Common Sense: Conventional Methods Reconsidered* by Judith Bruce and S. Bruce Shearer, 1979. It is a book on the increased acceptance of barrier contraceptives (condom, diaphragm, etc.) and their value in light of the risks involved with oral contraceptives and I.U.D.'s.

Resolve, Inc.
P. O. Box 474
Belmont, Mass. 02178

Resolve is a non-profit organization offering "counseling, referral and support groups for infertility." There are several local affiliates throughout the country. It is an excellent resource for couples with infertility problems. Literature available from Resolve includes: *Infertility: A Guide For The Childless Couple,* a book by Barbara Eck Menning (Prentice-Hall, 1977), a list of infertility resources, and information on adoption, artificial insemination and fertility drugs, as well as the "Resolve Newsletter," published six times yearly.

Publications On Family Planning And Related Topics

A Book About Birth Control, 1979 by Donna Cherniak and Shirley Gardiner, a 48-page booklet published by the Montreal Health Press, Inc., is an invaluable resource for patient education. It contains information on sexuality and reproduction as well as current information on contraception. Any nurse involved in family planning is urged to obtain this book for her/his clients. Copies are available for a minimal fee (the cost of postage and handling) for free distribution to clients. The Montreal Health Press also publishes a *VD Handbook* with a similar format to the birth control book and two series of five posters each, one on "Female And Male Reproduction," and the other on "Birth Control Methods." All of these materials are informative, interesting, and outstanding in the field. To order write: Montreal Health Press, Inc., P. O. Box 1000, Station G., Montreal, Quebec H2W 2N1, Canada.

A Clinical Guide To The Intra-Uterine Device And The Vaginal Diaphragm by Shirley Okrent, R.N., C.N.M., revised 1976 ($3.50 per copy), and *A Clinical Guide to Oral Contraception*, Shirley Okrent, R.N., C.N.M., revised 1975 ($2.50 per copy), are both written especially for nurse-practitioners, nurse-midwives, educators and students. They are excellent resources on these topics (bulk rates are available). Order from: Mrs. Shirley Okrent, R.N., C.N.M., 1262 Daffodil Lane, Wantagh, N.Y. 11793.

Family Planning Resume, published semi-annually, is an international journal for professionals working in family planning ($12 a year). Available from: Community And Family Study Center, University Of Chicago, 1411 East 60th Street, Chicago, Ill. 60637

Ortho Pharmaceuticals has available many educational materials for nurses working in family planning, including a diagrammatic presentation of the "Procedure for fitting the vaginal diaphragm," "Classification of Oral Contraceptive Side Effects," a handy reference, and several pamphlets on the different methods of birth control for patient education.

Resources On Natural Birth Control: *

Nofziger, Margaret, *A Cooperative Method of Natural Birth Control,* The Book Publishing Co., 156 Drakes Lane, Summertown, TN, 38482, $2.95, paperback.

Kippley, John and Sheila Kippley, *The Art of Natural Family Planning,* the Couple to Couple League International, P.O. Box 11084, Cincinnati, OH, 45211, $4.95.

References In Infertility

Bierkens, P. B. "Childlessness From The Psychological Point Of View," in the Bulletin of Menninger Clinic, 39 (2): 177–82, March, 1975.

Behrman, S. J., Kistner, R. S., eds.: *Progress In Infertility.* Boston, Little Brown and Co., 1975.

Conception: A Matter Of Timing, a book on human reproduction and infertility by Reproduction Research Associates, 535 Riverside Ave., Westport, Conn. 06880. The book includes information on the Ovu-Guide, a hand-calculator which determines the days when conception is most likely to occur for an individual woman. ($2.95 plus 50¢ postage for the book and $29.95 plus $3.00 postage, handling and insurance for the Ovu-Guide.)

Denber, H. C. "Psychiatric Aspects Of Infertility" in *Journal Of Reproductive Medicine,* 20:1, 23–9, January, 1978.

Menning, Barbara Eck, "RESOLVE—A Support Group For Infertile Couples," *American Journal Of Nursing,* February, 1976, 258–59.

Menning, Barbara Eck, "The Infertile Couple: A Plea for Advocacy," in *Child Welfare,* June, 1975, 454–460.

Shane, J. M., Schiff, I., and Wilson, E. H., *The Infertile Couple,* Ciba Clinical Symposia: 28, Number 5, 1976.

Taymor, M. L., *Infertility,* New York, Grune and Stratton, 1978.

Audiovisual Materials On Family Planning

"Family Planning: Children By Choice: a film describing

* *This material is adapted from* New Roots for the Northeast, *Nov./Dec., 1979,* © *1979, the Northeast Appropriate Technology Network, Inc., Box 548, Greenfield, Ma., 01302.*

methods of family planning and questions to ask one's self in deciding whether or not to have a child. American Educational Films.

"Planned Families," "Freedom From Pregnancy," and "Unwanted Pregnancy" are all for patient education on birth control methods, from Allend 'Or Productions.

"Contraception: Yesterday And Today," a patient education film, from Norwich-Eaton Pharmaceuticals.

"The Ins And Outs Of The Diaphragm," a film showing the types of diaphragms and how they work, from Perennial Education, Inc.

"Birth Control: The Choices," a film for patient education from Churchill Films.

"Methods Of Family Planning," an educational film from Paramount Communications.

"Happy Family Planning," an animated film, and "Margaret Sanger," a film biography of this birth control pioneer, both available from Planned Parenthood Of America Federation Film Library.

17 Resources in Sexuality

**American Association Of Sex Educators,
Counselors And Therapists (AASECT)**
5010 Wisconsin Avenue, N.W.
Suite 304
Washington, D.C. 20016

This is a non-profit, professional interdisciplinary organization for sex educators, counselors and therapists. AASECT certifies sex educators and therapists and functions in the areas of "training, education and research." Publications include a quarterly "Newsletter," the *Journal Of Sex Education And Therapy*, published semiannually ($6 a year), pamphlets on training sex educators and counselors, a bibliography of audiovisual materials for sex education, the *National Register (of) Certified Health Service Providers In Sex Education And Sex Therapy*, and reprints on sexuality, sex education and counseling.

National Sex Forum

The National Sex Forum sponsors two one-week-long programs annually on sexual attitude restructuring (SAR). These sessions include information and discussion on bisexuality, birth control, sex counseling with adolescents, transexualism and transvestism, incest and sexuality and its relation to the disabled. Among those who have found SAR of great value have been physicians, psychologists, psychiatrists, therapists, counselors, nurses, clergy, social workers, health educators, paraprofessionals and students in all the above areas. For further detailed information about these seminars write to:

National Sex Forum
1523 Franklin Street
San Francisco, California 94109

Reprinted from *National Resource Directory, 1979*, published by the National Spinal Cord Injury Foundation.

Sex Information And Education Council
Of The U.S. (SIECUS)
84 Fifth Avenue, Suite 407
New York, N.Y. 10011

SIECUS is a non-profit organization which serves as a resource center and provides educational materials for professionals and lay people on sexuality and sex education. Publications include: *Siecus Report,* a bimonthly publication on human sexuality; "Siecus Study Guides" on several topics (sex education, homosexuality, masturbation, sexual responses, etc.); *A Resource Guide In Sex Education For The Mentally Handicapped; Film Resources For Sex Education;* and other books on human sexuality. These publications may be ordered directly from the Human Sciences Press (see address under list of Publishers). For complete catalog of publications write SIECUS.

References On Human Sexuality And Sexual Counseling

Comfort, Alex, *The Joy Of Sex,* Crown Publishers, New York, 1972.

Comfort, Alex, *More Joy Of Sex,* Crown Publishers, New York, 1974.

Elder, Mary Scovill, "The Unmet Challenge . . . Nurse Counseling on Sexuality," *Nursing Outlook,* Vol. 18, No. 11 (Nov. 1970), p. 38–40.

Katchadourian and Lunde, *Fundamentals Of Human Sexuality,* Holt, Rinehart and Winston, Inc., New York, 1972.

Masters and Johnson, *Human Sexual Behavior,* Little Brown and Co., Boston, 1966.

Masters and Johnson, *Human Sexual Inadequacy,* Little Brown and Co., Boston, 1970.

McCary, James Leslie, *Human Sexuality,* Second edition, Van Nostrand Reinhold Co., New York, 1973.

Woods, Nancy Fugate, *Human Sexuality In Health And Illness,* Second edition, The C. V. Mosby Co., St. Louis, 1979.

Audiovisual Materials On Sexuality, Sex Education And Sexual Counseling

"Free," "Rich And Judy," "Sun Brushed" and "Unfolding" are films commissioned by the National Sex Forum. All are meant for educational purposes either for professionals or for use in sex therapy and all portray heterosexual activities including intercourse and oral sex. Multi Media Resource Center.

A series of patient education films on sex education and sex therapy is available from Professional Research, Inc.

"Human Sexuality And Nursing Practice," a series of eight filmstrips and sound cassettes on various aspects of sexuality, intended to help nurses to better interact with patients on these topics. From Concept Media.

A series of sex education sound filmstrips for elementary and junior high students is available from Perennial Education, Inc.

Tapes of sessions from the Annual Meeting of the National Sex Institute, covering a wide range of topics on sexuality, are available from the American Association Of Sex Educators, Counselors and Therapists.

"The Homosexuals" is a film from Carousel Films.

Films on homosexuality, sex education and sex therapy are available from Multi Media Resource Center.

"Human Sexual Disorders: Development, Diagnosis and Treatment" is a series of six cassette tapes from a conference at the College Of Physicians And Surgeons, Columbia University. Available from Communication Enterprises, Inc.

18 Nursing Records

What Is a Problem-Oriented Health Care Record?

The chief ingredient of a problem-oriented record is common sense. Therefore, it is within reach of any member of the health care team. Problem-oriented thinking leads to the reorganization of clinical records along lines first suggested by Dr. L. L. Weed. Used well, the system can facilitate smoother continuity of care, more efficient storage and retrieval of information, more effective audit and review.

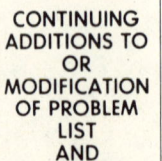

```
   DATA
   BASE
     ↓
  PROBLEM
   LIST
     ↓
   PLANS
     ↓
  PROGRESS
   NOTES
     ↓
 CONTINUING
 ADDITIONS TO
      OR
  MODIFICATION
  OF PROBLEM
     LIST
      AND
     PLANS
```

A problem-oriented record begins with information about the patient. Preferably, this is gathered systematically in a standardized way. It has been called the **data base**. From this a **problem list** is derived. All of the patient's significant problems are on the list, not just the "chief complaint" or "diagnosis." The problem list may change or grow as new data become available. Problems are numbered as they are identified, for easy reference. The problem list is the first page of the patient's record, or it is placed prominently where it can be referred to easily.

Information in the body of the record relates to one problem or another. **Progress notes** record current:

Subjective data:	complaints or statements of patient, family.
Objective data:	things actually observed or done by the provider; results of special studies, etc.
Assessment of the situation:	by the provider. Some prefer to use the marginal heading *Discussion* or *Impression*.
Care given:	Nurses and therapists find this a useful category.
Plans in relation to the above:	for further definition of the problem for patient care and treatment, for patient and family education.

This form of entry can be used by any provider, nurse, physician, therapist, social worker. Effectiveness is increased when providers in an organized setting can agree that all such entries should be made in one body of progress notes, not in separate parts of the chart.

When patients are discharged or transferred, problem-oriented summaries and referrals from one provider to another contribute to real continuity of care.

Most paper forms presently in use can continue to be used or can be adapted to accommodate problem-oriented thinking.

Reprinted with permission from *The Surgical Patient, behavioral concepts for the operating room nurse,* 2nd edition, Gruendemann, Barbara, Casterton, Shirley, Hesterly, Sandra, Minckley, Barbara, and Shetler, Mary, Copyright 1979, St. Louis, The C. V. Mosby Co.

SOAP

> **SOAP** notes are the written communication tool of the problem-oriented record. The components include:
>
> **S:** Subjective data consist of verbal information from client and significant others which may or may not be congruent with objective data.
>
> **O:** Objective data consist of information obtained about the client through observation or measurement. They include nonverbal behavior, laboratory data, and other measurements such as vital signs, height, and weight.
>
> **A:** Assessment is an analysis of the subjective and objective data and includes (*a*) rationale for problems, (*b*) the effect of medication and nursing intervention, (*c*) progress, and (*d*) prognosis.
>
> **P:** Plan of action includes specific plans for gathering further data and implementing diagnostic studies, treatment approaches, and client/family education.

Reprinted with permission from *Comprehensive Psychiatric Nursing*, Haber, et al., Copyright 1978, McGraw-Hill Book Co.

A Systematic Approach to the Nursing Care Plan
Marlene Glover Mayers
Second Edition, Copyright 1978, Appleton-Century-Crofts

This paperback book discusses in detail the purposes of care plans and how to formulate them. Sample care plans for different disease entities and clinical settings are included as well as information on the practical use of care plans and the evaluation of their effectiveness.

Resources on Nursing Records

Milcom Patient Care Systems
A Division Of Miller Communications, Inc.
322 Westport Avenue
Norwalk, Conn. 06856

Milcom offers a number of health care questionnaires for record keeping: a general health history questionnaire, and other specialized questionnaires such as occupational health, pediatrics (including a Spanish version), cardiovascular, gastrointestinal, OB/Gyn, and respiratory. Other products offered include medical record jackets, progress notes, treatment records, and chronic disease records.

19 Nursing Innovations

*Analysis and Planning for Improved Distribution of
Nursing Personnel and Services:
Inventory of Innovations in Nursing*
Edited by Sheila Kodadek, R.N.
Western Interstate Commission For Higher Education
(WICHE), 1976
DHEW Publication No. (HRA) 77-2
U.S. Department of HEW
Health Resources Administration
Division of Nursing
Bethesda, Maryland 20014

A valuable resource on current trends in nursing practice, this report is based on a study conducted by WICHE to evaluate existing utilization of nursing personnel and to plan for equitable distribution of personnel and services. The following excerpts from the Introduction of the book aptly describe its contents:

> The *Inventory* contains 159 descriptions of new and emerging roles, methods, practice sites, and payment mechanisms in nursing. The examples include both nursing practice and educational programs that prepare nurses for new roles and settings. They were collected as the result of a nationwide search.
>
> The *Inventory* examples include innovations in nursing roles—clinical nursing specialists, educators, patient/client advocates, administrators, and researchers. Such nurses are active in all settings, creating environments to allow the practice of professional nursing as they define it. Nurses in physicians' offices are providing health care that supplements medical care, rather than echoing it. Nurses in hospitals and in the community are in the vanguard of new approaches to caring for the terminally ill. Nurses in nursing-care homes, senior citizens' centers, and low-income housing complexes are providing care to the elderly to help them maintain their health and often their independence.

The *Inventory* is by no means an exhaustive catalogue of nursing innovations in the United States. But it will serve its purpose if it stimulates others to pursue new, more effective ways of making the American health-care system responsive to and supportive of nursing initiative.

This book is useful to all nurses interested in learning about current innovations in nursing and particularly "to nurse planners, administrators, and educators" involved in "meeting our Nation's nursing needs."

Leadership for Change:
A Guide for the Frustrated Nurse
Dorothy Brooten, Laura Hayman and Mary Naylor
Copyright 1978, J. B. Lippincott Company

This book discusses nursing leaders, both past and contemporary, and the ways in which they effected change. Emphasis is placed on the importance of group efforts in bringing about change. The authors point out areas in health care delivery where change is needed and realistic means of effecting this change. The book is thought provoking and a must for any nurse who has ever been frustrated by the resistance met when trying to change attitudes and policies on nursing care practices.

Audiovisual Materials on Nurses and Nursing

"The Involved Ones" is a film portraying nurses as dedicated and involved in community health issues, from Association-Sterling Films, Inc.

"Men In Nursing," "The Sign of Success" and "Why Stand Alone" are films and slide shows available from the National Male Nurse Association.

"Nursing: The Politics of Caring" is an extraordinary documentary film on the modern nurse from Ilex Films.

20 Transcultural Nursing

Challenges of Cross-Cultural Encounters

When working with individuals of another culture, the nurse is challenged to achieve the following objectives:

1. She must understand how the individuals perceive their health situation in terms of what they identify as health care needs and services desired.

2. She must appreciate cultural norms which influence communication patterns between the nurse and the individual or family.

3. She must implement nursing approaches to effect desired changes in health practices in a manner congruent with the cultural life style.

In addition to assessing the other person's cultural patterns, the nurse must realize that she brings her own cultural heritage to an interaction.

Thus it is essential that nurses recognize and assess their own cultural biases. The cultural impact on communication patterns cannot be treated lightly. It is the foundation upon which the nursing process develops from assessment, through implementing actions, to evaluation of the care delivered.

The nurse needs to understand that cultural groups will do what they feel works best or what brings them pleasure and success in daily living. For example, members of a particular culture may bind a newborn's umbilical cord and place oils or other substances on the area in the belief that this will promote healing. They will continue this practice until the nurses can prove to them that an alternative can also be successful. Proof is demanded in the form of a living example of a healthy infant whose umbilical area was exposed to air instead of being bound and treated with oils. All the nurse's explanations and pictures of infections will have no impact on the culture because these words and pictures are not an integral part of their process of daily living. Effecting change of a cultural pattern is a process that demands patience and perseverance. The desired changes may be manifested much later (e.g., in another generation's childbearing practices). The process is also time consuming because nursing actions must always reinforce cultural values rather than ridicule or label them as wrong. It is well to remember that one's culture serves to safeguard one's physical, emotional, and social health. Thus it is unrealistic to expect a person or a society to discard a cultural pattern until it can be replaced with a better one.

Reprinted by permission of F. A. Davis Co. from *Childbearing: A Nursing Perspective,* 2nd edition by Ann Clark and Dyanne Affonso, with Thomas Harris, © 1979 by F. A. Davis Co., Philadelphia.

Education in Transcultural Nursing

Formal education is now available in the expanding field of transcultural nursing, training nurses to work with people from varying cultural backgrounds. The University of Utah offers a doctoral program in this field and masters degree programs are offered at the University of Washington and Pennsylvania State University. Dr. Madeleine Leininger, dean at the University of Utah, is president of the Transcultural Nursing Society. For further information on the Society and educational programs in this field, contact her at the University of Utah, Department of Nursing, Salt Lake City, Utah.

This material is adapted from the *American Journal of Nursing,* January, 1980, Vol. 80, No. 1, p. 128–130.

The Nursing Clinics of North America, March, 1977, Vol. 12, No. 1, W. B. Saunders Co., is an excellent source for information on Transcultural Nursing. It contains information on cultural diversity and implications for health care and describes important cultural traits of several minority groups. Also included is an extensive bibliography on transcultural nursing.

21 Nursing Education

I. **Continuing Education**
II. **Special Education Programs for Nurses**
III. **Internships**
IV. **Doctoral Programs**
V. **Resources in Nursing Education**

Status of mandatory continuing education: States requiring mandatory continuing education (MCE) for R.N. relicensure and the dates by which R.N.s in those states must have completed a specified number of continuing education hours are:

California—July 1978

Colorado—1980

Florida—1980

Kansas—1978

Minnesota—1980 (probably)

In South Dakota and Louisiana, the state boards of nursing already have the legislative authority needed to mandate continuing education for R.N. relicensure.

In Connecticut, Illinois, Iowa, Massachusetts, New York, Pennsylvania (probably), and Texas, the state nurses' associations are planning to propose MCE legislation in the next few years.

Even if your state has not yet developed an MCE program, there's a good chance it will in the near future.

You will have to check with each particular state board in which continuing education is mandatory to find out the number of hours required for relicensure, because the requirements vary considerably.

Reprinted with permission of RN Magazine from *1979 Nursing Opportunities,* page 13, Copyright 1979, Litton Industries, Medical Economics Company, Oradell, N.J.

Continuing Education

One prime source of continuing education which is often overlooked—the colleagues we work with everyday—is pointed out by Gena Corea in *The Hidden Malpractice:*

"When she was a head nurse in a California hospital, (Kathleen) Mc Inerney arranged for aides, R.N.s and L.P.N.s to take turns giving seminars to each other. Each one had special talents and shared them with the others. Morale increased, she said, and workers requested transfers to her floor.

" 'We must begin to relate as peers and draw the best out of each other' she said. 'We need to learn from and support each other.' "

Reprinted with permission of William Morrow and Company, Inc. from *The Hidden Malpractice*, Gena Corea, Copyright 1977, William Morrow and Co., Inc.

An Example of Continuing Education in Practice

To provide continuing education for physicians and nurses in the use and interpretation of fetal monitoring equipment, Vanderbilt University established a program for hospitals throughout the state of Tennessee. The medical center provided a nurse trained in fetal monitoring to visit the hospitals to conduct workshops for the obstetrical personnel. She is available to return to the hospitals at various intervals, depending on their need, to provide further education for the staff.

Vanderbilt also conducts seminars in its own facilities on obstetrical topics. These seminars are open to personnel from the surrounding hospitals.

This is an example of how one medical center can share its knowledge and expertise with outlying health care facilities, a very important consideration in light of the trend toward increased regionalization.

Source: Haire, Mary, and Boehm, Frank, "A Statewide Program to Teach Nurses the Use of Fetal Monitors," *JOGN*, Vol. 7, No. 3, May/June, 1978.

Resources in Continuing Education

American Journal of Nursing
Educational Testing Service
Box 2842
Princeton, N.J. 08540

Nurses required to obtain a certain number of continuing education credits and others who simply wish to, may do so through home study of material published in the *American Journal of Nursing*. Periodically *AJN* publishes study guides for continuing education on various topics (past topics include, "The Person With a Spinal Cord Injury," "Congenital Cardiac Defects," "BCG in Cancer Therapy," and others). Nurses wishing to obtain continuing education units for studying these materials must send a registration fee (about $10.00) to the above address to obtain a test booklet and answer card. Consult current issues of *AJN* or write American Journal of Nursing Company for a listing of materials available for continuing education credits. (This material is adapted from *AJN*, September, 1978, "Continuing Education Through Home Study").

Health Education Seminars
P. O. Box 14472
San Francisco, CA 94114

Finding courses in continuing education which are directly relevant to the type of nursing one is doing is difficult and expensive. The Health Education Seminars offer an alternative in the San Francisco area to registered nurses and licensed practical/vocational nurses with state approved courses, which are somewhat unusual, taught by professionals. For example, courses offered include "The Value of Fasting," "Touch for Health," "Healing Herbs," and "Nursing and Wholistic Health: An Overview."

Nancy D. Sanford, R.N., M.S.
6246 Jackie Ave.
Woodland Hills, CA 91367
Phone: 213-992-7792

Nancy D. Sanford, R.N., M.S., is an independent nursing educator practicing in the state of California. She has excellent credentials in nursing education as well as in speaking and publishing.

Ms. Sanford's practice provides continuing education courses for nurses which are approved for six continuing education credit hours by the California Board of Registered Nursing. The courses are for a minimum of 15 nurses or allied health workers and are given on the premises of the hospital or agency requesting her services. The courses include a variety of topics covering practical aspects of nursing care as well as such topics as "Anxiety and Stress Reduction For Nursing Staff" and "Assertiveness Training."

To date Ms. Sanford has traveled mainly in California giving the continuing education courses but she is available for workshops in other states. For further information or to arrange for a workshop, contact Ms. Sanford at the above address.

Publications on Continuing Education

Nursing 78, Career Guide, "Mandatory Continuing Education: How Will it Affect You?", by Gloria Hochman and *Nursing 78,* in *Nursing 78,* November, 1978. This is a good overview of mandatory CE and what it means to nurses.

The American Nurses' Association has available three pamphlets on continuing education: "Continuing Education in Nursing, Guidelines for Staff Development," "Self-Directed Continuing Education in Nursing," and "Guidelines for Continuing Education in Developmental Disabilities."

"Why CEU?", "A Dialogue on Continuing Education," a pamphlet for practical/vocational nurses from the Education Department, National Federation of Licensed Practical Nurses (see address under "Nursing Organizations).

A Refresher Course for Registered Nurses
A Guide For Instructors and Students
DHEW Publication No. (HRA) 74-35, 1974, $3.20
Available from U.S. Government Printing Office
Superintendent of Documents
Washington, D.C. 20402

This is a refresher course for inactive registered nurses developed by the Arizona State Nurses' Association under a grant from the U.S. Public Health Service. It is a modular program using self instruction and individualized teaching.

Covering the basics in nursing care as well as recent innovations, it is meant to prepare a nurse for entering an orientation program in a hospital or agency. The course cannot be used without an instructor and a clinical setting must be available for practical experience.

Special Education Programs for Nurses: Career Mobility

The Edna McConnell Clark School of Nursing
of the Presbyterian Hospital
in the City of New York
179 Fort Washington Ave.
New York, N.Y. 10032

The Presbyterian Hospital offers a program whereby licensed practical nurses with at least one year's experience, may obtain an Associate Degree in nursing and be eligible to take the registered nurse licensure exam. The program consists of one fall, spring and summer semester and runs from September through June. Interested L.P.N.'s should write the above address for further information.

ACT Proficiency Examination Program (PEP)
P. O. Box 168
Iowa City, IA 52240

The American College Testing Program (ACT) administers proficiency examinations in nursing and other fields. Several colleges and universities grant college credit to individuals passing these exams. They are useful to L.P.N.'s and diploma school R.N.'s seeking credit for their previous education and experience. For information on the tests offered and the schools which grant credit for them, write the above address.

Directory of Career Mobility Programs in Nursing Education, National League for Nursing, New York, 1975, Pub. No. 19-1605.

This directory is useful to nurses and nursing students and teachers and counselors in nursing. It lists and describes schools and universities which give credit toward a nursing degree for previous education and experience. For example, L.P.N.'s seeking schools which will give them credit towards an R.N. degree or nurses with a diploma seeking credit towards a B.S. degree, will find schools which meet their needs listed here.

St. Joseph's College
North Windham, Maine
External Degree Center
107 Campbell Ave., S.W.
Roanoke, Virginia 24034

St. Joseph's College offers an "External Degree Program" (EDP) for registered nurses through which they can obtain a "Bachelor of Science in Professional Arts" by independent study with a modular system. The students in this external degree program study from their own locations throughout the country except for a three-week summer session on the College campus. For the College Bulletin describing the program in detail, write the External Degree Center at the above address.

Role Transformation Program For New Graduates
University of California at San Francisco
San Francisco, California

Background: A recent study found that one-third of the nurses that graduated and went to work in hospitals left nursing practice within four years. A large proportion of nurses also resolved the school-work conflict in ways that were considered unhealthy for the nurse and for nursing as a profession. A Role Transformation Program was established to equip nurses with the necessary skills to constructively resolve the professional-bureaucratic conflict between school and work.

Purpose: The program is expected (1) to decrease "reality shock" and equip nurses with the skill to resolve conflicts in a way that maintains their professional values, (2) to increase the tenure of the new staff nurse in her first job, thus decreasing turnover rate in hospitals, (3) to decrease the flight of nurses from nursing practice, and (4) to seed the system with bicultural nurses that may assist new nurses to put into practice the new ideas and concepts of nursing care.

The target population consists of graduates of nursing programs (within one year of graduation) who are in their first RN job experience and their respective head nurses. This research project involves eight medical centers throughout the country. The investigator is focusing on hospital nurses only, but believes that this has relevance for all practice situations.

Nursing Role: All the nurses involved are either in their first job experience or are head nurses in an inpatient (hospital) care setting.

Cost: Cost data have not been collected and analyzed to date. It is expected that the program will decrease the turnover rate and therefore decrease hospitals' cost to orient new staff nurses. This also will be dependent upon the cost to an institution to provide the Role Transformation Program.

Contact for Further Information:
Marlene Kramer, RN, Ph.D.
Professor of Nursing
University of California at San Francisco
School of Nursing N-631A
San Francisco, California 94143

Reprinted from *Analysis and Planning for Improved Distribution of Nursing Personnel and Services,* Sheila Kodadek, Ed., 1976, Division of Nursing, Health Resources Administration, U.S. Department of H.E.W.

Internship Programs

University of Florida School of Nursing
Gainesville, Florida

The University's School of Nursing, in conjunction with the Gainesville Veterans Administration, offers a 9-month long nursing internship program in which the intern receives post graduate credits which can be applied towards a master's degree. (Source: Carol J. Strauser, "An Internship With Academic Credit," in *AJN,* June, 1979.)

Hotel Dieu Hospital
2021 Perdido St.
P. O. Box 61262
New Orleans, LA 70161

The Hotel Dieu Hospital offers an internship program to help new graduates make the transition from student to practitioner. For further information write Brenda Washburn, Employment Manager, at the above address.

Doctoral Programs

Doctoral Programs in Nursing, 1979–80, © 1979 by the National League for Nursing. Pub. No. 15-1448. This booklet lists 21 institutions with doctoral programs in nursing, their addresses and types of programs offered. It also includes information on predoctoral and postdoctoral traineeships. NLN also has information on master's programs in nursing as well as all levels of undergraduate programs.

Summer Program of Doctoral Study at U-T, Austin, Texas

A summer doctoral program, intended for nurses holding faculty positions who can leave their jobs only during summer and for one academic year, is being offered by the University of Texas at Austin, School of Nursing.

Students will attend school for four summers and one academic year. Areas of study include adult health, psychiatric-mental health, maternal-child nursing, and research.

Write: Billye J. Brown, R.N., Dean, School of Nursing, University of Texas at Austin, 1700 Red River, Austin, Tex. 78701.

Reprinted from *American Journal of Nursing,* October, 1979, Vol. 79, No. 10, p. 1673, © 1979, The American Journal of Nursing Company.

Resources in Nursing Education

The Western Council on Higher Education for Nursing (WCHEN)
P. O. Drawer P
Boulder, CO 80302

WCHEN is a division of the Western Interstate Commission for Higher Education. Its functions include upgrading the status of nursing education in the thirteen participating Western states and promoting research into nursing education needs in the West. WCHEN has available many valuable publications of interest to nurse educators in the West and elsewhere.

Resource Guides for Preparing for Nurse Licensure Exams

The following books are review guides for students preparing for state boards and licensing exams for registered nurses and practical nurses:

How to Prepare for the Practical Nurse Licensing Exam, Hattie L. Allen and Vashti R. Curlin, © 1979, Barron's Educational Series, Inc., 113 Crossways Park Dr., Woodbury, N.Y. 11797 ($5.95).

Nursing Comprehensive Examination Review by George Horemis and Clemencia Matamors, 2nd Edition, © 1976, Arco Publishing Company, 219 Park Ave., South, New York, N.Y. 10003 ($5.00).

Nurse: Registered Nurse. Practical Nurse. Public Health Nurse, by David Turner, © 1975, Arco Publishing Co. (A Study Guide, $6.00).

Nursing Examination, Review in Basic Sciences, by George Horemis and Clemencia Matamors, © 1973, Arco Publishing Co.

Practical Nursing Review, by Sr. Mary Redempta Grawunder, © 1976, Arco Publishing Co. ($6.00).

Periodicals on Nursing Education

The Journal of Continuing Education in Nursing, from Charles B. Slack, Inc. This bi-monthly publication contains excellent articles on continuing education, information on current programs in this field, workshops and job openings. (Cost: $20.00/year, U.S., $24.00/year, Foreign.)

Journal of Nursing Education, from Charles B. Slack, Inc. This journal is published nine months/year and contains articles of interest to nurse educators.

Nurse Educator, from Concept Development, Inc. This bi-monthly journal is for all levels of nurse-educators. (Cost: $12.00/year, U.S., $15.00, Foreign.)

References on Scholarships and Grants for Nursing Education

"Scholarships And Loans For Beginning Education In Nursing," NLN Pub. No. 41-410, is available from the National League for Nursing.

"Scholarships, Fellowships, Educational Grants, and Loans For Registered Nurses," NLN Pub. No. 41-408, also is available from the National League For Nursing.

The Nurses Almanac, Howard S. Rowland, Aspen Press, 1978, page 189–202. This chapter contains helpful information on seeking funds, including sources for grants and loans.

22 Nursing Research

Regional Medical Libraries

Regions	Regional Medical Library
#1 New England	New England Regional Medical Library Service Francis A. Countway Library of Medicine 10 Shattuck Street, Boston, Ma. 02115 Tel: 617-732-2128; TWX: 710-338-6702 **(for: Connecticut, Maine, Massachusetts, New Hampshire, Rhode Island, Vermont)**
#2 New York & New Jersey	New York & New Jersey Regional Medical Library New York Academy of Medicine Library 2 East 103 Street, New York, N.Y. 10029 Tel: 212-876-8763; TWX: 710-581-6131 **(for: New Jersey, New York)**
#3 Mideastern	Mid-Eastern Regional Medical Library Service Library of the College of Physicians 19 South 22 Street, Philadelphia, Pa. 19103 Tel: 215-561-6050; TWX: 710-670-1646 **(for: Delaware, Pennsylvania)**
#4 Midatlantic	Mid-Atlantic Regional Medical Library National Library of Medicine 8600 Rockville Pike, Bethesda, Md. 20014 Tel: 301-496-5955; TWX: 710-824-9615 **(for: Maryland, North Carolina, Virginia, Washington, D.C., West Virginia)**
#5 East Central	Kentucky-Ohio-Michigan Regional Medical Library Program Shiffman Medical Library, Wayne State University 4325 Brush Street, Detroit, Mi. 48201 Tel: 313-577-1101 TWX: 810-221-5163 **(for: Kentucky, Michigan, Ohio)**
#6 Southeastern	Southeastern Regional Medical Library Program A.W. Calhoun Medical Library Emory University Atlanta, Ga. 30322 Tel: 404-329-5818; TWX: 810-751-8512 **(for: Alabama, Florida, Georgia, Mississippi, Puerto Rico, South Carolina, Tennessee)**
#7 Midwest	Midwest Health Science Library Network John Crerar Library 33 West 33 Street, Chicago, Ill. 60616 Tel: 312-225-2526 (x78); TWX: 910-221-5131 **(for: Illinois, Indiana, Iowa, Minnesota, North Dakota, Wisconsin)**

Continued on next page

#8 Midcontinental	Midcontinental Regional Medical Library Program Library of Medicine University of Nebraska Medical Center 42nd Street and Dewey Avenue, Omaha, Neb. 68105 Tel: 402-541-4646; TWX: 910-611-8353 **(for: Colorado, Kansas, Missouri, Nebraska, South Dakota, Utah, Wyoming)**
#9 South Central	South Central Regional Medical Library Program University of Texas Health Science Center 5323 Harry Hines Boulevard, Dallas, Tex. 75235 Tel: 214-688-2627; TWX: 910-861-4946 **(for: Arkansas, Louisiana, New Mexico, Oklahoma, Texas)**
#10 Pacific Northwest	Pacific Northwest Regional Health Sciences Library University of Washington Health Sciences Library Seattle, Wash. 98195 Tel: 206-543-8262; TWX: 910-444-1385 **(for: Alaska, Idaho, Montana, Oregon, Washington)**
#11 Pacific Southwest	Pacific Southwest Regional Medical Library Service Biomed Library, Center for the Health Sciences University of California, Los Angeles, Calif. 90024 Tel: 213-825-1200; TWX: 910-342-6897 **(for: Arizona, California, Hawaii, Nevada)**

Copyright 1978, American Journal of Nursing Company. Reprinted with permission from *MCN, The American Journal of Maternal Child Nursing*, September/October, Vol. 3, No. 5.

Resources in Nursing Research

American Nurses' Association Council Of Nurse Researchers
Department Of Research, Grants and Contracts
2420 Pershing Road
Kansas City, No. 64108

The Council of Nurse Researchers is a subdivision of the American Nurses' Association for members of the A.N.A. who have a master's degree or higher and who are involved in nursing research either directly or as consultants or teachers. Members receive the *CNR Newsletter* and the council holds meetings during the year to share research findings. The Council promotes research activities and provides information on funding sources for nursing research.

Division Of Research Resources
National Institutes Of Health
Bethesda, Md. 20014

This division of the NIH provides support and funding for medical research projects. It administers the General Clinical Research Centers Program which consists of 80 centers in hospitals and universities throughout the country with specialized research units. The Division publishes information on each of these centers and their activities in *General Clinical Research Centers: A Directory.* It is a good resource on the types of research currently underway. Copies may be obtained from the above address. Ask for DHEW Publication No. (NIH) 78-1433.

The Department of H.E.W. also has available Nurse Research Traineeships. For information on these write: Chief, Research Grants and Fellowships Branch, Division of Nursing, U.S. Public Health Service, Washington, D.C. 20201

Western Society For Research In Nursing
P. O. Box Drawer P
Boulder, Colo. 80302

This is a unit of the Western Council on Higher Education for Nursing. It conducts an annual "Communicating Nursing Research Conference" for nurse researchers and all interested persons. The conferences provide for sharing of current research, evaluation of the findings, and discussion on ways of applying them to patient care.

Periodicals on Nursing Research

Nursing Research

This bimonthly publication is sponsored by both the American Nurses' Association and the National League For Nursing. It is published by the American Journal Of Nursing Co. Its focus is new and current research practices.

Research In Nursing And Health

This is a quarterly journal on nursing research published by John Wiley and Sons, Inc. ($20 per year).

Western Journal Of Nursing Research
1330 South State College Boulevard
Anaheim, Calif. 92806

This is a quarterly journal for the sharing of current research. It includes articles on research being done, reviews of the research and practical information on conducting nursing research. The focus is on concerns of nursing researchers in the West, but the information is often applicable for all nurses involved in research ($15 U.S. and Canada, $20 foreign).

23 Independent Nursing Practice and The Expanded Role of the Nurse

Independent Nursing Practice

"My independent nursing practice is all about one professional nurse taking seriously the meaning of the words *professional, judgment, decision, authority, responsibility, accountability, truth, justice,* and *charity.* It is about one professional nurse who, after making a commitment and devising a way to meet that commitment, helps people who come to her for help. Finally, it is about one professional nurse helping other nurses to fructify their multiple talents to help many other people. This book presents the rationale for independent practice, for giving care, for putting nursing in its proper place in the health field as a practice discipline that is the extension of the person, the client." *

Independent Nursing Practice With Clients
by M. Lucille Kinlein, R.N.
Independent Generalist Nurse
J. B. Lippincott, 1977.

The preceding quote, taken from the introduction to Ms. Kinlein's book, is an apt description of the book and her work in independent nursing practice. The book describes her innovative and revolutionary approach to nursing and the independent practice she began in 1971. She makes the distinction between her practice and the traditional nursing approach by pointing out that in independent practice the nurse is an extension of the client rather than of the physician. As such he or she is free to give nursing care rather than to assist in medical care. The pur-

---

* *Reprinted with permission of J. B. Lippincott Co., from* Independent Nursing Practice With Clients, *by M. Lucille Kinlein,* © *1977, J. B. Lippincott Co.*

pose of nursing becomes meeting the "professional nursing needs" of the clients as they express them. The focus is on helping people achieve or maintain a state of health rather than on disease and there is an emphasis placed on the health assets of clients rather than deficits.

Ms. Kinlein is a true pioneer in the field of nursing. Her book is a great testimony to growth and to an individual nurse's ability to learn and grow. It is thought provoking and there is much to be learned from her experience by nurses in all fields of practice.

Organizing for Independent Nursing Practice
Ada K. Jacox and Catherine M. Novics
Copyright 1977, Appleton-Century-Crofts

Another resource on independent nursing practice, this book is a report of a two-day conference of nurses working independently which was funded by the Psychiatric Nursing Education Branch of the National Institute of Mental Health.

The brief descriptions of the participants in the conference serve as excellent examples of what nurses are doing in independent practice. The book goes on to relate papers presented at the conference and the discussions which followed.

Topics include reasons for going into private practice, how to set up a practice, relationships with other health professionals, descriptions of actual practices, research possibilities, and the future of nurses practicing independently.

The Expanded Role of the Nurse

"I dream that one day our expanded role will mean independent decision-making, total accountability, and patient-centered intervention—the responsibilities for which many of us have been well prepared and thousands of our colleagues are preparing themselves. When all of our assessments, all of our decisions, all of our interventions are judged for their benefit to the patient, our roles will automatically expand." *

* Reprinted with permission from Nursing Skillbook Assessing Vital Functions Accurately, Foreword by Frances Storlie, RN, MS, Ph.D, Copyright © 1978, Intermed Communications, Inc., Horsham, PA.

Nursing roles have expanded and are continuing to do so. The following is a listing of some of the many specialities or "expanded roles" now available to nurses:

- Adult Health Nurse Practitioner
- Cardiovascular Clinical Specialist
- College Health Nurse Practitioner
- Community Mental Health Nurse Practitioner
- Critical Care Nurse Practitioner
- Emergency Nurse Practitioner
- Enterostomal Therapist
- Family Health Nurse Practitioner
- Family Planning Nurse Practitioner
- Geriatric Nurse Practitioner
- Infection Control Nurse
- I.V. Therapist
- Maternal-Child Nurse Practitioner
- Medical-Surgical Nurse Practitioner
- Neonatal/Perinatal Nurse Practitioner
- Neurological Clinical Specialist
- Nurse-Anesthetist
- Nurse-Midwife
- Nurse Thanatologist
- Nursing Burn Specialist
- Occupational Health Nurse Practitioner
- Oncology Nurse Specialist
- Pediatric Nurse Practitioner
- Pediatric Oncology Nurse Specialist
- Primary Care Nurse Practitioner
- Psychiatric Clinical Specialist
- Rehabilitation Nurse
- Respiratory Nurse Specialist
- Rural Health Nurse Practitioner
- School Health Nurse Practitioner
- Trauma Nurse Specialist
- Women's Health Care Nurse Practitioner

Each of these expanded roles requires further training and education beyond the basic nursing preparation. Two excellent resources for information on these specialties and educational programs in them are:

1. "A Guide to Nursing Specialities," "A Nursing 78 Handbook," Part 1 in *Nursing 78,* October, 1978 (pp. 57–64), and Part

2 in *Nursing 78,* November, 1978 (pp. 49–56). This guide includes information on 24 nursing specialties, including the training necessary, where practitioners in each field work, salary levels, certification required and educational programs for each specialty.

2. *A Directory of Expanded Role Programs For Registered Nurses,* 1979, DHEW Publication No. HRA 79-10. Available from the Superintendent of Documents, U.S. Government Printing Office, Washington, D.C. 20402. This directory contains alphabetical listings by state of schools which offer expanded role training programs. It is divided into sections according to certificate, baccalaureate, and master's degree programs.

These two guides will be helpful to nurses interested in pursuing further training in an expanded role field. Other excellent sources for information on preparation for these roles are the nursing organizations for each specialty (see addresses in chapter on "Nursing Organizations"). For information on Pediatric Nurse Practitioner, Nurse-Midwifery, and Psychiatric Nurse-Practitioner Schools, see the chapters in this book on Pediatrics, Maternity Nursing, and Psychiatric Nursing, respectively.

Audiovisual Materials on the Expanded Role of the Nurse

"Portrait of A Nurse" is a film describing the role of a nurse practitioner in a joint practice with a physician and her work in primary care. From Butler Freedman Films.

"Nurse-Midwives in Practice" is a series of slides available from the American College of Nurse-Midwives.

"Nurse-Midwifery," a 16mm film and audiocassette which includes a history of obstetrics and midwifery as well as current practices, is available from the American Journal of Nursing Company.

24 Nursing and the Law

    I. **Malpractice—Negligence**

   II. **Liability Insurance**

  III. **Admission Consent Form**

  IV. **An Innovative Approach to Protecting Patients' Rights**

   V. **References**

  VI. **Audiovisual Materials**

GUIDELINES ON NEGLIGENCE PROFESSIONAL NEGLIGENCE IS MALPRACTICE		
Elements of liability	Explanation	Example – Giving medications
1. Duty to use due care (defined by the standard of care)	The care which should be given under the circumstances (what the reasonably prudent nurse would have done)	A nurse should give medications: • accurately and • completely and • on time
2. Failure to meet standard of care (breach of duty)	Not giving the care which should be given under the circumstances	A nurse fails to give medications: • accurately or • completely or • on time
3. Foreseeability of harm	Knowledge that not meeting the standard of care will cause harm to the patient	Giving the wrong medication or the wrong dosage or not on schedule will probably cause harm to the patient
4. Failure to meet standard of care (breach) *causes* injury	Patient is harmed because proper care is not given	Wrong medication causes patient to have a convulsion
5. Injury	Actual harm results to patient	Convulsion or other serious complication

Reprinted with permission of Aspen Systems Corporation from *Nursing and the Law*, 2nd edition, Charles J. Streiff and The Health Law Center, Copyright 1975, Aspen Systems Corporation.

Professional Liability Insurance Policy

A nurse who is covered by a professional liability insurance policy must recognize the rights and duties inherent in the policy. The nurse should be able to identify the risks that are covered, the amount of coverage, and the conditions of the contract.

Although coverage may vary in the policies of different insurance companies, the standard policy usually says the insurance company will "pay on behalf of the insured all sums which the insured shall become legally obligated to pay as damages because of injury arising out of malpractice, error, or mistake in rendering or failing to render nursing services."

A standard liability insurance policy has five distinct parts: (1) the insurance agreement; (2) defense and settlement; (3) policy period; (4) amount payable; and (5) conditions.

Many of the professional organizations in nursing specialties offer malpractice insurance at group rates to members. In addition, individuals may obtain professional and personal liability insurance from the following companies:

Professional Buyers Guild, Inc.
2517 Highway 35-Building D
Manasquan, N.J. 08736

Cotterell, Mitchell and Fifer, Inc.
151 William St.
New York, N.Y. 10038

Reprinted with permission of Aspen Systems Corporation from *Nursing and The Law,* 2nd edition, Charles J. Streiff and The Health Law Center, © 1975, Aspen Systems Corporation.

Explanation of Admission Consent Form

An admission consent form should be signed as part of the admission procedure. The admitting office personnel should specifically inform the patient of the need for the form. Both inpatients and outpatients should be required to sign the admission consent form upon admission for treatment.

The signing of the admission consent form may be dispensed with when

Continued on next page

a pregnant woman, already in labor, presents herself at the hospital for delivery of a child, because arrival at the hospital may be considered a voluntary submission to the medical and hospital routines and procedures usually associated with delivery of a child. Dispensing with the signing of a consent form is suggested in this instance because the patient may be in such pain as to be actually unaware of what she is signing, thus making the signed consent of no greater consequence than her submission to medical attention.

CONSENT UPON ADMISSION TO HOSPITAL AND MEDICAL TREATMENT

PATIENT: _____

DATE: _____ TIME: _____ A.M. / P.M.

1. I, (or _____ for _____) knowing that I, (or _____) am (is) suffering from a condition requiring hospital care do hereby voluntarily consent to such hospital care encompassing routine diagnostic procedures and medical treatment by Dr. _____ his assistants or his designees as is necessary in his judgment.

2. I am aware that the practice of medicine and surgery is not an exact science and I acknowledge that no guarantees have been made to me as to the result of treatments or examination in the hospital.

3. Check one:
   _____ A. I hereby authorize the _____ Hospital to preserve for scientific or teaching purposes or for use in grafts upon living persons, or otherwise dispose of the dismembered tissue, parts or organs resulting from the procedure authorized above.

   _____ B. I will be fully responsible for making other disposition arrangements. Removal of that part from the hospital will be accomplished within 5 days after discharge; failure to remove before 5 days have passed will constitute approval of disposition by _____ Hospital under (A).

4. This form has been fully explained to me and I certify that I understand its contents.

_____   _____
     Witness   Signature of Patient

(If patient is unable to consent or is a minor, complete the following):
Patient (is a minor _____ years of age) is unable to consent because _____
_____

_____   _____
     Witness   Closest relative or legal guardian

It should be noted that this exception to the general rule requiring an admission consent form does not apply when the patient is not in labor when admitted. Where delivery is to be by means of cesarean section, or labor is to be artificially induced after admission, or the patient requires other special procedures or anesthesia, the admission consent form should be signed when the patient is admitted to the hospital. In some of these situations, a special consent form may be required.

Paragraph 1. The consent form is designed to cover all procedures in the hospital which do not require a special consent form, including routine laboratory, diagnostic, and medical treatment as well as most outpatient care. It provides protection for procedures done by hospital personnel, attending physicians and assistants, or any other physicians called into the case. The form has the merit of providing personal coverage for all persons who have a legitimate reason for touching or ministering to the patient, thus protecting the hospital and the medical staff personnel. Blanks are provided for the name of anyone who consents on behalf of a patient who is physically unable or legally incompetent to consent. A blank is provided for the name of the attending physician. If two or more physicians are attending the patient, all names should be included. The form also provides coverage for the assistants and designees of the physician.

Paragraph 2. The courts have uniformly held that a patient can recover for damages, despite consent, if it can be shown that the physician guaranteed the success of the operation or treatment, and if the procedure was not successful. This paragraph provides evidence that no such guarantee was made.

Paragraph 3. These alternative paragraphs permit the hospital to carry out routine procedures for the disposal of specimens, tissues, and organs taken from the patient and also relieve the hospital of responsibility for their disposal.

Paragraph 4. This paragraph satisfies the requirement that the consent must be given with understanding; it does this by requiring the patient to agree only after proper disclosure that a variety of procedures may be performed.

Signature Block. Lines are provided for signature by the patient or someone authorized to consent for the patient. Space is also provided for the signing of a witness although no witness is required to make the consent effective. Obtaining a witness who can attest to the genuineness of the patient's signature and competency to sign the form is advisable. One witness would suffice to prove the circumstances of the signing. Formalizing the signing of the consent form by having more than one witness may introduce a degree of solemnity that may affect the patient's morale.

Reprinted with permission of Aspen Systems Corporation from *Nursing and the Law*, 2nd edition, Charles J. Streiff and The Health Law Center, Copyright 1975, Aspen Systems Corporation.

610

An Innovative Approach to Protecting Patients' Rights

Patient Service Officer
(Ombudsman)
Brentwood Veterans Hospital
Los Angeles, California

Purpose: The position of patient service officer was established at the Veterans Administration Hospital in late 1970. The position was created in response to the need to protect patients' statutory and constitutional rights and rights established through case law, such as informed consent and protection of suicidal patients. It was felt that hospital management has a duty to protect those rights and to prevent and eliminate abuses. It was also believed that management has a duty to protect patients from other kinds of abuses that tend to depersonalize them and rob them of their sense of dignity, self-respect, or self-esteem. This office was established in accordance with a mandate from the Veterans Administration central office to develop new programs to facilitate patient care.

Nursing Role: The patient service officer or ombudsman is a registered nurse who is also a lawyer. She actively responds to requests for help, complaints, and grievances from inpatients and outpatients and their families and from staff or friends on behalf of patients. If the request is appropriate for resolution by an existing unit, such as medical, administrative, nursing, or social service, the matter is referred to that service. Only if a problem cannot be resolved by the appropriate existing service is it handled by the patient service officer. If it is a reasonable request, a justified complaint, or a realistic grievance, the matter is investigated, and recommendations for resolution are made quickly to the appropriate service or division. A follow-up call or visit may be made to judge the extent and effectiveness of the resolution.

The nurse also helps improve the quality of administration by serving as a consultant and advisor to the director, bringing to his attention major problems and grievances of patients. She is responsible for helping the director supervise the overall function of the health-care facility by attempting to look at the system through the eyes of the patient and advising the director of the most effective procedures to follow.

The ombudsman serves as a lecturing consultant to many community groups and educational institutions. She lectures about new legal concepts that relate to health-care delivery, the role of the ombudsman, the legal aspects of nursing, and the legal rights of patients. The ombudsman has provided consultation and counseling to hospitals and clinics in the district and to state personnel representatives, legislators, and the State Department of Veterans Affairs.

Evaluation: An example of the program's accomplishments is the improved care provided by eliminating clinical practices that deprive patients of their rights. A policy was established requiring physicians to obtain proper consent for electro-convulsive treatment. A token economy program that was excessively punitive was modified, and wards are locked now only for therapy reasons, not for staff convenience. Administrative accomplishments include a policy allowing inpatients, outpatients, and ex-patients to rent post office boxes at the station and local post offices. A change was made in the patient-effects procedure that eliminated large losses of clothing and electrical and transistor items belonging to the patients. Finally, there have been fewer lawsuits against the hospital and personnel; this is believed to be a result of providing patients a forum for their complaints, with the resulting increased effectiveness of communications among patients, their families, and staff.

Reprinted from *Analysis and Planning for Improved Distribution of Nursing Personnel and Services,* Sheila Kodadek, Editor, 1976, Division of Nursing, Health Resources Administration, U.S. Department of H.E.W.

Contact for Further Information:
Wanda C. Nations, RN, LLB
Chief, Patient Relations, Brentwood Veterans Hospital
Wilshire and Sawtelle Boulevards
Los Angeles, California 90073

Selected References on Nursing and the Law

Hall, Virginia, *Statutory Regulation of the Scope of Nursing Practice—A Critical Survey,* Copyright 1975, the National Joint Practice Commission, 35 East

Wacker Drive, Suite 1990, Chicago, Ill. 60601. (Paperback, 51 pages, $2.50)

This book reviews the medical and nurse practice acts in each state. It is especially useful to nurses involved with trying to change their own state's nurse practice act to accommodate changes in nursing roles.

Mancini, Marguerite, "Documenting Clinical Records," in *AJN*, September, 1978, p. 1556.

Mancini, Marguerite, "What You Should Know About Malpractice Insurance," in *AJN*, April, 1979, p. 729.

Audiovisual Materials on Nursing and the Law

"Legal Responsibilities In the Health Care Institution," a filmstrip for nurses from Eye Gate Media.

The American Journal of Nursing Co. has several films and videocassettes available on nursing and the law. Sample titles include, "Nurse Practice Acts," "Malpractice," "Nursing Torts," "Rights Of Patients-1," "Rights of Patients-11," and "Ethical-Legal Aspects of Nursing Practice."

25 Military Nursing

Military Nursing Opportunities

Bethea Brost, RN, BSN *

Many individuals have misconceptions concerning military nursing. One can live his/her own life-style, when a member of one of the three branches recruiting military nurses—The Army, Navy and the Air Force. Basically, one works a forty-hour week, as with any civilian job, and off-duty time is free to do as one pleases. Living quarters are often available on the military installation, but the nurse can also choose to live within the local community. The officer rank enables the military nurse to become a member of an officer's club, which usually offers excellent dining and dancing, as well as swimming, tennis, and golfing facilities. Most military installations offer a variety of services for their people at reasonable rates such as hobby shops, equipment rental, photo shops, movie theaters, bowling, horseback riding, flying and many others. Along with this is the eligibility to shop in the commissary (grocery store) and the exchange (department store) for their lower-priced items. Advantages of military nursing include:

Job satisfaction with varied clinical areas and geographical locations from which to choose.

Opportunities for professional growth and advanced education.

Free medical and dental benefits.

Opportunity for world-wide duty assignments or free travel on military aircraft.

All moving and travel expenses are paid when entering, transferring or departing from the military.

A tax-free extra housing allowance above the basic pay if one chooses to live off the military base.

Thirty days of paid vacation each year.

Hospital uniforms and laundering are provided free of charge. A $300 allowance is given for other duty uniforms.

Periodic raises in salary plus promotions.

Life insurance policy.

A retirement plan is offered if one should choose to make a career of the military.

The initial obligation to the Army, Navy or Air Force is for three years. This period begins with travel to the specific branch's orientation course. These courses are designed to familiarize nurses with military history, customs, courtesies, leadership, and to provide orientation to military medicine. Each branch has its own individual orientation course format.

The introduction to the Army Nurse Corps is given during a five week orientation course held at Fort Sam Houston, San Antonio, Texas, at the Army's Academy of Health Sciences.

The Naval Officer and Education Training Center, Newport, Rhode Island, holds a five-and-one-half-week Officer Indoctrination Program.

The Nurse Orientation Course for the Air Force is held at Sheppard Air Force Base, Wichita Falls, Texas, for a two-week period.

Opportunities for professional growth and advanced education in the military are numerous. Each branch has its own specialty courses in areas such as Nurse-Midwifery, Pediatric, Adult, and Family-Practice Practitioners, Anesthesia, Psychiatry, Community Health and many other areas. Some lead to a Master of Science Degree in Nursing.

Continuing education at nearby colleges and universities is encouraged. Tuition assistance, as high as 75 percent of the costs, is available with an additional commitment attached.

Following two years of active duty, it is possible, if qualified, to attend an accredited school or university full time towards a higher degree. All fees will be paid in addition to full salary.

For more specifics concerning the Army, Navy or Air Force nursing programs or qualifications, contact the local recruiter through the yellow pages or contact the following:

Army Nurse Opportunities
Box 4444
Mt. Vernon, New York, 10551
800-431-1234

Navy Opportunity Information Center
P. O. Box 2000
Pelham Manor, New York 10803
800-841-8000
(Georgia 800-342-5855; Hawaii 533-1871; call collect in Alaska, 272-9133 and Puerto Rico, 724-4525

Air Force Nursing
Box 1776
Valley Forge, Pennsylvania 19481
800-523-5000
(Pennsylvania, 800-362-5696)

* Bethea Brost served as an Army nurse. She is currently completing studies at Seton Hall University, South Orange, N.J., for a master's degree in pediatric nursing.

26 Job Hunting

Practical Tips for Job Hunting

Sample Cover Letter

Mrs. Mildred White, RN
Director of Nursing
Fernwood Medical Center
2611 Hilldater Drive
San Francisco, CA 92623

June 4, 1977

Dear Mrs. White,

    I am responding to the "Job Opportunity" you placed in *Pediatric Nursing* for a pediatric nurse practitioner (PNP) position in your pediatric neurology clinic. I have a Masters degree in child development from the University of California and five years' experience working with general pediatric patients, ages birth through 18 years.

    For the last two years I have been working as a PNP with Dr. Wm. Shakespear in the care of children with learning disorders and other neurological problems. We work with 85 to 100 patients and their families in diagnosis, drug therapy, school liaison, home behavior modification paradigms, parent support groups, and educational workshops for the community. I think my education and experience are appropriate to meet your position's requirements. I enjoy this area of pediatrics immensely and wish to stay within the field.

    I will be moving to your area within a month and would like to interview for the position at your earliest convenience. I have taken the liberty of sending you a resumé which contains my home and work addresses and phone numbers. Please do not hesitate to contact me at home or work as I am very interested in the position.

                                        Sincerely,

                                        Maria Sanchez Patterson

Reprinted with permission from "What Is A Good Resume?" by Karen Fond in *Pediatric Nursing*, January/February, 1978.

Sample Resume*

Professional Career Goal: To provide direct patient care to pediatric patients in ambulatory settings. Secondary plans are to conduct patient care research and teach in an academic setting.

Demographic Data

Name	Maria Sanchez Patterson
Home Address and Telephone	4529 Miller Lane Los Angeles, CA 90046 (213) 857-3756
Employer Address and Telephone	Childrens Little Hospital Division of Neurology 496 Mountain Road Los Angeles, CA 90053 (213) 450-5724
Date of Birth	September 3, 1946
Marital Status	Married
Special Skills	Fluent in Spanish and Sign Language

Education

A. *Formal*

College: University of California at Los Angeles, School of Nursing, Los Angeles, California, 1968, Bachelor of Science in Nursing, Deans List (GPA 3.8)

Graduate School: University of California, Berkeley
Department of Psychology—Child Development
Berkeley, California 1972
Master of Science
Thesis: Behavior Modification and the use of sign language in Deaf children.

Nurse Practitioner:
University of Arizona, Department of Nursing, Phoenix, Arizona, 1975 Pediatric Nurse Practitioner Certificate, Preceptor: Dr. Bill Sharp.

B. *Continuing Education*
Role Transitions in Advanced Clinical Practice, Nurse Practitioner Seminar, University of Arizona, Phoenix, Arizona, 1975.

Behavior Modification and Dyslexia
a 4-day workshop
Department of Psychology and School of Medicine
University of California at Los Angeles
Los Angeles, California, 1975

Common Pediatric Neurological Defects, PNP Continuing Education Lecture, Loma Linda University, Loma Linda, California, 1976

Learning Disorders: Current Trends
1 semester course School of Nursing and Medicine
California State University, Long Beach
Long Beach, California 1976

Professional Credentials

RN License California #C 123654 Expires May 25, 1979

PNP Certificate University of Arizona, 1975

National Board of Pediatric Nurse Practitioners and Associates Certification as a Pediatric Nurse Practitioner, 1977

Professional Experience

Staff Nurse, Charge Nurse
  Medical-Surgical ICU: 6/68–6/70

    Good Samaritan Hospital, Los Angeles, California. Evening charge nurse for 10 bed critical care unit, staffing and supervisory responsibilities. Left to attend graduate school.

Public Health Nurse II

    Well and Sick Child Clinics, Los Angeles County Health Department, El Monte Health Center, El Monte, California. Caseload of 190 patients, 6 clinics including communicable disease, chronic disease within the division of Maternal and Child Health. Left to accompany husband in residency and to attend nurse practitioner program. 8/72 to 6/74.

Pediatric Nurse Practitioner

    Childrens Little Hospital
    Division of Neurology
    Los Angeles, California
    10/75 to present
    Caseload of 85 to 100 patients in multiphasic care paradigms including extensive diagnostic evaluation, experimental and traditional drug therapy regimens, psychological support through behavior modification, home program, parent groups, educational and liaison responsibilities with the community, schools, parent groups, pediatric associations.

Professional Organizations, Honor Societies

    Sigma Theta Tau, 1968
    California Nurses Association, member, 1968 to present
    American Nurses Association, member, 1968 to present
    National Association of Pediatric Nurses Associates and Practitioners, member, 1973 to present. Public Relations Committees, 1974–75.

Publications, Paper and Lectures Presented

Sanchez, Maria, "The Use of Behavior Modification Techniques in Teaching Deaf Children," unpublished Masters Degree Thesis, University of California, Berkeley, California, 1972.
Sancheez-Patterson, Maria, "Parent Support Groups," *Nursing Clinics of North America,* vol. 6, No. 2, April, 1976.

Community Involvement

Listing provided upon request or during interview.

References

Listing provided upon request or during interview.

Reprinted with permission from "What Is A Good Resume?" by Karen Fond in *Pediatric Nursing*, January/February, 1978.

1979 Nursing Opportunities, published by *RN* Magazine, Litton Industries, Oradell, N.J., 1979. (300 pages, cost: $3.50).

This book is an annual guide to nursing jobs available in hospitals throughout the country. It gives detailed information on the hospitals, including positions available, and offers advice on seeking a job, including interviewing, writing an application and resume, and obtaining a license in another state. It is especially useful to new graduates.

New Career Guide Now Available from NSNA

The National Student Nurses' Association has published its first annual *Career Planning Guide*.

The guide contains articles on career choices and self-assessment, help in decision making, coping with a career, and surviving reality shock.

To assist in job hunting, the guide also features over 50 career opportunity profiles of hospitals across the country.

The guide is published in the September issue of *Imprint*, NSNA's magazine and may be purchased for $2.00 from NSNA, 10 Columbus Circle, New York, N.Y. 10019.

Reprinted from *The American Journal of Nursing*, December, 1979, Vol. 79, No. 12, p. 2074, © 1979, The American Journal of Nursing Co.

27 Nursing Abroad

Sources of Information on Employment Opportunities in International Nursing

1. *Technical Assistance Information Clearing House, 200 Park Avenue South, New York, N.Y. 10003.* A publications list is available that includes a directory of U.S. organizations in development assistance abroad and reports of development projects by country. *A Listing of U.S. Nonprofit Organizations in Medicine and Public Health Assistance Abroad* became available in June.

2. *Nursing Abroad.* Available free from the International Council of Nurses, Box 42, 1211 Geneva 20, Switzerland. Describes the services offered by ICN member associations in arranging salaried employment and/or study abroad.

3. *Option, P.O. Box 81122, San Diego, California 92138.* This agency is a source of information on volunteer and salaried employment in areas of need, both domestic and international; a monthly newsletter and yearly catalog describing opportunities are available.

4. *Job Opportunities Bulletin.* Available free from the New Transcentury Foundation, 1789 Columbia Rd., N.W., Washington, D.C. 20009. Lists and describes current openings in private and voluntary organizations working in third world development.

5. *International Voluntary Services, Inc., 1717 Massachusetts Ave., N.W., Suite 605, Washington, D.C. 20036.* IVS recruits skilled volunteers to work in developing countries in the broad area of rural development, which includes health.

6. *Intercristo, P.O. Box 9323, Seattle, Washington 98109.* An information center on worldwide Christian service; phone 800-426-0507 to receive further information on nursing opportunities.

7. Classified ads in major newspapers are the best source of information on overseas employment with multinational corporations. Recruitment may be direct or through an overseas placement agency.

8. Many international health organizations recruit nurses through advertisements in professional journals, letters to schools of nursing, and recruitment meetings or displays at nursing conventions.

9. Nurses should write directly to organizations in which they have a specific interest. This initial contact may lead to others with equally promising opportunities for employment.

Reprinted with permission from *American Journal of Nursing,* July, 1979, page 1245, Copyright 1979, American Journal of Nursing Co.

28 Miscellaneous Nursing Information

Foreign Nurses Wishing to Work in the United States

In order to enter the U.S. and work as a professional nurse in this country, a foreign nurse must have been petitioned for by a particular employer and must present evidence that she/he can work immediately upon entering this country.

There is currently a regulation pending which will require foreign nurses to pass an exam given by the Commission on Graduates of Foreign Nursing Schools (CGFNS) before they can enter this country. This Commission was established with support of the A.N.A. and N.L.N. to prevent exploitation of foreign nurses who arrive in the U.S., take nursing State Board exams and fail, and then are not able to work as nurses. The exam does not replace State Board exams but it gives foreign nurses an indication of their likelihood of passing State Boards. It is given twice a year, in April and October, in 33 locations throughout the world. It is the first step for foreign nurses in coming to the U.S. to practice.

After passing the CGFNS qualifying exam and having proof that she/he will be employed upon entering the U.S., a foreign nurse must pass the State Board exam in the state where the nurse will be employed.

For applications for the CGFNS qualifying exam and further information, write:

Commission on Graduates of Foreign Nursing Schools
3624 Market St.
Philadelphia, Pa. 19104
U.S.A.

(Source: "Guidebook For Applicants," © 1978, Commission on Graduates of Foreign Nursing Schools.)

For background information on foreign nurse immigration, see "Immigration of Graduates of Foreign Nursing Schools," Report of the Conference on Immigration of Graduates of Foreign Nursing Schools, June, 1975, DHEW Pub. No. (HRA) 76–84, available from the Superintendent of Documents, U.S. Government Printing Office, Washington, D.C. 20402.

Writing for Nursing Publications
Andrea B. O'Connor
Charles B. Slack, Inc.
Thorofare, New Jersey 08086
(99 pages, paperback)

An encouraging book on the why's and how's of writing for nursing journals, this book is useful to nurses interested in publishing. Aimed at beginning nurse-writers, it covers the basics of writing for journals. Advice is given on choosing a subject, approaches to writing, the mechanics of writing the manuscript, preparing it for submission to a publisher, and on the advisability of querying a publisher as to interest in the manuscript before submitting it.

Ms. O'Connor recommends the use of resource books for grammar and spelling accuracy but emphasizes that books can't teach someone how to write; the best teacher is experience. She stresses the need to just "sit down and write."

The "rights and responsibilities of authors and editors" are described and a "glossary of publishing terms and proofreader's marks" is included, as well as an index to Nursing Journals.

Guide to Publishing Opportunities For Nurses
Edited by Ida Marie Martinson, Ph.D
Revised 1979. ($3.00)
The University Of Minnesota, School Of Nursing
Research Center
3313 Powell Hall
500 Essex Street, S.E.
Minneapolis, Minnesota 55455

This guide is an excellent source for nurses interested in writing articles for publication. It contains annotated listings of journals in the United States and foreign publications, including the editor and address, the types of articles published, the form for submitting manuscripts, and special instructions for each journal. A total of 88 journals are listed.

Fundraising

American Eagle Company
1130 E. Big Beaver Road
Troy Commerce Center
Troy, Mich. 48084

American Eagle Company provides groups such as local chapters of nursing organizations and student nursing groups with complete packaged fundraising sales of nursing T-shirts. The shirts are printed with slogans such as, "Love A Nurse P.R.N." For further information on this fundraising opportunity contact American Eagle at the above address.

Grantsmanship: It Can Be Learned

Robert A. Saunders, M.S.

Part I

Free money! Something for nothing! That's what grant money seems like to many people who feel that once you get a grant you can just put your feet up and relax until the grant money has run out. Unfortunately, this is not true.

A grant is money given by a government agency, a corporation, or a foundation to a worthy non-profit organization. Rarely are grants given directly to individuals. If the grant is for a specific project, it may be earmarked for use by a particular person (such as a Program Director) within a recipient organization, but the organization must apply for, and accept responsibility for the use of the grant money. Usually, the only stipulation is that the money be used solely for the purpose for which it was given. This restriction is applied in various degrees of detail depending on the grantor, but it carries the force of law.

How do you take advantage of grant generosity? Applying for and managing grant money takes work, and there is considerable competition for grants. But the procedures are basically simple and straightforward.

You must start by deciding precisely why you need the grant money; find the appropriate organizations to apply to; follow their procedures for style and protocol for the application; use the money for the purposes it is given; show the grant giver how well it was used; and maintain good relations with the grantor. The first task may seem the simplest, but in actuality requires the most decisions. In effect, your organization must ask itself: why would anyone want to give us money? What can this organization accomplish so that a grantor would want to give us financial support?

What Kinds of Grants Are Available?

To help answer this question, let us look at three general categories of grants.

- Do you need to *supplement the normal operating budget* of your organization? For example, the Metropolitan Opera in New York City solicits contributions from corporations just to keep going year after year.
- Do you need money for a *building fund for new construction*? A home for the elderly may seek federal funds for a new wing.
- Are you planning a *special project* that would be new to your organization? Many professional associations would like to institute continuing education programs if they could get some financial assistance.

In general, potential grantors see a real difference among these three types of needs. Since many consider only requests in one or two categories, you should carefully identify your needs and the considerations of potential grantors before you even make your requests.

Developing a Grant Request

Once your type of need has been decided, a more detailed plan is needed. Break down your operations, building program or special project into an outline showing each objective to be accomplished in the proper order. At this point, involve the people who will participate in carrying out the project for which you are seeking a grant. The more they contribute to the planning, the more stake they have in its success. From this outline, the personnel and resources necessary for each step can be determined. An estimate of all costs can then be made, and a budget developed. Exhibit A shows what a portion of such a budget breakdown might look like. This initial outline shows prospective

Continued on next page

grantors the logic and thoroughness of your plans. It makes sure that the full costs of a project have been considered in advance. Finally, it helps you decide whom to approach for a possible grant.

Finding the Right Grantor

A basic sourcebook on government grants is the *Catalog of Federal Domestic Assistance*. This is available at many public and university libraries. It may also be purchased for $20.00.* Indices arranged by subject help match your need to the proper supporting agency. Detailed information is given on each funding program, including eligibility requirements. From these listings, you should be able to find out where and how to apply or at least where to ask for more information. Although this catalog is the best general sourcebook, other more specialized ones may be more appropriate for your needs. If you have frequent dealings with a particular agency which gives grants, make inquiries there. Having common concerns with a potential grantor may predispose them in your favor.

Unfortunately, there is no such central reference for individual states. Each state is organized differently. But each state has departments that deal with education and with various social services. Inquiries at these agencies may yield information about whom to contact. Usually a request for information — without mentioning money — will be more likely to help you locate the proper contacts. The same procedure applies to local community governments.

If you are planning to approach a foundation, finding the right one (or ones) may take longer, since there are an estimated 25,000 foundations in this country. The non-profit Foundation Center**, in New York City, collects and publishes information about foundations and will direct you to the publications and services which will be most useful to you. The Foundation Center's own publications, especially the *Foundation Directory*, are the best information sources for grant applicants. The *Directory* lists 2,818 of the largest foundations. Its subject index helps you to match your needs with interested grantors and lists detailed information about each foundation.

The Foundation Center also makes available information on grants from *all* foundations recognized by the Internal Revenue Service and helps prospective grant seekers to find exactly the right places to apply. Since foundations vary widely in their requirements and interests, it is absolutely necessary to get this advance information.

If you are seeking a grant from a corporation, you may find that its granting process, if any, may not be as well established or systematic and the grant decision makers may not be as accessible. A helpful guideline in considering potential corporation grantors is that companies most likely to give financial aid to your organization are those with a definite stake in your community; those who need its goodwill and/or the goodwill of those who would benefit from your project. Contact your local (or state) Chamber of Commerce or the librarian at your public library to help you find corporations to contact. Once you have some possibilities, learn as much as you can about each **business. Find out who makes the financial decisions, especially grant decisions.** While the public relations department of a corporation may disburse the grant money, usually it is others who make the crucial decisions. If possible, find out who the key decision-makers are, even if this means calling the corporation and asking questions.

Once you have the names of some possible grantors to approach — government, foundation, or corporation — research each one thoroughly. Find out the types and sizes of grants given in the past. Perhaps a grantor is interested only in certain specialized fields. Another grantor may give grants in amounts greater than you feel justified in asking for or so small that you would need other support. A third may have requirements for eligibility that your organization cannot meet. Research can save a lot of time and effort by eliminating impossible alternatives. By concentrating on those grantors who have previously supported organizations or projects similar to yours, you will be dealing with people more likely to be knowledgeable and sympathetic to your ideas.

Guidelines for Grant Applications

Once you have decided where to apply for a possible grant, contact each organization. Find out if particular forms for applying are needed, what the deadline for applications is, what else is required for application and whom to contact with your application.

Once you know the procedures required by the grantors you have chosen, prepare your formal proposals. Since you worked out the basic ideas in your initial outline, the details can now be added easily, and written up in the required format. The credibility of your organization should be established and supported throughout every one of your applications. You must show what you plan to do and how you plan to do it, should you be given the grant money.

Most proposals contain two major parts — a technical proposal and a business proposal. The first part of each proposal consists of four logical steps: an explanation of the specific community need that you are addressing; a plan of action to satisfy that need; a demonstration that you have the resources and experience to carry out this plan, and a detailed discussion of what you expect to accomplish. Whether the money will be used for normal operating expenses, for construction, or for a special project, your presentation must detail each of these steps.

The complexity of the application will depend on the size and type of the grant, as well as on the requirements of the proposal application. If you are trying to raise money for the construction of a nursing home, it may be necessary to include blueprints in your submission. For a nurse training program, it would be well worth including proposed curricula, drawn up by consulting experts. Remember, your idea will be reviewed by experts in the field. By giving them all the required information, you will be more likely to attract their interest. Grantors are quick to spot impractical requests and poorly prepared plans.

**The Foundation Center, 888 Seventh Avenue, New York, New York 10019. Telephone: (212) 975-1120.

You must also address yourself to what will happen to those benefiting from your project when the original grant funding runs out. Has your organization made provisions for funding after the grant money has been spent? Could you afford to staff and maintain a building after the grantor has paid for its construction?

The unique abilities and resources of your organization must be emphasized in the application. Give a brief history of your organization, including any similar accomplishments in the past. Show your financial stability, and your ability to handle money. If the project will require people with special experience, you should include resumes of the backgrounds of these key people. In many cases, a potential donor will require your latest audited financial statement. All this is necessary and serves to build your organization's credibility.

Grantsmanship: It Can Be Learned
Robert A. Saunders, M.S.
Part II

The second major section of the application is the business or financial one — the budget. Even more than your credibility is at stake here. The budget will be examined by experts, and it will be measured against hard reality. Underestimating costs could hurt you financially later. Overestimating could raise questions concerning your credibility in a potential donor's mind. The budget must, therefore, be estimated carefully and realistically.

Knowing the total amount of money you will require helps in the search for a grantor. Most grantors have determined what size grant is best for them. If the funding you need is greater than a particular grantor's range, you will know in advance to seek more than one source. Asking for the appropriate amount increases your chances of getting the grant.

Making up the budget should be as logical and thorough a process as putting together the technical proposal. Remember that a budget is an estimate of the costs necessary to accomplish certain objectives. Developing the technical proposal will clarify and detail those objectives.

But you must also make allowances for possible future changes in your plans. For instance, in setting up a teaching program, you may find that certain subjects will require extra review. Your students might need special tutoring or a special guest teacher in order to understand material that proves particularly difficult. In another case, the roof of a building might be constructed in one of two ways, depending on which of two proposed building regulations is passed by the local legislature. Some flexibility must, therefore, be built into your plans, and the proper allowances made in the budget preparation.

Once the objectives are known, the necessary resources and their costs can be calculated. For a non-profit organization, especially one in the health care field, the primary resource is usually personnel. This includes the salaries of the people directly involved in the work, and possibly a portion of the salaries of the supporting staff. It also includes fringe benefits, a term encompassing the related expenses that employers pay, such as sick leave, vacation pay, pension payments, health and life insurance, and disability and unemployment insurance. For most companies, fringe benefits add 15 to 25% to the basic salary expenses. Neglecting to include these expenses in your budget could be financially disastrous.

Other costs could include specialized equipment and supplies, building materials necessary for construction, expenses for insurance, recruiting costs, lawyers' or architects' fees, advertising or consulting fees, and travel expenses. Try to estimate every possible expense in advance.

Determining the cost of housing a project can cause complex problems. If there will be a distinct building for the project, with rent, utilities and insurance to be paid separately, it is easy to calculate the expenses to be charged to the grant. More often, however, facilities are shared, so a basis must be found to determine what percent of these costs apply to the grant-supported project. This gets into the frequently encountered concept of "indirect costs."

Expenses for a given specific project are called direct costs. Expenses which cannot be clearly separated from the expenses of the organization but are shared with it are considered "indirect costs" for each project. Suppose, for example, that you have two grants of different sizes, both handled by one of your organization's accountants. A portion of his or her salary should be split between the two grants, and the rest allotted to the organization's budget. Since it is often difficult to divide these costs precisely, some grantors work out a percentage which can be charged to the grant. This indirect cost rate is similar in concept to the markup or overhead rates used by stores. When making up the budget, therefore, it is a good idea to check with the potential grantors to see how they figure indirect costs. How you estimate and indicate these costs will depend on the requirements of the contributor and the sophistication of your accounting system.

Once the budget has been worked out, the technical and financial parts put together, and the necessary copies made, the proposal is submitted. If you have not received an acknowledgement within a month, you can make a follow-up call to be sure the application was received intact and contained all the required information. This may be your last contact with the potential grantor.

When Grant Applications Require More Information

For certain grant applications, an interview may be required at which time you will be expected to explain your application further. You may meet with only a single staff member or with a committee of experts. If the application was carefully prepared, you will have no problem explaining it and you can use the interview as another opportunity to "sell" your organization.

For some grants, especially those awarded by large contributors such

Continued on next page

as the Federal government, a site visit will be part of the application process. Experts and staff members of the grantor will tour your facilities and talk over your proposal. Such a site visit calls for careful preparation, a briefing of your entire staff and possibly a dress rehearsal for your key personnel. Try to remember, however, that a site visit is an educational experience for *both* parties involved. Your organization has a chance to learn what really interests this grantor, and the grantor can learn all about your organization and its capabilities. Together you might even explore a project of mutual interest that would be better for you than your originally proposed project.

The entire application process outlined above takes work and time. Once this is completed you must wait for an award or a rejection.

Before this occurs you may receive a preliminary letter from the grantor telling you that, "you have been recommended for an award by the review committee," or "an award will be forthcoming." At this point, it is important *not* to spend any money until you have received the actual reward document, contract, or authorizing letter, and the grantor is now legally obligated to cover stipulated expenses. Most grantors, especially the government, do *not* repay expenditures made before the date that the grant becomes effective.

Once You Get the Grant

Once you receive the award notice, READ IT CAREFULLY! There is no ruder shock than spending $24,000 for a piece of equipment, only to discover later that the grantor won't cover that particular expense. All restrictions and limitations must be checked out carefully at the start and made known to everyone affected. If you have any questions concerning specific regulations, ask the grantor. Certain regulations may be written into a grant because of legal restrictions; in other cases, only financial considerations apply. Foreknowledge at this point is better than regret at a later time.

Right now you must also determine whether the records of income and expenses of the grant must be kept separate from other income and expenses of your organization. If you may simply record the grant as a gift, you could just add it to your regular revenues. If grant monies are given for a specific limited purpose, and the grantor requires financial reporting, all receipts and costs must be recorded separately. Your accounting system for a grant must then be set up so that grant expenditures can be identified and distinguished from regular expenses.

Salaries are one of the major expenses of any non-profit organization. Since some employees may be working on their regular work as well as on the work of the grant, money paid out for grant time must be split out from money paid for regular time. In the case of other expenses where grant and non-grant expenses cannot be separated, a portion must be allocated to indirect cost. A separate bank account is only rarely required for grant funds, as long as your accounting system meets with the approval of the grantor.

A well-designed accounting system can also be utilized to keep track of accomplishments. The ideal accounting system does more than record monetary transactions — it should link expenditure levels with the attainment of appropriate targets. Has 60% of the money been spent, yet the project is only one-third finished? Has the money slated for the first three weeks of class already been spent, but the program is still recruiting students? A manager provided with this kind of information knows when to take corrective action.

The actual administration of the grant project may be simple or difficult. One false economy is to hire less-than-the-best people for any job. Competent people who have been seriously consulted in formulating the original plans usually commit themselves wholeheartedly to its successful completion. Most of the time they will stay committed if they are paid what they are worth. It is wise to remember that your personnel is your most important asset and that a core of capable, dedicated employees are essential to your project's success.

Specific, detailed systems can now be developed to keep track of the progress of your project. For many projects these are obvious — the new building must have a floor before the roof is put up. Other projects require special parameters — a new program for teaching handicapped adults might be measured by the number of students placed in jobs after graduating. But a more subtle indicator might be the turnover rate among the staff.

Continuous checking against your original objectives may help you keep on the right track; however, the experience of working on the grant project may call for changes. Deviations from the original plans are not necessarily undesirable — as long as you are aware of each change, understand the reasons for making it and can anticipate the effect of each change.

If time is a major consideration, it, too, may be used to advantage in planning. Each step in the project may be assigned a certain maximum time limit. If there are significant variances from the schedule, appropriate steps can be taken at an early stage. If, for example, a construction job that must be completed by July is running behind schedule, it would be much better to know this in January than in June so that you could then authorize more overtime to complete the job by the deadline. In some very sophisticated systems, time-money tradeoffs are constantly calculated by computers to complete a project in the least time and at the least expense. The level of control will, of course, depend on the needs of your own particular organization.

No matter how efficient your monitoring system is, it is only as good as the person to whom the resultant information is supplied. To a committee, the data is useless. If the system informs a responsible person empowered with the authority to make necessary changes, the grant will be properly administered. With dedicated, high-quality personnel, backed by good administrative support, a grant-funded project should be successful.

At the completion of the project, the final report should be prepared. Since the grantors have involved themselves so deeply, courtesy alone demands that they should be told how their money was spent. The grantor will usually specify the form (and amount of detail desired) for the final report. If this is not the case, a financial report can be submitted similar in form to the budget submitted in the original application. The technical side of the report may be less structured, but must address the needs and objectives originally stated. Once again, the objective is to show that the grantor's money was used successfully for the purposes for which it was given.

Detailed financial records must back up these expenditure reports. Many grantors, especially the government, send their own auditors to examine your books. Other grantors only require that you supply them with a copy of your CPA-approved financial statements. Since most organizations require CPA audits anyway, this should not be an added burden. It is prudent, however, to know in advance of the grant's completion exactly how far back in time your records and files should be kept.

Once the project has been completed, don't forget your old friends — the grantors. Try to maintain contact with them, particularly with small foundations and local businesses who are especially concerned with the work of your organization. Send them a short report each year showing how well your organization, and the work for which their grant money paid, are doing. After all, these grantors have invested their money and their interest in your organization. They are entitled to your continued courtesy.

Researching, obtaining and managing grant monies takes considerable time and work. The keynotes are thorough planning, careful researching and continued thoughtful commitment from everyone concerned. □

A Sample Worksheet: Turning Your Objectives Into a Concrete Budget

Objective	Resource	Cost
B. Registration of Students		
1. Preregistration counseling by phone	1. Registration counselor	$150.00/week x 8 weeks + 20% for fringe benefits = $1440.00
	2. Telephone line	$ 30.00/month x 2 months + $60.00 installation = $120.00
	3. Office	$175.00 rental/month x 2 months = $350.00
	4. Desk	$140.00
	5. Chair	$ 60.00
	6. Office supplies	$ 30.00
2. Registration Night	1. Registration clerks	4 @ $20.00 each + 20% fringe benefits = $96.00
	2. Room for Registration	$ 20.00/night = $20.00
	3. Registration forms, preprinted	$ 40.00 minimum order = $40.00
	4. Supplies — pens, papers, etc.	$ 36.00
	5. Books for students	$ 18.00/student x 100 students = $1800.00
	6. Furniture (borrowed)	$ 0.00

Reprinted from *The Journal of Practical Nursing*, May, 1979, by Robert A. Saunders, reprinted with permission of the author and publisher.

ANA Publishes Ethics Handbook

A 32-page handbook on nursing ethics, *Ethics In Nursing: References and Resources,* was published this fall by the American Nurses' Association.

The document is the result of the work of the 1978-1980 ANA Committee on Ethics, chaired by Kathleen M. Sward, director of the nursing program at Elmira College, N.Y.

The six-member committee compiled the reference book "to assist the nurse in decision making when she is faced with an ethical dilemma," according to the preface.

The handbook, in addition to providing pertinent bibliographies, also lists national and regional organizations concerned with nursing ethics as well as resource persons.

The handbook (ANA Publication No. G-137) may be obtained for $2 by writing ANA Publications, 2420 Pershing Road, Kansas City, Mo. 64108.

Reprinted from *The American Journal of Nursing*, December, 1979, Vol. 79, No. 12, p. 2087, © The American Journal of **Nursing** Co., 1979.

29 Nursing Organizations

Chronology of Nurse Associations

1893 American Society of Superintendents of Training Schools for Nurses founded (Renamed—National League of Nursing Education in 1912)

1897 Nurses Associated Alumnae of the United States and Canada founded (Renamed—American Nurses' Association, 1911)

1900 American Federation of Nurses organized

1908 National Association of Colored Graduate Nurses organized

1912 A.F.N. (dissolved)—National Organization of Public Health Nursing founded

1931 American Association of Nurse Anesthetists organized

1932 Association of Collegiate Schools of Nursing organized

1942 American Association of Industrial Nurses organized

1950 National Association of Colored Graduate Nurses merged with A.N.A.

1952 National League for Nursing organized
National Organization of Public Health Nursing
National League of Nursing Education
Association of Collegiate Schools of Nursing
} Reorganized into the National League for Nursing

1954 Association of Operating Room Nurses founded

1955 American College of Nurse Midwives organized

1968 American Association of Nephrology Nurses and Technicians founded
American Association of Neurosurgical Nurses founded
Nurses Association of the American College of Obstetricians and Gynecologists founded

1970 Emergency Department Nurses' Association founded

1972 American Indian Nurses' Association founded
Association for Practitioners of Infectious Control founded
Orthopedic Nurses' Association founded
National Black Nurses' Association founded

1973 Gay Nurses' Alliance founded
Nurses Concerned for Life founded
Federation of Nurse Specialty Groups and the A.N.A. organized

1974 Association of Pediatric Oncology Nurses organized
Association of Rehabilitation Nurses founded

From Miller, Michael H.: "Special Interest Groups of the A.N.A.: An Analysis." In Miller, Michael H., and Flynn, Beverly C.: *Current Perspectives in Nursing: Social issues and Trends,* Vo. I, © The C. V. Mosby Co., 1977, St. Louis.

Nursing Organizations

The following are specialty organizations in nursing and the allied health fields which are open to nurses.

American Association for Rehabilitation Therapy, Inc. (AART)
P.O. Box 93
North Little Rock, Arkansas 72115

AART is an organization for professionals working in rehabilitation. It promotes the advancement of medical rehabilitation and sets standards for practice. Publications include "American Archives for Rehabilitation Therapy," the "Rehabilitation Therapy Bulletin," pamphlets on rehabilitation, and a "Registry of Medical Rehabilitation Therapists and Specialists."

American Association Of Critical-Care Nurses (AACN)
P. O. Box C19528
Irvine, Calif. 92713

This is the professional organization for registered nurses working with the critically ill in a variety of settings (coronary care, burn units, emergency rooms, etc.). AACN provides continuing education for members through national and regional teaching institutes and disseminates information on recent practices in critical care. The organization publishes literature on critical care nursing; *Heart And Lung, The Journal Of Critical Care,* a bi-monthly journal; and *Focus,* a bi-monthly newsletter. Associate membership is available for LPN/LVN's and R.N. and LPN/LVN nursing students. (Membership: $30 a year, $35 for members from foreign countries.)

American Association Of I.V. Therapy, Inc.
National Headquarters
Two Elm Square
Andover, Mass. 01810

The Association Of I.V. Therapy is an organization for professionals working in I.V. therapy. The group promotes high standards of practice, disseminates information on I.V. therapy, promotes further education in the field, and provides for a sharing of knowledge among I.V. therapists and allied health professionals. (Membership: $30 a year.)

American Association Of Nephrology Nurses And Technicians (AANNT)
Two Talcott Road, Suite 8
Park Ridge, Ill. 60068

AANNT is the professional organization for nurses and technicians working with patients with kidney disease. It provides for continuing education, promotes research, and sets standards for care in this field. Publications include a newsletter, published ten times a year, and a quarterly journal, *AANNT*. (Annual dues: $25.)

American Association Of Neurosurgical Nurses
625 North Michigan Avenue, Suite 1519
Chicago, Ill. 60611

This is a professional organization for nurses involved in neurosurgical nursing. Publications include *The Core Curriculum For Neurological Nursing; The Journal Of Neurosurgical Nursing;* "Synapse," a bimonthly newsletter; "Standards For Neurological and Neurosurgical Nursing Practice." (Published in conjunction with the American Nurses' Association.) Membership is $35 a year.

American Association Of Nurse Anesthetists
111 East Wacker Drive
Chicago, Ill. 60601

This is the national professional organization for certified registered nurse anesthetists. It functions as an accrediting organization for schools of nurse anesthesia and sets educational standards. The AANA publishes the *Journal Of The American Association Of Nurse Anesthetists* six times a year.

American Association Of Occupational Health Nurses, Inc.
575 Lexington Avenue
New York, N.Y. 10022

This is the professional organization for nurses working in occupational health, with local, state, and regional affiliates.

AAOHN sets standards of practice for occupational health nursing and conducts educational programs for nurses. The annual conference of AAOHN is held in conjunction with the American Occupational Medical Association and is called the American Occupational Health Conference.

Publications of the Association include: *Occupational Health*

Nursing, a monthly journal; *A Guide For The Preparation Of A Manual Of Policies And Prodecures For The Occupational Health Service; The Nurse In Industry; A History Of The American Association Of Occupational Health Nurses, Inc.;* and several other informative guides for occupational health nurses.

American Board For Occupational Health Nurses, Inc.
Executive Secretary
P. O. Box 638
Thousand Palms, Calif. 92276

This board functions as an agent for examination and certification of occupational health nurses. It maintains a "Directory Of Certified Occupational Health Nurses." Write for eligibility requirements for certification.

American College Of Nurse-Midwives (ACNM)
1021 Fourteenth Street, N.W.
Washington, D.C. 20005

The ACNM is the professional organization of nurse-midwives. It sets standards for care and for the education of nurse-midwives and promotes improved maternity care. Publications include: "What Is A Nurse-Midwife?", a pamphlet; "Statements Of Functions, Standards And Qualifications For The Practice Of Nurse-Midwifery;" "Survey Of Legislation Pertaining To The Practice Of Nurse-Midwifery;" and the *Journal Of Nurse-Midwifery,* a quarterly publication of interest to all nurses working in maternal-child care.

American College Of Nursing Home Administrators
4650 East-West Highway
Washington, D.C. 20014

This is the professional organization for administrators of long-term health care facilities. It provides educational programs and professional development. Publications include *Journal Of Long-Term Care Administration,* a quarterly journal, *Long-Term Care Administrator,* a semimonthly newsletter, and several books and booklets on administration of nursing homes.

American Indian/Alaska Native Nurses Association, Inc.
P. O. Box 1588
Norman, Okla. 73070

An association of professional nurses who are Native Americans, this group functions to promote good health for American

Indians, to recruit more American Indians into the nursing profession, and to provide educational information on the health needs of Native Americans. There are over 600 members. The association sponsors an American Indian Nurses Association/Allstate Scholarship for American Indian nursing students attending associate degree programs. (Annual dues: $15, $20 for non/Indian associate members, $1 for student members.)

American Nurses' Association (A.N.A.)
2420 Pershing Road
Kansas City, Mo. 64108

The A.N.A. is the national professional organization for registered nurses encompassing members from all areas of nursing specialties. It is composed of affiliates from each state, Guam, the District Of Columbia and the Virgin Islands.

A.N.A. works toward improving standards of health care for all people, promotes the needs and concerns of nurses through educational programs for professional development, and works toward improved working conditions for nurses. The organization sets standards of practice for each of its five Divisions on Nursing Practice (Community Health, Gerontological, Maternal and Child Health, Medical/Surgical, and Psychiatric and Mental Health Nursing Practice).

A.N.A is active in lobbying for legislation on health care and nursing. The "political action arm" of the organization is N-CAP (Nurses Coalition for Action in Politics, Suite 408, 1030 Fifteenth Street, N.W., Washington, D.C. 20005). N-CAP, funded by contributions of A.N.A members, seeks to make nurses politically aware and active and to support candidates who promote issues affecting nurses and health care. Booklets on political involvement are available from the N-Cap office.

A.N.A. members and associate members who hold a master's degree or higher and are active in the field of research may join the American Nurses' Association Council of Nurse Researchers. The Council promotes research in nursing and publishes the *CNR Newsletter* for members. It works in conjunction with the A.N.A. Commission on Nursing Research.

Other subdivisions of the A.N.A. include the Commission on Human Rights, the Commission on Nursing Education, and the Commission on Nursing Services.

A.N.A has available many publications on all aspects of nursing. These include *Facts About Nursing,* a yearly book of nursing statistics; *The American Nurse,* A.N.A.'s newspaper; and the official monthly journal of the A.N.A., *The American Journal Of Nursing* ($12 a year for non-members, $8 a year for members). Write for a free copy of A.N.A.'s "Publications" list for information on the association's many other materials.

A history of the A.N.A., *One Strong Voice: The Story Of The American Nurses' Association,* compiled by Lyndia Flanagan, 1976, is available from the Lowell Press, Kansas City, Missouri. (Annual dues for the A.N.A. are $35 plus state and local dues for each locality.)

American Public Health Association
1015 Eighteenth Street, N.W.
Washington, D.C. 20036

A.P.H.A. is a national interdisciplinary organization for public health professionals which promotes public health through setting standards for care, education, research, and interdisciplinary exchange. Publications include: *The American Journal Of Public Health,* published monthly; *The Nation's Health,* a monthly newspaper; *Washington Newsletter,* containing information on public health legislation; and a variety of books on public health, communicable diseases and mental health.

American School Health Association
P. O. Box 708
Kent, Oh. 44240

This is an organization for all health professionals involved in the health care of school-aged children. It promotes health education and services for children. Publications include: *The Journal Of School Health,* published ten times yearly; *Guidelines For The School Nurse In The School Health Program,* a manual for school nurses; *Directory Of National Organizations Concerned With School Health,* eighth edition; and guides on health education. (Membership: $30 per year.)

American Society Of Allied Health Professions
One Dupont Circle
Washington, D.C. 20036

This is an organization with members from all of the allied health professions, whose goal is to further health care education and practice by upgrading standards of education and certification for health professionals. The organization has information available on education and career programs in the health fields. Publications include "Allied Health Trends," a monthly newsletter, and a quarterly journal, the *Journal Of Allied Health.*

American Society For Nursing Service Administrators Of The American Hospital Association
840 North Lake Shore Drive
Chicago, Ill. 60611

This is the national professional organization for nursing administrators and is an affiliate of the American Hospital Association. It provides for communication between nursing administrators and the dissemination of literature on nursing administration. Publications include *Nursing Service Administration,* a newsletter, and various "Position Papers."

American Urological Association Allied
c/o Alice Morel, R.N.
National Membership and Promotion Chairman
111 East 210 Street
Bronx, N.Y. 10467

This is a professional organization for nurses and allied health personnel working in urological care. It offers continuing education programs for urology specialists and is planning to produce films on urologic nursing care. Certification exams for urologic specialists are available.

The Association Of Operating Room Nurses, Inc.
10170 East Mississippi Avenue
Denver, Colo. 80231

The A.O.R.N. is a national "organization of registered professional nurses concerned with care of the patient before, during and after surgery." Membership is through local chapters (there are 240 in the U.S.) or individually if there is no chapter in the area. The Association promotes continuing education for operating room nurses. Publications include the monthly journal, *AORN Journal* ($24 a year to non-members), which features information and articles of interest to surgical nurses; the "AORN Standards Of Practice"; and books on topics of interest to nurses in this field. (Membership is $25 a year.)

Association Of Pediatric Oncology Nurses (APON)
c/o Lorraine Bivalec, R.N.
Pacific Medical Center
P. O. Box 7999
San Francisco, Calif. 94120

APON is a professional organization of nurses working with children with cancer. Its goals include providing a means of communication between members and setting standards of care. The organization publishes a quarterly newsletter. (Annual dues: $15.)

Association For Practitioners In Infection Control
P. O. Box 546
Palatine, Ill. 60067

An interdisciplinary organization for health professionals involved with infection control, this Association promotes communication among infection control specialists, and educational and research programs in the field. Publications include the *APIC Journal.* (Annual dues: $25.)

Association Of Radical Midwives
17 Fairfax Road
Derby, England

The A.R.M. is an organization of student and practicing midwives in England. It was founded as a support group for midwives frustrated with recent changes in the role of midwives and the increasing depersonalization of maternity care. With advanced technology and a trend toward more hospital deliveries in England, the role of the midwife in providing continuity of care to families has been eroded. This group seeks to restore the role of the midwife as prime advocate and care giver to mothers and infants. A.R.M. publishes a "Newsletter" with information on its activities and information of interest to maternity nurses and midwives.

Association Of Rehabilitation Nurses (ARN)
Suite 470
1701 Lake Avenue
Glenview, Ill. 60025

The international professional organization for rehabilitation nurses, ARN offers educational opportunities for nurses working in rehabilitation and promotes sharing of information within the field. Publications include the *ARN Journal,* published bimonthly, and "Standards of Rehabilitation Nursing Practices" (published in conjunction with the American Nurses' Association).

Emergency Department Nurses Association (EDNA)
666 North Lake Shore Drive, Suite 1729
Chicago, Ill. 60611

EDNA is the national professional organization for emergency nurses. It offers continuing education programs and works toward improved patient care in emergency nursing. Publications include the *EDNA Continuing Education Curriculum,* the "Standards Of Emergency Nursing Practice" (published in conjunction with the American Nurses' Association), and *JEN, The Journal Of Emergency Nursing,* published bimonthly. (Annual dues: $35.)

International Committee Of Catholic Nurses (C.I.C.I.A.M.S.)
Palazzo S. Callisto
00120 Citta de Vaticano
Rome, Italy

This international organization of Catholic nurses is made up of several national member organizations from throughout the world. There is currently no national organization for Catholic nurses in the United States but Catholic nurses in the U.S. who wish to join the international group may become corresponding individual members and as such will receive the "CICIAMS News."

International Council Of Nurses (ICN)
P. O. Box 42
1121 Geneva 20/ Switzerland

ICN is the international federation of national nurses associations. The member association from the United States is the American Nurses' Association. The ICN aids countries in establishing national nursing organizations and works toward improving the status of nursing and standards of nursing care in member countries. Publications include the *International Nursing Review,* the prestigious bimonthly journal ($15 a year), and literature on nursing care, nursing ethics, and other aspects of international nursing.

National Association Of Pediatric Nurse Associates And Practitioners (NAPNAP)
North Woodbury Road
Box 56
Pitman, N.J. 08071

Active membership in NAPNAP is open to pediatric nurse practitioners and associates, family nurse practitioners and school nurse practitioners. Associate membership is open to anyone interested in supporting this professional organization. NAPNAP offers continuing education for members and works to improve health care for infants and children. Publications include *Pediatric Nursing,* an excellent bimonthly journal ($12 per year), and "Pediatric Nurse Practitioner Newsletter," published bimonthly. (Annual dues: $25.)

National Association Of Physicians' Nurses
9401 Lee Highway, Suite 210
Fairfax, Va. 22030

This is the professional organization for nurses and medical assistants employed by physicians. It conducts educational workshops and seminars and publishes a monthly newsletter, *The Nightingale.*

National Association For Practical Nurse Education And Service, Inc. (NAPNES)
122 East 42nd Street
New York, N.Y. 10017

NAPNES is a national organization devoted to practical nursing which develops and maintains standards of education for practical nurses. It accredits schools of practical nursing and approves programs in continuing education. Publications include *The Journal Of Practical Nursing,* a monthly periodical devoted to "continuing education and clinical needs of LP/VN's." (Cost: $12 a year, U.S.; $13 a year, foreign.)

National Association Of School Nurses, Inc.
An affiliate of the National Education Association
1201 Sixteenth Street, N.W.
Washington, D.C. 20036

This is a professional organization for registered nurses working as school nurses. It promotes the advancement of school nursing and the health care of school-aged children. Publications include a quarterly journal, *The School Nurse,* "Standards For School Nurse Services"; "The School Nurse Specialist Packet" and "Nutrition In Today's Education As A School Nurse Sees It."

National Association Of Spanish Speaking, Spanish Surnamed Nurses
12044 Seventh Avenue, N.W.
Seattle, Wash. 98177

This is a professional organization of Hispanic nurses which promotes quality health care for Hispanics in this country. The Association publishes a *Newsletter* for members, a "Directory Of Hispanic Nurses In The United States," and holds a biennial National Conference.

National Black Nurses Association, Inc.
425 Ohio Building
175 South Main Street
Akron, Oh. 44308

This is an organization for bringing together black nurses and promoting good health for Black people. Membership is open to all R.N.'s, L.P.N.'s, L.V.N.'s and nursing students. Members join through local chapter affiliates or individually if no local chapter exists. (Annual dues: $25 a year, $10 for students.)

National Center For Nursing Ethics
P. O. Box 2237
Cincinnati, Oh. 45201

This non-profit organization is devoted to the study of nursing ethics. Publications include "Update On Ethics," a newsletter, and the *Journal Of Nursing Ethics*.

National Federation Of Licensed Practical Nurses, Inc.
888 Seventh Avenue, 18th Floor
New York, N.Y. 10019

This is the "national professional organization for licensed practical/vocational nurses and practical nursing students in the United States." Membership is through local and state affiliates. The organization serves as the voice of practical vocational nurses and promotes high standards of nursing education and patient care. It has a data bank of continuing education units for members which keeps track of their continuing education units received from programs approved by NFLPN.

The group maintains representation in Washington, D.C., to lobby for its interests.

The official publication is *The Journal Of Nursing Care,* published monthly. (Members obtain it as part of their dues, non-members' fee is $9 a year.) Annual membership fee is $25.

National Intravenous Therapy Association, Inc.
850 Third Avenue, 11th Floor
New York, N.Y. 10022

N.I.T.A is a professional organization for health care workers involved with I.V. therapy. Members include registered nurses, L.P.N.'s, technicians and pharmaceutical representatives. The organization "is a member of the Federation of Specialty Nursing Organizations and the A.N.A."

N.I.T.A establishes standards of care, promotes quality patient care in the field of I.V. therapy, provides information on this field and promotes quality education for I.V. therapists. It has local chapter affiliates throughout the United States.

Publications include *NITA,* the official publication of the association, published six times yearly by the J. B. Lippincott Co.

National Joint Practice Commission
35 East Wacker Drive, Suite 1990
Chicago, Ill. 60601

This is an organization of practicing nurses and physicians established by the American Medical Association and American Nurses' Association to promote the collaboration of nurses and doctors to improve patient care. Publications include *National Joint Practice Commission Bulletin,* and *Together: A Casebook Of Joint Practice in Primary Care* (paperback, $5.95).

National League For Nursing, Inc. (NLN)
10 Columbus Circle
New York, N.Y. 10019

NLN is a non-profit organization uniting nursing leaders in the fields of nursing education and nursing services with other health professionals. NLN has both individual members (registered and practical nurses, allied health workers and others interested in promoting good nursing care) and agency members (educational institutions, hospitals, public health agencies, and others).

The organization accredits nursing education programs (A.D., B.S., diploma, practical nursing and master's programs). It offers consultation to nursing schools and provides continuing education seminars and workshops.

In its Nursing Services division the NLN is composed of the Council Of Home Health Agencies and Community Health Services, the Council Of Hospital And Related Institutional Nursing Services, and the National Forum For Administrators Of Nursing Services. Through these Councils, the NLN offers consultation and education in each area of interest.

NLN offers tests for admission to nursing schools and is the testing agency for the State Board Test Pool Examination for registered and practical nurses.

NLN has a Division Of Research which conducts surveys and other research.

Through its Public Affairs Committee, NLN studies issues in health policy and promotes health care legislation.

The League Exchange is a subgroup of the NLN which publishes and distributes materials for the sharing of knowledge and skills among nurses. Nurses having reports or materials which other nurses could learn from, may submit them for consideration for publication to the League Exchange.

The publications available from NLN are many and include: *Nursing Outlook,* the official monthly journal of the organization, geared toward leaders in nursing and covering topics such as current trends in health care, education for health professionals, and legality; *NLN News,* a newsletter; publications on NLN programs and services; information on accreditation of programs; information on nursing and nursing education (including names and addresses of schools for each level of nursing education); testing information; nursing services information; and record forms for health agencies and nursing schools. Write for a copy of *NLN Publications Catalog* for detailed listings. (Annual membership dues for NLN: $25.)

National Male Nurse Association
2309 State Street, West Office
Saginaw, Mich. 48602

This association promotes the entrance of men into the field of nursing and provides a voice for male nurses. Membership is open to R.N.'s and L.P.N.'s, licensed psychiatric attendants, and student nurses, of both sexes. Publications include brochures on men in nursing and a bimonthly newsletter, "Men In Nursing." (Annual dues: $20 for active nurses, $10 for students and retired nurses.)

National Nurses for Life, Inc.
P. O. Box 75
Allison Park, Pa. 15101

This is an organization for nurses interested in the "pro-life movement," especially those against abortion and euthanasia. The group provides educational material on these topics and works to protect nurses who refuse to take part in abortions or euthanasia from losing their jobs.

National Perinatal Association
800 Madison Avenue
Memphis, Tenn. 38163

This is a multi-disciplinary organization of members of state or regional perinatal associations and members-at-large. It promotes optimum perinatal health and health care through education of professionals and health care receivers and promotes perinatal health care legislation. The Association serves as a resource for local groups or individuals interested in establishing a perinatal group. It publishes *Perinatal Press,* ten times a year ($10 per year in U.S., $12 in Canada and Mexico, $13.50 all other countries, with reduced rates for members.)

National Student Nurses Association, Inc.
10 Columbus Circle
New York, N.Y. 10019

This is the organization for students in programs preparing for R.N. licensure and is composed of state and local chapters. The Association publishes *Imprint,* a quarterly magazine for nursing students ($5 a year for non-members, no charge for members), and several other publications of interest to students on such topics as career choices within nursing. Scholarships, malpractice insurance, and reduced rates for the *American Journal Of Nursing* and the A.N.A. convention are available to members. (Annual dues: $10.)

Nurses Association Of The American College
Of Obstetricians And Gynecologists (NAACOG)
One East Wacker Drive, Suite 2700
Chicago, Ill. 60601

NAACOG is a professional organization of nurses and allied health care workers employed in obstetric, gynecologic and neonatal nursing. Active membership is open to R.N.'s in the field and associate membership is available to licensed practical/vocational nurses and allied health personnel.

NAACOG offers a certification program for inpatient obstetric nurses, OB/Gyn nurse practitioners and neonatal intensive care nurses. It also conducts seminars and workshops and continuing education programs.

Publications include: *The Journal Of Obstetric, Gynecologic and Neonatal Nursing,* published bimonthly ($15 a year to non-members); *NAACOG Bulletin* (published monthly, for members only); books on standards of care in the field and on family centered care; and technical bulletins on aspects of nursing care of interest to the OB/Gyn nurse.

Nurse Consultants' Association (N.C.A.)
℅ Susan Lee, R.N., Secretary N.C.A.
87 East Hamilton Avenue
Englewood, N.J. 07631

This is a new professional organization for registered nurses who serve as consultants and liaisons between the nursing professional and the health care manufacturing industry, promoting optimal patient care. Membership is open to nurses employed as consultants to companies in the health care industry.

Nurse Healers Professional Associates Cooperative
Box 7
70 Shelley Avenue
Port Chester, N.Y. 10573

This is a non-profit organization for nurses involved in alternative healing practices, focusing on a holistic approach rather than the traditional treatment-of-illness approach. The group serves as a forum for sharing research and skills and as a resource for information on health professionals working in alternative healing practices who are available for workshops and seminars.

Nurses House, Inc.
Room 1616
60 East 42nd Street
New York, N.Y. 10017

Nurses House is a national non-profit organization which assists registered nurses in financial need due to illness or disability. It is composed of members who join to support this function. A nurse need not be a member to receive aid from the organization. Nurses who are in temporary financial need and require assistance may apply for aid themselves or be referred by another nurse. All nurses interested in helping other nurses are urged to join Nurses House since it is the contributions of members which make it possible to provide financial assistance to nurses who need it.

Nurses in Transition
P.O. Box 14472
San Francisco, CA 94114

This is a local support group for nurses which also assists nurses in other locations in establishing similar support groups. Publications include a "Nurses in Transition Newsletter" ($5.00/year). (This material is adapted from *Medical Self-Care*, Number 7, 1979, p. 60, © 1979, *Medical Self-Care*).

Oncology Nursing Society (ONS)
P. O. Box 33
Oakmont, Pa. 15139

Established in 1975, this organization of oncology nursing specialists works toward increasing knowledge on the prevention and treatment of cancer, sharing this knowledge with others working in the field of malignant diseases, fostering educational programs in this nursing specialty, and establishing standards for nursing care. The ONS publishes a quarterly journal, the *Oncology Nursing Forum*. (Annual dues: $25.)

Orthopedic Nurses Association, Inc.
1938 Peachtree Road, N.W., Suite 501
Atlanta, Georgia 30309

This is the national professional organization for R.N.'s and L.P./V.N.'s involved in orthopedic nursing. It sets standards for practice, offers exchange of information and continuing education. O.N.A. publishes a monthly journal, *Orthopedic Nurses Association, Inc. Journal* and has available orthopedic manuals and audiovisual aids of use to nurses in this field. (Annual dues: $15 plus local chapter fee.)

Self Care Associates
P. O. Box 161
Boulder Creek, Ca. 95006

This is a group of nurses working together to promote preventive health practices and self care. A book service is available, offering books on self care as well as a newsletter for the sharing of ideas in this field, and classes on self care. The group is new and growing and welcomes input from nurses working in preventive health and self care. (This material is adapted from *Medical Self-Care*, Number 8, 1980, p. 58, © 1980, *Medical Self-Care*.)

30 Sources of Equipment and Supplies of Use to Nurses and Their Clients

With more nurses practicing independently, and with nurses having an increased say in the administration of some health care institutions, it is useful for nurses to have knowledge of sources for equipment and supplies.

The following companies manufacture products of use to nurses and their clients. The information on the companies and their products is adapted from their catalogs and promotional brochures. The companies are listed alphabetically in the following general categories: Patient Care, Obstetrics, Surgery, Urological and Ostomy Supplies, Teaching Aids, and Uniforms and Supplies for Nurses. Write directly to the companies for information on local distributors, detailed product information, price lists and any other products they may carry.

I. Types of Tape and Their Uses
II. Stethoscopes and Sphygmomanometers
III. Sources for Patient Care Equipment and Supplies
IV. Sources for Obstetric Equipment and Supplies
V. Sources for Surgical Equipment and Supplies
  Surgical Instruments and Their Care
IV. Sources for Urological and Ostomy Appliances
  Characteristics of Ostomy Appliances
VII. Sources for Teaching Aids
VIII. Sources for Uniforms and Other Supplies For Nurses
  Nursing Uniforms—Yesterday—And Today

Stethoscopes

For an excellent guide to the types of stethoscopes available and which one best suits your needs, see "For the Last Word On Stethoscopes Listen Here!" by Estelle Beaumont, RN, in *Nursing*

78, November, 1978, pp. 32–37. This article describes the various types of stethoscopes and their uses, and lists sources for obtaining them, including estimated costs of purchase.

Sphygmomanometers

A similar article rating sphygmomanometers appeared in *Consumer Reports,* March, 1979. For a copy of the issue send $1.00 to: Consumer's Union, 256 Washington St., Mt. Vernon, N.Y. 10550.

This material is adapted from *Medical Self-Care,* Number Six, Fall, 1979, p. 54.

Types of tape and their uses

HYPOALLERGENIC ADHESIVE

BACKING	MOST COMMON USES
Paper	Light dressings for wounds with drains, such as appendectomies.
Taffeta	Medium to heavy dressings for draining wounds, such as from a cholecystectomy, requiring frequent dressing changes; Montgomery straps.

REGULAR * ADHESIVE (rubber base)

BACKING	MOST COMMON USES
Plastic	Securing IVs and catheters.
Cotton cloth ("adhesive tape")	Support and immobilization; dynamic strapping (ankle taping).
Elastic cloth (similar to an elastic bandage, but with adhesive backing)	Dynamic strapping, as for fractured ribs; pressure dressings. Not usually applied directly to skin. Generally applied over a layer of gauze, as when taping ribs, or over a combine dressing.

Reprinted by permission from *RN Magazine,* May, 1979, page 32.

Sources for Patient Care Equipment and Supplies

Acme Medical Scales
P. O. Box 8601
Emeryville Station
Oakland, Calif. 94662

Acme manufactures in-bed scales, digital bedside scales, chair scales for the ambulatory and partially disabled, and wheelchair weighing ramps.

Aeroceuticals, Division of ATI, Inc.
P. O. Box 4
49 John Street
Southport, Conn. 06490

Aeroceuticals manufactures a disposable flotation system—a hydrostatic mattress for one-time adult use.

It also manufactures aerosol sprays for a variety of purposes: first aid for burns, topical anesthesia, antiseptic spray, adhesive tape remover, alcohol sprays, skin conditioner, eyeglass cleaner, air sterilizers, and disinfectants. Sterilization trays and instrument racks and holders are also available.

Ames Company
Division Miles Laboratories, Inc.
Elkhart, Ind. 46514

Ames offers a variety of in vitro diagnostic products such as reagent strip tests, blood analyzers, automated urinalysis instruments and slide stainers.

BAXA Corporation
1968 Raymond Drive
Northbook, Ill. 60062

Baxa manufactures an oral liquid dispenser for pediatric patients, along with a bottle adaptor, an I.V. additive cap, and a narcotic accounting system. The company also distributes the following products manufactured by Burron Medical Products: a filter straw, a vacuum transfer tube, and a vented piggyback I.V. set.

Becton-Dickinson
Division of Becton, Dickinson and Company
Rutherford, N.J. 07070

B-D manufactures single-use and reusable hypodermic equipment, fever thermometers, elastic support products, laboratory products and specialty instrumentation products for I.V. therapy, anesthesiology, and biopsy needles.

Beiersdorf, Inc.
P. O. Box 529
South Norwalk, Conn. 06854

Beiersdorf makes adhesive dressings in sixteen different sizes and shapes including special bandages for the large and small digits, the knuckle, toes and eyes.

Be OK
Self-Help Aids
Fred Sammons, Inc.
Box 32
Brookfield, Illinois 60513

Fred Sammons, Inc. carries a large line of "Be OK Self-Help Aids" for the handicapped. Products available include aids for eating, dressing, homemaking, wheelchair accessories, and many others. The products are sold to health professionals and institutions only, though they may order for their clients.

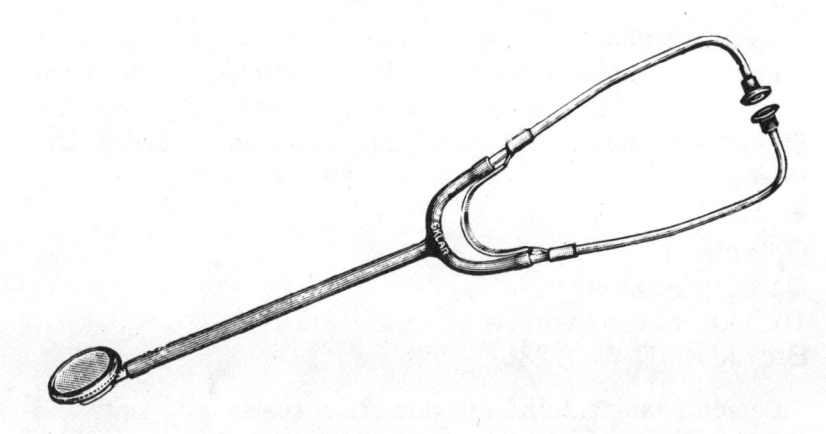

Reprinted by permission of J. Sklar Co. from *Sklar Products Surgical Instruments* (Catalog), 19th edition, © 1978.

Burron Medical Products, Inc.
824 12th Avenue
Bethlehem, Pa. 18018

Burron manufactures disposable I.V. additive products for filtration needs, including: a filter needle, a double filtered I.V. set, an extension set which features a five micron conical filter plus flashbulb and slide clamp, a vented needle, a primary solution I.V. set, and a secondary I.V. set.

Carolyn Health Care Products
800 Chatham Road
Winston-Salem, N.C. 27107

Carolyn Health Care Products has a special bandage to aid in the application of nitroglycerine ointment, support hosiery, and elastic bandages.

Cincinnati Sub Zero Products, Inc.
2612 Gilbert Avenue
Cincinnati, Ohio 45206

This company manufactures a hyper-hypothermia system: blankets, disposable covers, and instrumentation for remote reading of temperature.

Daisy Manufacturing Co.
39 Bridge Street
South Hadley Falls, Mass. 01075

Daisy manufactures patient positioners, wheelchair rests, walker pouches, bibs, wheelchair foam cushions, assorted body holders, supports and belts, hamper bags, stands and caps. Products are sold directly to nursing homes and hospitals. Buy directly from the manufacturer for a 20% discount.

Detecto
Detecto Scales
103-00 Foster Avenue
Brooklyn, N.Y. 11236

Detecto manufactures a talking scale, scales for infants, and other clinical scales including digital ones for doctors and hospitals. The scales may be purchased from surgical supply dealers.

Diatek, Inc.
3910 Sorrento Valley Boulevard
San Diego, Calif. 92121

Diatek manufactures electronic thermometers.

Dyna Med, Inc.
6200 Yarrow Drive
Carlsbad, CA 92008

Dyna Med manufactures all types of emergency health care equipment and supplies. Products available include equipment for resuscitation, transport, first aid and patient monitoring, and such unique items as a "medi-vest" for emergency workers to wear to hold their supplies, and simulation kits and models (such as the "Resusci-Anne") for practicing first aid measures and delivery procedures, anatomical charts, and books on emergency care.

Edwards Laboratories
Division of American Hospital Supply Corporation
P. O. Box 11150
17221 Red Hill Avenue
Santa Ana, Calif. 92711

Edwards offers prostheses, cardiac catheters, and a variety of electronic equipment such as a thermodilution cardiac output computer.

Everest and Jennings, Inc.
1803 Pontius Avenue
Los Angeles, Calif. 90025

Everest and Jennings, Inc. manufactures suction equipment (floor and portable models), stretchers, power wheelchairs, patient lifts and other patient aids such as commodes, shower chairs, walking aids, overbed tables, patient operated stretchers, moist heat treatment pads and whirlpool bath units.

Distribution centers are located in Los Angeles, Murray Hill, N.J., Bensenville, Ill., Atlanta, Ga., and Grand Prairie, Tex.

Extracorporeal Medical Specialties, Inc.
Royal and Ross Roads
King of Prussia, Pa. 19406

Extracorporeal manufactures dialysis products, vascular access devices, dialysate delivery systems, products for I.V.

therapy, tracheostomy and endotracheal tubes, cardiovascular and surgical products.

Fashion Able
Rocky Hill, N.J. 08553

Fashion Able carries a wide variety of products for the handicapped including special clothing and self-help aids to daily living.

Geddis, Inc.
Box 1262
Dunedin, Fla. 33528

Geddis distributes a hydraulic lift bath tub chair for Trevo, Inc.

Gerber Family Health Care
Division of Gerber Products Company
445 State Street
Fremont, Mich. 49412

Gerber makes products for incontinency, snap-on cotton/vinyl stretch pants, and a disposable absorbent pad, in sizes for adults and children. Available by direct order only, they are not sold in retail stores. Special prices are available for institutions.

Green Mountain Products, Inc.
Muller Park
Norwalk, Conn. 06852

Green Mountain offers home health care aids such as furniture leg extenders, a product called Reach and Grip which has a retrieving hook and a magnetic loop to make reaching easy, and a lighted cane.

Health and Safety Products
P. O. Box 778
Palm Harbor, Fla. 33563

This company makes a stethoscope that blocks out 90% of outside noises that interfere with sound acuity. Useful for tests in ambulances, planes and other moving vehicles.

Healthco, Inc.
Medical Supply Division
25 Stuart Street
Boston, Mass. 02116

Healthco manufactures physician's supplies and equipment, including: furniture for reception and business area, examining and treatment rooms, waiting and consultation rooms, instruments such as neurological hammers, stethoscopes, head mirrors, eye test charts, catheters and pessaries; laboratory equipment and supplies; dressings; and such products as tongue depressors, ear basins, silver nitrate applicators, door signs, urine specimen bottles, and others.

Heelbo Corporation
5745 West Howard Street
Niles, Ill. 60648

Heelbo offers decubitus protector pads, slippers, and patient positioners.

Hill-Rom Company, Inc.
A Hillenbrand Industries Co.,
Batesville, Ind. 47006

Hill-Rom provides hospital beds, bedside cabinets, safety lights, reclining chairs and overbed tables, and a centralized vertical column which provides critical patient care incorporating electric switches, medical gases, receptacles, lighting potentials, and a nurse call system, clock, night light, telephone and emergency power receptacles.

Hollister, Inc.
211 East Chicago Avenue
Chicago, Ill. 60611
or
Hollister, LTD.
322 Consumers Road
Willowdale, Ontario M2J 1P8
Canada

Hollister makes many ostomy products such as stoma bags and drains, and a variety of other products including birth certificates, a circumcision tray, umbilical cord clamp, on-patient identification, signs for doors, beds and walls, and newborn and pediatric urine specimen collectors.

Identical Form, Inc.
17 West 60th Street
New York, N.Y. 10023

This company offers identical breast forms for mastectomy patients.

IVAC Corporation
11353 Sorrento Valley Road
San Diego, Calif. 92121

Mail: P. O. Box 2385
La Jolla, Calif. 92038

IVAC offers parenteral medication delivery systems, an electronic clinical thermometer, and system programs for I.V. therapy and clinical thermometry.

Jobst Institute, Inc.
Box 653
653 Miami Street
Toledo, Ohio 43694

Jobst offers a variety of custom-made venous-pressure supports for arms, legs, hands and for use in pregnancy. The company also has a jolastic washing solution and general body lotion, a hydro-float pad for wheelchairs, anti-burn/scar supports, mastectomy products, anti-embolism extremity pumps, commode pads, water beds and anti-shock airpants.

Ken McRight Supplies, Inc.
7456 South Oswego
Tulsa, Okla. 74136

This company offers anti-decubitus air cushions that equalize pressure, seat cushions and pneumatic mattress units.

F & F Koenigkramer
96 Caldwell Drive
Cincinnati, Ohio 45216

Among the products manufactured by F & F Koenigkramer are examination and treatment chairs, tables, wall units and instrument stands, adjustable stools, and surgery and treatment tables.

Lumex, Inc.
Medical Equipment and Patient Aids
100 Spence Street
Bay Shore, N.Y. 11706

and

2960 Leonis Boulevard
Los Angeles, Calif. 90058

Lumex offers the following products: footstools, I.V. stands, trapeze bars, grab bars, overbed tables, bedrails, recliners, canes and crutches, commodes, shower and bath aids, safety rests and body holders, and wheelchair seat pads.

Maddak, Inc.
Pequannock, N.J. 07440

Maddak's products for home health care and aids for daily living include: walkers, wheelchair accessories, exercise and recreation equipment, heat/cold therapy products, communication aids such as a breath operated call signal for calling a nurse or aide, furniture, bathroom and toilet aids, reading aids such as page turners and book holders, writing aids, dressing aids, grooming aids, eating and drinking aids, kitchen and household aids (including a special potato peeler and jar opener), cushions and pillows, automotive and garden aids, diagnostic testing products such as a finger-muscle tester, and laboratory products including microscope covers and utility bags. These products are available through surgical dealers.

Marion Scientific Corporation
A Marion Laboratories Company
9233 Ward Parkway
Kansas City, Mo. 64114

Marion manufactures ammonia inhalants, a variety of first aid kits, an emergency resuscitator, a scrub applicator for use in skin prep procedures, a transparent isolation unit for both primary and secondary isolation of anaerobic bacterial specimens, a disposable environmental system designed to maintain a CO_2-enriched environment, and a number of microbiological collection products.

Mason Rubber Company
Division of MRC Industries, Inc.
115 West 27th Street
New York, N.Y. 10001

Mason offers wheelchair cushions in varying sizes.

Medex Products Corporation
323 Niagara Street
Buffalo, N.Y. 14201

Medex offers form-cut plastic bandages, available in fingertip sizes, strips, patches and spots, and plastic surgical tape in rolls of 40 yards.

Metropolitan Wire Corporation
Wilkes-Barre, Pa. 18705

This company makes wire shelves for storage, laundry, dietary, pharmacy and operating rooms. Also available is a group of utility carts with open wire or solid stainless steel shelves, or a combination of both.

Monoject
Division of Sherwood Medical
St. Louis, Mo. 63103

Monoject manufactures a blood collection system and laboratory products such as collection tubes, collecting needles, metal hubs, plastic hubs, needle holders, syringes, lancets, culture tubes, delivery trays, disposable boxes for contaminated materials, oral medication syringes, surgeon's gloves, utility gloves, glove racks, and a number of prepackaged procedure trays (for lumbar puncture, gastroanalysis, fetal blood sampling, spinal anesthesia, and others).

Nelson Medical Products
5690 Sarah Avenue
Sarasota, Fla. 33583

This company has available a variety of self help devices and automotive aids, including: hand controls for accelerator and brakes in automobiles; a spinner bar for those with difficulty grasping a steering wheel; wheelchair ramps; special food utensils; dressing aids such as a long reach zipper pull and shoe remover; doorknob levers; electric razor holder; chair leg extenders; external catheters and accessories; enema kits; incontinent pants; bathroom aids; foot, heel and elbow protectors; hydraulic bath lift; phone holders for quadriplegics; home blood pressure kits; canes, crutches and walkers, and knee separators. A unique item from Nelson's is their bowling ball holder and a bowling stick for wheelchair bowlers.

Neutrogena Corporation
5755 West 96th Street
Los Angeles, Calif. 90045

Neutrogena makes soaps, bath gels, shampoos, and skin care products such as hand cream and body oil.

Norton Health Care Products
P. O. Box 350
Akron, Ohio 44309

Norton manufactures monitoring and administration tubing in a variety of lengths. Sales offices are also in New York City; Atlanta, Ga.; Rolling Meadows (Chicago), Ill.; Houston, Tex.; and Irving (L.A.) Calif.

N/R Laboratories
900 East Franklin Street
Centerville, Ohio 45459

N/R Laboratories makes a no-rinse shampoo, a hair conditioner, and a body bath, that require no water for usage. They are useful for bedridden or convalescing patients.

Oem Medical, Inc.
29 Meridian Road
Edison, N.J. 08817

Oem offers the following inhalation therapy products: oxygen outlets, flowmeters, airway emergency packs, nebulizers, disposable corrugated tubing, vinyl face masks, nasal cannula, a neonatal resuscitator and a disposable sealing mouthpiece.

Omnimed, Inc.
Cooper Street and Rt. 130
Burlington, N.J. 08016

and

8765 Lankershim Blvd.
Sun Valley, Calif. 01352

Omnimed offers the following items: chart accessories, I.V. holders, identification bracelets, emergency drug kits, birth records, dye/disinfectant for umbilical stumps, witch hazel pads, anesthetic sprays, plastic zip bags, arm slings, safety jackets, vests and belts, body holders, cervical collars, cushions and pillows, surgeon's masks, and a variety of restraints and limb holders.

J. T. Posey Company
5635 Peck Road
Arcadia, Calif. 91006

Posey manufactures safety vests, belts, limb holders, plastic cuffs, foot care products, limb protectors, wheelchair accessories, physical therapy products, orthopedic products, slings, bed accessories, pediatric, emergency, and surgical products. Posey maintains warehouses in many states.

Principle Business Enterprises, Inc.
Pine Lake Industrial Park
Dunbridge, Ohio 43414

PBE manufactures laundry bags, hamper stands, restraints, bibs and slippers. The products are marketed through surgical laundry and linen supply dealers throughout the U.S. and Europe.

Rajowalt Company, Inc.
Atwood, Ind. 46502

Rajowalt offers fracture and rehabilitation equipment, including: a hair-rinser for chair-bound patients, cervical and lumbar traction units, folding wheelchairs, splints, knee caps, slings, collars, belts, immobilizers, traction accessories, walkers, post-op shoes, crutches, canes, bath accessories, and exercisers.

Raymo Products, Inc.
212 South Blake
Olathe, Kansas 66061

The following products are available from Raymo: a mobile medication chart, walker trays, reading rack and lap tray, medication card time racks, diet card racks (as well as the cards themselves), medication and thermometer trays, chart holder wall racks, shampoo-rinse trays, and record racks for beds. Custom-made racks and trays will be produced to fit customers' special needs.

Roehampton Medical Supply Co., Ltd.
271 Dewey Avenue
Rochester, N.Y. 14608

This company makes a silver swaddler to prevent hypothermia in the newborn. They also offer a polyurethane foam dressing for use in the care of burns, and an emergency squad kit for fire departments, ambulance units, police cars, and industrial first-aid and fire stations.

Sage Products, Inc.
1300 Morse Avenue
Elk Grove Village, Ill. 60007

Sage offers a full range of specimen collection containers

such as a midstream urine collection kit, a 24-hour urine collection cooling wrap, a 24-hour specimen collection container, and a calculi strainer.

Sclano, Inc.
5 Mansard Court
Wayne, N.J. 07470

Sclano manufactures a T.B. skin test which is a sterile multiple-puncture device containing a tuberculin PPD used for identification of individuals who have a delayed hypersensitivity to tuberculin. It uses a spring device to avoid excess pressure or accidental twisting.

Sigmamotor, Inc.
14 Elizabeth Street
Middleport, N.Y. 14105

Sigmamotor manufactures a volumetric I.V. pump which may be acquired through purchase, lease or a trade-in program.

Smithkline Diagnostics
880 West Maude Avenue
P. O. Box 1947
Sunnyvale, Calif. 94086

Smithkline offers diagnostic culturing systems for throat infections, gonorrhea, trichomonal infections, staphylococcus aureus, and others. The company also offers a test for fecal occult blood. It has distribution offices around the U.S.

Sterling Name Tape Company
177 Depot Street
Winsted, Conn. 06098

This company manufactures washproof sew-on name tapes, with lettering in black, blue or red, on white tape.

Surgical Products Company
P. O. Box 369
Needham, Mass. 02192

This company makes elastic hosiery for above and below the knee, with full foot or open toe; elastic and support panty hose; and ankle, knee and wrist braces. There are special values for irregulars.

Teledyne Water Pik
1730 East Prospect Street
Fort Collins, Colo. 80525

Teledyne makes products for dental use such as rechargeable automatic toothbrushes, and an oral irrigator. Other products include shower massages, water filters, smoking withdrawal systems, smoke alarms, foot massagers, permanent weight loss systems, baby food makers and warmers, baby spoons, tumblers, and overall bibs.

Three-M Company
Surgical Products Division
3-M Center
St. Paul, Minn. 55101

3-M offers tapes and dressings, rehabilitation products, diagnostic instruments, ECG products, radiation therapy products, critical care and diagnostic products, clinical lab services, sterilization equipment, sterile packaging, and protective masks. Products are available through local representatives.

The Vollroth Company
1236 North 18th Street
Sheboygan, Wisc. 53081

Vollroth makes reusable and autoclavable patient care products such as bed pans, wash basins, soapdishes, emesis basins, sponge bowls, urinals, thermometer and forceps jars, and bedside trays including pitchers and cups. Products for patient treatment include dressing jars, solution bowls, sterilization units and instrument trays. Products for patient service include insulated servers, tea or coffee pots, menu holders and beverage servers. Laboratory products include beakers, funnels, and graduated measures. Operating room products include I.V. stands, instrument tray stands, solution bowl stands, buckets and bucket covers and stands. Vollrath has several sales representatives in all sections of the U.S.

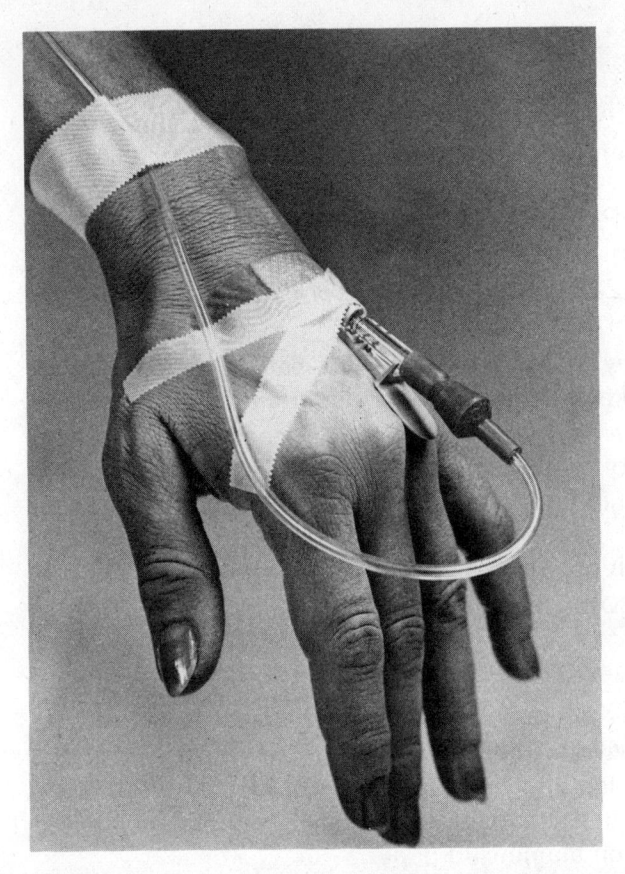

"Gordon 'IVs' Intravenous Stabilizer" in place on patient's hand. This is used for "securely locking IV catheters in place." Photo courtesy of Whitman Medical Corporation, 990 Raritan Rd., Clark, N.J. 07066. Reprinted by permission. For further information on the Stabilizer, write Whitman Medical Corporation.

Sources for Obstetrics Supplies and Equipment

Cascade Birthing Supplies
Paul and Donna Ruscher
109 NW 35th St., #N
Corvallis, OR 97330

A wide variety of birthing supplies including birthing kits and fetoscopes is available from Cascade Birthing Supplies. Write for free brochure.

This information is adapted from "Napsac News," Winter, 1979, Vol. 4, No. 4, published by the International Association of Parents and Professionals for Safe Alternatives in Childbirth.

Evenflo
771 North Freedom Street
Ravenna, Ohio 44261

Evenflo manufactures a breast pump kit.

Health Care Products, Inc.
9597 W. Ohio Avenue
P. O. Box 26221
Denver, Colorado 80226

This company offers a lambskin for babies to sleep on or under, said to keep babies warm in winter and cool in summer; the lambskin can be washed by hand or machine. Health Care Products also offer a washable sheepskin used for the prevention of decubiti in bedridden patients.

Obstetrics Diversified
31983 Emerson Lane
P. O. Box 797
Cottage Grove, Oreg. 97424

This company offers an electronic instrument to record and print continuous fetal heart data, without the necessity of straps or apparatus being attached to the baby or mother. Information is funneled by the attendant, synchronized by mini-computer, and visualized on aluminized paper.

Obstetrics Diversified also manufactures an obstetrical delivery pan, with special features including: a dip for extension of the infant's head, allowing for deep suctioning if necessary; hand grips; and a basin for body fluids and placenta (the height of the basin allows for delivery of the shoulders).

Far Right;
Stethoscope for Auscultation of Fetal Heart

Left;
Grave's Speculum

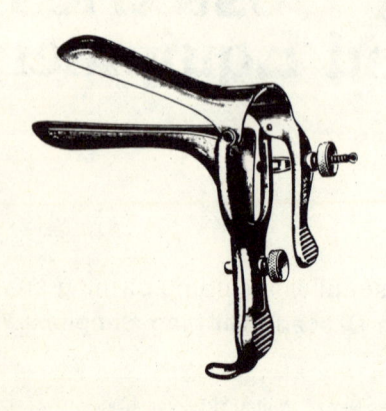

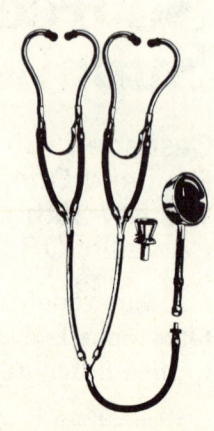

Reprinted by permission of J. Sklar Co. from *Sklar Products Surgical Instruments* (Catalog), 19th edition, © 1978.

Snugli Cottage Industries
1150 Colorado Highway 74
Evergreen, Colo. 80439

Snugli makes a baby carrier that is used in hospitals for premature infants to increase the amount of physical contact and stimulation provided these infants. It can also be used in pediatrics with infants with failure-to-thrive syndrome, for treatment of colic, and for congenital hip disorder. When ordering, be sure to distinguish between regular and premie snuglis, or regular will be shipped. Hospitals and medical facilities may purchase snuglis singly or in any quantity at wholesale prices.

The J. B. Williams Company, Inc.
Diagnostic Division
767 Fifth Avenue
New York, N.Y. 10022

This company manufactures an in-home pregnancy test.

Sources for Surgical Equipment and Supplies

Anchor Products Company
52 Official Road
Addison, Ill. 60101

Anchor manufactures surgical needles of varying sizes, disposal and packed in cartons of 20 and 144. Reusables are also available. They may be ordered from local distributors.

Baka Manufacturing Co.
7-11 Cross Street
Plainville, Mass. 02762

Baka manufactures the Dale line of medical products which includes abdominal binders, catheter tube holders, rib belts, and a hospital utility grip for organizing and holding O.R. equipment such as suction tubes, I.V. tubing, and cautery leads. Products available from hospital supply dealers.

Beaver
Rudolph Beaver, Inc.
480 Trapelo Road
Belmont, Mass. 02178

Beaver offers a variety of surgical blades including a periodontal knife kit, orthopedic and podiatry blades and handles. Orders may be placed with any local Beaver dealer.

BG Bio Clinic Co.
Division of Medidyne, Inc.
59 East Orange Grove Avenue
Burbank, Calif. 91502
and

70 State Road
Media, Pa. 19063

This company offers operating room protectors and positioners, including foam towels and pads, cushions and wedges for various parts of the body.

Chaston Medical and Surgical Products
3 Huntington Quad
Melville, N.Y. 11746

Chaston offers a soapless, non-irritating, non-alkaline microbicidal health care personnel handwash in bar form containing povidone-iodine U.S.P. 5%. It also makes a surgical scrub solution, dispensers, swabsticks, an ointment, and a concentrate.

Dover Products
Will Ross, Inc.
Milwaukee, Wisc. 53212

Dover Products include items for urology, anesthesiology, and surgical specialties. They make catheters, catheter trays, drainage bags, tracheostomy cleaning trays, and both adult and pediatric tracheostomy tubes.

Gilbert Surgical Instruments, Inc.
115 Harding Avenue
Bellmawr, N.J. 08031

Gilbert manufactures trachea tubes, laryngectomy tubes, and miscellaneous instruments such as suction tubes, uterine sounds and curettes.

MDT Corporation
Medical Division

MDT Corporation products are manufactured at:

Sterilization Systems Group
15025 South Main Street
Gardena, Calif. 90248

and

Examining Equipment Group
19365 S.W. 89th Avenue
Tualatin, Oreg. 97062

MDT sells surgical lamps, sterilizers and accessories, chairs and stools.

Medicom Instruments
3188 Doolittle Drive
Northbrook, Ill. 60062

Medicom manufactures a large variety of surgical instruments for all types of surgery and dentistry.

National Catheter Co.
A Division of Mallinckrodt, Inc.
Hook Road
Argyle, N.Y. 12809

This company makes a sterile disposable tracheal tube for adults and children. It also makes an endotracheal tube which provides directional tip control for difficult nasal intubation, and another model of tracheal tube with a double lumen for irrigation purposes, gas sampling or pressure monitoring of the trachea. These devices may be sold only by order of a physician, according to Federal Law.

Olympus Corporation of America
4 Nevada Drive
New Hyde Park, N.Y. 11042

The Medical Instrument Division of Olympus manufactures fiberscopes, endophotographic systems, and camera adaptors, along with standard accessories.

Perry
A Division of Affiliated Hospital Products, Inc.
1875 Harsh Avenue, S.E.
Massillon, Ohio 44646

Perry offers surgeons' gloves, medical gloves, sterile tubing, tourniquets, catheters and instrument detergents. Orders should be placed through franchised distributors.

The Purdue Frederick Company
Norwalk, Conn. 06856

This company manufactures microbicidal antiseptics for infection control programs, including a surgical scrub, a skin cleanser, a vaginal gel, and an aerosol spray, as well as an antiseptic gauze pad, a microbicidal applicator, swabsticks, and other cleansing and disinfecting agents.

Quinton Instrument Co.
2121 Terry Avenue
Seattle, Wash. 98121

Quinton manufactures A-V cannula systems, gastrointestinal biopsy instruments, portable oxygen meters, anthropometric instruments, and other miscellaneous accessories.

Richard-Allen Medical Industries
P. O. Box 351
Richland, Mich. 49083

Richard-Allen sells microscope slides, cover-glasses, cytology fixatives, surgeons' blades, blade handles, and a blade dispenser box.

Richards Manufacturing Company, Inc.
1450 Brooks Road
Memphis, Tenn. 38116
and
Richards Surgical, Ltd.
7524 Bath Road
Malton, Ontario L4T 1L2

Richards manufactures implants for the human body along with supplementary instruments. They also make instruments for a variety of surgeries, and cervical collars, slings and splints.

Richards products are sold exclusively through factory-to-you distributors. Contact the Customer Service Department for address of local representatives.

J. Sklar Mfg. Co., Inc.
Long Island City, N.Y. 11101

J. Sklar manufactures suction and pressure apparatus, and a large variety of diagnostic (including stethoscopes and vaginal speculums) and surgical instruments. Sklar products are sold through authorized Surgical Supply Distributors.

Storz Instrument Company
3365 Tree Court Industrial Blvd.
St. Louis, Mo. 63172

Storz manufactures a variety of surgical microscopes and photographic and television systems, anatomical models, lamps, and a variety of surgical instruments. Storz representatives are available in major metropolitan areas throughout the U.S.

Stryker Corporation
420 Alcott Street
Kalamazoo, Mich. 49001

Stryker offers surgical instruments, transport stretchers, surgical beds, cast cutters, cervical collars, orthopedic tables, and products for decubiti prevention.

3-M
Surgical Products Division
15 Henderson Drive
West Caldwell, N.J. 07006

3-M's surgical division offers surgical drapes, sponge brushes, masks, wound closures, and electrosurgical products.

Your Surgical Instruments & Their Care
TROUBLE SHOOTING CHART

PROBLEM	NATURE	SOLUTION
Spotting	Mineral deposits left by slow or improper drying of instruments.	1. Check operating instruments and operation of autoclave. 2. Use chloride-free solutions for sterilization, disinfecting, rinsing and cleaning. Distilled or mineral free water preferred (pH approx. 7.0).

Continued on next page

PROBLEM	NATURE	SOLUTION
Rust (corrosion)	Film left by steam	1. Check purity of water supply. 2. If water softeners are used, check for composition. 3. Purge steam pipes, especially new installations.
	Deposit	1. Do not mix stainless steel with other metals (especially where there is evidence of defective plating). 2. Rinse with distilled water particularly important where tap water may have high metallic content. 3. Remove all debris from lock areas, teeth, etc. 4. Dry all instruments thoroughly in autoclave. Use full time cycle. This is most important when in packs. 5. Thoroughly clean all walls of autoclave.
Pitting	Chemical and electronic attack of surfaces	1. Rinse instruments thoroughly immediately after use. 2. Avoid long exposure to chlorides and acids. 3. Do not use detergents having high levels of pH. 4. Do not mix metals in ultrasonic cleaners.
Staining	Black to purple	1. Avoid exposure to ammonia in solutions and cleaning compounds. 2. Rinse instruments thoroughly (distilled water preferred)
	Brown	1. Check water supply in sterilizer. 2. Check cleaning compounds and detergents. Avoid excessive use.
	Gray-Blue	1. Use fresh cold sterilizing solutions and follow manufacturers suggestions for use.

Reprinted by permission of J. Sklar Co. from *Sklar Products Surgical Instruments*, (Catalog), 19th edition, 1978.

WARNING!

Because of the presence of water in alcohol, instruments immersed in it for extended periods of time may spot or discolor. To minimize this, it is suggested that a little soda be added.

Another word of caution—do not expose stainless steel for more than four hours to any of the chemicals listed at right in alphabetical order:

If you must use any of these, clean immediately after use. Never put the instruments away without thorough cleaning.

Aluminum Chloride
Barium Chloride
Bichloride of Mercury
Calcium Chloride
Carbolic Acid
Chlorinated Lime
Citric Acid (Boiling)
Dakin's Solution
Ferrous Chloride

Lysol
Mercuric Chloride
Mercury Salts
Phenol
Potassium Permanganate
Potassium Thiocyanate
Sodium Hypochlorite
Stannous Chloride
Tartaric Acid

Reprinted by permission of J. Sklar Co. from *Sklar Products Surgical Instruments*, (Catalog), 19th edition, 1978.

Sources for Urological and Ostomy Supplies

Bard Hospital Division
C. R. Bard, Inc.
Murray Hill, N.J. 07974

Bard manufactures urological products such as catheters, medical tubing, urological kits, trays, and other case goods. Order from your Hospital-Surgical Supply Dealer.

Diamed
A Division of Illinois Tool Works, Inc.
830 Lee Street
Elk Grove Village, Ill. 60007

Diamed manufactures urethral catheter kits for men and women, with or without specimen reservoir, gloves, underpads, and alcohol handiwipes. These cannot be sold directly to patients but the company will honor orders from pharmacies or home care centers.

Diamond Shamrock Medical Products, Inc.
6235 Packer Drive
P. O. Box 1101
Wausau, Wisc. 54401

Diamond Shamrock distributes ostomy products (for Marsan) and Stomagrad products, manufactured by Doval Laboratories of St. Louis, Missouri, such as ostomy rings, adhesive squares, and drainable pouches. All products may be ordered through Diamond Shamrock.

Greer Ostomy Appliances
530 East 12th Street
Oakland, Calif. 94606

Greer makes pouches, pads, belts, and irrigation appliances for the ostomy patient, as well as appliances and accessories for urinary diversion.

Gricks
Division of 2-T Products, Inc.
Hollis, N.Y. 11423

Gricks supplies ostomy appliances including Karaya gum and

appliances and accessories for colostomy, ureterostomy, ileostomy, ileal bladder, irrigators and adhesive drains. Products may be purchased directly or through your hospital. Hospital orders receive a 25% discount.

Marlen Manufacturing and Development Co.
5150 Richmond Road
Bedford, Ohio 44146

Marlen supplies appliances and accessories for ileostomy, colostomy, ureterostomy, and ileal bladder operations.

Mason Laboratories, Inc.
P. O. Box 344
Horsham, Pa. 19044

Mason makes appliances and supplies for colostomy, ileostomy, urostomy, and fistula operations.

Medical Dynamics, Inc.
Ostolite
Building 75
14 Inverness Drive East
Englewood, Colo. 80112

Ostolite carries faceplates, urinary pouches, ileostomy pouches, colostomy bags, adhesive discs and removers, cleansing agents, elastic binders, and irrigation sleeves and tubes.

Mentor Corporation
Biomedical Systems
1499 West River Road, North
Minneapolis, Minn. 55411

Mentor makes a male external catheter and a one-time use catheter designed for self-catheterization for women. These may be ordered directly from the company.

Nu-Hope Laboratories, Inc.
2900 Rowena Avenue
Los Angeles, Calif. 90039

Nu-Hope manufactures ileostomy appliance kits, ureterostomy bags, ileostomy bags and accessories for ileal-bladder products. They also offer skin treatment products, deodorizers and appliance cleansers, incontinence appliances and leg bags, supplemental vitamins and minerals, colostomy irrigation sets and dressing pads, and post-op bags for children and adults.

The Perma-Type Company, Inc.
P. O. Box 448
Farmington Industrial Park
Farmington, Conn. 06032

Perma-Type manufactures face plates, synthetic ileostomy and colostomy pouches, karaya washes, and ostomy accessories.

United
Division of Howmedica Inc.
11775 Starkey Road
P. O. Box 1970
Largo, Fla. 33540

United makes products for colostomy, ileostomy, urinary diversion, transverse loop, and ostomy care accessories. Their catalog is tri-lingual: English, French and Spanish.

Characteristics for Urostomy Appliances

	LIFE OF APPLIANCE
Permanent	One to three years depending on care and type of urine. Cost $30, $100 per year.
Semipermanent	Permanent faceplate (five years plus) with disposable pouches (two to eight weeks). Cost: $30, $50 per year.
Disposable	Easiest to use. Cost: $30, $150 per year.
	TYPE OF MATERIAL
Vinyl	Odor resistant, easy to maintain, inexpensive.
Rubber	Durable, develops odor and calcium deposits producing maintenance problems, allergies to rubber, expensive.
	NUMBER OF PIECES
One	No assembly, rubber or totally disposable, larger pouch necessitates larger faceplate.
Two	Rubber or vinyl, may change pouch independently of faceplate, pouch size and faceplate size independent, must be assembled.

Continued on next page

	FACEPLATE
Flexible	Most easily worn, least likely to be loosened by fat folds, activity, etc., flexibility varies.
Rigid	Variety of convexities to choose from for depressed stomas, flabby musculature, oval stomas, etc.
Size	The smaller the diameter, the easier it is to find a spot on the abdomen which avoids scars, folds, incisions, bony prominences.
	METHOD OF ADHERENCE
Adhesive Discs	Easy to use, many manufacturers, some allergies develop with time.
Cement	Seal is generally most durable, many manufacturers, many people develop allergies, more difficult to use.
Relia-Seal	Easy to use, many outlast adhesive discs, manufacturer claims no allergies, expensive.
Karaya	Urine causes rapid disintegration.

Reprinted by permission of Appleton-Century-Crofts from *Cancer Care Nursing* by Donovan and Pierce, Copyright 1976, Appleton-Century-Crofts.

Sources for Teaching Aids

Carolina Biological Supply Company
Main Office and Laboratories
Burlington, N.C. 27215

or

Powell Laboratories Division
Gladstone, Oreg. 97027

This company sells viral cultures, living animals and plants, preserved animals and plants, biological mounts, skeletons, microscope slides, books, filmstrips, models, charts, optical instruments, chemicals, teaching materials and other products.

Educational and Scientific Plastics, Ltd.
76 and 78 Holmethorpe Avenue
Redhill, Surrey RHI 2PF
Great Britain

This company manufactures anatomical models for nurse training, including muscles of the female pelvic floor, a flexible obstetric pelvis, neonatal endotracheal intubation heads, obstetric pelvis with fetal skulls mounted on a stand, female urogenital organs, fetal dolls, fetal head for palpation, composite pelvis and pelvic floor, placental circulation, and anatomical models of other parts of the body (foot, brain, ear, heart, jaw, kidney, intestines, and others).

Simulaids
269 Tinker Street
Woodstock, N.Y. 12498

Along with manufacturing a line of medical equipment, Simulaids makes first aid and emergency medical teaching and training aids. The company offers casualty simulation kits with make-up blood, assorted lacerations, fractures, gunshot wounds, and an abdominal wound with protruding intestines. Also offered is a life-sized manikin which provides a number of first aid emergency situations including mouth-to-mouth resuscitation, broken bones and bleeding. Other products include an obstetrical manikin (a life-sized pelvic section, umbilical cord, placenta, interior canals for simulated blood and amniotic fluids, and a fetus).

Winning At Wellness
4207 Woodlawn Avenue, N.
Seattle, Wash. 98103

"Winning At Wellness" is a board game and educational tool for teaching people to make positive health choices. Physical fitness, nutrition, stress management, self-responsibility and accident/illness prevention are concepts that come under discussion in this game for ages ten and above. It is useful for schools, health departments, outpatient facilities, mental health clinics and senior citizens centers.

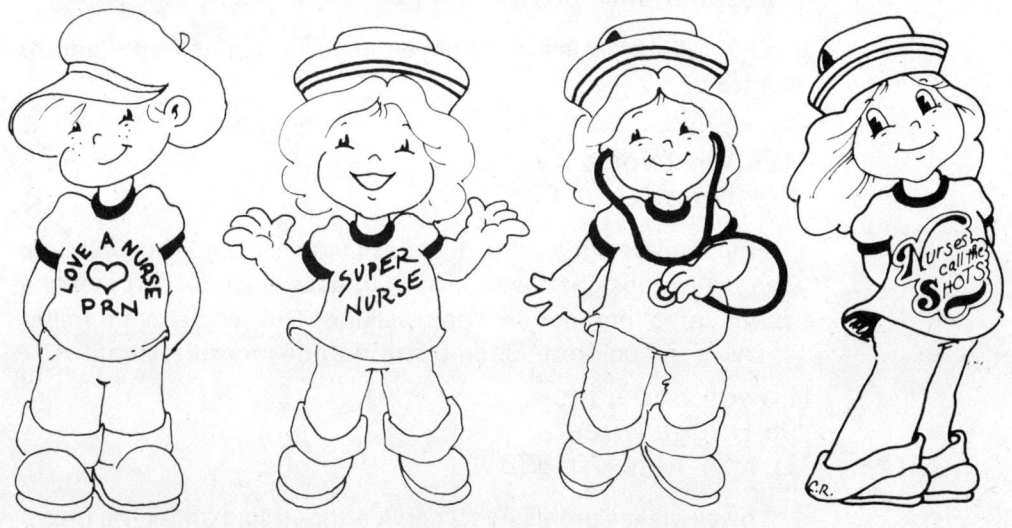

Drawings by Chris Reagen, courtesy of American Eagle Company, Troy, Michigan.

Sources for Uniforms and Other Supplies for Nurses

Bencone Uniforms
121 Camer Avenue
Westwood, N.J. 07675

Bencone has uniforms for nurses, including dresses, pantsuits, lab coats and jackets, smocks, t-shirts, and shoes. Write for catalog to order by mail.

Budget Uniform Center
941 Mill Road
Cornwell Heights, Pa. 19020

Budget makes a variety of uniforms for nurses, including dresses, pantsuits, smocks, lab coats and shoes.

The Clinic Shoe
7912 Bonhomme
Suite 206, Guild Building
St. Louis, Mo. 63105

The Clinic Shoe offers a variety of shoes for nurses, including a shoe with conductive soles and heels to eliminate static electricity, especially useful in operating and delivery rooms.

Duty Shoes, Inc.
721 Olive Street
St. Louis, Mo. 63101

Duty offers professional shoes made of leather with side or center tie.

Famolare
198 Westwood Avenue
Westwood, N.J. 07675

Famolare designs a line of shoes made especially for walking. The heel is designed with a wave to absorb shock and create a continual rolling motion when walking. They come in a number of styles and colors, including one in white for professional use.

Lowell Shoe, Inc.
95 Bridge Street
Lowell, Mass. 01852

Lowell makes professional service shoes sold under the brand names of "Nurse-Mates" and "Day-Lites." They are sold at the retail level and may be found in uniform and shoe stores throughout the country.

Old Pueblo Traders
600 South Country Club Road
P. O. Box 27800
Tucson, Ariz. 85716

Old Pueblo Traders makes "The Solvang Clog," a lightweight, no-nail construction shoe in perforated leather. The clog has a cork-like wedge laminated to the rubber soles. It comes in white, red or camel.

J. C. Penney Company, Inc.
Catalog Division
11800 West Burleigh Street
Milwaukee, Wis. 53201

Penney's has a special catalog of uniforms for professional and career men and women which includes dresses, pantsuits, and separate pants, jackets and other tops for nurses, shoes for men and women, and coffee mugs with nursing slogans printed on them.

Professional Uniforms and Accessories
19 Booker Street
Westwood, N.J. 07675

Professional has a catalog full of nursing uniforms including dresses, pantsuits, jackets and shoes. They also offer stethoscopes, electronic thermometers, watches, and a variety of novelty items such as t-shirts, coffee mugs, and tote bags with slogans on them.

Reeves Company, Inc.
225 O'Neil Boulevard
Attleboro, Mass. 02703

Reeves manufactures name-pins in a choice of all metal, metal-framed, plastic laminated, or molded plastic. They also carry enameled pins with insignia (R.N., L.P.N., etc.), cap totes, pocket savers, shoulder bags, tote bags, and capes.

Whitehouse Manufacturing Co.
Division of Opelika Mfg. Corp.
361 West Chestnut Street
Chicago, Ill. 60610

Whitehouse offers surgical gowns and scrub dresses, jackets and pants, scrub shirts, x-ray examining gowns, patient hospital gowns and children's pajamas, linens for hospital beds and operating rooms (including towels and drapes), and hamper bags and covers. Sales are made directly to the institution through the purchasing department, the company does not sell to individuals.

Nursing Uniforms Yesterday And Today

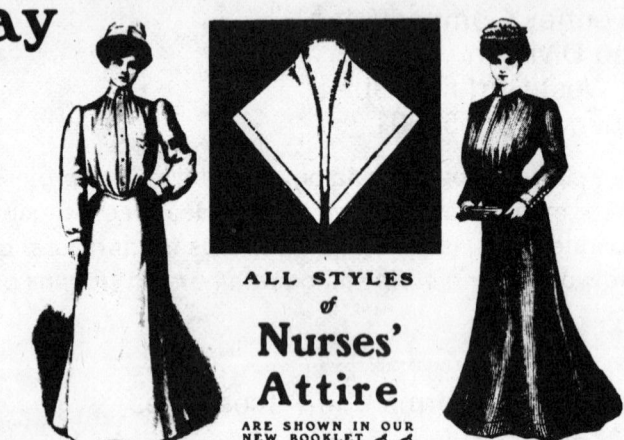

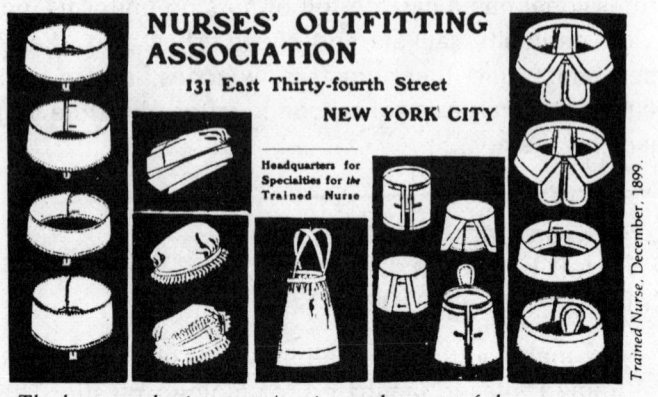

The latest styles in nurses' attire at the turn of the century.

Source: *Trained Nurse*, December, 1899, as reprinted in *The Advance of American Nursing*, Philip Kalisch and Beatrice Kalisch, © 1978, Little Brown and Company, Boston.

677

JCPenney® Uniform Catalog

PROFESSIONAL AND CAREER WEAR FOR WOMEN AND MEN

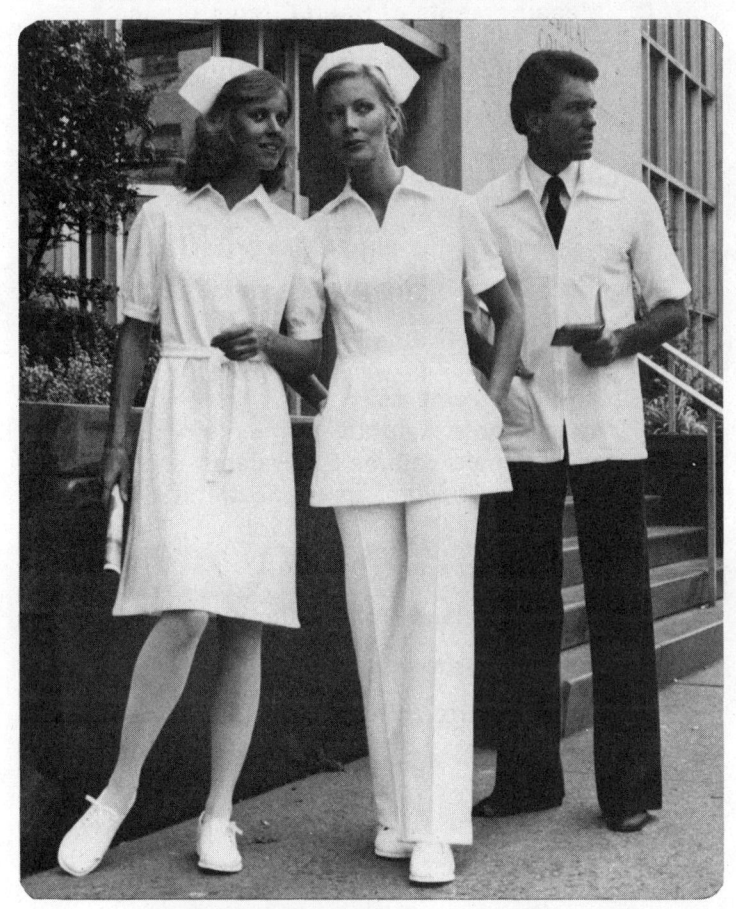

SPRING AND SUMMER 1979
WE'RE PROUD OF OUR PRICES. WE URGE YOU TO COMPARE!
PRICES ARE SUBJECT TO CHANGE AFTER JULY 21, 1979

Copyright J. C. Penney Company, Inc. 1979. Reproduced by permission from *J. C. Penney Uniform Catalog,* Spring and Summer, 1979.

31 Appendix

A. Conversion of Pounds and Ounces to Grams

B. Average Height and Weight For Children

C. Measurements of Head Circumference

D. Percentile Charts for Measurement

Infant Girls
Girls Ages 2–13
Infant Boys
Boys Ages 2–13

E. Desirable Weights of Men and Women, Ages 25 and Over

F. Equivalents

Metric Equivalents
Approximate Weight Equivalents
Approximate Volume Equivalents
Common Conversions to the Metric System

G. State Boards of Nursing

H. Largest Poison Control Centers

I. State Departments of Vocational Rehabilitation

J. State Welfare Offices

K. Sources for Audiovisual Aids

L. Index of Publishers

M. Abbreviations in Common Use

CONVERSION OF POUNDS AND OUNCES TO GRAMS

POUNDS \ OUNCES	0	1	2	3	4	5	6	7	8	9	10	11	12	13	14	15
0	—	28	57	85	113	142	170	198	227	255	283	312	340	369	397	425
1	454	482	510	539	567	595	624	652	680	709	737	765	794	822	850	879
2	907	936	964	992	1021	1049	1077	1106	1134	1162	1191	1219	1247	1276	1304	1332
3	1361	1389	1417	1446	1474	1503	1531	1559	1588	1616	1644	1673	1701	1729	1758	1786
4	1814	1843	1871	1899	1928	1956	1984	2013	2041	2070	2098	2126	2155	2183	2211	2240
5	2268	2296	2325	2353	2381	2410	2438	2466	2495	2523	2551	2580	2608	2637	2665	2693
6	2722	2750	2778	2807	2835	2863	2892	2920	2948	2977	3005	3033	3062	3090	3118	3147
7	3175	3203	3232	3260	3289	3317	3345	3374	3402	3430	3459	3487	3515	3544	3572	3600
8	3629	3657	3685	3714	3742	3770	3799	3827	3856	3884	3912	3941	3969	3997	4026	4054
9	4082	4111	4139	4167	4196	4224	4252	4281	4309	4337	4366	4394	4423	4451	4479	4508
10	4536	4564	4593	4621	4649	4678	4706	4734	4763	4791	4819	4848	4876	4904	4933	4961
11	4990	5018	5046	5075	5103	5131	5160	5188	5216	5245	5273	5301	5330	5358	5386	5415
12	5443	5471	5500	5528	5557	5585	5613	5642	5670	5698	5727	5755	5783	5812	5840	5868
13	5897	5925	5953	5982	6010	6038	6067	6095	6123	6152	6180	6209	6237	6265	6294	6322
14	6350	6379	6407	6435	6464	6492	6520	6549	6577	6605	6634	6662	6690	6719	6747	6776
15	6804	6832	6860	6889	6917	6945	6973	7002	7030	7059	7087	7115	7144	7172	7201	7228
16	7257	7286	7313	7342	7371	7399	7427	7456	7484	7512	7541	7569	7597	7626	7654	7682
17	7711	7739	7768	7796	7824	7853	7881	7909	7938	7966	7994	8023	8051	8079	8108	8136
18	8165	8192	8221	8249	8278	8306	8335	8363	8391	8420	8448	8476	8504	8533	8561	8590
19	8618	8646	8675	8703	8731	8760	8788	8816	8845	8873	8902	8930	8958	8987	9015	9043
20	9072	9100	9128	9157	9185	9213	9242	9270	9298	9327	9355	9383	9412	9440	9469	9497
21	9525	9554	9582	9610	9639	9667	9695	9724	9752	9780	9809	9837	9865	9894	9922	9950
22	9979	10007	10036	10064	10092	10120	10149	10177	10206	10234	10262	10291	10319	10347	10376	10404

Average Height and Weight for Children

Age (Years)	Boys Height ft	Boys Height in	Boys Height cm	Boys Weight lb	Boys Weight kg	Girls Height ft	Girls Height in	Girls Height cm	Girls Weight lb	Girls Weight kg
Birth	1	8	45.7	7 1/2	3.4	1	8	50.8	7 1/2	3.4
1/2	2	2	66.0	17	7.7	2	2	66.0	16	7.2
1	2	5	73.6	21	9.5	2	5	73.6	20	9.1
2	2	9	83.8	26	11.8	2	9	83.8	25	11.3
3	3	0	91.4	31	14.0	3	0	91.4	30	13.6
4	3	3	99.0	34	15.4	3	3	99.0	33	15.0
5	3	6	106.6	39	17.7	3	5	104.1	38	17.2
6	3	9	114.2	46	20.9	3	8	111.7	45	20.4
7	3	11	119.3	51	23.1	3	11	119.3	49	22.2
8	4	2	127.0	57	25.9	4	2	127.0	56	25.4
9	4	4	132.0	63	28.6	4	4	132.0	62	28.1
10	4	6	137.1	69	31.3	4	6	137.1	69	31.3
11	4	8	142.2	77	34.9	4	8	142.2	77	34.9
12	4	10	147.3	83	37.7	4	10	147.3	86	39.0
13	5	0	152.4	92	41.7	5	0	152.4	98	45.5
14	5	2	157.5	107	48.5	5	2	157.5	107	48.5

(From *Handbook of Medical Treatment,* 16th edition. M. J. Chatton (ed.). Jones Medical Publications, Greenbrae, California, 1979.)

Head Circumference

Girls	10		50		90	
Age in years	In.	Cm	In.	Cm	In.	Cm
0·25	15·0	38·1	15·6	39·7	16·1	40·9
0·50	16·2	41·2	16·9	42·9	17·4	44·2
0·75	17·0	43·2	17·6	44·6	18·1	46·2
1	17·5	44·4	18·0	45·7	18·6	47·2
2	18·1	46·2	18·9	48·0	19·4	49·3
3	18·5	47·1	19·4	49·2	19·9	50·5
4	18·9	48·0	19·6	49·9	20·2	51·4
5	19·1	48·6	19·8	50·4	20·4	51·9
6	19·3	49·1	20·0	50·8	20·6	52·2
7	19·5	49·5	20·1	51·1	20·7	52·5
8	19·6	49·8	20·2	51·3	20·8	52·8

Boys	10		50		90	
Age in years	In.	Cm	In.	Cm	In.	Cm
Birth	13·1	33·5	13·8	35·0	14·1	36·0
0·25	15·5	39·3	16·0	40·6	16·6	42·1
0·50	16·5	42·0	17·2	43·8	17·7	45·0
0·75	17·1	43·6	18·0	45·7	18·6	47·2
1	17·5	44·5	18·4	46·8	19·1	48·5
2	18·5	47·1	19·3	49·1	20·0	50·9
3	19·0	48·2	19·8	50·2	20·5	52·0
4	19·3	48·9	20·0	50·8	20·7	52·5
5	19·4	49·4	20·2	51·3	20·9	53·0
6	19·6	49·9	20·4	51·8	21·0	53·4
7	19·8	50·3	20·5	52·1	21·1	53·8
8	19·9	50·6	20·6	52·4	21·3	54·2

* Through the courtesy of Professor J. M. Tanner.

Reprinted by permission of Churchill Livingstone from *The Normal Child*, 6th edition, Ronald S. Illingworth, Copyright 1975, Churchill Livingstone.

PERCENTILE CHART FOR MEASUREMENTS OF INFANT GIRLS

THIS CHART provides for infant girls standards of reference for body weight and recumbent length by month from birth to 28 months and for head circumference by week from birth to 28 weeks. It is based upon repeated measurements at selected ages of a group of more than 100 white infants of North European ancestry living under normal conditions of health and home life in Boston, Mass. The distribution of the measurements obtained from the infants at each age is expressed in percentiles, each percentile giving a value which represents a particular position in the normal range of occurrences. The number of the percentile refers to the position which a measurement of the given value would hold in any typical series of 100 infants. Thus, the 10th percentile gives the value for the tenth in any hundred; that is, 9 infants of the same sex and age would be expected to be smaller in the measurement under consideration while 90 would be expected to be larger than the figure given. Similarly the 90th percentile would indicate that 89 infants might be expected to be smaller than the figure given while 10 would be larger. The 50th percentile represents the median or midposition in the customary range. Here, the 10th and 90th percentiles are presented in heavy lines to show the limits within which most infants remain. The lighter lines in the graphs divide the distributions into segments for ready recognition and description of individual differences as well as of the "regularity" of progress. The 3rd and 97th percentiles represent unusual though not necessarily abnormal findings.

In line with common usage in the United States, the charts are ruled on a scale in pounds to represent weight. They are ruled, however, in centimeters to represent length and head circumference, because this scale facilitates accuracy in measuring and recording and centimeter rules and tapes are readily available. For the convenience of those preferring them, scales for kilograms and inches are placed outside of the principal scales and paralleling them. Therefore, if weights are taken in kilograms and lengths and head circumferences in inches, they may be plotted directly without conversion by placing a ruler at the appropriate points on the outer scales of the charts.

To determine the percentile position of any measurement at a given age, the vertical age line is located and a dot is placed where this intersects the horizontal line representing the value obtained from the measurement. Vertical lines give age by one-month intervals for weight and length and one-week intervals for head circumference; horizontal lines give ½-pound, 1-cm. and 0.5-cm. intervals respectively. This permits by interpolation accurate placement for age to weeks, for weights to 2 ounces and for centimeters to 0.5 cm. Recognition of the position within or outside of the range held by an infant in respect to each measurement recorded calls attention to the relative size and build of the individual at the time. More importantly, comparisons of percentile positions held by these measurements at repeated periodic examinations indicate adherence to or possibly significant deviation from previous percentile positions. Under normal circumstances, one expects an infant to maintain a similar position from age to age — that is, on or near one percentile line or between the same two lines. Occasional sharp deviations or gradual but continuing shifts from one percentile position to another call for further investigation as to their causes. In all cases, readings of measurements should be checked and care should be taken to secure the same position of the infant at all examinations. The following procedures were used in obtaining these norms and therefore are recommended:

Body Weight — The infant is weighed without clothing, preferably on special infant scales.

Recumbent Length — The infant lies relaxed on a firm surface parallel to a centimeter rule or on a special infant measuring board which permits the following procedure. The soles of the feet are held firmly against a fixed upright at the zero mark on the rule, and a movable square is brought firmly against the vertex. Care must be taken to secure extension at the knees, and the head should be held so that the eyes face the ceiling.

Head Circumference — This measurement is more satisfactory if taken with the infant lying on his back. The tape is passed around the head from above and placed anteriorly over the lower forehead just above the supraorbital ridges. With the position of the tape thus fixed anteriorly, the largest circumference is obtained by passing it posteriorly over the most prominent part of the occiput.

The following four graphs are reprinted by permission from the Department of Maternal and Child Health, Harvard School of Public Health, Boston, Mass.

Percentile Chart for Measurements of . . .

INFANT GIRLS

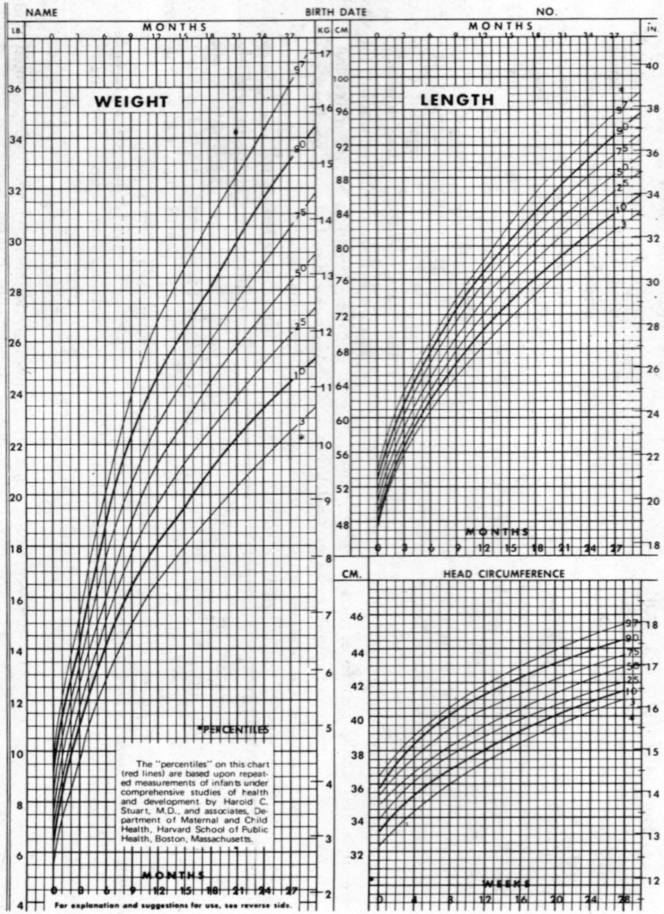

GIRLS AGES 2–13

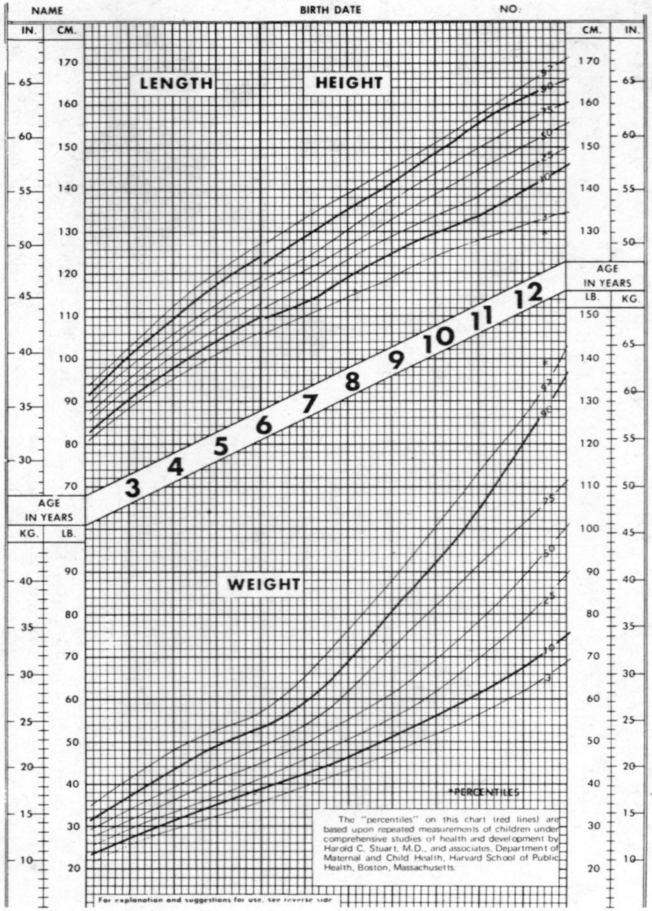

Percentile Chart for Measurements of...

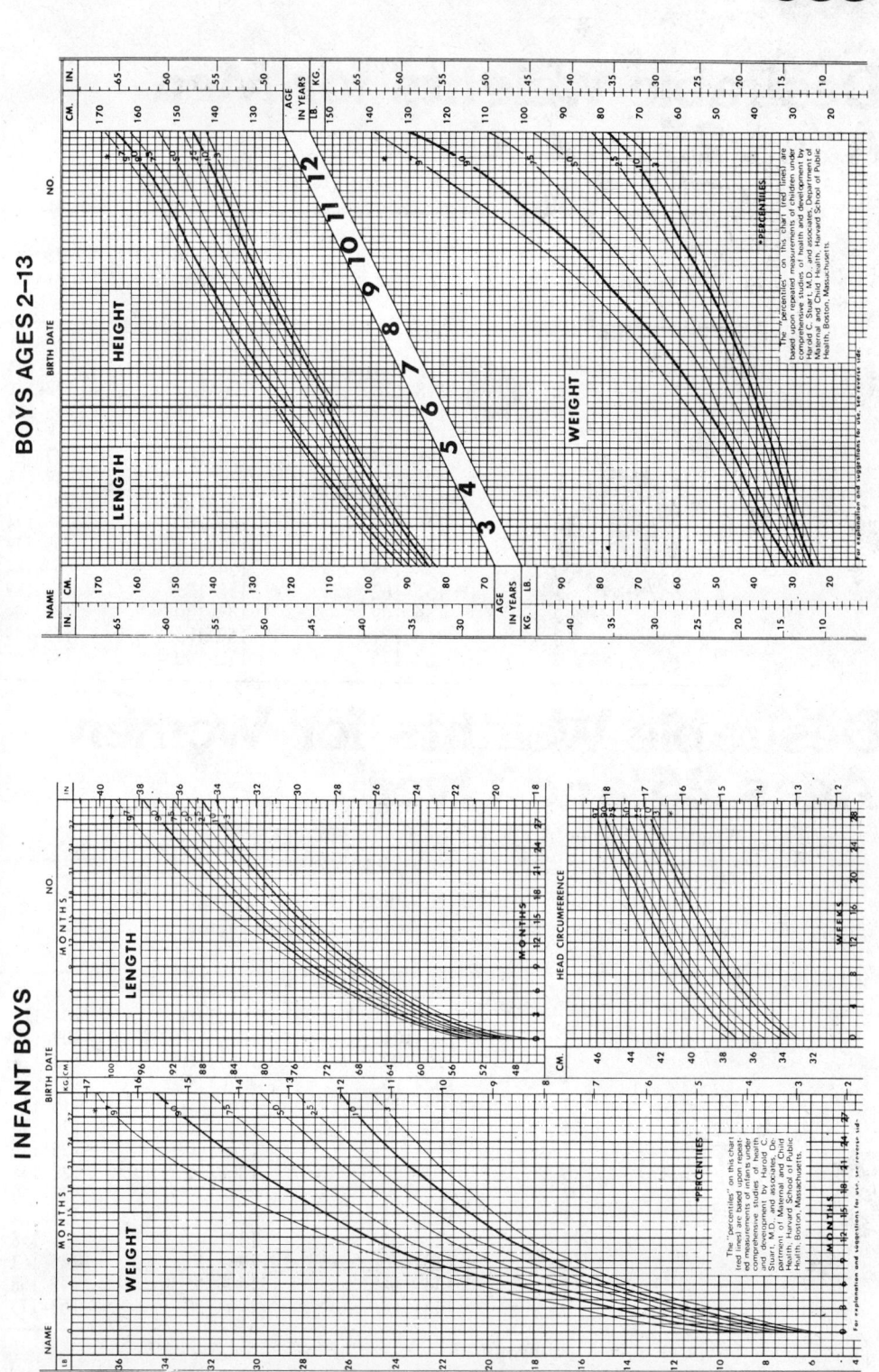

INFANT BOYS

BOYS AGES 2-13

Desirable Weights for Men Ages 25 and Over*

Weight in Pounds According to Frame (In Indoor Clothing)

Height (with shoes on) 1-inch heels Feet / Inches	Small Frame	Medium Frame	Large Frame
5 2	112–120	118–129	126–141
5 3	115–123	121–133	129–144
5 4	118–126	124–136	132–148
5 5	121–129	127–139	135–152
5 6	124–133	130–143	138–156
5 7	128–137	134–147	142–161
5 8	132–141	138–152	147–166
5 9	136–145	142–156	151–170
5 10	140–150	146–160	155–174
5 11	144–154	150–165	159–179
6 0	148–158	154–170	164–184
6 1	152–162	158–175	168–189
6 2	156–167	162–180	173–194
6 3	160–171	167–185	178–199
6 4	164–175	172–190	182–204

Desirable Weights for Women Ages 25 and Over*

Weight in Pounds According to Frame (In Indoor Clothing)

Height (with shoes on) 2-inch heels Feet / Inches	Small Frame	Medium Frame	Large Frame
4 10	92– 98	96–107	104–119
4 11	94–101	98–110	106–122
5 0	96–104	101–113	109–125
5 1	99–107	104–116	112–128
5 2	102–110	107–119	115–131
5 3	105–113	110–122	118–134
5 4	108–116	113–126	121–138
5 5	111–119	116–130	125–142
5 6	114–123	120–135	129–146
5 7	118–127	124–139	133–150
5 8	122–131	128–143	137–154
5 9	126–135	132–147	141–158
5 10	130–140	136–151	145–163
5 11	134–144	140–155	149–168
6 0	138–148	144–159	153–173

*Reprinted with permission of Metropolitan Life Insurance Company, New York.
For girls between 18 and 25, subtract 1 pound for each year under 25.

Equivalents

Metric Equivalents

Weights

1 picogram	= 10^{-12} gm
1 nanogram	= 10^{-9} gm
1 microgram	= 10^{-3} mg = 10^{-6} gm
1 milligram	= 1000 micrograms = 10^{-6} gram
1 centigram	= 10 milligrams = 10^{-1} decigrams = 10^{-2} gram
1 decigram	= 100 milligrams = 10 centigrams = 10^{-1} gram
1 gram	= 1000 milligrams = 100 centigrams = 10 decigrams
1 kilogram	= 1000 grams

Volume

1 milliliter	= 1 gram
1 liter	= 1 kilogram = 1000 grams (milliliters)

Approximate Weight Equivalents: Metric and Apothecaries' Systems

Metric	Apothecaries'	Metric	Apothecaries'
0.1 mg	1/600 grain	60 mg	1 grain
1.12 mg	1/500 grain	100 mg (0.1 gm)	1 1/2 grains
0.15 mg	1/400 grain	150 mg (0.15 gm)	2 1/2 grains
0.2 mg	1/300 grain	200 mg (0.2 gm)	3 grains
0.25 mg	1/250 grain	300 mg (0.3 gm)	5 grains
0.3 mg	1/200 grain	400 mg (0.4 gm)	6 grains
0.4 mg	1/150 grain	500 mg (0.5 gm)	7 1/2 grains
0.5 mg	1/120 grain	600 mg (0.6 gm)	10 grains
0.6 mg	1/100 grain	1 gram	15 grains
0.8 mg	1/80 grain	1.5 gm	22 grains
1 mg	1/60 grain	2 gm	30 grains
1.2 mg	1/50 grain	3 gm	45 grains

Continued on next page

1.5 mg	1/40 grain	4 gm	60 grains (1 dram)
2 mg	1/30 grain	5 gm	75 grains
3 mg	1/20 grain	6 gm	90 grains
4 mg	1/15 grain	7.5 gm	120 grains (2 drams)
5 mg	1/12 grain	10 gm	2½ drams
6 mg	1/10 grain	30 gm	1 ounce (8 drams)
8 mg	1/8 grain	500 gm	1.1 pounds
10 mg	1/6 grain	1000 gm	2.2 pounds (1 kilogram)
12 mg	1/5 grain		
15 mg	1/4 grain		
20 mg	1/3 grain		
25 mg	3/8 grain		
30 mg	1/2 grain		
40 mg	2/3 grain		
50 mg	3/4 grain		

Approximate Volume Equivalents: Metric, Apothecaries', and Household Systems

Metric	Apothecaries'	Household
0.06 ml	1 minim ( )	1 drop (g +)
0.3 ml	5 minims	
0.6 ml	10 minims	
1 ml	15 minims	15 drops
2 ml	30 minims	
3 ml	45 minims	
4 ml	60 minims (1 fluid dram)	60 drops (1 tsp)
8 ml	2 fl. drams (f)	2 teaspoons
15 ml	4 fl. drams	4 tsp. (1 tbsp)
30 ml	8 fl. drams (1 fl. ounce) (f)	2 tablespoons

Appendices

Metric	Apothecaries	Household
60 ml	2 fl. ounces	
90 ml	3 fl. ounces	
200 ml	6 fl. ounces	1 teacup
250 ml	8 fl. ounces	1 large glass
500 ml	16 fl. ounces (1 pint)	1 pint
750 ml	1½ pints	
1000 ml (1 liter)	2 pints (1 quart)	1 quart
4000 ml	4 quarts	1 gallon

Reprinted by permission of Addison-Wesley Publishing Co. from *Fundamentals of Nursing* by Kozier and Erb, © 1979, Addison-Wesley Pub. Co.

Some Common Conversions to the Metric System of Measurement

Length

1 foot	= 30.48 centimeters	3.28 feet	= 1 meter
1 inch	= 2.54 centimeters	39.37 inches	= 1 meter
1 inch	= 25.4 millimeters	1.09 yards	= 1 meter
		1 mile	= 1.61 kilometers

Weight

1 pound	= 454 grams
2.2 pounds	= 1 kilogram
1 ounce	= 28.35 grams

Liquid

1.06 quarts	= 1 liter
2.1 pints	= 1 liter

Reprinted from *New American Pocket Medical Dictionary*, Nancy Roper, editor, adapted by Jane Clark Jackson, Copyright 1978, Churchill Livingstone.

688
State Boards of Nursing*

Below are the addresses of each of the state boards of nursing, the fees they charge, and the principal requirements for endorsement and licensure. Examination fees and endorsement fees are identical unless otherwise noted.

ALABAMA Board of Nursing, State of Alabama, Montgomery 36130. Fee: $40. Foreign nurses need official nursing school transcript.

ALASKA State Board of Nursing, Department of Commerce and Economic Development, Pouch D, Juneau 99811. Application packets with guidelines available.

ARIZONA State Board of Nursing, 1645 West Jefferson, Room 254, Phoenix 85007. Write for information regarding application, fees, and examination dates.

ARKANSAS State Board of Nursing, 4120 West Markham, Suite 308, Little Rock 77205. Fee: $40; Temp. permit: $3. Charge for verifying original license to another state: $15. Endorsement fee: $40.

CALIFORNIA Board of Registered Nursing, 1020 N Street, Sacramento 95814. Fee: $35. All applicants need nursing school transcript. Foreign nurses must pass S.B.T.P.E.

COLORADO State Board of Nursing, 1525 Sherman Street, Denver 80203. Fee for examination, $40; endorsement, $30. Permit issued for four months to nurses currently licensed in another state while application is processed. Permit to new graduates pending results of first examination. No permit issued to applicants from countries outside the U.S. and territories.

CONNECTICUT Board of Examiners for Nursing, 79 Elm Street, Room 101, Hartford 06115. Fee: $30. Temporary permit issued only to new graduates pending results of first exam given by board following date of graduation. Foreign nurses must pass the S.B.T.P.E. in some states of the U.S. and meet minimum state education requirements.

DELAWARE Board of Nursing, Cooper Building, Room 234, Dover 19901. Fee: $30. Foreign nurses not licensed by examination in another state must file for licensure by S.B.T.P.E. Persons seeking endorsement must, if inactive in nursing for 5 or more years, show evidence of participation in a refresher type program.

DISTRICT OF COLUMBIA Nurses Examining Board, 614 H Street N.W., Room 112, Washington 20001. Fee for examination or endorsement: $50; for verifying original license to another state, $10.

FLORIDA Board of Nursing, 6501 Arlington Expressway, Bldg. B, Jacksonville 32211. Fee for examination, $50; endorsement, $30. All applicants need certificate of physical and mental health; nurses licensed after Jan. 1, 1951, must have psychiatric nursing. No temporary permits. Foreign nurses need school transcripts, must pass S.B.T.P.E. Beginning in 1979, each licensed nurse shall participate in a minimum of 15 hours per annum of appropriate continuing education for licensure renewal. These requirements shall be met before renewals are issued.

GEORGIA Board of Nursing, 166 Pryor Street, N.W., Atlanta, 30303. Registration without examination (endorsement) $50. References required by endorsement. Application by examination, $30 examination, fee and $15 registration fee. School transcript required. Foreign nurses require verification of registration, school transcript, references, and must take written examination.

HAWAII Board of Nursing, Box 3469, Honolulu 96801. Fee: $30. New graduates of state accredited schools of nursing are eligible for a temporary permit when they have been accepted for the Hawaii board exam. Foreign nurses need nursing school transcript, proof of proficiency in English; must pass all five tests in

Reprinted with permission of RN Magazine from *1979 Nursing Opportunities*, page 13.
Copyright 1979. Litton Industries, Medical Economics Company, Oradell, N.J.

S.B.T.P.E.; are not eligible for temporary or work permits.

IDAHO State Board of Nursing, 413 West Idaho Street, Room 203, Boise 83702. Fee for examination $65 for R.N., $50 for P.N. Fees for endorsement: $50; $5 fee for verification of original license to another state. All nurses need nursing education transcript, references, and if licensed, satisfactory reference from previous employer. By examination—applicants need nursing education transcripts. By endorsement—applicants must have license in good standing and satisfactory reference from previous employer.

ILLINOIS Department of Registration and Education, Nurse Section. Fourth Floor, 628 East Adams Street, Springfield 62786. Fee: $25; no charge for verifying original license to another state. Exam given in Illinois. All applicants for endorsement need proof of current registration (or proof of inactive status).

INDIANA State Board of Nurses' Registration and Nursing Education, 700 North High School Road, Indianapolis 46224. Fee: $40 for examination; $25 for endorsement. Applicants for endorsement need verification of license from original board.

IOWA Board of Nursing, 300 Fourth Street, Des Moines 50319. Fee: for examination, $40; for endorsement, $25; for verification of an Iowa license to another board, $5. Applicants for endorsement need birth certificate, nursing transcript, evidence of high school graduation or the equivalent. Foreign nurses need additional credentials. Information may be obtained from Iowa Board of Nursing.

KANSAS State Board of Nursing, Box 19235, Topeka 66601. Information sent at the time of application.

KENTUCKY Board of Nursing, 6100 Dutchmans Lane, Louisville 40205. Fee: for examination, $48; for endorsement, $20; for verification of Kentucky license to another state, $4. Foreign graduates must meet the same educational standards required of Kentucky nursing school graduates. No temporary permits for foreign nurses until they have passed licensure requirements.

LOUISIANA State Board of Nursing. 150 Baronne Street, Room 907, New Orleans 70112. Fee for examination, $55; registration by endorsement, $25. Fee for verification of licensure to another board: $10. Applicants for endorsement need verification of license from original board, personal and work references, and school data form. (A temporary permit may be issued while application is being processed.) Foreign nurses need nursing school transcript, language certificate, must pass S.B.T.P.E. or C.N.A.T.S., earning a score of 350 or above in each area.

MAINE State Board of Nursing, 295 Water Street, Augusta 04330. Fee: for examination, $40; for endorsement, $40. Authorization to practice may be issued pending results of examination and pending completion of licensure by endorsement. Applicants for endorsement need verification of license from original board.

MARYLAND Board of Examiners of Nurses, 201 West Preston Street, Baltimore 21201. Fee: $35. No temporary permits. Applicants for endorsement no longer need proof of H.S. graduation or equivalency (since July 1, 1975).

MASSACHUSETTS Board of Registration in Nursing, 1509 Leverett Saltonstall Building, Boston 02202. Fee: $50 for endorsement; $30 for examination; $2 for verification. No temporary permits. All applicants need proof of high school graduation or equivalent plus (in some instances) transcript from nursing school. Applicants for endorsement must meet curriculum requirements in effect in Massachusetts at time of their graduation. U.S. board-constructed exams accepted for endorsement if passed before Massachusetts adopted S.B.T.P.E. Foreign nurses must pass S.B.T.P.E.

MICHIGAN Board of Nursing, 905 Southland, Lansing 48926. Fee: $45 for licensing exam; $20 for reexamination and $25 for licensure by endorsement. Temporary permit may be issued while endorsement application is being processed if all cre-

Continued on next page

dentials are received. Send no money or documents until Board requests them. Applicants whose original license was obtained in another country may be required to pass an English competency test and all are required to write the S.B.T.P.E.

MINNESOTA Board of Nursing, 717 Delaware Street S.E., Minneapolis 55414. Fee: $35. For further information, write the Board.

MISSISSIPPI Board of Nursing, 135 Bounds Street, Suite 101, Jackson 39206. Fee: $50. All applicants need nursing school transcript, character references from two R.N.s (or one R.N., one M.D.). Temporary (45-day) permit issued while endorsement application is being processed. Foreign nurses must pass both C.G.F.N.S. and S.B.T.P.E. except Canadian R.N.s who have passed the C.N.A.T.S. exam in English with 350 or above score may be endorsed.

MISSOURI State Board of Nursing, P.O. Box 656, Jefferson City 65101. Fee: $25 (subject to change). Graduates from schools outside Missouri can write the examination only if space is available after Missouri school candidates have been accommodated. Temporary permits will be considered on an individual basis. Foreign applicants should contact board of nursing for licensure requirements.

MONTANA Board of Nursing, La Londe Building, Last Chance Gulch, Helena 59601. Fee: $35. No charge for verifying original license to another state. Foreign nurses must pass S.B.T.P.E.

NEBRASKA State Board of Nursing, Box 95065, State House Station, Lincoln 68509. Fee: $50. All applicants need nursing school transcript, references.

NEVADA Board of Nursing. 1201 Terminal Way, Room 203, Reno 89502. Fee: for examination, $60; for endorsement, $45. All applicants need references from employers.

NEW HAMPSHIRE Board of Nursing-Education and Nurse Registration. 105 Loudon Road, Concord 03301. Fee: $40. All applicants need nursing school transcripts and must be currently licensed in some state and show evidence of having passed a written state licensing examination.

NEW JERSEY Board of Nursing, 1100 Raymond Boulevard, Room 319, Newark 07102. Fee: for examination, $35; for endorsement, $25. All applicants need nursing school transcript, high school diploma, and references. Temporary permits are issued to endorsement candidates pending verification of records and/or completion of educational deficiencies. Foreign nurses must take test of English competency, pass S.B.T.P.E.

NEW MEXICO Board of Nursing, 2340 Menaul N.E., Suite 112, Albuquerque 87107. Fee: endorsement $62, initial licensure $75. Temporary licenses given immediately to R.N. graduates of U.S. schools holding a current license from another state issued on basis of having passed S.B.T.P.E. Graduates of foreign schools need certified transcript, and must pass S.B.T.P.E. given in English.

NEW YORK Division of Professional Licensing Services, State Education Department, 99 Washington Avenue, Albany 12230. Write for information and application forms for license either as a registered professional nurse or as a licensed practical nurse.

NORTH CAROLINA Board of Nursing, Box 2129, Raleigh 27602. Fee: for examination, $27; for endorsement, $30. All fees are subject to change. No temporary permits. All applicants need character and health references. Foreign nurses who have not passed S.B.T.P.E. must do so in North Carolina.

NORTH DAKOTA Board of Nursing, 420 North Fourth Street, Bismarck 58505. Fee: $50. Foreign nurses must take the licensing examination.

OHIO Board of Nursing Education and Nurse Registration, 180 East Broad Street, Suite 1130, Columbus 43215. Fee: $30. All applicants need proof of high school graduation or its equivalent; nurses educated outside U.S. must pass S.B.T.P.E. Language proficiency examination required of nurses from non-English speaking countries.

OKLAHOMA Board of Nurse Registration and Nursing Education, 4030 Lincoln Boulevard, Suite 76, Oklahoma City 73105. Fee: $55. Foreign nurses must provide evidence of high school graduation or equivalent, nursing school transcript, evidence of score of 80 on ELS English Language Proficiency examination, proof of visa, etc.

OREGON State Board of Nursing, 1400 Southwest Fifth Avenue, Room 555, Portland 97201. Fee for examination: $45; endorsement, $35. Applicants for endorsement need current valid license and endorsement from another state. No temporary permits. The board obtains work references from previous employers submitted by nurses. All graduates of schools of nursing outside U.S.A. will be required to take and pass the S.B.T.P.E. for Registered Nurses unless the applicant holds a current valid license in another U.S.A. jurisdiction and obtained that license by examination. In such cases, the foreign nurse applicant will follow the procedure for licensure by endorsement.

PENNSYLVANIA State Board of Nurse Examiners, Box 2649, Harrisburg 17120. Fee: $24; no charge for verifying Pennsylvania license to other boards. Certificate of Preliminary Education from Department of Education required for foreign nurses graduating from hospital programs. Applicants for endorsement required to have been registered by examination in original state of licensure. Foreign nurses must take S.B.T.P.E.

PUERTO RICO Board of Nurse Examiners, Ponce de León Avenue, Stop 19, Box 9342, Santurce, 00908. Fee for examination: $5. No charge for verifying original license to another board. All nurses need proof of high school or equivalent education, nursing school diploma. All nurses must pass the S.B.T.P.E. Provisional licenses are granted to nurses who studied in Puerto Rico or the U.S. Foreign nurses must first pass the exam.

RHODE ISLAND Board of Nurse Registration and Nursing Education, Cannon Building, 75 Davis Street, Providence 02908. Fee: $30. R.N.s licensed in another state can work as registered nurses for up to three months provided they apply for a Rhode Island license within that time. Foreign nurses (except Canadians) must take S.B.T.P.E.

SOUTH CAROLINA State Board of Nursing, 1777 St. Julian Place, Suite 102, Columbia 29204. Fee: $50. All nurses need evidence of current licensure in one state, birth certificate, evidence of good health. For an additional $5.00, a temporary permit may be issued for eight (8) weeks.

SOUTH DAKOTA Board of Nursing, 304 South Phillips Avenue, Suite 205, Sioux Falls 57102. Fee: $55. Applicants for endorsement need high school or equivalent education, graduation from an approved school of nursing. Must be a citizen or resident alien of the United States. Nurses licensed after January 1, 1951, must have psychiatric nursing.

TENNESSEE Board of Nursing, State Office Building, Ben Allen Road, Nashville 37219. Fee: $50. No fee for verifying original license to another state. Nurses may need nursing school transcript, record from previous employer, proof of good health. Endorsement applications evaluated on an individual basis.

TEXAS Board of Nurse Examiners, 7600 Chevy Chase Dr., Suite 502, Austin 78752. Fee: $30. All applicants for examination need nursing school transcript. Foreign nurses must take S.B.T.P.E.

UTAH Department of Registration, Board of Nursing, 330 East Fourth South, Salt Lake City 84111. Fee: $30. All applicants for endorsement must have current license, need health certificate (certificate is on form issued with application). Out of state R.N.s who have been inactive five or more years must work four months on probation before being licensed, or complete a State Board approved refresher course. Canadian R.N.s are eligible for endorsement if they have passed S.B.T.P.E. or Canadian Nurses' Association's current licensure exam in all 5 areas with no less than 350 SS, Utah's passing score.

Continued on next page

VERMONT Board of Nursing, 10 Baldwin Street, Montpelier 05602. Fee $25. No temporary permits. Completed application and fee must be received before beginning practice.

VIRGINIA Board of Nursing, Department of Health Regulatory Boards, 3600 West Broad Street, Suite 453, Richmond 23230. Fee: $30. Charge for verifying Virginia license to another state: $3. Nurses holding a current license in another state may practice for 30 days in Virginia pending processing of their endorsement application. Foreign nurses must write and pass licensing exam.

WASHINGTON Board of Nursing, Box 9649, Olympia 98504. Fee: $25. All applicants must submit written official evidence of diploma or degree from approved school of nursing and other official records specified by the board. Foreign nurses shall meet all qualifications required and shall pass examinations as determined by the board.

WEST VIRGINIA Board of Examiners for Registered Nurses, 922 Quarrier Street, Suite 309, Embleton Building, Charleston 25301. Fee: $40 for examination, $30 for endorsement in and out. All nurses need high school or equivalent (GED) diploma. Foreign nurses must pass S.B.T.P.E. Temporary permits issued only to graduating students who have had no opportunity to take licensing exam.

* (S.B.T.P.E. = State Board Test Pool Exam.)

WISCONSIN State Board of Nursing. 1400 East Washington Avenue, Madison 53702. Fee for registration by examination, $50; by endorsement, $50. All applicants need proof of general and professional educational qualifications.

WYOMING Board of Nursing, Room 523, Hathway Building, Cheyenne 82002. Fee: $50. A 90-day permit may be issued at the board's discretion to nurses currently registered in another state while licensure application is being processed. Fee for temporary permit: $20 plus licensure fee, payable at time of application. Not refundable. New law provides for temporary permit for students who meet state requirements. No charge for new graduate temporary permit. Licensure fee payable before temporary permit is issued. Foreign nurses must prove English proficiency by passing test of English as a foreign language (T.O.E.F.L.) with a minimum score of 500, including a minimum of 50 in listening comprehension and 50 in reading comprehension (or a total of 100 with a plus or minus 5 in either area). Record of nursing school is required. Nurse must pass S.B.T.P.E. and meet other requirements of the Wyoming Nursing Practice Act.

Largest Poison Control Centers

New England

Poison Center
Children's Hospital Medical Center
300 Longwood Ave.,
Boston, MA 02115
Phone: (617) 232-2120

Middle Atlantic

New York City Poison Center
455 First Ave., Rm. 123
New York, N.Y. 10016
Phone: (212) 340-4495

Strong Memorial Hospital
260 Crittenden Blvd.
Rochester, N.Y. 14620
Phone: (716) 275-5151

Pittsburgh Poison Center
Children's Hospital of
Pittsburgh
125 De Soto St.
Pittsburgh, Pa. 15213
Phone: (412) 681-6669

Children's Hospital
111 Michigan Ave., N.W.
Washington, D.C. 20010

South

Orange Memorial Hospital
Emergency Room
1416 S. Orange Ave.
Orlando, Fl. 32806
Phone: (305) 841-8411 Ext. 656

Grady Memorial Hospital
80 Butler St., S.E.
Atlanta, Georgia 30303
Phone: (404) 588-4400

Poison Information Center
Children's Hospital
1601 6th Ave., S.
Birmingham, AL 35233
Phone: (205) 933-4050

Maryland Poison Information
Center
University of Maryland at
Baltimore
School of Pharmacy
636 W. Lombard St.
Baltimore, MD 21201
Phone: (301) 528-7701

Duke University Poison Center
Duke University Hospital
Durham, N.C. 27710
Phone: (919) 684-8111

Midwest

Poison Control Center
Children's Mercy Hospital
24th St. and Gilham Rd.
Kansas City, MO 64108
Phone: (816) 471-0626

St. Louis Poison Center
Cardinal Glennon Memorial
Hospital for Children
1465 S. Grand Blvd.
St. Louis, MO 63104
Phone: (314) 865-4000 Ext. 417

Poison Information Center
Children's Memorial Hospital
44th St. and Dewey Ave.
Omaha, NE 68105
Phone: (402) 553-5400

Children's Hospital
17th at Livingston
Columbus, Ohio 43208
Phone: (614) 228-1323

Milwaukee Poison Center
Milwaukee Children's Hospital
1700 W. Wisconsin Ave.
Milwaukee, WI 53233
Phone: (414) 931-1010

Poison Control Center
Rush-Presbyterian-St. Lukes
Medical Center
Pharmacy Dept.
1753 W. Congress Parkway
Chicago, IL 60612
Phone: (312) 942-5969

Southwest

New Mexico Poison and Drug
Information Center
Bernalillo County Medical Center
2211 Lomas Blvd. N.E.
Albuquerque, N.M. 87106
Phone: (505) 843-2551

Oklahoma State Dept. of Health
N.E. 10th St. and Stonewall
Oklahoma City, Oklahoma
Phone: (405) 271-5454

Southeast Texas Poison Center
University of Texas
Medical Branch Hospitals
8th St. and Mechanic St.
Galveston, TX 77550
Phone: (713) 765-1420

W. I. Cook Children's Hospital
1212 W. Lancaster Ave.
Fort Worth, TX 76102
Phone: (817) 336-5521 Ext. 17

Rocky Mountain

Rocky Mountain Poison Center
Denver General Hospital
West 8th Ave. and Cherokee St.
Denver, CO 80204
Phone: (303) 629-1123

Intermountain Regional Poison
Control Center
University of Utah Medical
Center
50 N. Medical Dr.
Salt Lake City, Utah 84132
Phone: (801) 581-2151

Pacific

Anchorage Poison Center
3200 Providence Dr.
Anchorage, Alaska 99504
Phone: (907) 274-6535

Children's Hospital of Los
Angeles
P.O. Box 54700
4650 Sunset Blvd.
Los Angeles, CA 90054

Central Emergency Medical
Services
County Health Dept.
135 Polk St.
San Francisco, CA 94102
Phone: (415) 431-2800

Santa Clara Valley Medical
Center
751 S. Bascom Ave.
San Jose, CA 95128
Phone: (408) 393-0262

San Diego Poison Information
Center
University Hospital
225 W. Dickinson St.
San Diego, CA 92103
Phone: (714) 294-6000

Poison Information Center
Children's Orthopedic Hospital
and Medical Center
4800 Sandpoint Way, N.E.
Seattle, WA 98105
Phone: (206) 634-5252

Pediatrics Dept.
University of Oregon Medical
School
3181 S.W. Sam Jackson
Park Rd.
Portland, Oregon 97201
Phone: (503) 225-8500

Source: The *National Clearinghouse for Poison Control Centers Bulletin: Directory,* August, 1978, U.S. Department of H.E.W., Public Health Service, Food and Drug Administration.

Reprinted with permission from *1979 Nursing Opportunities,* © 1979 by Litton Industries.

State Departments of Vocational Rehabilitation

ALABAMA
Vocational Rehabilitation
2129 E. South Boulevard
Montgomery, Alabama 36111
205-281-8780

ALASKA
Office of Vocational Rehabilitation
Pouch F, Mail Station 0581
Juneau, Alaska 99811
907-586-6500

ARIZONA
Rehabilitation Services Bureau
Dept. of Economic Security
1400 W. Washington Street
Phoenix, Arizona 85007
602-271-3332

ARKANSAS
Dept. of Social & Rehabilitation
   Services
1801 Rebsamen Park Road
P.O. Box 3781
Little Rock, Arkansas 72203
501-371-2571

CALIFORNIA
Dept. of Rehabilitation
830 K Street Mall
Sacramento, California 95814
916-445-3971

COLORADO
Division of Rehabilitation
Dept. of Social Services
1575 Sherman Street
Denver, Colorado 80203
303-892-2285

CONNECTICUT
State Dept. of Education
Division of Vocational Rehabilitation
600 Asylum Avenue
Hartford, Connecticut 06105
203-566-7329

DELAWARE
Dept. of Labor
Division of Vocational Rehabilitation
1500 Shallcross Avenue
P.O. Box 1190
Wilmington, Delaware 19899
302-571-2860

DISTRICT OF COLUMBIA
Social & Rehabilitation Administration
Dept. of Human Resources
122 C Street, N.W. - 8th Floor
Washington, D.C. 20001
202-629-5896

FLORIDA
Office of Vocational Rehabilitation
Dept. of Health & Rehabilitative
   Services
1323 Winewood Boulevard
Tallahassee, Florida 32301
904-488-6210

GEORGIA
Dept. of Human Resources
Division of Vocational Rehabilitation
47 Trinity Avenue
Atlanta, Georgia 30334
404-656-2621

GUAM
Dept. of Vocational Rehabilitation
P.O. Box 10-C
Agana, Guam 96910
472-8806

HAWAII
Division of Vocational Rehabilitation
Dept. of Social Services & Housing
Room 216, Queen Liliuokalani Building
P.O. Box 339
Honolulu, Hawaii 96809
808-548-6367

IDAHO
State of Idaho
Division of Vocational Rehabilitation
1501 McKinney
Boise, Idaho 83704
208-384-3390

ILLINOIS
Division of Vocational Rehabilitation
623 East Adams Street
P.O. Box 1587
Springfield, Illinois 62706
217-782-2093

INDIANA
Indiana Rehabilitation Services
1028 Illinois Building
17 W. Market Street
Indianapolis, Indiana 46204
317-633-5687

IOWA
State of Iowa
Dept. of Public Instruction
Rehabilitation Education & Service
  Branch
507 10th Street - Fifth Floor
Des Moines, Iowa 50309
515-281-4311

KANSAS
Division of Vocational Rehabilitation
Dept. of Social & Rehabilitative
  Services
5th Floor, State Office Building
Topeka, Kansas 66612
913-296-3911

KENTUCKY
Bureau of Rehabilitative Services
Capital Plaza Office Tower
Frankfort, Kentucky 40601
502-564-4440

LOUISIANA
Division of Vocational Rehabilitation
State of Louisiana
Dept. of Health and Human Services
Office of Rehabilitation Service
1755 Florida Boulevard
P.O. Box 44371
Baton Rouge, Louisiana 70804

MAINE
Bureau of Rehabilitation
32 Winthrop Street
Augusta, Maine 04330
207-289-2266

MARYLAND
Division of Vocational Rehabilitation
Box 8717, Baltimore-Washington
  International Airport
Baltimore, Maryland 21240
301-796-8300

MASSACHUSETTS
Rehabilitation Commission
296 Boylston Street
Boston, Massachusetts 02116
617-727-2172

MICHIGAN
State of Michigan
Dept. of Education
Vocational Rehabilitation Service
P.O. Box 30010
Lansing, Michigan 48909
517-373-3390

MINNESOTA
Division of Vocational Rehabilitation
Dept. of Economic Security
390 North Robert Street, 5th Floor
St. Paul, Minnesota 55101
612-296-5619

MISSISSIPPI
Vocational Rehabilitation Division
550 High Street
Walter Sillers Building
P.O. Box 1698
Jackson, Mississippi 39205
601-354-6825

MISSOURI
State of Missouri
Dept. of Elementary and Secondary
  Education
Division of Vocational Rehabilitation
3523 North Ten Mile Drive
Jefferson City, Missouri 65101
314-751-3251

MONTANA
State of Montana
Social & Rehabilitation Services
Rehabilitative Services Division
P.O. Box 4210
Helena, Montana 59601
406-449-2590

NEBRASKA
Dept. of Education
Division of Rehabilitative Services
301 Centennial Mall - 6th Floor
Lincoln, Nebraska 68508
402-471-2961

NEVADA
Dept. of Human Resources
Kinkead Building, Fifth Floor
505 E. King Street
Carson City, Nevada 89701
702-885-4440

NEW HAMPSHIRE
State Department of Education
Division of Vocational Rehabilitation
105 Loudon Road, Building No. 3
Concord, New Hampshire 03301
603-271-3121

NEW JERSEY
Division of Vocational Rehabilitation
  Services
Labor and Industry Building, Rm. 1005
John Fitch Plaza
Trenton, New Jersey 08625
609-292-5987

NEW MEXICO
Department of Education
231 Washington Avenue
P.O. Box 1830
Santa Fe, New Mexico 87503
505-827-2266

NEW YORK
The University of the State of New York
The State Education Department
Office of Vocational Rehabilitation
99 Washington Avenue
Albany, New York 12230
518-474-3941

NORTH CAROLINA
Division of Vocational Rehabilitation
  Services, Dept. of Human Resources
State Office
620 N. West Street, Box 26053
Raleigh, North Carolina 27611
919-829-3364

NORTH DAKOTA
Division of Vocational Rehabilitation
1025 N. 3rd Street, Box 1037
Bismarck, North Dakota 58501
701-224-2907

OHIO
Rehabilitation Services Commission
4656 Heaton Road
Columbus, Ohio 43229
614-466-5157

OKLAHOMA
Dept. of Institutions, Rehab Services
Social & Rehabilitative Services
Division of Rehabilitative and Visual
  Services
P.O. Box 25352
Oklahoma City, Oklahoma 73125
405-521-3374

OREGON
Vocational Rehabilitation Division
Dept. of Human Resources
2045 Silverton Road, N.E.
Salem, Oregon 97310
503-378-3850

PENNSYLVANIA
Bureau of Vocational Rehabilitation
Labor and Industry Building
7th and Forster Streets
Harrisburg, Pennsylvania 17120
717-787-5244

PUERTO RICO
Dept. of Social Services
P.O. Box 1118
Hato Rey, Puerto Rico 00919
809-725-1792

RHODE ISLAND
Vocational Rehabilitation
40 Fountain Street
Provdence, Rhode Island 02903
401-421-7005

SOUTH CAROLINA
Vocational Rehabilitation Department
3600 Forest Drive
P.O. Box 4945
Columbia, South Carolina 29240
803-758-3237

SOUTH DAKOTA
Dept. of Vocational Rehabilitation
Division of Rehabilitative Services
State Office Building, Illinois Street
Pierre, South Dakota 57501
605-224-3195

TENNESSEE
Division of Vocational Rehabilitation
Suite 1400 - 1808 W. End Building
Nashville, Tennessee 37203
615-741-2521

TEXAS
Texas Rehabilitation Commission
7745 Chevy Chase Drive
Austin, Texas 78752
512-447-0100

UTAH
Division of Rehabilitation Services
250 East Fifth South
Salt Lake City, Utah 84111
801-533-5991

VERMONT
Vocational Rehab Division
State Office Building
Montpelier, Vermont 05602
802-244-5181

VIRGINIA
Dept. of Vocational Rehabilitation
4901 Fitzhugh Avenue
P.O. Box 11045
Richmond, Virginia 23230
804-786-2091

VIRGIN ISLANDS
Dept. of Social Welfare
Division of Vocational Rehab
P.O. Box 539
St. Thomas, Virgin Islands 00801

WASHINGTON
State Office
Division of Vocational Rehabilitation
Dept. of Social and Health Services
P.O. Box 1788 (Mail Stop 311)
Olympia, Washington 98504
206-753-2544

WEST VIRGINIA
Division of Vocational Rehabilitation
P&G Building, Washington Street
Charleston, West Virginia 25305
304-348-2375

WISCONSIN
Ken McClarnon
Acting Administrator
131 West Wilson Street
Madison, Wisconsin 53702
608-266-1683

WYOMING
Division of Vocational Rehabilitation
Hathaway Building, West
Cheyenne, Wyoming 82002
307-777-7387

TRUST TERRITORY
Office of the High Commissioner
Trust Territory of the Pacific Islands
Saintan, Mariana Island 96550
9422

AMERICAN SAMOA
Palauni Puiasosopo
Assistant to the Governor of
   American Samoa
Pago Pago, American Samoa 96799
633-0116

Reprinted from *National Resource Directory, 1979*, published by the National Spinal Cord Injury Foundation.

State Welfare Office Listings

ALABAMA
Bureau of Public Affairs
Office of External Administration
64 N. Union St.
Montgomery 36130
(205) 832-6011

ALASKA
Director
Division of Social Services
Pouch H-05
Juneau 99811
(907) 465-3085

ARIZONA
Richard Bistirtz, Chief
Assistance Programs Bureau
Program Operations Division
P.O. Box 6123
Phoenix 85005
(602) 258-6361

ARKANSAS
Administrator
Financial Assistance Section
P.O. Box 1437
Little Rock 72203
(501) 376-2041

CALIFORNIA
AFDC Program Management Branc
Dept. of Benefit Payments
744 P St.
Sacramento 95814
(916) 322-9900

COLORADO
Division of Title XX Services
1575 Sherman St.
Denver 80203
(303) 839-2524

CONNECTICUT
Genevieve Elliott
Information and Inquiry Section
Dept. of Social Services
110 Bartholomew Ave.
Hartford 06115
(203) 566-2550

DELAWARE
Administrator
Family Services Section
Division of Social Services
P.O. Box 309
Wilmington 19899
(302) 762-6860

DISTRICT OF COLUMBIA
Administrator
Payments Assistance Admin.
500 First St., N.W. Rm. 9000
Washington 20001
(202) 724-5506

FLORIDA
Staff Director
Social & Economic Services Office
4311 Winewood Blvd.
Tallahasse 32301
(904) 487-2380

GEORGIA
Director
Specialized Services Section
Div. of Family & Children Services
47 Trinity Ave., S.W.
Atlanta 30334
(404) 656-4462

HAWAII
Administrator
Public Welfare Division
P.O. Box 339
Honolulu 96809
(808) 548-5908

IDAHO
Chief
Bureau of Financial Assistance
Division of Welfare
Statehouse
Boise   83720
(208)   377-7000

ILLINOIS
Supervisor
Inquiries and Referral Service
316 S. Second St.
Springfield   62762
(217) 782-0963

INDIANA
Division of Public Assistance
State Office Bldg., Rm. 701
100 N. Senate Ave.
Indianapolis   46204
(317) 633-4000

IOWA
Division of Community Services
3619 Douglas Ave.
Des Moines   50310
(515) 281-5758

LOUISIANA
Assistant Secretary
Office of Family Services
P.O. Box 44065
Baton Rouge   70804
(504) 342-3950

MAINE
Income Maintenance Unit
Bureau of Social Welfare
State House
Augusta   04333
(207) 289-2415

MARYLAND
Chief, Division of Policy
Social Services Admin.
11 South St.
Baltimore   21202
(301) 234-2222

MASSACHUSETTS
Office of Assistance Payments
Dept. of Public Welfare
600 Washington St.
Boston   02111
(617) 727-7537

KANSAS
Public Assistance Section
Division of Social Services
State Office Bldg., 5th Fl.
Topeka   66612
(913) 296-3959

KENTUCKY
Commissioner
Bureau for Social Insurance
275 E. Main St.
Frankfort   40601
(502) 564-3703

MICHIGAN
Director, Bureau of Assistance
  Payments
Citizen Services Administration
300 S. Capital Ave.
Lansing   48926
(517) 373-1837

MINNESOTA
Assistant Commissioner
Bureau of Community Services
Centennial Office Bldg. - 4th Fl.
St. Paul   55155
(612) 296-6117

MISSISSIPPI
Director, Div. of Assistance Payments
P.O. Box 4321, Fondren Station
Jackson   39216
(601) 956-8713

MISSOURI
Social Services Section
Division of Family Services
Broadway State Office Bldg.
Jefferson City   65101
(314) 751-3221

MONTANA
Economic Assistance Division
P.O. Box 4210
Helena   59601
(406) 449-3952

NEBRASKA
Division of Income Maintenance
P.O. Box 95026
Lincoln   68509
(402) 471-3121

NEVADA
Administrator, Welfare Division
251 Jeanell Dr.
Carson City   89710
(702) 885-4771

NEW HAMPSHIRE
Public Information Officer
Division of Welfare
8 Loudon Rd.
Concord   03301
(603) 271-2382

NEW JERSEY
Chief
Bureau of Policy & Standards Develop.
Division of Public Welfare
3525 Quakerbridge Rd.
Trenton 08625
(609) 890-9500

NEW MEXICO
Director, State Welfare Agency
P.O. Box 2348
Santa Fe 87503
(505) 827-2376

NEW YORK
Executive Communications Unit
Dept. of Social Services
40 N. Pearl St.
Albany 12243
(518) 474-2121

NORTH CAROLINA
Assistant Director
Programs and Policy
Division of Social Services
325 N. Salisbury St.
Raleigh 27611
(919) 733-4759

NORTH DAKOTA
Director of Community Services
Social Service Board
State Capitol
Bismark 58505
(701) 224-2310

OHIO
Division of Social Services
Office of Programs
30 E. Broad St., 31st Fl.
Columbus 43215
(614) 466-2360

OKLAHOMA
Director
Dept. of Institutions, Social and
  Rehabilitative Services
Attn: Division of Assistance Payments
P.O. Box 25352
Oklahoma City 73125
(405) 521-3374

OREGON
Manager, Assistance Program Unit
Public Welfare Division
Public Service Bldg., Rm. 318
Salem 97310
(503) 378-2720

PENNSYLVANIA
Deputy Secretary
Office of Social Programs
P.O. Box 2675
Harrisburg 17120
(717) 787-1870

RHODE ISLAND
Assistance Administrator
Assistance Payments
Division of Managment Services
600 New London Ave.
Cranston 02920
(401) 943-3000

SOUTH CAROLINA
Commissioner's Office
Dept. of Social Services
P.O. Box 1520
Columbia 29202
(803) 758-3244

SOUTH DAKOTA
Division of Social Welfare
Attn: Inter-Agency Inquiry
State Office Bldg.
Illinois St.
Pierre 57501
(605) 773-3491

TENNESSEE
Director of Public Assistance
Department of Human Services
State Office Bldg.
Nashville 37219
(615) 741-2917

TEXAS
Division of Special Services
John H. Reagan Bldg.
Austin 78701
(512) 475-5615

UTAH
Director
Division of Family Services
P.O. Box 2500
Salt Lake City 84110
(801) 486-1811

VERMONT
Director
Social Services Division
Dept. of Social & Rehabilitation
  Services
81 River St.
Montpelier 05602
(802) 828-3401

VIRGINIA
Office of Communications
Dept. of Welfare
8007 Discovery Dr.
Richmond 23229
(804) 786-8772

703

...unseling and
...-42 ...Center
8504 ...mit Avenue, Suite 710
034 ...th, Tex. 76102

...GINIA
. Pol...el Films
...of Broadway
...ash... York, N.Y. 10036

J. B. Fleet Co., Inc.
P. O. Box 1100
Lynchburg, Va. 24505

Centre Films, Inc.
1103 N. El Centro Avenue
Hollywood, Calif. 90038

Childbirth Education Associates
108 Natchez Drive
Hendersonville, Tenn. 37075

Child Care Information Service
532 Settlers Landing Road
P. O. Box 548
Hampton, Va. 23669

Churchill Films
662 North Robertson Boulevard
Los Angeles, Calif. 90069

Ciba-Geigy
Medical Education Division
P. O. Box 195
Summit, N.J. 07901

Cinema Medica
664 N. Michigan Avenue
Chicago, Ill. 60611

Columbia Special Products
CBS Records
A Division of CBS, Inc.
51 W. 52nd Street
New York, N.Y. 10019

Communication Enterprises, Inc.
936 Courthouse Road, Suite 3
Gulfport, Miss. 39501

Concept Media
P. O. Box 19542
Irvine, Calif. 92714

Concern For Dying
250 W. 57th Street
New York, N.Y. 10019

Corometrics Medical Systems, Inc.
473 Washington Avenue
North Haven, Conn. 06473

EDC Distribution Center
39 Chapel Street
Newton, Mass. 02160

Eli Lilly and Company
Audio-Visual Film Library
Indianapolis, Ind. 46206

Ethicon, Inc.
Route 22
Somerville, N.J. 08876

Eye Gate Media
146-01 Archer Avenue
Jamaica, N.Y. 11435

Films Incorporated
733 Green Bay Road
Wilmette, Ill. 60091

Green Mountain Post Films
P. O. Box 177
Montague, Mass. 01351

Hartley Productions
Films For A New Age
Cat Rock Road
Cos Cob, Conn. 06807

Health Sciences Communications Center
Marketing Division, Room WA-6725
Case Western Reserve University
University Circle
Cleveland, Oh. 44106

Hoechst Pharmaceuticals, Inc.
Route 202-206 North
Somerville, N.J. 08876

ICEA Publication/Distribution Center
P. O. Box 9316, Midtown Plaza
Rochester, N.Y. 14604

ICEA Bookcenter
P. O. Box 70258
Seattle, Wa. 98107

Ilex Films
P. O. Box 226
Cambridge, Mass. 02138

International Film Bureau, Inc.
332 South Michigan Avenue
Chicago, Ill. 60604

Jay Hathaway Production Services
4846 Katherine Avenue
Sherman Oaks, Calif. 91423

Johnson and Johnson
Baby Products Company
Piscataway, N.J. 08854

Joseph T. Anzalone Foundation
P. O. Box 5206
Santa Cruz, Calif. 95063

Juvenile Diabetes Foundation
Greater Washington Area Chapter
P. O. Box 48
Silver Spring, Md. 20907

Kartemquin/Haymarket Films
1901 West Wellington Avenue
Chicago, Ill. 60657

Keith Merrill Associates
2068 Cynthia Way
Los Altos, Calif. 94022

La Leche League International, Inc.
9616 Minneapolis Avenue
Franklin Park, Ill. 60131

Lederle Laboratories
Film Library
A Division Of American Cyanamid Company
1 Casper Street
Danbury, Conn. 06810

Leukemia Society Of America, Inc.
211 East 43rd Street
New York, N.Y. 10017

Lippincott's Audio Visual Media
J. B. Lippincott Company
East Washington Square
Philadelphia, Pa. 19105

Marshfilm Enterprises, Inc.
P. O. Box 8082
Shawnee Mission, Kans. 66208

Mary Jane Company
P. O. Box 736
North Hollywood, Calif. 91609

McGraw-Hill Films
Film Library
1221 Avenue Of The Americas
New York, N.Y. 10020

Media For Childbirth Education
P. O. Box 2092
Castro Valley, Calif. 94546

Mental Health Media Evaluation Project
P. O. Box 1548
Springfield, Va. 22151

Merck, Sharp and Dohme
Division Of Merck and Company, Inc.
West Point, Pa. 19486

Michael Chait
P. O. Box 1959
Grand Central Station
New York, N.Y. 10017

Milner-Fenwick, Inc.
3800 Liberty Heights Avenue
Baltimore, Md. 21215

Modern Talking Picture Service
2323 New Hyde Park Road
New Hyde Park, N.Y. 11042

Monterey Laboratories, Inc.
c/o Joyce Abrams
P. O. Box 15129
Las Vegas, Nv. 89114

Motion, Inc.
4437 Klingle Street, N.W.
Washington, D.C. 20016

Motorola Teleprograms, Inc.
4825 N. Scott Street
Schiller Park, Ill. 60176

Multi Media Office
Mt. San Jacinto College
21400 Highway 79
San Jacinto, Calif. 92383

Multi Media Resource Center,
540 Powell Street
San Francisco, Calif. 94108

Music Therapy Center
251 West 51st Street
New York, N.Y. 10019

Narcotics Education, Inc.
P. O. Box 4390
6830 Laurel Street, N.W.
Washington, D.C. 20012

National Association For Retarded Citizens
2709 Avenue E., East
P. O. Box 6109
Arlington, Tex. 76011

National Center On Child Abuse And Neglect
U. S. Children's Bureau
Administration For Children, Youth And Families
U. S. Department Of H.E.W.
P. O. Box 1182
Washington, D.C. 20013

National Clearinghouse For Drug Abuse Information (NCDAI)
P. O. Box 1909
Rockville, Md. 20850

National Dairy Council
6300 North River Road
Rosemont, Ill. 60018

National Film Board Of Canada
16th Floor, 1251 Avenue Of The Americas
New York, N.Y. 10020

National Society For The
Prevention Of Blindness, Inc.
Public Relations Department
79 Madison Avenue
New York, N.Y. 10016

New Times Films, Inc.
1501 Broadway, Suite 1904
New York, N.Y. 10036

New Yorker Films
16 West 61st Street
New York, N.Y. 10023

NIDA Resource Center
National Institute On Drug Abuse
Room 10A-54 Parklawn Building
5600 Fishers Lane
Rockville, Md. 20857

Norwich-Eaton Pharmaceuticals
(East of the Rockies)
Norwich-Eaton Film Library
17 Eaton Avenue
Norwich, N.Y. 13815

Annapolis, Md. 21404

Occidental Publishing
Company
P. O. Box 9620
Stanford, Calif. 94305

Paramount Communications
5451 Marathon Street
Hollywood, Calif. 90038

Parenting Pictures
A Division Of Courter Films
And Associates
R.D. #1, Box 355B
Columbia, N.J. 07832

Parents' Magazine Films, Inc.
52 Vanderbilt Avenue
New York, N.Y. 10017

Perennial Education, Inc.
477 Roger Williams
P. O. Box 855, Ravinia
Highland Park, Ill. 60035

Photoview Instructional Aids
27935 Roble Alto
Los Altos Hills, Calif. 94022

Physicians For Automotive
Safety
Communications Department
5 Eve Lane
Rye, N.Y. 10580

Pictura
Films Distribution Corporation
111 Eighth Avenue
New York, N.Y. 10011

Planned Parenthood
Federation Of America, Inc.
Film Library
470 Park Avenue, South
New York, N.Y. 10016

Polymorph Films
331 Newbury Street
Boston, Mass. 02115

Professional Research, Inc.
12960 Coral Tree Place
Los Angeles, Calif. 90066

Pyramid Films
Box 1048
Santa Monica, Calif. 90406

Robert J. Brady Company
A Prentice-Hall Company
Bowie, Md. 20715

Soundwords, Inc.
56-11 217th Street
Bayside, N.Y. 11364

Stethophonics
P. O. Box 122
Wellesley Hills, Mass. 02181

Suzanne Arms Productions
151 Lytton Avenue
Palo Alto, Calif. 94301

Syntex Laboratories, Inc.
Professional Services
Department
3401 Hillview Avenue
Palo Alto, Calif. 94304

Teach'em, Inc.
c/o Aaron Cohades
625 North Michigan Avenue
Chicago, Ill. 60611

The Graphic Curriculum, Inc.
P. O. Box 565
Lenox Hill Station
New York, N.Y. 10021

Trainex Corporation
P. O. Box 116
Garden Grove, Calif. 92642

Tricontinental Film Center
333 Avenue Of The Americas
New York, N.Y. 10014

or

Tricontinental Film Center
P. O. Box 4430
Berkeley, Calif. 94704

United Cerebral Palsy
Associations, Inc.
66 East 34th Street
New York, N.Y. 10016

University of California*
Extension Media Center
2223 Fulton Street
Berkeley, Calif. 94720

University of Wisconsin-Milwaukee
Media, School of Nursing
P. O. Box 413
Milwaukee, Wisconsin 53201

Upjohn
Upjohn Professional Film Library
7000 Portage Road
Kalamazoo, Mich. 49001

U. S. Department of H.E.W.
Public Health Service
Health Services Administration
5600 Fishers Lane
Rockville, Md. 20852

UW-Extension, Department
Of Nursing
424 Lowell Hall
610 Langdon Street
Madison, Wi. 53706

Wayne State University
c/o Frederick J. Margolis, M.D.
Project Director
Systems Distribution and
Utilization Department
Center For Instructional Technology
Detroit, Mich. 48202

West Glen Films
West Glen Communications, Inc.
565 Fifth Avenue
New York, N.Y. 10017

Westwood Pharmaceuticals, Inc.
468 Dewitt Street
Buffalo, N.Y. 14213

Women Make Movies, Inc.
257 West 19th Street
New York, N.Y. 10011

World Health Organization Films
WHO Regional Office
For The Americas
525 23rd Street, N.W.
Washington, D.C. 20037

Zipporah Films
54 Lewis Wharf
Boston, Mass. 02110

* *Titles of films from the University Of California Extension Media Center, originally appeared in the University Of California Extension Media Center publication, Films 1977–78, copyright 1977 by the Regents of the University Of California. This is a comprehensive bulletin describing more than 4,000 films in dynamic areas of national interest. Portions reprinted here by kind permission of the University Of California Extension Media Center, Berkeley, Calif. 94720.*

Audiovisual Equipment

The following companies have audiovisual equipment available for sale along with the films and other aids listed previously. (See directory of audiovisual resources above for addresses of the companies.)

Cinema Medica

Materials available: Video recorders, projectors, and all brands of video equipment. Special rates are available on equipment purchased with Cinema Medica video cassettes or Super 8 cartridges.

Communication Enterprises, Inc.

Materials available: Cassette tape recorders, blank cassettes and cassette storage boxes.

Marshfilm

Materials available: Dukane 35mm sound filmstrip projectors for use with cassettes or records.

Professional Research, Inc.

Materials available: Technicolor film projectors, both portable and console models.

Government Catalogs

The National Medical Audiovisual Center Catalog contains over 300 pages of listings of audiovisual materials available for free short-term loan from the Center in Atlanta, Ga. The catalog (Dept. of H.E.W. Publication No. (NIH) 77-506) may be purchased for $4.25 per copy, from the Superintendent Of Documents, U. S. Government Printing Office, Washington, D.C. 20402.

A listing of nursing information audiovisual materials produced by or for the Federal government may be obtained by contacting the General Services Administration, National Archives And Records Service, National Audiovisual Center, Washington, D.C. 20409. This list includes films on all aspects of nursing care and is particularly useful to nursing educators.

Guide To Audiovisual Aids For Spanish-Speaking Americans, a 37-page booklet, is available from the U.S. Department of H.E.W. Public Health Service. It is free of charge and includes annotated listings of the films and addresses of the film distributors. (DHEW Publication No. (HSA) 74-30.)

Index of Publishers

The following Publishers are sources for books and periodicals named elsewhere in this book, and for other publications of interest to nurses. For a complete listing of current publications available from each, write for catalog.

Addison-Wesley Publishing Co.
Sand Hill Rd.
Menlo Park, CA 94025

Alfred A. Knopf, Inc.
201 East 50th St.
New York, N.Y. 10022

Allyn and Bacon, Inc.
470 Atlantic Ave.
Boston, Mass. 02210

American Journal of Nursing Co.
10 Columbus Circle
New York, N.Y. 10019

American Medical Association
535 North Dearborn St.
Chicago, Illinois 60610

And/Or Press, Inc.
P.O. Box 2246
Berkeley, CA 94702

Appleton-Century-Crofts
292 Madison Ave.
New York, N.Y. 10017

Arlington House Publishers
New Rochelle, N.Y.

Aspen Systems Corporation
20010 Century Boulevard
Germantown, Maryland 20767

Bantam Books
666 5th Ave.
New York, N.Y. 10022

Beacon Press
25 Beacon St.
Boston, Mass. 02108

Bobbs-Merrill
4 West 58th St.
New York, N.Y. 10019

California Health Publications
P.O. Box 963
Laguna Beach, CA 92652

Charles B. Slack, Inc.
6900 Grove Rd.
Thorofare, N.J. 08086

Charles Scribner's Sons
597 5th Ave.
New York, N.Y. 10017

Churchill Livingstone Inc.
19 West 44th St.
New York, N.Y. 10036

CIBA
Medical Education Division
Summit, N.J. 07901

Clarkson N. Potter
One Park Ave.
New York, N.Y. 10016

Concept Development, Inc.
12 Lakeside Park
607 North Ave.
Wakefield, Mass. 01881

Coward, McCann and
Geoghegan, Inc.
200 Madison Ave.
New York, N.Y. 10016

Crown Publishers
One Park Ave.
New York, N.Y. 10016

The C. V. Mosby Co.
11830 Westline Industrial Dr.
St. Louis, Missouri 63141

Doubleday and Co., Inc.
245 Park Ave.
New York, N.Y. 10017

Ed-U Press
760 Ostrom Ave.
Syracuse, N.Y. 13210

Elsevier North-Holland
52 Vanderbilt Ave.
New York, N.Y. 10017

Faber and Faber, Ltd.
3 Queen Square
London WC1 England

F. A. Davis Co., Publishers
1915 Arch St.
Philadelphia, Pa. 19103

Fawcett Publications, Inc.
P.O. Box 1014
Greenwich, Conn. 06830

G. P. Putnam's Sons
200 Madison Ave.
New York, N.Y. 10016

Grosset and Dunlap, Inc.
51 Madison Ave.
New York, N.Y. 10016

Grune and Stratton Corporation
111 5th Ave.
New York, N.Y. 10011

Harcourt Brace Jovanovich
757 Third St.
New York, N.Y. 10017

Harper and Row Publishers, Inc.
2350 Virginia Ave.
Hagerstown, Md. 21740

Holt, Rinehart and Winston, Inc.
383 Madison Ave.
New York, N.Y. 10017

Houghton, Mifflin, Inc.
2 Park St.
Boston, Mass. 02107

Human Sciences Press
72 Fifth Ave.
New York, N.Y. 10011

or

Human Sciences Press
3 Henrietta St.
London, WC2E 8LU England

Intermed Communications, Inc.
132 Welsh Rd.
Horsham, Pa. 19044

Irvington Publishers, Inc.
551 Fifth Ave.
New York, N.Y. 10017

J. B. Lippincott Co.
East Washington Square
Philadelphia, Pa. 19105

Jones Medical Publications
355 Los Cerros Drive
Greenbrae, CA 94904

The Johns Hopkins University Press
Baltimore, Md. 21218

John Wiley and Sons, Inc.
1 Wiley Dr.
Somerset, N.J. 08873

Lange Medical Publications
Drawer L
Los Altos, CA 94022

Lea and Febiger
600 South Washington Square
Philadelphia, Pa. 19106

Little, Brown and Co.
34 Beacon St.
Boston, Mass. 02106

Macmillan Publishing Co., Inc.
866 Third Ave.
New York, N.Y. 10022

Masson Publishing U.S.A., Inc.
14 East 60th St.
New York, N.Y. 10022

McGraw-Hill Book Co.
1221 Ave. of the Americas,
New York, N.Y. 10020

Mc Mahon Publishing Co.
83 Peaceable St.
Georgetown Station, Conn. 06829

Medical Economics Co.
A Litton Division
Oradell, N.J. 07649

Med/Law Publishers, Inc.
P.O. Box 293
Westville, N.J. 08093

National Academy of Sciences
2101 Constitution Ave.
Washington, D.C. 20418

National League for Nursing
10 Columbus Circle
New York, N.Y. 10019

The New American Library, Inc.
1300 Ave. of the Americas
New York, N.Y. 10019

Northeast Appropriate Technology Network, Inc.
Box 548
Greenfield, MA 01302

Nursing Publications, Inc.
Box 218
Hillsdale, N.J. 07642

Oxford University Press
200 Madison Ave.
New York, N.Y. 10016

Paddington Press
30 East 42nd St.
New York, N.Y. 10036

Plenum Publishing Corporation
227 West 17th St.
New York, N.Y. 10011

Pocket Books, Division of Simon
and Schuster, Inc.
635 5th Ave.
New York, N.Y. 10022

Prentice-Hall
Englewood Cliffs, N.J. 07632

Princeton University Press
Princeton, N.J. 08540

Random House, Inc.
201 East 50th St.
New York, N.Y. 10022

Rawson Associates Publishers, Inc.
630 3rd Ave.
New York, N.Y. 10017

Redgrave Publishing Co.
A Division of Docent Corporation
430 Manville Rd.
Pleasantville, N.Y. 10570

Roche Laboratories
5 Johnson Dr.
Raritan, N.J.

Rodale Press, Inc.
Organic Park
Emmaus, PA 18049

Running Press
38 South 19th St.
Philadelphia, PA 19103

Simon and Schuster, Inc.
1230 6th Ave.
New York, N.Y. 10019

Springer Publishing Co.
200 Park Ave. South
New York, N.Y. 10003

Superintendent of Documents
Government Printing Office
Washington, D.C. 20402

Van Nostrand Reinhold Co.
450 West 33rd St.
New York, N.Y. 10001

The Viking Press
Viking Penguin, Inc.
625 Madison Ave.
New York, N.Y. 10022

W. B. Saunders Company
West Washington Square
Philadelphia, PA 19105

William Morrow and Co., Inc.
105 Madison Ave.
New York, N.Y. 10016

Williams and Wilkins
428 East Preston St.
Baltimore, Md. 21202

Another source for books for nurses, along with the Publishers listed above, is the Nurses' Book Society. It functions as other book clubs do, offering current books at lower prices. For further information write:

The Nurses' Book Society
Front and Brown Streets, P.O. Box 6666
Riverside, N.J. 08370

Abbreviations in Common Use

ABBREVIATION	MEANING
a.a.	of each
A.A.	Alcoholics Anonymous
abd	abdomen
a.c.	before meals
Ac.	acid
ACTH	adrenocorticotropin
ADL	activities of daily living
ADP	adenosine diphosphate
ad lib	as desired
adm	admission
alk.	alkaline
A.M.	morning
AMA	against medical advice
amp	ampule
amt	amount
ANS	autonomic nervous system
ante	before
AP	anteroposterior
aq	water
AROM	artificial rupture of membranes
ASHD	arteriosclerotic heart disease
ASD	atrial septal defect
ATP	adenosine triphosphate
A-V	atrio-ventricular
A & W	alive and well
BCP	birth control pills
B.E.	barium enema
b.i.d.	twice a day
BM	bowel movement
BMR	basal metabolic rate
BP	blood pressure
BRP	bathroom privileges
BS	blood sugar
BSE	breast self examination
BSP	bromosulfophthalein
BT	bleeding time
BUN	blood urea nitrogen
Bx	biopsy

ABBREVIATION	MEANING
C	centigrade
c̄	with
Ca	calcium
CA, Ca	cancer
Cal	calorie
cap	capsule
cath	catheter
C.B.C	complete blood count
CBD	common bile duct
C.B.R.	complete bedrest
cc	cubic centimeter
CC	chief complaint
C.C.U.	coronary care unit
CF	cystic fibrosis
CHF	congestive heart failure
CHO	carbohydrate
chol.	cholesterol
ck	check
cm	centimeter
CMV	cytomegalo virus
CNM	Certified Nurse Midwife
CNS	central nervous system
c/o	complains of
C.O.	cardiac output
comp	compound
contra	against
CPD	cephalopelvic disproportion
C & S	culture and sensitivity
CS	cesarean section
CSF	cerebrospinal fluid
CSS	central sterile supply
CST	convulsive shock therapy
cu. mm.	cubic millimeter
CVA	cerebrovascular accident
CVP	central venous pressure
CVS	cardiovascular system; clean voided specimen
Cx	cervix
cysto	cystoscopy
d.c.	discontinue
D & C	dilation and curettage

ABBREVIATION	MEANING
DD	differential diagnosis
diff.	differential
dig.	digitalis
dil.	dilute
disch.	discharge
DNA	deoxyribonucleic acid
DOA	dead on arrival
DOB	date of birth
DOE	dyspnea on exertion
DPT	diphtheria, pertussis, tetanus
dr	dram
Dr.	doctor
D.R.	delivery room
drsg, dsg	dressing
DSD	dry sterile dressing
DT's	delirium tremens
DTR	deep tendon reflexes
D/W	dextrose and water
D-5-W	5% dextrose in water
Dx	diagnosis
ECG, EKG	electrocardiogram
ECT	electroconvulsive therapy
EDC	estimated date of confinement
EEG	electroencephalogram
EENT	eye, ear, nose and throat
e.g.	for example
elix.	elixir
E.R.	emergency room
E.S.P.	extrasensory perception
et al.	and others
ext.	extract
f	frequency
F	fahrenheit
F.B.S.	fasting blood sugar
F.D.A.	Food and Drug Administration
Fe	iron
FH	family history
FHR	fetal heart rate
fld	fluid
FNP	family nurse practitioner
G	gravida

ABBREVIATION	MEANING
gal	gallon
GC	gonococcus
GH	growth hormone
GI	gastrointestinal
Gm	gram
G.N.	graduate nurse
GP	general practitioner
gr	grain
gtt	drops
GTT	glucose tolerance test
GU	genitourinary
Gyn	gynecology
h (hr)	hour
Hb (Hgb)	hemoglobin
HCL	hydrochloric acid
Hct	hematocrit
H.E.W.	Health, Education and Welfare
Hg	mercury
MHD	hyaline membrane disease
HMO	health maintenance organization
h/o	history of
HO	house officer
HPI	history of present illness
H.R.	heart rate
h.s.	hour of sleep
ht	height
HT	hypertension
Hx	history
IBC	iron-binding capacity
ICF	intracellular fluid
ICU	intensive care unit
ID	intradermal
I & D	incision and drainage
i.e.	that is
I.M.	intramuscular
inj	injection
I & O	intake and output
IPPB	intermittent positive pressure breathing
IQ	intelligence quotient
irrig	irrigation
IU	international unit

ABBREVIATION	MEANING
IUD	intrauterine device
IV	intravenous
IVP	intravenous pyelogram
K	potassium
Kg	kilogram
L	left; liter
Lab	laboratory
Lap	laparotomy
lb	pound
LE	lupus erythematosus
LGA	large for gestational age
LH	luteinizing hormone
liq	liquid
LLQ	left lower quadrant
LMP	last menstrual period
LOA	left occiput anterior
LOP	left occiput posterior
LOT	left occiput transverse
LP	lumbar puncture
LPN	licensed practical nurse
LUQ	lift upper quadrant
LVN	licensed vocational nurse
l & w	living and well
lymph	lymphocyte
m	meter
MCV	mean corpuscular volume
MD	muscular dystrophy; medical doctor
meds	medications
mEq	milliequivalent
mEq/L	milliequivalent per liter
mg	milligram
MI	myocardial infarction
mid	middle
min	minute; minim
mixt	mixture
ml	milliliter
mm	millimeter
MOM	milk of magnesia
MS	multiple sclerosis
MSU	midstream urine
multip	multipara, pregnant woman who has previously borne children

ABBREVIATION	MEANING
NA	nurse anesthetist
NB	note carefully; newborn
neg	negative
neuro	neurology
N-G	nasogastric
nil	none
no.	number
noct	at night
non rep.	do not repeat
NPO	nothing by mouth
NS	normal saline
NSVD	normal, spontaneous, vaginal delivery
nullip	nullipara, a woman who has never borne child
N & V	nausea and vomiting
O_2	oxygen
OA	occiput anterior
OB, Obs	obstetrics
O.C.	oral contraceptive
od	daily
OD	right eye; overdose
OOB	out of bed
Op	operation
OP	occiput posterior
OPD	outpatient department
Ophth	ophthalmology
O.R.	operating room
Ortho	orthopedics
os	opening
OS	left eye
osteo	osteomyelitis
OT	occupational therapy
oz	ounce
$\bar{p}$	after
P	para; pulse
PA	physician's assistant
Pap	Papanicolaou smear
Para	number of pregnancies
Path	pathology
PBI	protein bound iodine
p.c.	after meals
PCO_2	partial pressure of carbon dioxide

ABBREVIATION	MEANING
PE	physical examination
Peds	pediatrics
PERLA	pupils equal and reactive to light and accommodation
P.H.	past history
pH	hydrogen ion concentration
PI	present illness
PID	pelvic inflammatory disease
PKU	phenylketonuria
p.m.	afternoon
PNP	pediatric nurse practitioner
p.o.	by mouth
PO$_2$	partial pressure of oxygen
P.O.R.	problem oriented record
pos	positive
postop	postoperative
preop	preoperative
prep	preparation
p.r.	per rectum
p.r.n.	when needed
pro time	prothrombin time
PSP	phenolsulfonphthalein
PSRO	Professional Standards Review Organization
psych	psychology; psychiatry
Pt	patient
PT	physical therapy
PTA	prior to admission
PVC	premature ventricular contraction
q.	every
q.d.	every day
q.h.	every hour
q2h., etc.	every 2 hours, etc.
q.h.s.	at bedtime
q.i.d.	4 times a day
q.o.d.	every other day
qt	quart
R, Rt	right
RBC	red blood cell
RDS	respiratory distress syndrome
REM	rapid eye movement

ABBREVIATION	MEANING
Rh	Rhesus factor
RHD	rheumatic heart disease
RLQ	right lower quadrant
RN	registered nurse
RNA	ribonucleic acid
R/O	rule out
ROA	right occiput anterior
ROM	range of motion
ROP	right occiput posterior
ROT	right occiput transverse
RR	respiratory rate; recovery room
RUQ	right upper quadrant
Rx	therapy; treatment
$\bar{s}$	without
sc	subcutaneous
SD	standard deviation
sg	specific gravity
SGA	small for gestational age
SIDS	sudden infant death syndrome
sig	label
SLE	systemic lupus erythematosus
S.N.	student nurse
S.O.A.P.	subjective, objective, assessment plan
SOB	shortness of breath
SOS	once if necessary
spec	specimen
SR	sedimentation rate
$\bar{ss}$	one half
SSE	soap suds enema
staph	staphylococcus
stat	immediately
STS	serologic test for syphilis
strep	streptococcus
subcu; sub q	subcutaneous
supp	suppository
susp	suspension
SVD	spontaneous vaginal delivery
Sx	symptoms
T & A	tonsillectomy and adenoidectomy
TB	tuberculosis
Tbsp, T.	tablespoon

ABBREVIATION	MEANING
t.i.d.	three times a day
tinc	tincture
TL	team leader
TLC	tender loving care
t.o.	telephone order
TPR	temperature, pulse and respiration
tsp	teaspoon
TUR	transurethral resection
Tx	treatment
U	unit
U/A	urinalysis
ung	ointment
URI	upper respiratory infection
UTI	urinary tract infection
vag	vaginal
VD	venereal disease
VDRL	venereal disease research laboratory
Vit	vitamin
v.o.	verbal order
vol	volume
VS	vital signs
WBC	white blood cell
WC	wheelchair
WDWN	well developed, well nourished
WNL	within normal limits
wt	weight

Index of Associations and Organizations

Academy of Holistic Medicine, Inc., 551
Action on Smoking and Health (ASH), 229
Administration for Children, Youth and Families, 193
Administration on Aging, 193, 465
Alan Guttmacher Institute, 574
Al-Anon Family Group Headquarters, 525
Alcohol, Drug Abuse and Mental Health, 193
Alcoholics Anonymous, Inc., 524–525
Alexander Graham Bell Association for the Deaf, 231
American Academy for Cerebral Palsy and Developmental Medicine, 444
American Academy of Husband-Coached Childbirth, 355–356
American Academy of Pediatrics, 426
American Art Therapy Association, Inc. (AATA), 521
American Association for Rehabilitation Therapy, Inc., 631
American Association of Blood Banks, 185
American Association of Critical-Care Nurses, 631
American Association of I.V. Therapy, Inc., 631
American Association of Nephrology Nurses, 632
American Association of Neurosurgical Nurses, 632
American Association of Nurse Anesthetists, 632
American Association of Occupational Health Nurses, Inc., 632–633
American Association of Ophthalmology, 232
American Association of Sex Education, 579
American Association of Suicidology, 528
American Association on Mental Deficiency (AAMD), 440

American Board for Occupational Health Nurses, Inc., 633
American Burn Association, 166
American Cancer Society, Inc., 204
American Civil Liberties Union, 3
American Coalition of Citizens with Disabilities, Inc., 218
American College Health Association (ACHA), 185–186
American College of Home Obstetrics, 351
American College of Nurse-Midwives (ACNM), 633
American College of Nursing Home Administrators, 633
American College Testing Program (ACT), 593
American Dance Therapy Association, 521
American Diabetes Association, Inc., 211
American Dietetic Association, 274
American Foundation for the Blind, 233
American Health Care Association, 465–466
American Heart Association, 186
American Hospital Association, 186
American Humane Association, 436
American Indian/Alaska Native Nurses Association, Inc., 633–634
American Journal of Nursing Educational Testing Service, 591
American National Red Cross, 186–187
American Nurses' Association (ANA), 634–635
American Nurses' Association Council of Nurse Researchers, 600
American Occupational Medical Association, 213
American Physical Therapy Association, 196
American Printing House for the Blind, Inc., 233

American Psychological Association, 522
American Public Health Association, 635
American School Health Association, 635
American Society for Nursing Service Administrators of the American Hospital Association, 636
American Society for Psychoprophylaxis, 356
American Society of Allied Health Professions, 635
American Society of Group Psychotherapy and Psychodrama, 522
American Society of Hospital Pharmacists, 126
American Speech-Language-Hearing Association, 231
American Urological Association, 636
Amputee Shoe and Glove Exchange, 218
Anorexia Nervosa and Associated Disorders (ANAD), 522
Arthritis Foundation, the, 187
Association for Childbirth at Home International, 351
Association for Holistic Health, 552
Association for Humanistic Psychology, 522–523
Association for Practitioners in Infection Control, 637
Association for the Advancement of Health Education, 187
Association for the Care of Children in Hospitals, 445
Association for Voluntary Sterilization, Inc., 574
Association of Operating Room Nurses, Inc., the, 636
Association of Pediatric Oncology Nurses (APON), 636–637
Association of Radical Midwives, 637
Association of Rehabilitation Nurses (ARN), 637
Asthma and Allergy Foundation of America, 187

Better Vision Institute, Inc., 233
Biofeedback Society of America, 552
Birth Day, 351
Boston Women's Health Book Collective, 561
Bureau of Education for the Handicapped, 192

CALM. Child Abuse Listening Mediation, Inc., 436
Cancer Information Clearinghouse, 205–206
Cancer Counseling and Research Center, 205
Candlelighters Foundation, the, 446
Center for Attitudinal Healing, 446–447
Center for Chinese Medicine, 552
Center for Disease Control, 193
Center for Inner Motivation and Awareness, 552
Center for Integral Medicine, 553
Center for Medical Consumers and Health Care, 226
Center for Science in the Public Interest (CSPI), 274
Childbirth Without Pain Education League, Inc., 356
Child, Inc., 426
Children in Hospitals, Inc. (CIH), 445
Closer Look, 441
Coalition for Children and Youth, 426
Coalition for the Medical Rights of Women, 561
Coalition for the Reproductive Rights of Workers, 213
Common Focus, the Center for Early Adolescence, 433
Compassionate Friends, Inc., 447
Concern for Dying, 478
Consumer Coalition for Health, 226
COPE, Coping with the Overall Pregnancy/Parenting Experience, 353–354
Council for Exceptional Children (CEC), 441–442
C. Sec. Inc. (Cesareans/Support, Education and Concern), 349
Cystic Fibrosis Foundation, 438–439

DES Action, Inc., 206
Division of Research Resources, 600–601
Do It Now Foundation, 525

East West Academy of Healing Arts (EWAHA), 553
Emergency Department Nurses Association (EDNA), 637–638
Emory University-Grady Memorial Hospital Family Planning Program, 574
Environmental Action, 214
Epilepsy Foundation of America, 188

Families Anonymous, 433
Federation for Children with Special Needs, 442
Food and Drug Administration, 192

Health Activation Network, 226–227
Health Care Financing Administration, 192
Health Education Seminars, 591
Health/PAC, 227
Health Resources Administration, 192
Healthright, 561–562
Health Services Administration, 193
HEW agencies, 191–193
HEW/Office for Civil Rights, 193
Holistic Life University, 553–554
H.O.M.E. (Home Orientated Maternity Experience), 352
Homebirth, 352
Human Lactation Center, the, 348
Human Life and Natural Family Planning Foundation, 575

Industrial Health Foundation, Inc., 214
Informed Homebirth, 352
International Association for Enterostomal Therapy, Inc., 188
International Association for Suicide Prevention, 528
International Association of Laryngectomees, 207
International Childbirth Education Association (ICEA), 345–346
International Committee of Catholic Nurses (CICIAMS), 638
International Council of Nurses (ICN), 638
Industrial Health Foundation, Inc., 213

International Society for Burn Injuries, 203

Joslin Diabetes Foundation, Inc., 211
Juvenile Diabetes Foundation (JDF), 446

La Leche League International, Inc., 348
Leukemia Society of America, Inc., 207–208
Living with Cancer, 208

Make Today Count, 478
Mandala Society, the, 555
Maternity Center Association, 346–347
Medic Alert Foundation International, 188
Men's Reproductive Health Clinic, 567
Milcom Patient Care Systems, 584
Muscular Dystrophy Association (MDA), 442

Naim Conference, the, 479–480
Nancy D. Sanford's Continuing Education Courses, 591–592
Narcotics Education, Inc., 526
National Association for Mental Health, 523
National Association for Music Therapy, Inc., 523
National Association for Practical Nurse Education and Service, Inc., 639
National Association for Retarded Citizens (NARC), 442–443
National Association of Parents and Professionals for Safe Alternatives in Childbirth (NAPSAC), 347
National Association of Patients on Hemodialysis and Transplantation, 189
National Association of Pediatric Nurse Associates and Practitioners, (NAPNAP), 638–639
National Association of Physicians' Nurses, 639
National Association of School Nurses, Inc., 639

National Association of Spanish Speaking and Spanish Surnamed Nurses, 639
National Asthma Center at Denver, 189
National Black Nurses Association, Inc., 640
National Center for Nursing Ethics, 640
National Center for the Prevention and Treatment of Child Abuse and Neglect, 436-437
National Center on Child Abuse and Neglect, 436
National Childbirth Trust, 356
National Clean Air Coalition, 214
National Clearinghouse for Alcohol Information, 525
National Clearinghouse for Drug Abuse Information (NCDAI), 526
National Committee for Prevention of Child Abuse, 437
National Council for Homemaker, Home Health Aid Services, 543
National Council of Senior Citizens, 466
National Council on Alcoholism, Inc., 526
National Council on Family Relations, 523
National Council on the Aging, 466
National Council on Wholistic Therapeutics and Medicine, 554
National Dairy Council, 274
National Easter Seal Society, 443
National Federation of Licensed Practical Nurses, Inc., 640
National Fire Protection Association, 203-204
National Foundation for Ileitis and Colitis, Inc., 189
National Foundation, the,/March of Dimes, 439
National Genetics Foundation, Inc., 349-350
National Health Federation, 227
National Hemophilia Foundation, Inc., 439
National Hospice Organization, 480
National Institute for Occupational Safety and Health (NIOSH), 214
National Institute of Mental Health, 524
National Institutes of Health, 192
National Interagency Council on Smoking and Health, 229-230
National Intravenous Therapy Association, Inc., 640-641
National Joint Practice Commission, 641
National Kidney Foundation, 189-190
National League for Nursing, Inc., 641-642
National Library Service for the Blind and Physically Handicapped, 233
National Male Nurse Association, 642
National Multiple Sclerosis Society, 190
National Nurses for Life, Inc., 642
National Nurses Society on Alcoholism, 526
National Perinatal Association, 642-643
National Psychiatric Association, 524
National Safety Council, 190
National Save-a-Life League, 528
National Self-Help Clearinghouse, 227-228
National Sex Forum, 579
National Sickle Cell Disease Program, 190
National Society for the Prevention of Blindness, 233
National Spinal Cord Injury Foundation, 219
National Student Nurses Association, Inc., 643
National Sudden Infant Death Syndrome Foundation, 447
National Tay/Sachs and Allied Diseases Association, Inc., 439-440
National Women's Health Network, 562
Neurotics Anonymous International Liaison, Inc., 524
Northeast Invitational Healers' Workshop, 554-555
Nurse Consultants' Association (NCA), 644
Nurse Healers Professional Associates Cooperative, 644
Nurses Association of the American College of Obstetricians and Gynecologists, 643

Nurses Environmental Health Watch, 644
Nurses House, Inc., 644
Nurses in Transition, 644–645
Nutrition Today Society, 275

Office of Human Developmental Services, 193
Omega Institute for Holistic Studies, 555
Oncology Nursing Society (ONS), 645
Orthopedic Nurses Association, Inc., 645

Parents Anonymous (PA), 437
Parkinson's Disease Foundation, 191
Pharmaceutical Manufacturers Association, 191
Planned Parenthood Federation of America, Inc., 575
Population Council, Inc., 575
Post-Cana, 480
Primary Nursing Development, 559
Professional Health Services, Inc. (PHS), 215
Psychiatric Nurses Association of Canada, 524
Public Health Service, 192

Recording for the Blind, Inc., 234
Rehabilitation International, USA, 220
Resolve, Inc., 575
Resources in Human Nurturing, 347

Seeing Eye, Inc., the, 234
Self Care Associates, 645

Sex Information and Education Council, 580
Shanti Project, 479
Sigma Theta Tau, 198
Sister Kenny Institute, 220
Smokenders, 230
Society for Adolescent Medicine, 433
Society for Occupational and Environmental Health, 215–216
Society for Public Health Education, Inc., 543
Society for the Right to Die, Inc., 478
Spina Bifida Association of America, 440
Synthesis Graduate School for the Study of Man, 555

Type II Association, 562

United Cerebral Palsy Associations, Inc., 443
United Ostomy Association, Inc., 191
University Hospital's Cancer Center At-Home Rehabilitation Project, 205

Wellness Resource Center, 555
Western Council on Higher Education for Nursing (WCHEN), 597
Western Society for Research in Nursing, 601
World Health Organization (WHO), 543–544
Women's Occupational Health Resource Center, 216

Index

Abbreviations in common use, 714–722
Abdomen
 differential diagnosis of pain in, 61–63
 palpation of, 46
Abducens nerve, 31
Abortion, resources for, 565
Abscess, lung, 59
Accidents. *See also* First aid.
 children and, 380–381, 432–433
 prevention of, 190
Acetaldehyde, 180
Acetaminophen (Tylenol), 91–92
Acetazolamide (Diamox), 113
Acetic anhydride, 180
Acetone, urine, normal values, 15
Acetyldigitoxin (Acylanid), 104
Acetylene, 180
Acetylsalicylic acid (ASA), 91
Acid-base imbalance, assessment of, 57–58
Acne, 435
Acoustic nerves, 32
Acrolein, 180
Acupuncture, 552, 553, 556
Additives, food, safety of, 243–246
Administration, nursing, 197, 198, 199, 633, 636
Adolescence
 accidents in, 381
 drug abuse in, 506, 516–519, 435
 pregnancy in, 295–302, 435
 resources on, 433–435
 social growth and development, 507
Adriamycin (doxorubicin), 109
Aging, changes due to, 193, 459–460, 466–467
Agranulocytosis, 120
Airway obstruction, 132–136, 202–203
Albumin, normal values, 14
Alcohol abuse, 124
 in pregnancy, 302–304, 365
 resources, 193, 524–528
Alkylating agents, in chemotherapy, 111–112
Allergies, 187–195
Allyl Chloride, 180
Alpha-l-fetoprotein (AFP), 309
Amino acids, essential, 255–256
Aminophylline, 86

Ammonia, 180
Amniocentesis, 308–314
Amobarbital (Amytal), 100
Amobarbital sodium (Amytal Sodium), 100
Amoxicillin, 115, 119
Amphetamines, 124, 518
Ampicillin (Polycillin, Penbriten), 86, 115, 119
Amputees, resources for, 218, 220, 225
Amyl nitrite, 123
Analgesics, 90–92
Androgens, in chemotherapy, 110
Anemia
 aplastic, 120
 drug therapy for, 96–97
 hemolytic, 120–121
 megaloblastic, 121
Anesthesia, 93–95, 363
Anesthetists, nurse, 632
Aniline, 180
Anorexia nervosa, 522
Antibiotic therapy, 109–110, 115
Anticoagulants, 88
Antidepressants, 121–122
Antihistamines, 122
Antihypertensive agents, 98, 121
Antimetabolites, in chemotherapy, 108–109
Antipsychotic drugs, 99
Antispasmodics, 122
Apgar score, 327
Apothecaries measurements, equivalents, 685–686
Appendicitis, acute, 61
Aprobarbital (Alurate), 100
Arrhythmias, cardiac, 39–40, 195
Arsenic, 86, 180
Arthritis, resources on, 187
Art therapy, 521, 531, 535
Asbestos, 180
Associations, nursing, 630
Asthma, 187, 189
Atropine, 86, 107
Audiovisual aids, sources for, 701–708
Audiovisual equipment, sources for, 708–709
Autism, 452
Auscultation, of the heart, 37, 76, 194

Babinski reflex, 34
Barbital, 100
Barbital sodium, 100
Barbiturates, 88, 100–103, 122
  abuse of, 124, 518
Battered child syndrome. See Children, abuse of.
BCG vaccine, in chemotherapy, 112
Behavioral modification, 260, 261, 506, 549–551
Bence-Jones protein, normal values, 15
Benedict's test, 23
Benzene, 180
Bereavement
  nursing approach, 129–130, 473–474, 483
  support groups, 480, 483
Beryllium, 180
Bile duct, ascariasis, 61
Bilirubin, normal values, 18
Bill of rights, patient's, 2–3, 283–285, 470–471
Biofeedback, 550, 552, 556
Biopsy procedures, 46–47
Biotin, 241
Biparietal diameter, fetal, measurement of, 20
Birth defects, resources on, 438–440
Birthing room, 285, 287
Bleeding time, normal values, 11
Bleomycin (Blenoxane), 110
Blindness, resources on, 232–234
Blood
  ABO typing system, 26
  hematocrit, normal values, 17
  hemoglobin, normal values, 17
  normal laboratory values, 11–15, 17–19
  sampling techniques, 151
  transfusions. See Transfusions.
Blood pressure recording, 43
Blood sugar, normal values, 18
Body language, 534
Body water balance, 138, 196
Bone-marrow biopsy, 47
Bone scan, 54
Bottlefeeding, 348–349
Breast
  nodules, differentiation of, 71
  self-examination, 210, 566
Breastfeeding, resources on, 338–341, 348–349, 364
Bronchiectasis, 59

Burn care
  chemical lesions, 165
  educational programs and materials on, 166
  in children, 413
  methods of treatment, 166
  resources on, 203–204
Busulfan (Myleran), 112
Butabarbital sodium (BBS, Butacaps, Butisol Sodium), 100
Butyl alcohol, 180

Caffeine, 123, 243
Calcium, 18, 239, 242
Calcium chloride, 107
Calories, 258
Cancer
  audiovisual materials on, 209–210
  in children, 446, 448, 636
  psychiatric problems in, 490–491
  resources on, 204–209, 551, 636–637, 645
Cannabis, 125
Cantharis (Spanish fly), 122
Carbenicillin, 119
Carbohydrates, 237, 242, 258
Carbon dioxide, 12
Carbon disulfide, 180
Carbon monoxide, 86
Carbon Tetrachloride, 180
Carcinoma. See Cancer.
Cardiac arrest
  adult risk factors, 42–43
  cardiopulmonary resuscitation, 131–132
  emergency equipment for, 107, 137–138
Cardiac emergencies, drugs for, 104–106, 107
Cardiac glycosides, 104–106
Cardiac monitoring. See Electrocardiogram.
Cardiopulmonary resuscitation
  audiovisual aids, 202, 265
  equipment for, 137–138, 396
  nurse opinion on, 478
  pediatric, 365, 396, 400–401, 450
  technique, 131–132
Cardiovascular disorders
  differential diagnosis, 64
  drugs for, 104–106, 107
  in children, 452
  in infants, 403–404
  radiology, 51
  resources, 186, 195, 201

risk factors, 42-43
stress and, 550
Care plans, 583
Cast, care of, 168-169
Catheterization, urinary, 157-159, 195
Cat odor syndrome, 56
Central nervous system, assessment, 28, 29, 147
Cerebellar function, tests of, 29
Cerebral embolism, 66
Cerebral function, tests of, 28
Cerebral ischemia, focal, 66
Cerebral palsy, 443, 444, 452
Cerebral thrombosis, 66
Cerebrovascular accidents, 65-66, 221
Cervix, dilation in labor, 319, 320, 359
Cesium 137 (137Cs), 117
Chaddock's sign, 34
Chemotherapy
  drugs used in, 108-112
  nursing interventions in, 162-164
Cheyne-Stokes breathing, 44
Chickenpox, 382
Child abuse. *See* Children, abuse of.
Childbirth. *See also* Labor; Maternity care; Pregnancy.
  anesthesia for, 363
  cesarean, 349, 362, 363, 364
  emergency, 328-330, 363
  exercises for, 358
  family-centered, 286-288
  father's role in, 298-299, 365
  fetal monitoring in, 322-327, 364
  home delivery, 350-352
  hospital admission procedures for, 607-609
  preparation for, 293, 295, 355-358
  resources on, 355-358, 361-363
Childbirth educator, role of, 293
Child psychiatry, 531
Child-rearing, education for, 421-424
Children, 369-425
  abuse of, 332, 415-424
    resources, 425, 436-437, 452-453
  accidents and, 380-381, 432-433
  burn care in, 413
  cancer in, 446, 448, 636
  cardiovascular disorders in, 452
  choking in, 134-136, 202-203
  computation of drug dosages for, 78-79
  death of, 414, 446-448, 453, 481, 482, 484
  disturbed, 414-415
  gifted, 442
  growth and development, 371-379, 431, 450
    average heights and weights, 679
    of language, 378-379
    percentile charts for, 681-683
    social, 507
  handicapped, 440-444
  head circumference, 680
  hospitalization of, 385-391, 394
    resources, 445-451
  immunization, 381-382
  injection sites, 83, 392
  intravenous therapy for, 413-414
  learning disabilities in, 440, 444
  molestation of, 452
  normal laboratory blood values, 17-19
  normal resting pulse rate in, 35
  nutrition of, 242, 276-277
  physical assessment of, 371, 450
  prenatal classes for, 294-295
  preventive dentistry, 383-385
  resuscitation of, 396, 450
  surgery, 395-396
Chloquine (Aralen), 112
Chloral, 88
Chloramphenicol, 86
Chloride, normal values, 18
Chlorine, 180
Chloroform, 180
Chlorpromazine (Thorazine), 88, 99
Chlorprothixene (Taractan), 99
Choking, first aid for, 132-136, 202-203
Cholecystitis, acute, 61
Cholelithiasis, 61
Cholesterol, blood, 12, 42
Cholinesterase inhibitors, 85
Chromium, 181
Chromosomes, number and karyotype in clinical conditions, 25
Circulatory overload, 154
Clark's rule, 78
Clofibrate, 88
Clonus reflex, 34
Clotting time, 11
Cloxacillin (Tegopen), 119
Cobalt 60 (60Co), 117
Cocaine, 95, 124, 518
Codeine sulfate, 90
Code, nursing, 1
Cold applications, 143
Colic, renal, 62
Colitis, ulcerative, 189

College health care, 185–186, 635, 639
Coloring, artificial in food, 243
Coma, diabetic, 68
Communicable diseases, 210–211, 382, 437–438
Communication skills, 200
Comprehensive Psychiatric Nursing, 520–521
Consent, patient, 2, 607–609
Constipation, 196
Consumer-oriented health care, 226–229
Contraception. *See* Family planning.
Contraceptives, oral, 569–572, 576
Copper, 341
Coronary care unit, 176, 198, 201
Corticosteroids, in chemotherapy, 110
Counselling
  family relations, 523, 532
  in adolescent pregnancy, 298–299
  in Sudden Infant Death Syndrome (SIDS), 447
  peer, 172
Cranial nerve, function tests, 28–29, 31–32
Crash cart, equipment for, 137–138
Creatine phosphokinase (CPK), 12
Creatinine, normal values, 12, 16, 21
Creosol, 181
Cri-du-chat syndrome, 25
Critical care nursing, 197, 198, 200, 201, 631
Cultural bias in nurses, 271–273, 587–588
Cyanide, 86
Cyclophosphamide (Cytoxan), 111
Cyclopropane, 94
Cystic fibrosis, 438–439
Cytosine arabinoside (Ara C, cytosar), 109

Dactinomycin (actinomycin D; Cosmegen), 110
Dance therapy, 521, 535
Deafness. *See* Hearing disorders.
Death, 470–484
  audiovisual materials on, 484
  children and, 414, 446–448, 453, 481, 482
  holistic view of, 472–473, 481
  hospices, 480, 481
  infant, 409–413, 447
  nurse reaction to, 475, 481, 482
  nurse-specialists in, 471–483
  patient support, 471, 474–475, 479
  resources on, 478–484
  rights of dying patient, 470–471, 478–479
  separation and loss, crisis of, 473–477
  stages in the acceptance of, 472
Denial, as ego defense mechanism, 472, 509
Dentistry, preventive, pediatric, 383–385
Depression, 534
DES, 110, 206, 561, 562, 563
Deslanoside (Cedilanid-D), 104
Developmental testing, resources for, 431
Diabetes mellitus
  audiovisual materials on, 212
  diet in, 253
  juvenile, 67, 446, 451
  insulin reaction vs. diabetic coma, 68
  pregnancy and, 320, 355
  resources on, 211–212
  stages of, 23, 56
Diagnosis, differential, 55–74
  abdominal pain, 61–63
  dyspnea, 64
  pyrexia, 59–60
Diagnostic procedures. *See also* Physical assessment.
  biopsies, 46–47
  isotopic, 52–55
  laboratory. *See* Laboratory, normal values.
  radiological, 48–51
  resources, 75–76
  tests, 20–25. *See also under specific tests*.
Dialysis. *See* Hemodialysis.
Diaphragm, vaginal, 576, 578
Dichloroethyl Ether, 181
Dicloxacillin (Dynapen; Pathocil; Veracillin), 119
Diet(s). *See also* Nutrition.
  bland, 251–252
  in diabetes, 253
  Jewish laws of, 272–273
  liquid, 247–249
  low calories, 261
  low carbohydrate—high protein, 261
  low fat, 252
  low fiber, 250–251
  low sodium, 250, 276

oriental, 271-272
pregnancy and lactation, 242, 254, 353
  cultural variants, 271-272
  vegetarian, 257-258
  protein sparing modified fast (PSMF), 260, 262-270
  recommended daily allowances (RDA), 242
  vegetarian, 254-258
Digitalis, 41, 88
Digitalis glycosides mixture (Digiglusin), 104
Digitalis leaf, powdered (Digifortis; Pil-Digis), 104
Digitoxin (Crystodigin; Digitaline; Nativelle; Purodigin), 104-105
Digoxin (Lanoxin), 104
Dimethyl Sulfate, 181
Diphenoxylate hydrochloride (Lomotil), 92
Diphtheria, 382
Disasters, nursing role in, 203
Displacement, as ego defence, 508
Diuretics, 113-114
Down's syndrome, 25
Doxorubicin (Adriamycin), 109
Drug(s)
  abuse
    common terminology, 518-519
    effect on neonate, 365
    in adolescence, 435, 506, 516-518
    in nurses, 527
    pharmaceutical characteristics, 103, 124-125
    resources on, 525-528
      audiovisual, 527-528
  administration
    calculating flow rate, 79-80
    dosages, computation of, 78-79
    injection sites, 81-84, 392, 393
    related to meals, 84-85
  blood dyscrasias due to, 120-121
  effects on ECG, 41
  effects on sexuality, 121-123
  effects on urine color, 26
  incompatibilities, 86-87
  interactions, 88-89, 126
  resources, 126
  teratogenic, 307
  toxic, antidotes for, 85-86, 432
DTIC (dimethyltriazenomicarboxamidedacarbazine), 112
Duodenal ulcer, perforation of, 61
Dying. See Death.

Dyspnea, differential diagnosis of, 64

Eclampsia, 316-317
Education, nursing, 589-598
  burn care programs, 166
  career mobility programs, 593-595
  continuing, 589-590, 592
    resources, 591-592
  doctoral programs, 596
  exam preparations, 597
  external degree programs, 594
  from peers, 590
  geriatric nursing, programs in, 467-469
  graduate transition programs, 594-596
  grants and scholarships for, 529, 560, 598
  internship programs, 595-596
  midwifery programs, 366-368
  pediatric nursing programs, 453-457
  primary nursing, 560
  psychiatric nursing programs, 529-530
  research, 599-601
  resources in, 597-598, 641-642
  teaching aids, 672-673
  transcultural nursing, 588
Ego defense mechanisms, 508-509
Electrocardiogram
  arrhythmias, 39-40, 195
  chest leads, positioning, 39
  drug effects on, 41
  electrolytes, effect on, 41, 268, 269
  limb lead positioning, 38
  resources, 195
Electrolytes, effects on ECG, 41, 268, 269
Embolism
  cerebral, 66
  during IV therapy, 150
  fat, 169-170
  pulmonary, 169
Emergency nursing, 637-638
Encephalitis, 60
Enflurane (Ethrane), 93
Enterostomal therapy, 188, 191, 653, 669-671
Environmental health, resources in, 213-215, 217, 644
Eosinophils, normal laboratory values, 11, 19
Epilepsy, 70, 188
Epinephrine (Adrenalin), 107

Equipment for patient care, sources, 648–661
Equivalents
  metric, 679, 685–686, 687
  volume, 686
  weight, 685–686
Erikson's theory of social growth and development, 507
Erythrocytes, normal values, 11
Estriol, urinary, normal values, 16, 20
Estrogen therapy, 110, 564
Ethacrynic acid (Edecrin), 114
Ether, 94
Ethics in nursing, 629, 640
Ethnic groups, dietary habits of, 271–273
Ethyl alcohol, 122
Euthanasia, 478, 484, 642
Examination, positions for, 139
Exercise
  for childbirth, 358
  for joint flexibility, 140, 169
  in prevention of heart disease, 201
  obesity and, 260

Facial nerve, 32
Family-centered maternity care, 286–288
Family planning, 569–578
  adolescents and, 298
  natural, 575, 577
  resources in, 574–578
Fasting, 260, 262–270
Fat, dietary, 237, 252, 258, 265
Fat embolism, 169–170
Fentanyl (Sublimaze), 95
Ferrocholinate (Chel-iron; Ferrolip; Kelex), 96
Ferrous fumarate (Eldofe; Feostat; Fumasorb; Fumerin; Ircon; Laud-Iron; Palmiron; Span-FF; Toleron), 96
Ferrous gluconate (Fergon; Ferralet), 96
Ferrous sulfate (Fero-Gradumet; Mol-Iron), 96–97
Fetal alcohol syndrome, 302–303, 365
Fetus
  alcohol, effects on, 302–303, 365
  biparietal diameter, 20
  distressed, 325
  drugs affecting, 307
  gestational age, assessment of, 310
  head compression, 322–323
  heartrate, 21, 322–323, 324
  intrauterine growth retardation, 315
  isoimmunization, 309
  LOA position, 321
  maturity, assessment of, 310
  monitoring, 322–327, 364
  status, assessment of, 20–21
Fever, differential diagnosis of, 59–60
Fiber, dietary, 250–251
Fibrinogen, normal values, 18
Financial assistance for nurses, 644
First aid
  resources, 186–187, 431–433
    audiovisual, 202–203
  techniques, 131–138
Fish odor syndrome, 57
Flavorings, artificial, safety of, 243–246
Fluorocarbons, 124–125
5 Fluorouracil (5FU; Efudex; Fluoroplex), 108
Fluphenazine (Permitil; Prolixin), 99
Fluoride, in preventive dentistry, 384
Foley catheters, 158–159
Folic Acid (Folacin), 240, 242
Food additives, safety of, 243–246
Forearm, superficial veins of, 148
Foreign nurses, qualifications required in U.S., 623–624
Fractures, complications of, 169–170
Friction rub, pleural, 45
Fried's rule, 78
Fundraising, 625
Fungus, 181
Furosemide (Lasix), 114

Gangrene, gas, 170
Gastric bypass surgery, 259
Gastroenteritis, acute, 62
Gastrointestinal tract
  acute obstruction, 62
  isotopic procedures, 54
  parasites of, 62
  radiology of, 49–50
Genetics, resources on, 349–350, 438–444
Geriatric care, 193, 458–465. See also Aging; Death.
  educational programs in, 467–469
  innovations in, 460–465
  resources on, 465–467
Gerontological nursing. See Geriatric care.
Gestalt therapy, 534
Gestational age, 310
Gitalin (Gitaligin), 104
Glandular fever, 382
Globulin, normal values, 14
Glossopharyngeal nerve, 32

Glucose
    intolerance, 43
    intravenous, drugs incompatible with, 86-87
    normal laboratory values, 13, 16, 23
    tolerance test, oral, 22
    urine tests for, 23
Glycosides, cardiac, 104-106
Gold 198 (198Au), 117
Gonorrhea, 115, 210-211, 576
Gordon's sign, 34
Gramp, 475-477
Grand mal, 70
Grants
    administration of, 628-629
    applications for, 626-628
    availability, 625, 626
    for nursing education, 529, 560, 598
Granulocytopenia, 120
Grief, 473-478, 484
Griseofulvin, 88
Group work, 496-506
    concepts in, 497-499
    discussion groups, 500-501
    resources, 504-506, 522, 532
    specific task groups, 501

Hallucinogens, 123, 124, 519
Haloperidol (Haldol), 99
Halothane (Flothane), 93
Hand, superficial veins of, 148
Handicapped
    audiovisual materials on, 224-226
    children, 440-444, 452
    financial resources for, 221-222
    higher education and, 223-224
    mental, 440, 442-443, 452
    resources on, 218-226, 233
    sexuality and, 220, 222, 225
    supplies and equipment, sources for, 649, 652, 655, 656, 658
Head
    circumference in children, 680
    compression in the fetus, 322-323
    injury, assessment of, 160-161
    lice, 438
Healing process in wounds, 142
Health care
    history taking, 5-10
    records of, 582-583, 584
Health care industry, nurse liason with, 644
Health education, resources in, 187, 191, 201, 226
Health history, 5-10
Hearing disorders, resources, 231-232, 225-226

Heart
    auscultation of, 37, 76, 194
    clinical assessment of, 37-43
    emergency drugs, 107
    fetal, 21, 322-323, 324
    transplants, 201
Heart attack
    adult risk factors, 42-43, 201
    cardiopulmonary resuscitation, 131-132
    emergency equipment for, 107, 137-138
Heimlich maneuver, 132-136, 202-203
Hematocrit, normal values, 17, 19
Hematology. *See* Blood.
Hemodialysis
    nursing role in, 155-156
    resources, 189, 197, 202
Hemoglobin, normal values, 17, 19
Hemophilia, 439
Hemorrhage, cerebral, 65-66
Hepatitis, infectious, 60
Heroin, 123, 518. *See also* Drug abuse.
Herpes Simplex virus Type II, 562
Hexobarbital (Sombulex), 100
Hoffman's sign, 34
Holistic health, 545-556
    mind-body relatedness, 549-551
    resources in, 426, 551-556, 644
        audiovisual, 556
    role of nurse in, 545-546
    therapeutic touch, 546-549, 556
Home birth, resources for, 350-352
Home Care for the Dying Child, 414
Homosexual, rights of in hospital, 515-516, 581
Hormones, 110-111, 122
Hospices, 480-481
Hospitalization of children. *See* Children, hospitalization of.
Hot applications, uses of, 143
Hydralazine hydrochloride (Apresoline), 98
Hydrocarbons, 124-125
Hydroxyurea (Hydrea), 109
Hydroxyzine (Atarax; Vistaril), 99
Hypercalcemia, 41
Hyperkalemia, 269
Hyperlipoproteinemia diet, 252
Hypertension
    coronary risk associated with, 42
    drug therapy, 88, 98, 121
    phases of, 167
    resources, 194, 201
Hyperventilation, 44

Hypocalcemia, 41
Hypoglossal nerve, 32
Hypokalemia, 41
Hypotensive agents, 88, 98, 121
Hysterectomy, 563, 564, 566

Icterus index, normal laboratory values, 13
Identification, as ego defense mechanism, 508
Immunization, pediatric, 381, 382, 437–438
Independent nursing practice, 602–603
Independent Nursing Practice with Clients, 602–603
Industrial agents, effects on workers, 180–182
  resources, 213–215
Infants
  death in, 409–413, 447
  dental hygiene for, 384
  growth and development in, 353, 371–376, 431, 450, 507
  high-risk, 449
  immunization, 381–382
  nutrition, 276
  resources, 352–353, 365
Infection
  associated with surgery, 141
  urinary tract, 59, 565
Infection control, resources, 637
Infectious diseases, 210–211, 382, 437–438
Infertility, resources in, 575–576, 577
Injection sites
  in children, 83, 392
  in diabetics, 211–212
  in neonates, 393
  intramuscular, 81–83
  subcutaneous, 84
Innovar, 95
Insulin, 68, 85, 116
Insurance, liability, 495, 511, 512, 607, 612
International nursing, 622
Internship programs, 595–596
Intraoperative care, clinical nurse specialists in, 184–185
Intrauterine device, 573, 576
Intravascular monitoring techniques, 151–152
Intravenous therapy
  cardiac assessment during, 146
  cerebral nervous system, assessment during, 147

  complications of, 149–150
  pediatric, 413–414
  renal function, assessment, 145
  resources, 197, 198, 202, 631, 640–641
  superficial veins of hand and arm, 148
Introjection, as ego defense, 508
Iodine, 13, 241, 242
  radioactive, 117
Iridium 192 (192 Ir), 117
Iron, normal laboratory values, 13, 85, 239, 242
Iron dextran (Imferon), 97
Iron Oxide, 181
Iron sorbitex (Jectofer), 97
Ischemia, focal cerebral, 66
Isoflurane (Forane), 94
Isolation, as ego defence, 508
Isoproterenol (Isuprel), 107
Isotopic procedures, 52–55

Jejunoileal bypass surgery, 259
Jews, dietary laws of, 272–273
Job hunting, 616–621
  resources, 620–621
  sample applications, 616–620
Joints, exercises for, 140, 195

Kanamycin, 87
Ketamine (Ketalar), 94
Kidney, anatomy of, 202
Kleinefelter's syndrome, 25

Labor. *See also* Childbirth; Maternity care; Pregnancy.
  audiovisual aids for, 363–364
  cervical dilation in, 319, 320, 359
  emergency management, 328–330, 363
  fetal monitoring, 322–327, 364
  mechanisms of, 321
  normal, 319
  umbilical cord occlusion in, 322–323
  uteroplacental insufficiency in, 322–323
Laboratory, normal values, 11–19
Lactation, dietary requirements during, 254
Lanatoside C (Cedilanid), 106
Language, development of, 371, 378–379
Laryngectomy, 207
Law, nursing and. *See* Legal aspects of nursing.

L-Dopa, 123
Lead, 13, 16, 86, 181, 218
Leadership For Change, 586
Learning disabilities in children, 440, 444
Lecithin/sphingomyelin ratio (L/S), 20, 310
Legal aspects of nursing, 606–612
  audiovisual materials, 612
  emergency room nursing, 197
  malpractice, 606
  patient consent, 21, 607–609
  resources, 611–612
Leopold's maneuvers, 292, 363
Leptospirosis, 60
Leukemia, 207, 210, 448
Leukocytes, normal values, 11, 19
Leukopenia, 120
Levarterenol (Levophed), 107
Liability insurance, 495, 511, 512, 607, 612
Libido, 511, 512
Lice, head, 438
Lidocaine (Xylocaine), 95, 107
Lipids, 13
Liver
  biopsy, 47
  function tests, 24, 54
LSD, 123, 124
Lumbar puncture, 47
Lung
  abscess, 59
  assessment of, 44–45, 64
  bronchogram of, 51
  isotopic procedures, 53
  neonatal disorders of, 401–402

Magnesium, 18, 241, 242
Malaria, 60
Male health
  audiovisual material on, 568
  desirable weights, 684
  resources on, 567–568
Male nurses, 586, 642
Malignant hypertension, 167
Malpractice, guidelines on, 606
Manganese, 181
Maple syrup urine disease, 56
Marijuana, 123, 125, 519
Mastectomy, resources on, 208, 653
Mastitis, acute, 60
Maternity care, 280–368. *See also* Childbirth; Fetus; Labor; Neonate; Pregnancy.
  audiovisual aids, 361–366
  family-centered, 286–288

home visiting services, 342, 344
innovations in, 342–344
resources, 345–368, 643
sources of supplies and equipment, 661–663
Measles, 59, 382
Mechlorethamine hydrochloride (Nitrogen mustard; Mustargen), 111
Medical libraries, regional, 599–600
Medical-Surgical nursing, 127–234
  audiovisual materials, 200–203
  resources, 185–234
Meditation, 550
Melphalan (L-phenylalanine mustard; L-PAM; Alkeran), 111–112
Meningitis, epidemic, 60
Menopause, 565
Menstruation, 513
Mental handicaps, 440, 442–443, 452
Mental health, resources in, 521–535
Meperidine hydrochloride (Demerol), 90
Mephobarbital (Mebaral; Menta-Bal), 101
Mercaptomerin sodium (Thiomerin), 113
6-mercaptopurine (6-MP; Purinethol), 109
Mercury, 86, 181
Mesoridazine (Serentil), 99
Metabolic acidosis, 57
Metabolic alkalosis, 57
Metaraminol (Aramine), 107
Methadone, 122
Methanol, 85
Metharbital (Gemonil), 101
Methicillin (Staphcillin), 87, 118
Methohexital sodium (Brevital sodium), 101
Methotrimeprazine (Levoprome), 91
Methyldopa, 98
Methyldopate hydrochloride (Aldomet), 98
Methysergide maleate (Sansert), 92
Metric conversions, 679, 685–686, 687
Mica, 181
Midwifery. *See also* Maternity care.
  educational programs in, 366–368
  resources, 605, 633, 637
Military nursing, 613–615
Mind-body relatedness, 549–551
Minds, Mothers and Midwives, 344–345
Minerals, sources and functions, 241, 242

Miotitic inhibiting drugs, in chemotherapy, 109
Mithramycin (Mithricin), 110
Monoamine oxidase inhibitors, 88
Monocytes, normal laboratory values, 11, 19
Monosodium Glutamate (MSG), 244
Morphine, 89, 90, 123
Mothering, 332, 422–424
Motor functions, assessment of, 29
Mourning, 473–478
MTX (methotrexate), 108–109
Multiple sclerosis, 190
Mumps, 382
Muscle relaxants, 89
Muscular dystrophy, 442
Music therapy, 523, 535
Myocardial infarction, 42–43, 201, 490

Nafcillin (Unipen), 119
Narcotics, 89, 123, 518
　and neonates, 365, 449
Negligence, guidelines on, 606
Neonate
　apgar scoring, 327
　assessment of, 327, 334, 338, 397, 398
　　resources, 366, 450
　birth defects, resources on, 438–440
　cardiovascular disorders in, 403–404
　common variations in, 335–337, 359
　drugs affecting, 307
　gestational age, assessment of, 333–335, 365
　head circumference, 680
　high risk, 338
　　parental support for, 404–408
　injection sites, 393
　narcotic addiction in, 365, 449
　normal laboratory values, 17–19
　normal resting pulse rate in, 34
　premature, characteristics of, 398–399
　reflexes of, 397
　resources, 365–366, 449, 642–643
　respiratory distress in, 401–402
　resuscitation of, 365, 396, 400–401, 450
　small-for-dates, 398–399
　suctioning methods, 401
Neoplasms, benign vs. malignant, 73–74

Nephrology nursing, 632
Nerves, cranial, clinical examination of, 31–32
Nervous system, 28–35, 48–49
Neurological examination, 28–35
　in acute head injury, 161
　in the neonate, 334, 397
Neurosurgical nursing, 632
Neutrophils, normal laboratory values, 11, 19
Niacin, 238, 242
Nickel, 181
Nitrobenzene, 181
Nitrogen dioxide, 181
Nitrosoureas, 112
Nitrous oxide, 93
Nocturnal emissions, 512
Nurse, licensed practical
　exam preparation, 597
　resources, 593, 639, 640
Nurse practitioners, 604–605
　for the dying, 471–483
　in gerontology, 461–462, 463, 464, 467–469
　in intraoperative care, 184–185
　in maternity care, 341–343, 366–368
　in public health nursing, 537–538
　in psychotherapy, 493–495
　psychiatric liaison, 486–492, 529–530
Nursing code, 1
Nursing homes, primary medical care in, 460–463
Nursing, international, 622
Nursing organizations, 630–645
Nursing periodicals, 196–200
Nursing practice
　independent, 602–603
　innovations in, 585–586, 603–605
Nutrition, 235–279
　dental health and, 383–384
　desirable weights, 684
　in pregnancy, 242, 254, 353
　resources, 274–279

Oasthouse urine disease, 56
Obesity, treatment for, 259–270
Obstetric nursing. *See* Childbirth; Maternity care; Pregnancy.
Obstetric supplies, sources of, 661–663
Occupational health, resources in, 180–182, 213–217, 632–633
Oculomotor nerve, 31
Odors, unusual, diseases associated

with, 56–57
Olfactory nerve, 31
Ombudsman, 610–611
Oncology nursing, resources in, 204–209, 636–637, 645
Ophthalmology, 232
Opiates, 85, 92, 124
Opium (Paregoric), 92
Oppenheim's sign, 34
Optic nerve, 31
Organizations, for nurses, 630–645
Organizing for Independent Nursing Practice, 603
Orgasm, 512, 513
Orientals, dietary habits of, 271–272
Orthopedics, 168–170
  resources, 199, 645
Ostomy appliances, sources of, 653, 669–671
Ouabain (G-Strophanthin), 106
Oxacillin (Prostophilin; Resistopen), 119
Oxygen
  arterial saturation, normal values, 13
  methods of administration, 144
Oxytocin challenge test, 21

Pain, 143
  abdominal, differential diagnosis, 61–63
  resources, 202, 209
  therapeutic touch and, 546–549, 556
Palsy, cerebral, 443, 444, 452
Pancreatitis, acute, 62
Pancytopenia, 121
Pantothenic acid, 241
Parasites, 62, 181
Parental support groups, 404–408, 447
Parenting
  disorders, of, 332, 416
  programs in, 421–424, 429–430
  resources, 428–430, 561
Parkinson's disease, 191
Patient
  education, 130
    resources, 194, 195, 226–229, 672–673
  preoperative assessment, 183
  rights of, 2–3, 283–285, 470–471
    informed consent, 2, 607–609
    protection of, 610–611
    resources, 3, 193, 612
Patient service officer, 610–611

PCO_2, whole blood, normal values, 14, 18
PCP, 124
Pediatric nursing, 369–425. *See also* Children; Infant; Neonate.
  audiovisual aids, 450–453
  educational programs in, 453–457
  resources in, 426–457, 638–639
Penicillin, 89
Penicillin G, 87, 118
Penicillin V (phenoxymethyl penicillin; Compocillin V), 118
Penis, 513
Pentazocine (Talwin), 90
Penthrane, 93
Pentobarbital sodium (Nebralin; Nembutal sodium), 101–102
Peptic ulcer, perforation of, 61
Perphenazine (Trilafon), 99
Petit mal, 70
Petroleum products, carcinogenic effects, 181
PH, whole blood, normal values, 14, 18
Pharmacology. *See* Drugs.
Phenethicillin (Syncillin; Chemipen; Darcil), 118
Phenobarbital (Eskabarb; Hypnette; Luminal; Pheno-Squar; Solfoton), 102
Phenobarbital sodium (Luminal sodium), 102
Phenol, 181
Phenolphthalein (PSP), 16
Phenothiazines, 99
Phentolamine (Regitine), 98
Phenylalanine, normal values, 14
Phenylbutazone, 89
Phenylketonuria, 56
Phenytoin, 89
Phosphorus, 18, 32, 117, 241, 242
Physical assessment, 4–76
  audiovisual materials, 76
  neonatal, 327, 334, 338, 397, 398
  of children, 371, 450
  resources, 75–76, 366, 450
PKU deficiency, 452
Placenta, 322–323, 330
Platelets, normal values, 11
Pneumonia, lobar, 59, 63
PO_2, whole blood, normal values, 14, 18
Poison control centers, 692–694
Poisoning, antidotes, 85–86, 432
Poliomyelitis, 382
Potassium, 14, 18, 269

Potassium chloride, 87
Potassium nitrate (Saltpeter), 122
Practical nurses, licensed. *See* Nurses, licensed practical.
Preeclampsia, 316-317
Pregnancy. *See also* Childbirth; Fetus; Labor; Maternity care.
   adolescent, 295-302, 435
   alcohol and, 302-304
   amniocentesis, 308-314
   audiovisual aids on, 366
   diabetes and, 320, 355
   diagnosis of, 289
   diet in, 242, 254, 353
      cultural variations, 271-272
      vegetarian, 257-258
   ectopic, 63
   estriol, normal values in, 16
   examination techniques, 292
   fetal position in, 321
   fundal heights in, 291
   high risk, 304-306
   intrauterine growth retardation, 315
   nutrition in. *See* Diet.
   patient rights in, 283-285
   preeclampsia-eclampsia in, 316-317
   resources on, 353-358, 361-363
   termination of, 565, 642
   weight gain in, 290
Preservatives, in food, safety of, 243-246
Primary nursing, 557-560
   resources in, 559-560, 605
Probenecid, 115
Problem-oriented health care record, 582-583
Procaine hydrochloride (Novocaine; Ethocaine), 95
Procaine penicillin G, 115
Procarbazine (Matulane; Natulan), 112
Prochlorperazine (Compazine), 99
Progestins, in chemotherapy, 111
Projection, as defense mechanism, 508
Pro-life movement, 642
Promazine (Sparine), 99
Propranolol, 89
Protein, 14, 237, 242, 255-256, 258, 263
Protein Sparing Modified Fast, 260, 262-270
Psychiatric liaison nurse, 486-492
Psychiatric nursing, 485-521

   acceptance of client, 515-516
   certification, 494-495
   educational programs in, 529-530
   group therapy, 496-506
   liability insurance, 495
   liaison nurse, 486-492
   of professional client, 510-511
   psychotherapy, private practice of, 493
   public health nurses, role in, 540-541
   resources in, 521-535
   self-acceptance and, 506-507
Psychomotor seizures, 70
Psychotherapy, private nursing practice in, 493
Puberty, resources on, 434
Publications, nursing, guide to writing for, 624
Public health nursing, 536-544
   affiliation with group physician practices, 539-541
   mental health care, 540-543
   resources in, 543-544, 635
   specializations, 537-538
Publishers, addresses of, 710-713
Puerperal fever, 60
Pulse points, 36
Pulse rates, normal, 35

Quinacrine (Atabrine), 112
Quinine, 41, 243

Radiation, 177-179
   audiovisual resources, 217-218
   contamination, protocol for, 178-179
   exposure, permissible levels, 177
   terminology, 177
Radioisotopes, 117
Radiology, common procedures, 48-51
Radium 226 (226 Ra), 117
Radon 222 (222 Rn), 117
Rales, 45
Rancid butter odor syndrome, 57
Rape, 452, 563, 566
Rationalization, as ego defense mechanism, 509
Reaction formation, as ego defense mechanism, 508
Records, nursing, 582-584
   resources, 584
Rehabilitation, 170-172
   resources, 218-226, 637

vocational, state departments of, 695–698
Reflexes
 deep tendon, 33
 neonatal, 397
 pathological, 30, 34–35
 superficial, 30
 tests of, 30
Regression, as ego defense mechanism, 508
Renal disorders
 radiology of, 51
 resources, 189–190, 202
Repression, as ego defense mechanism, 508
Research, nursing, 599–601
 resources, 600–601
Reserpine (Serpasil), 98
Respiration, abnormalities in rate and rhythm, 44–45, 58
Respiratory acidosis, 58
Respiratory alkalosis, 58
Respiratory disorders
 differential diagnosis of, 44–45, 58, 64
 in the neonate, 401–402
 isotopic diagnosis, 53
 radiology, 51
 resources, 195, 202
Resume, sample, 617–620
Resuscitation, cardiopulmonary
 equipment for, 137–138, 396
 nurse opinion on, 478
 pediatric, 365, 396, 400–401, 450
 technique, 131–132
Reticulocytes, normal values, 19
Rheumatic diseases, 59, 187
Rh hemolytic disease, 355
Rhonchi, 45
Riboflavin, 238, 242
Rubella, 382

Saccharin, 243
Safety, resources on, 431–433
Salicylates, 89
Salpingitis, acute, 63
Scabies, 438
Scarlet fever, 59
Schistosomiasis, acute, 60
Schizophrenia, 534
Scholarships, for nursing education, 529, 560, 598
School health care, 185–186, 635, 639
Secobarbital (Seconal), 103
Secobarbital sodium (Seconal Sodium), 103

Seizures, 70
Selenium, 123
Self-acceptance, 506–507
Self-defense, 566
Self-help, resources on, 226–229, 645
Sensory function, assessment of, 29–30
Septicemia, 60
Serum, normal chemistry, 12
Sex education, resources on, 579–581
Sexual assault, 563, 566
Sexuality
 audiovisual materials on, 580–581
 drug effects on, 121–123
 dysfunction, 513–514, 581
 in the handicapped, 222, 224
 myths concerning, 511–513
 resources, 533, 579–581
Shock, 55, 150, 200, 282, 331
Shock hazards, from monitoring equipment, 326–327
Sickle cell disease, 190
Silica, 181
Sister Stella's Babies, 344–345
Smoking, resources on, 229–231
Snake test, 21–22
Sodium
 dietary restriction, 250, 276
 normal blood values, 14, 18
Sodium bicarbonate, 87, 107
Sodium chloride, 246
Sodium ethacrynate (Sodium Edecrin), 114
Spanish language, health care resources in, 196
Spectinomycin dihydrochloride (Trobicin), 115
Speech disorders, resources in, 231–232
Sphygmomanometers, 647
Spina bifida, 440
Spinal accessory nerve, 32
Spinal cord lesions
 equipment for, 172–175
 functional goals, 172–175
 rehabilitation, 170–172
 resources, 218–226
 sexuality and, 222, 224
Spironolactone (Aldactone), 113
State Boards of Nursing, 688–692
 mandatory continuing education requirements, 589–590
State vocational rehabilitation departments, 695–698
State Welfare offices, 698–701

Status epilepticus, 70
Sterilization, voluntary, 568, 574
Stethoscopes, 646
Stool, drugs affecting color of, 26
Streptozotocin, 110
Stress, 530, 534, 550
Strokes, 65-66, 221
Strychnine, 122
Sublimation, as ego defense mechanism, 509
Substitution, as ego defense mechanism, 509
Sudden Infant Death Syndrome, 409-413, 447
Suicide, 509-510, 528-529
Superfemale, 25
Supermale, 25
Supplies for patient care, sources of, 648-661
Surgical instruments, care of, 667-668
Surgical nursing
  intraoperative care, 184-185
  preoperative patient assessment, 182-183
  resources, 200, 636
  sources for supplies and equipment, 663-668

Tachypnea, 44
Talbutal (Lotusate), 103
Tape, types and uses, 647
Tay-Sachs disease, 439-440
Teaching aids, sources of, 672-673
Testes, self-examination, 568
Testing, developmental, resources, 431
Tests, diagnostic. *See* Laboratory diagnosis, *and under specific tests*
Tetanus, 170
Tetracycline, 115
Tetraethyl Lead, 182
Thallium, 182
Thanatologists, nurse, 471-483
Therapeutic touch, 546-549, 556
Thiamin (B1), 238, 242
Thiamylal sodium (Surital Sodium), 103
Thiazide diuretics, 89
Thiopental sodium (Pentothal Sodium), 94, 103
Thioridazine (Mellaril), 99
Thio-Tepa, 111
Thiothixene (Navene), 99
Thoracentesis, 47

Thrombocytopenia, 121
Thrombophlebitis, 69, 149
Thrombosis, cerebral, 66
Thyroid gland, isotopic procedures, 52
Thyroxine (T4), 15
Toluene, 182
Toxic drugs, 85-86, 432
Transcultural nursing, 199, 587-588
  dietary habits, 271-273
  educational programs in, 588
Transfusions
  reactions
    allergic, 154
    bacterial, 153-154
    hemolytic, 153
  resources, 185
Transplants, 201
Trauma, management, 160-161
Trichloroethylene, 182
Trifluoperazine (Stelazine), 99
Trigeminal nerve, 31
Triiodothyronine (T3), normal values, 14
Trisomy, 25
Trochlear nerve, 31
Tuberculosis, 59
Tubocurarine, 89
Turner's syndrome, 25, 57
Typhoid, 60

Ulcer
  decubitus, 196, 202
  duodenal, 61
Ultrasound, in pregnancy, 20
Umbilical cord, occlusion of, 322-323
Undoing, as ego defense mechanism, 508
Uniforms, nursing, sources of, 674-677
Urea (Ureaphil), 113
Urea nitrogen, normal values, 15, 16, 18
Uric acid, normal values, 16
Urinary catheterization, 157-159
Urinary tract, infections of, 59, 565
Urine
  color, drugs affecting, 27
  normal chemistry, 15-16
  tests for glucose in, 23
Urological nursing, 636
  supplies, sources of, 669-671
Urostomy appliances, 671-672
Uteroplacental insufficiency, 322-323

Vaginitis, 565

Vagus nerve, 32
Vasectomy, 568, 574
Vegetarian diets, 254-258
Veins, hand and arm, 148
Venereal disease, 115, 210-211, 576
Ventricular hypertrophy, left, 43
Vinblastine (Velban), 109
Vincristine (Oncovin), 109
Vinyl Chloride, 182
Vinyl ether (Vinethene), 93
Vitamin(s)
  A (Retinol), 237, 242
  B1, 238, 242
  B6, 240, 242
  B12, 240, 242
  C (Ascorbic Acid), 238, 242
  D, 240, 242
  E, 123, 240, 242
Vocational rehabilitation, State departments of, 695

Volume equivalents, 686

Warfarin, 86
Weights
  average pediatric, 679, 681-683
  desirable adult, 684
  equivalents, 685-686
Welfare, state offices, 698-701
Well Elderly Clinics, 464-465
Women's health. *See also* Family planning; Maternity care; Pregnancy.
  desirable weights, 684
  resources in, 561-566
Wound healing process, 141-142

Yohimbine, 122
Young's rule, 78

Zinc, 241, 242